# Forensic Vision

## With Application to Highway Safety

Third Edition

Marc Green, Ph.D.
Merrill J. Allen, O.D., Ph.D.
Bernard S. Abrams, O.D.
Leslie Weintraub, O.D.

**Contributor**
J. Vernon Odom, Ph.D.

**Lawyers & Judges Publishing Company, Inc.**
Tucson, AZ

**Lawyers & Judges Publishing Company, Inc.**

P.O. Box 30040 • Tucson, AZ 85751-0040
(800) 209-7109 • FAX (800) 330-8795
e-mail: sales@lawyersandjudges.com
www.lawyersandjudges.com

Library of Congress Cataloging-in-Publication Data

Forensic aspects of vision and highway safety / Marc Green ... [et al.]. -- 3rd ed.
p. cm.
Includes bibliographical references and index.
ISBN-13: 978-1-933264-54-7 (hardcover : alk. paper)
ISBN-10: 1-933264-54-3 (hardcover : alk. paper)
1. Forensic ophthalmology. 2. Automotive medicine. 3. Automobile driving. 4. Traffic accident investigation. I. Green, Marc.
RA1062.5.F67 2008
614'.1--dc22

2008009189

ISBN 13: 978-1-933264-54-7
ISBN 10: 1-933264-54-3
Printed in the United States of America
10 9 8 7 6 5 4 3 2

# Contents

# Preface: From Judkin's Law To Daubert Criteria

Marc Green, Ph.D.

*"When you believe in things you don't understand, then you suffer."*
—Stevland Hardaway Judkins, aka Stevie Wonder

## A Tale Of Two Experts

The great German scientist Hermann Helmholtz (1821–94) was the first forensic vision expert. A local court asked Helmholtz to give an opinion in a burglary case. The plaintiff testified that the defendant had broken into his home in the middle of the night, struck him in the head and stolen some property. Even though it had been pitch black, the plaintiff claimed that he could identify the defendant without any doubt. At the time, there was no consensus on the relationship between light and perception, but a popular theory suggested that light radiated outward from the viewer's eyes rather than entered into the eyes from the world.[1] The idea seemed plausible because everyone knew that a blow to the head could make you see light ("stars" as we would say). The plaintiff claimed that when struck on the head, his eyes generated enough light to see the defendant clearly.

The court asked Helmholtz if this could be true. Helmholtz returned to his lab, turned off the lights, and sat his assistant in a chair. Helmholtz then proceeded to bang on the unfortunate assistant's head with a mallet. Meanwhile, Helmholtz watched to see if any light shot out from the assistant's eyes. Of course none did, so Helmholtz returned to court and testified that the plaintiff's statement had no credibility. The court acquitted the defendant.

Subsequent forensic vision experts have not always fared as well. The notable Antarctic explorer Sir Ernest Shackleton testified on iceberg visibility at an inquiry on the Titanic sinking. Shackleton gave expert opinion on how the crew could have failed to see an object as big as an iceberg. The court listened to Shackleton and then dismissed his testimony. They noted that the Titanic had struck an iceberg in the North Atlantic while Shackleton had experience with icebergs in the Southern Ocean that surrounds Antarctica. This was thousands of miles away, so his testimony was not relevant.

The difference between Helmholtz and Shackleton is instructive. Helmholtz would probably pass Daubert, but Shackleton would not. He was a domain expert while Helmholtz was a scientific expert, with years of experience in basic sensory science. (In fact, he probably invented sensory science.) Shackleton's expertise lay in his experience within some specific area of work. The court ruled that his domain knowledge from the Southern Ocean did not transfer to the domain of the North Atlantic. It was highly situation specific. In contrast, Helmholtz's testimony was based on fundamental scientific principles and on empirical research observation. It didn't matter whether he banged on his assistant's head in the basement of his laboratory, in the victim's bedroom or on Mt. Everest. It didn't matter whether he used a mallet, sledgehammer or waffle iron. The basic principle was independent of the specific situation.

Perhaps Sir Ernest would have fared better if he had been a scientist. (Admittedly, light measurements would have been impossible since an accident recreation was out of the question.) He could have explained the principles of vision and how they would operate in iceberg detection. He could have explained that we carry our visual systems around in our heads and that it operates similarly when viewing icebergs in the Southern Ocean or in the North Atlantic.

## Changes To The Third Edition

I raise these historical examples in order to prepare the reader for some changes in this new edition of *Forensic Vision.* While the second edition was only a very slight deviation from the first, this third edition is significantly different in several ways.

### 1. More Basic And Explanatory Science

Science in general and scientific opinion in particular fall into two broad categories: "explanatory science" and "cookbook science" (Gale, 1979). "Cookbook science" uses a set of rules, i.e., "IF this is true THEN that is true." In cognitive psychology, this is called "heuristic" or "shallow knowledge" because there is no deep understanding. A person using cookbook science knows *that* but not *why*. For example, an expert might say *that* driver reaction time is 1.5 seconds because he heard it in a lecture, or class, read it in an accident reconstruction book, or as so often happens, simply believes it to be the "accepted value." Such a person cannot explain *why* 1.5 is the right value, describe how it arose or extrapolate or interpolate it based on situational variables. He doesn't know what the number 1.5 actually represents. He is a candidate for Judkins' Law.

"Explanatory science" uses "deep knowledge" or "first principles." There is an understanding of *why* rather than merely an application of *that.* A person who states that normal driver reaction time is 1.5 seconds is not giving an explanatory scientific opinion unless he can explain scientifically *why* 1.5 seconds is the correct estimate. This would require familiarity with the basic reaction time phenomenon and theory, the research literature and the actual data. He preferably has actually conducted behavioral experimentation so that he can read and interpret the research studies.

The cookbook science approach may suffice on the routine problems in simple domains. When encountering a problem, the optimal solution is a single, all-purpose number: neat, efficient and requiring a minimum amount of time to obtain and mental resource to apply. Many fields have books of tables, regulations, recommendations and standards. There's no need to understand; just turn the cookbook to the right recipe.

However, cookbook science fails in more complex or extreme problems or when there is a shift in the context. To illustrate with an analogy, using bird migrations might provide a good rule for when to plant crops. It may work beautifully, so there is no need to understand weather patterns, soil conditions, etc. However, if the birds changed their patterns, or became extinct or if you moved to a different hemisphere, the rules would no longer work. You only know *that* but not *why*. If you understood weather and soil, however, then you could still know when to plant. You can extrapolate current data to new situations. Vision, as this book will demonstrate, is a very complex and context-dependent phenomenon, so cookbook science is often inadequate. Most regulations, for example, are only minima. Actual conditions might require a different standard.

This edition focuses more on basic, explanatory science. The previous editions focused more narrowly on vision in the roadway environment. The focus is still on the roadway environment, but the book is about vision *per se*, and not just about vision on the roadway or even just about forensic vision. People carry their visual systems around with them, so the same visual science that applies to analyzing road accidents also applies to accidents in aviation and marine environments. It is also relevant to non-transportation accidents such as falls, medical errors, warnings and eyewitness identification as well as to other areas of law such as intellectual property. Chapter 4 touches on some of these topics. Perhaps the fourth edition, if there is one, will cover these domains in some detail.

Somewhat paradoxically, however, this edition is also more applied than the previous edition. While the book begins with basic science, it ends with a series of "how to" chapters on analyzing specific accident scenarios involving visibility, pedestrian accidents and roadway collisions as well as a chapter on use of pictorial evidence in the courtroom. It also includes practical material from the previous edition on the pragmatics of testifying about vision in court (Chapter 19).

**2. More Psychology And Human Factors**

Writing is never neutral. All books, fiction and nonfiction alike, have a viewpoint and a theme. It's best to make this clear upfront in order to orient the reader, especially if the viewpoint is novel. Most readers will find the viewpoint here unfamiliar because it departs from the more common engineering and medical forensic writing on vision and human factors. Much of the book is written by experimental psychologists (Green and Odom), so many chapters have a strong psychological orientation. Since experimental psychologists are trained in science, the psychological and scientific orientations go hand-in-hand.[2]

While there is some overlap, the experimental psychologists learn a different viewpoint from medical professionals and from engineers. Seeing involves much more than the registration of an image on the retina. Vision includes cognitive processes, such as attention, learning, memory and decision-making. The viewer has goals and expectations that influence where he looks, what he notices and how he interprets. Vision is a psychological phenomenon. Moreover, there are no clear delineations among the specific topic of vision and the more general topics of psychology, the basic science, and human factors, the application of psychology. (Attorneys are also often surprised to learn that psychologists are human factors experts. In fact, the largest membership group of the *Human Factors and Ergonomics Society*, the major human factors professional group in America, is experimental psychologists.)

In sum, when an experimental psychologist looks at vision, he sees the entire behaving organism and not just an eye. The initial chapter explains the classic information processing model that forms the connection between eye and mind and between the two fundamental visual processes, sensation and perception.

*I know what you are thinking*. It's the same question as the attorney who called me while I was typing this very page. He wanted to talk about a road accident. After discussing the case for a while, he asked me about my background. I told him that I'm an experimental psychologist by training. Silence. Long silence. He eventually asked me what a psychologist has to do with vision and human factors. This question is not unusual, and I imagine that many readers are already asking themselves the same.

Many are often surprised to learn that psychology is one of the foundational vision sciences. The abilities to see, as well as to remember, to make decisions and to respond, are natural phenomena that can be studied scientifically like any other natural phenomena. For the study of topics such as visibility, reaction time, conspicuity, judgments of speed, distance, time, size, etc., it is *the* foundational field, and most of the basic and much of the applied research appears in psychology books and journals. The references cited in this book highlight psychology's centrality to vision. Most forensic vision discussions will cite *Society of Automotive Engineers*, *Transportation Research Record*, *Automotive Engineering*, etc. This book cites these sources, too, but it also cites core scientific research from many psychology journals, such as *American Journal of Psychology, Applied Psychology, Ecological Psychology, Journal of Experimental Psychology, Annual Review of Psychology, Perception & Psychophysics, Psychonomic Science, Psychological Science,* and *Quarterly Journal of Experimental Psychology*. Other relevant psychology research is published in interdisciplinary journals such as *Science, Nature, Vision Research, Human Factors* and *Journal of the Optical Society of America*.

Experimental psychology's absence from popular conceptions of science stems from several causes. Most people believe that all psychologists are "shrinks," which is only natural because the pop culture of TV and movies portrays all psychologists that way. In fact, only slightly more than half of all Ph.D. psychologists are clinical psychologists. Further, most people have large misconceptions about science. If asked to define "science," most people will give an incorrect answer. Some will say that science is a systematic body of knowledge. By this definition, political science, library science and poultry science are all sciences. I doubt this is an acceptable Daubert interpretation. A more common answer defines science as a set of topics, chemistry, biology, geology, astronomy, physics, etc. This is also incorrect because specific topics are not scientific or unscientific. "String theory," so popular in physics, is clearly an unscientific notion, but it does not make physics as a whole unscientific. Similarly, much of psychology is not scientific but that does not make psychology as a whole unscientific.

The correct answer is that science is a *method* of learning about the world through systematic, controlled observation. Science is not a set of facts about a particular topic but rather a method used to collect facts on any topic. Further, any research using this method is by definition scientific research. Certainly, different sciences have their own detailed procedures, but everyone follows the same, general "scientific method."

The Daubert criteria underscore the importance of methodology by requiring that scientific evidence be based on accepted method. The ruling quite properly recognizes that the methodology used to collect the facts is as important as the facts themselves. Moreover, this Daubert criterion further implies that qualification as a scientific expert requires a thorough understanding of methodology. In order to interpret research data (his own or others) and to extrapolate them to the real world, the expert must know the methodology underlying the data.

Anyone wishing to become an expert in vision, or any other scientific topic, should resist the urge to skip the "boring" methodology discussions. Two chapters in this edition focus heavily on methodology. Chapter 2 outlines "psychophysics," the field and methodology used in most research on visual capabilities. Chapter 17, *Methodological Analysis of Driver Perception-Brake Times*, discusses the different reaction time values obtained under different conditions and different methodologies. Discussion of methodological effects on contrast detection, measurement of conspicuity, etc. appear at various points throughout the book.

**What's In This Book?**

To sum up the changes in this edition, there is more basic visual science and methodology, citation of basic research data, cognitive psychology, and human factors. It is more about explanatory visual science and covers its entire span, from photoreception of quanta to decision-making and to response. The subtext is the importance of basic visual science for forensic application.

This third edition reflects the changes in two obvious ways. First, the first two editions were entitled *Forensic Aspects of Vision and Highway Safety*. This edition has a subtle change to "*Forensic Vision*"; and *With Application To Highway Safety* is only a subtitle. Second, the book has a new structure, which moves from mostly basic science to increasingly applied topics:

I Basic Vision—the operation of normal vision;
II Clinical Vision—impairments of vision due to disease and aging;
III Roadway Vision—factors affecting vision in the roadway environment; and
IV Forensic Vision—application of the preceding material to accident analysis.

About two-thirds of the book is new. Section I is a mini-course in basic vision, although each chapter of the four chapters also discusses applied topics. There will be much discussion of unfamiliar topics, such as "psychophysics," "naïve realism" and "information processing" that feature prominently in understanding vision in general and forensic vision in particular. Section II covers visual deficits due to eye disease. The chapters are mostly revisions of similar chapters from the previous edition. However, a new chapter on "Aging Vision" outlines losses in the elderly and their effects on older drivers. The Section III chapters focus specifically on vision in driving and are reprinted directly from the previous edition. Section IV contains new chapters on forensic analyses of visibility, collision, pedestrian accidents, and pictorial evidence. These chapters, especially the ones on visibility analysis, are highly technical. Another chapter is an article on driver perception-reaction reprinted from *Transportation Human Factors,* 2000. Supplemental comments update and amplify the discussion. The final chapter, "The Forensic Vision Toolkit," is an amalgam of four chapters of practical advice appearing in the previous edition. Lastly, the book has seven appendices, some new and some reprinted from the previous edition.

What can a reader reasonably expect to gain from reading this book? It will not, by itself, make him an expert. Vision is too large and complex a topic to cover in any one book. Reading a text certainly can't make anyone a scientist—only doing scientific research can. For those wishing to become experts, however, it is a starting point that describes basic concepts, provides fundamentals and explains several common analyses. For attorneys, it offers useful background for asking the right questions and for finding the right expert. For everyone, it inoculates against Judkins' Law.

Marc Green, Ph.D.
Toronto, January 2008

## Endnotes

1. This notion is not completely dead. It lives on as the "attentional spotlight" metaphor discussed in Chapter 4.

2. Of course, engineers and medical people may incorporate some psychology into their viewpoint. The difference is more a matter of emphasis and depth of background.

# Chapter 1

# Introduction to Vision

Marc Green, Ph.D.

*"We see our world of organized scenes and moving objects by combining information from the light which reaches our eyes with knowledge stored in memory about the structure and identity of objects and scenes. We understand our surroundings partly by seeing them but also by inferring what is there...Vision is therefore a genuine cognitive function, not merely a sensory one."*

—Hampson and Morris (1996)

***Synopsis***



## 1.1 Introduction

Vision is the most complex task that humans perform. This may seem an absurd statement because vision is so easy and effortless. We just open our eyes and see. The apparent ease and simplicity, however, is illusory.

As a beginning professor, I quickly learned that none of my students had ever asked herself, "How do I see?" Most people just implicitly assume the "homunculus theory" of vision (Figure 1.1). The eyes are cameras projecting an image onto an internal screen that is viewed by the homunculus, a little man in the head.[1] In fact, explaining vision to any layperson is daunting because most aren't even aware that there is anything to explain. I can assure the skeptical, however, that the 70 percent of the human brain involved in vision is doing *something*.

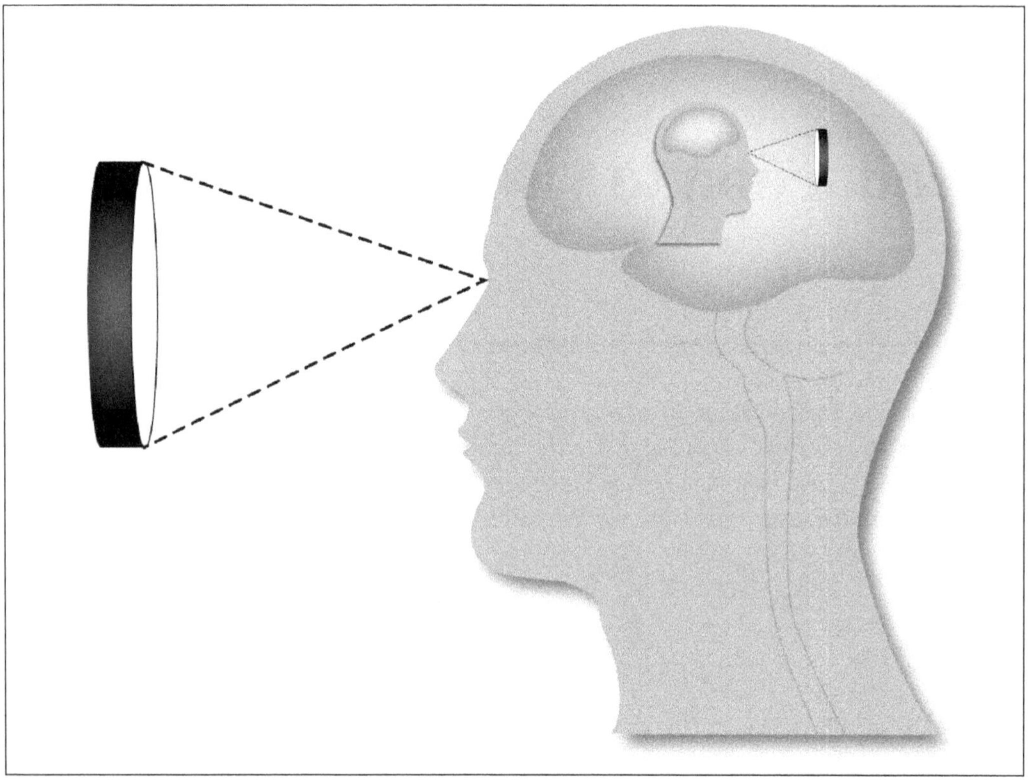

***Figure 1.1*** *The homunculus views the inner screen.*

Below, I discuss this *something* and provide a general overview of factors that contribute to vision. The discussion will surprise those who naïvely view vision as separate from other aspects of behavior. Vision exists to provide information that people may use to act intelligently and adaptively. Vision is not just about the eyes but also about attention, memory, decision-making and other cognitive functions. Moreover, vision and action are closely bound, so motor control and response are also factors in vision. One major school of vision, ecological optics (Gibson, 1979), rests on the belief that vision's main purpose is to guide action. There is no clear separation between seeing and behavior in general, so the topic of vision segues smoothly into human factors. In fact, much of this initial chapter *is* human factors.

The discussion provides perspective by placing vision in the broader context of normal human behavior. Context is key, since vision is highly context-dependent. It cannot be disembodied from the exact circumstances that a person experiences and has experienced. This context consists of many components, including the present physical circumstances, human abilities, limitations and predispositions. It also consists of the past and future. People carry the past with them, since it created knowledge about the world and a set of expectations. The future is both the predictions that the expectations create as well as the desired goals and aims that the person wants to achieve.

The discussion begins by explaining the fundamental distinction between sensation and perception, and the role of attention as gatekeeper between the two. The ensuing section focuses on the close connection between vision and action by contrasting open-loop and closed-loop behavior. I next introduce the classic "information processing" model, which is one of the most important concepts in this book. It shows the relationships among the basic components of behavior, visual input, attention, memory and response. The ensuing section expands the information-processing model into seven stages in a typical behavioral sequence. The final section describes the information-processing model at work in a typical accident scenario, the underride collision.

## A. Vision = Sensation + Perception (+Attention)

Traditionally, scientists decompose vision into two components: "sensation" and "perception," which are separated by the "attentional filter." Another mechanism, "saccadic eye movements," sometimes helps tie the other three components together.

### 1. Sensation

Sensation is the detection of energy from the environment. Visual processing starts when light energy creates an image that stimulates the eye's photoreceptors, specialized nerve cells that convert light energy into electrical energy and eventually into nerve impulses. When the brain receives enough electrical impulses, the sensation reaches "sensory threshold," and the viewer detects the image and indirectly the object that created it.

The primary scientific disciplines that study these processes are physiology and psychophysics. Physiology studies mechanical, physical, and biochemical functions. "Psychophysics" mixes physiology with psychology and physics to examine how the light and other forms of energy translate into sensations. For forensic analysis, psychophysics is generally more directly relevant than physiology. Physiological mechanism may underlie vision, but legal matters depend on functionality—what a viewer could see. In some limited cases, physiology provides guidance, but in many cases it does not.

The most important sensation is not light *per se* but rather contrast, the difference between an object and its background. In a real sense, it is misleading to say that the eye sees light. Unless illumination level is extremely low, the eye functions as an edge-detector whose principle job is to detect contrast borders that define shapes and to make them stand out from the background. There are several types of contrast, but brightness[2] contrast is by far the most important. In some situations, however, color, texture or motion contrast may be relevant.

### 2. Attention

The "attentional filter" lies between sensation and perception. At any given moment, the senses are bombarded by so much input that it may be impossible to fully process everything. Attention acts like a gatekeeper, allowing some information through to perceptual processing while blocking the rest. The attentional filter's selection rules are critical in determining conspicuity. Many people mistakenly believe that attention makes its decision based solely on sensations such as flicker, motion and color. As I will explain in Chapter 4, attention has one foot in sensation and the other in perception, as it can filter using either sensory quality or cognitive meaning.

### 3. Perception

Perception is the cognitive process of organizing and attaching meaning to sensation that has penetrated the attentional filter. The viewer draws on memory, inference and other psychological processes in order to make sense of what he sees. As the Hampson and Morris (1996) quote says, perception is a cognitive function that operates by interpreting images based on both the image and on stored knowledge. Viewers use this knowledge to evaluate the image information in terms of the current context. This context lies both inside the person and in the physical environment. Moreover, the context is not only the present, but also the past and the future.

*The present* consists of both the current environment and the set of human mental and physical abilities and predispositions that are wired into the viewer. The current environment affords a set of physical circumstances that place constraints on possible behavior. There is only so much light, time, distance, etc. People also have obvious mental and physical limitations. Everybody appreciates that people can only see so well, respond so fast, etc. People also have many hard-wired predispositions and limitations, however, that are not so obvious. Evolution has equipped humans with a set of generally useful, but infallible, tendencies. Some are purely mental, such as "heuristics" and "biases," while others, such as "stimulus-response compatibility," constrain action.

We need these inborn tendencies because human mental abilities are limited. In many situations, there is simply no time to completely analyze what is happening. Moreover, people may generally want to make intelligent, rational decisions, but they seldom have all the information needed to act in "perfect rationality." Instead, people typically act in a state of "bounded rationality"(Simon, 1956; Sivak, 2002) where they must interpret events and select responses based on partial information. In emergencies and other stressful situations, people "perceptually narrow," (Estabrook, 1959) further reducing the amount of information used in decision-making.

As partial compensation for bounded rationality, humans have evolved many useful rules of thumb, called "heuristics," to help make quick, efficient decisions based on limited information. Some of the more prominent heuristics include "availability heuristic," "representativeness heuristic," "homogeneity bias," and "small sample bias." The most powerful of all is "confirmation bias," the tendency to seek out and accept evidence that confirms a previously held belief and to ignore and dismiss evidence that contradicts it. Heuristics are valuable but not infallible. They represent a tradeoff among the demands of accuracy, speed and simplicity. They are generally beneficial but may encounter unusual circumstances where they fail.

*The past* also provides a context for behavior. People are not blank slates. People start every situation with expectations, assumptions and extensive general knowledge about how the world works. They have learned this knowledge from previous experience extending into the distant past. Drivers, for example, have learned that other vehicles on their side of the roadway will travel in the same direction and at about the same speed, that STOP signs will only appear at intersections, that pedestrians do not typically walk in front of cars, etc. Road safety experts acknowledge the significance of driver experience in the doctrine of "positive guidance" (Lunenfeld and Alexander, 1990), which stresses the importance of designing roadways and signage to conform with driver expectation.

People also experience a recent past that supplies information about the current, unfolding situation. Accidents usually do not occur instantaneously but rather evolve over a brief time period that can last from milliseconds to seconds. Perceptions of one moment trigger the interpretations of new information seen the next. For example, a driver seeing a "School Ahead" sign is more likely to interpret the object seen a few seconds later as a child. This is an example of the psychological phenomenon called "priming." Memory is associative, so activating part of a schema (school) makes the rest of the schema (schools have students, students are often children…) more available in memory. Schemata are organized knowledge structures, as discussed below.

*The future* also acts as context. Unlike machines, people have goals and purposes. Their attention and perceptions partly depend on what they hope to achieve. Everyone has had the experience of going to meet a friend and thinking that you see him, only to realize that it is someone else who resembles the friend. A driver at an intersection who wishes to turn right will direct his attention leftward because that is where the threatening traffic is coming from. This is one reason vehicles turning right frequently collide with bicycles approaching from the right (Summala, Pasanen, Räsänen and Sievänen, 1996).

Unfortunately, accident analyses frequently overlook context in assigning blame. People almost never set out to cause an accident, so their behavior must have seemed reasonable at the time (Dekker, 2002). It is often only in hindsight that the behavior seems blameworthy or careless. Hindsight all too easily dismisses errant behavior as "stupid," but this merely applies a label and fails to explain anything. Oftentimes, an examination of the contextual factors will turn apparent stupidity into intelligent and adaptive behavior. Or not.

## B. Vision Is Complex, Naïve Realism Is Simple

By now, it should be clear why vision is such a complex topic. It involves the past and the future as well as the present. It involves behavior and psychology, plus some physics and physiology. It involves not just the eye, but also attention, memory, and learning. Moreover, it involves an intelligent reasoning process that occurs without conscious awareness or volition. In sum:

> We do not see what we sense. We see what we think we sense. Our consciousness is presented with an interpretation, not the raw data. Long after presentation, an unconscious information processing has discarded information, so that we see a simulation, a hypothesis, an interpretation; and we are not free to choose. (Norretranders, 1998)

This and the Hampson and Morris (1996) quote that began this chapter highlight vision's fundamental nature. It starts with the detection of raw sensation, but this is just grist for the mill. The viewer takes highly ambiguous sensations and actively organizes and interprets them based on assumptions, expectations, general knowledge, heuristics and goals plus some innate, hard-wired tendencies. This perceptual process occurs automatically without conscious control using incomplete information and is limited by a bounded rationality. Helmholtz called this "the doctrine of unconscious inference."

Lest anyone believe that this discussion is purely theoretical and has no practical value, it has at the very least served three purposes. First, it alerts the reader that this book will deal with issues that would seem far removed from everyday notions of vision and that much of the discussion will be counterintuitive. Second, it warns the reader that explaining vision in court can be a very difficult job. Like introductory perception students, judges and jurors simply accept the homunculus theory and have never really asked themselves how vision works. Of course, they might not know how they see, but they know what they see. Chapter 18 will explain that they are often wrong about this too, at least with regard to pictorial and graphic evidence.

Third, it dispels common fallacies about vision. The homunculus theory is only one example of a more general set of beliefs called "naïve realism" (e.g., Smallman and St. John, 2005), the false notion that commonsense perception reveals the world as it is. Two other main fallacies are completeness and objectivity. People tend to believe that vision is complete and that they see everything. In reality, they are unaware that they are unaware of almost everything. The other fallacy is objectivity, the belief that vision presents a hard reality that exists independently of their expectations, beliefs and goals.

Naïve realism is the reason that explaining vision is so difficult. It is also the reason that jurors place so much faith in eyewitness testimony. They believe that the witness is reporting objective reality. In fact, the witness is, at best, reporting an interpretation of a subset of information that was present at the time. Vision and memory are both largely a function of belief and expectation. It is often said that *seeing is believing*, but it is perhaps more accurate to say that *believing is seeing*.

## 1.2 Embedding Vision In Behavior

Vision is integrated into overall behavior. It both affects and is affected by many other cognitive and motor functions. The next few sections demonstrate this integration by unfolding the role of vision through a series of increasingly detailed descriptions of normal human behavior and the underlying mental processes that guide it.

### A. Open-Loop and Closed-Loop Behavior

Vision's primary purpose is to provide a meaning that can guide action. Figure 1.2 is the popular man-machine depiction showing how a person might relate what he sees to what he does. As in many systems, from computers to digestion, functioning occurs in three stages: input, processing and output.

- Input (Sensation): Energy from the environment enters the eyes, ears, etc. and stimulates the senses' neural mechanisms. If the stimulation is sufficiently high, then the sensation reaches threshold and is detectable.[3]
- Information Processing (IP): The person applies knowledge stored in memory to the sensation in order to interpret the meaning and to decide whether action is required. If so, then the person forms an intent to respond.
- Output (Motor Response): If the intent successfully results in muscle activation, then there is a response that changes some aspect of the environment.

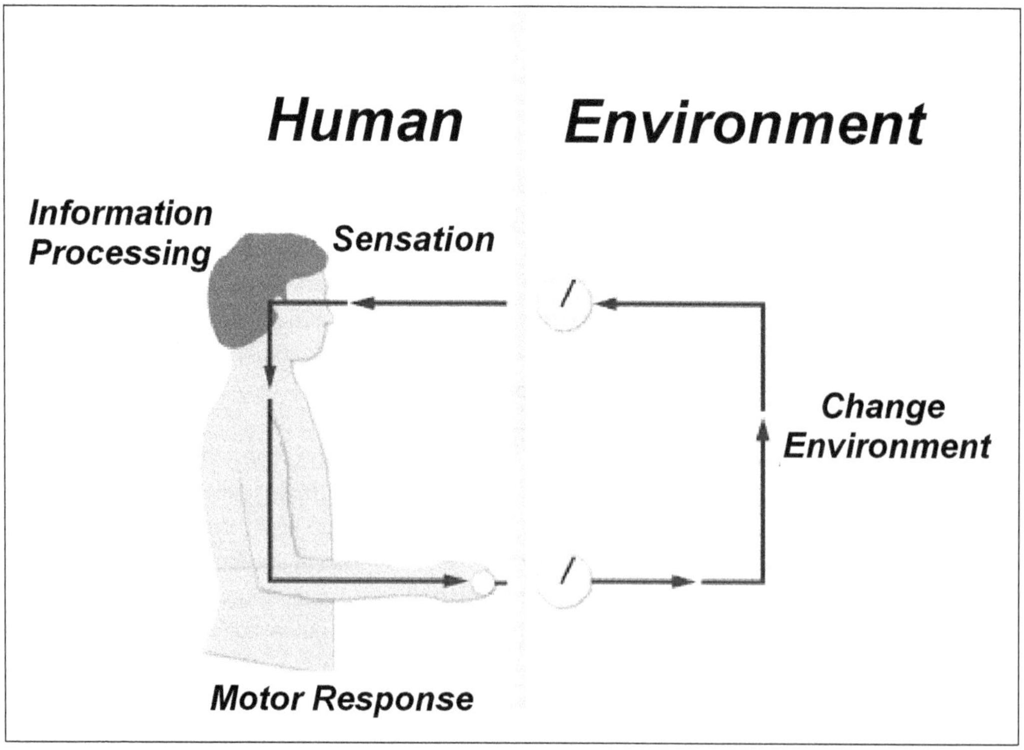


**Figure 1.2** *Human interaction with the environment.*

This figure highlights the distinction between two general classes of behavior: open-loop and closed-loop. In some cases, the action changes the sensory input, which triggers more information processing and possibly another response. The behavior becomes "closed-loop" because the output of the first time through the sequence provides the feedback used in the next iteration. Behaviors such as wayfinding and driving are visually guided and closed-loop. For example, imagine a driver steering a car into a turn. He views the road to gauge the sharpness of the turn, mentally figures the required steering wheel movement and then moves his hands to make it so. This changes the scene ahead so that there is a new view, a new sensation and more information processing that might suggest turning the wheel more or might suggest returning the wheel to the centered position. In closed-loop behavior, perception and action are tightly coupled. This is most obvious in Gibson's (1979) theory of ecological perception and $\tau$ (Lee, 1976) discussed in Chapter 16. As Lee (2006) says, "perception and movement are mutually dependent: perception requires movement and movement requires perception."

In other cases, the person does not cycle through the sequence. In this "open-loop" behavior the viewer sees the world and responds but makes no further attempt to obtain feedback in order to fine-tune the response. The driver, for example, might be so close to a collision that he turns the wheel as fast and as hard as possible. The driver's action, once initiated, is no longer sensitive to feedback and cannot be corrected if in error. Open-loop behavior is especially common in highly-practiced and automatic behavior, such as walking and descending stairs, tasks where control is proprioceptive (feedback from the internal world of muscles and joints, etc.) rather than exteroceptive (feedback from the external world of vision, audition, etc.).

## B. Cognitive Information Processing

Figure 1.3 demonstrates an engineering approach to behavior. It looks at a person's interaction with the world from the outside in purely functional terms. A more scientific analysis examines behavior from the inside by looking at the actual mental processing mechanisms that produce the behavior. Figure 1.3 shows the standard cognitive information-processing model that psychologists use to represent the mechanisms' underlying behavior. The picture depicts open-loop behavior. For closed-loop, a line would run from response to the start.

The model has five basic components: three memories, attention and response. Each component decomposes further into subsystems. I'll ignore this decomposition, except for a detailed examination of attention in Chapter 4.

In normal operation, images (sounds, smells, etc.) from the world strike receptors in the senses. Each sense has its own memory, with vision having an "iconic memory," hearing having an "echoic memory," etc. Sensory memory is very large, holding everything that the senses receive at a given moment, but has a brief duration of perhaps less than a second. Iconic memory is responsible for the "persistence of vision," the sensory memory that allows the eye to integrate a series of still pictures into a smoothly continuous movie.

*Attention* blocks the vast majority of sensory input; people are oblivious to most of their surroundings at any given time. (The "late selection" and "early selection" attentional filter models are discussed in Chapter 4.) This notion is counterintuitive to most people, but it is easy to prove. Feel the touch of your sole on your shoe. Listen to the background noise. Notice the up-down movement of your chest while breathing. Most common sensations are unnoticed because attention has learned that they are irrelevant. This is a key observation because there is no fundamental difference between attentional filtering of information from the soles of the feet and the filtering of the pedestrian that is about to cross the road at an unexpected location.

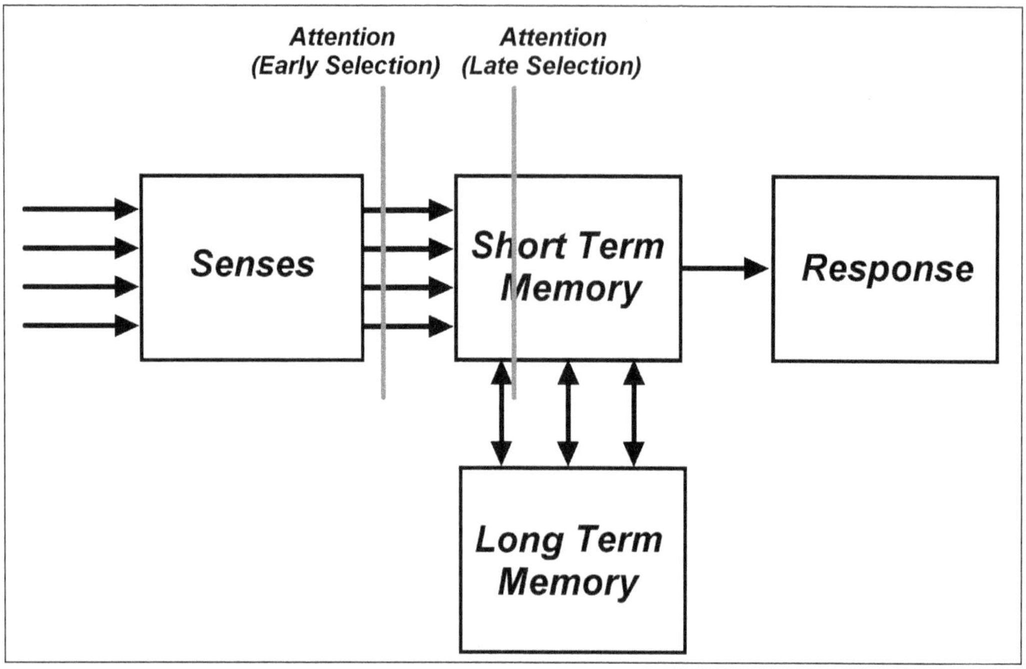


***Figure 1.3*** *Cognitive Information Processing Model.*

The classic "cocktail party" phenomenon nicely demonstrates the relationship among sensation, perception and attention and the importance of meaning. A guest at a cocktail party is having a conversation with the host. He understands the host's words but may be vaguely aware of the buzz of other, unintelligible conversations. The buzz is unanalyzed sensation that may exist at some dim level of awareness, but the listener does not have the capacity to simultaneously interpret both the host's sounds as well as those of other conversations. He is only able to analyze one stream of sensation and to process it for meaning.

The guest can then decide to mentally scan the room, switch attention to someone else and understand that conversation. However, the partner's words disappear or become a meaningless buzz, demonstrating again that attention is limited to one stream at a time. If someone behind him says his name, however, this breaks through the attentional filter, automatically attracting attention to that conversation. All other sounds disappear or join the meaningless buzz.

The cocktail party phenomenon demonstrates many important properties of attention. First it shows that attention is essentially limited to a unitary stream of consciousness that may be either controlled by our conscious effort or involuntarily attracted by some outside influence. Further, it shows that even though we are not consciously aware of what is being said in the background, we must be monitoring it at some unconscious level in order to pick out our name from the buzz. This further demonstrates that most of our perceptual processing occurs outside of awareness.

Similar effects occur in vision. Everyone experiences the unitary nature of consciousness when watching a sports station like ESPN. People can consciously direct attention to the game or the scores scrolling across the display at the bottom. It you are looking for a particular score that you don't want to miss, your attention focuses even tighter and the game picture entirely disappears.

The automatic attraction of attention to meaningful input also occurs frequently in everyday life. When reading the newspaper, I normally only notice the print that is near my focus of attention. However, the letter string "Pitt" often pops out of the background somewhere on the page and draws my attention. I'm from Pittsburgh and went to university at Pitt so the sensation is meaningful. Someone who is from Philadelphia and who went to college at Drexel would probably not notice. This example explains one reason that witnesses so often disagree; they have somewhat different experiences and may notice different aspects of a scene and have different perceptions.

*Short-term memory* receives the sensory information penetrating the attentional filter. It is the mental scratch pad where the real action occurs: the viewer consciously perceives and interprets the sensory input by drawing on *long-term memory*, the repository of stored knowledge. In most cases, the viewer accesses long-term memory very quickly and automatically. In a few instances, the viewer must actively search long-term memory. ("What was his name, again?") There are also cases, such as "affordances" discussed below, in which the interpretation is hard-wired genetically into us so memory is seemingly unnecessary.

Short-term memory is itself a bottleneck because it has both small capacity and short duration. The capacity is low but difficult to quantify. The oft-cited capacity of 7 +/- 2 chunks (Miller, 1956) is vague because the definition of a 'chunk' is unclear. Experts, for example, learn to form large chunks and hold more in working memory than novices (e.g., Green, 1992).

Short-term memory's maximum duration is about 30 seconds. If the information is not rehearsed, refreshed (the viewer continues to look at it) or consolidated into long-term memory, it is lost. New information flowing into short-term memory pushes old, unconsolidated information out. Everyone is familiar with the experience of hearing someone say a phone number, only to discover that by the time you hear the last few digits, the first few are gone from memory—it is just too much to hold in short-term memory at one time.

The same phenomenon happens on the roadway. For example, people have very poor recollection for road signs. In several studies (e.g., Macdonald and Hoffman, 1991), researchers have stopped drivers only a few seconds after passing a sign and asked them what it said. Most drivers could not remember seeing the sign. Presumably, they saw the sign and then the torrent of new visual input pushed it out of working memory. (It is possible that some of these people simply failed to notice the sign. The two events, never seen and seen but lost from working memory, create the same result—no memory.) Motorists remember some signs, however, much better than others. The best remembered contain relevant information, imperatives likely to command immediate action. This is evidence that both attention and retention are based on meaning, not just sensation.

*Long-term memory* is an organized body of stored knowledge. People who encounter the same situation repeatedly typically develop "schemata" and "scripts." A schema (Bartlett, 1932) is a mental model of an object or environment. People create schemata in order to organize complex situations and as a cognitive shortcut; there is no need to reinterpret common situations on every encounter. A script is a stereotyped sequence of events that normally occurs when acting in the schema. Each script has "props," standard objects that are used in a particular way. Viewers are less likely to notice an object that does not belong in the script or occurs at the wrong place or time. A pedestrian, vehicle or sign at an unusual location will not be in the driver's schema and may be less noticeable.

Schemata and scripts distort memory as well as perception. Over time, eyewitnesses tend to 'normalize,' making their recollections consistent with the dominant schema (e.g., Holst and Pezdek, 1992). The same cognitive factors, attention, expectation, confirmation bias, etc., that affect perception all affect memory.

*Response* is the final process. There is a distinction, however, between forming an intent to respond and actually moving the muscles. The intent does not always dictate the actual movement.

Any response, however, changes the world and can initiate a new round of closed-loop processing. The next section elaborates the entire sequence from sensation to response into a seven-stage behavior sequence.

**Table 1.1**
**Stages in a Typical behavioral Sequence**

| | Processing Stage | Question | Example |
|---|---|---|---|
| In | 1. Search and Vigilance | "Where should my eyes point?" | Focus of expansion: the road at the horizon. |
| | 2. Detection | "Is something there?" | Light from the trailer hits eye. |
| IP | 3. Attention and Conspicuity | "Is it worth noticing?" | Something is there. |
| | 4. Recognition | "What is it?" | It's a trailer. |
| | 5. Situation awareness | "What is happening? What will happen next?" | Heading for a collision. |
| | 6. Response Selection | "What should I do?" | Steer immediately. |
| Out | 7. Response | Do it! | Turn the wheel. |

## C. Behavioral Sequences

Human behavior occurs in a sequence that begins with sensation and ends with a muscle movement. Each stage answers a specific question about the world. Vision results from sensation flowing upward from the most peripheral part of the visual system, the eye, to meet cognition flowing downward from the most central part of the visual system, the brain.[4] As a result, each stage is characterized by whether it is driven "bottom-up" by sensation and/or "top-down" by cognition.

### 1. Search and Vigilance

Vision depends on where the viewer points his eyes. The viewer can see only information that falls within the visual field. Even then, the viewer is less likely to see information that falls in the "corner of the eye."

The eye operates somewhat like a camera, with optics focusing an image on a light sensitive "film" called the retina. Unlike camera film, however, the retina is not uniform. If the viewer looks directly at the object, the image forms on the fovea, the retinal area that permits sharpest vision. (See Chapter 3.)

When a person repeatedly performs a task, such as driving, he learns where to point the retina for important information. People learn the regularities in the environment and spend the most time looking where experience has found the greatest benefit. Vehicle drivers typically spend most of their time looking for information helpful in steering. On straight roads, this is a point called the "focus-of -expansion" (FOE) usually located where the road meets the horizon. Drivers can maintain course by driving straight toward the FOE because it is the only stationary point in the visual field. On curves, drivers typically look at the road's tangent point (Land and Lee, 1994).

If the viewer is uncertain or merely wishes to search or to look around, then he must move the eyes. The fovea is very small and does not cover much of the visual world. Even search over small areas of a scene requires eye movements in order to bring different parts on to the fovea for clarity. The viewer normally moves the eyes in a series of "saccades," sharp, quick movements that occur 2–3 times a second. We seldom notice these movements, but normal viewing is a series of snapshots that the eye-brain somehow integrates into an illusion of a coherent and continuous world.

In typical search, the eye makes a saccade, stops and fixates for a brief "dwell time" and then moves on if there is nothing interesting to see in that part of the scene. If the viewer finds an object of interest, he may make several short saccades within a single object. Dwell times are usually about 200–250 msec. (quarter of a second) but are longer in low visibility or when the viewer sees a situation that is ambiguous or potentially has special meaning. A "glance" is the sum of one or more fixations on a single object.

Saccades, like attention, operate under two sources of control (Posner, 1980). One is conscious: "endogenous" control. People may make controlled eye movements for many reasons (Land, 1999): locate objects (where is the exit ramp), direct the hand or object in the hand to a new location (hold out the hand to catch the ball), guide one object to another (put the key in the ignition), or check the state of some variable (examine the gas gauge).

The other is involuntary (exogenous) attraction to a conspicuous object, as when a flashing light by the roadside attracts a driver's attention or when "Pitt" catches my eye. Exogenous control can play an important role in connecting sensation to perception. When a sensation located outside the fovea in the visual periphery attracts attention, the viewer makes an involuntary saccadic eye movement in order to bring the image on to the fovea.

A viewer may also turn the head as well as the eyes to inspect sensations that are in the periphery. Most saccadic movements are 15° or smaller. To see more peripheral objects, a viewer will likely move his head as well as his eyes. When targets are more than 40° in the periphery, head turns are almost a certainty.

When searching, viewers do not sample the scene randomly. Rather, they look where they expect to find task-relevant information. Neisser (1976) suggested a "perceptual cycle (Figure 1.4) that guided eye movements. Viewers start with a schema about each common environment. For example, a road schema might suggest that pedestrians cross at intersections. This directs the driver's eyes to sample locations where a pedestrian would likely be located at intersections. If the driver repeatedly fails to see pedestrians in the actual environment, then the viewer modifies the schema, i.e., the viewer concludes that pedestrians don't cross in this location. The next time the driver reaches that location, the schema will not include pedestrians so the driver will not look for them. Although not shown, the perceptual exploration also depends on goals. If the viewer is looking for a particular street, then he samples areas where street signs are located (according to his schema).

The driving schema, however, can produce sampling errors in unusual environments. The first time I drove the Autobahn, I was whizzing along at 85 mph, checked the rear-view mirror and saw the tiny dot of a car in the far distance behind me. I unconsciously applied my driving schema and concluded the car was no concern because I was traveling fast and because most vehicles travel at about the same speed. The car was so far away, in both distance and time, that I need not keep track of its location. I then decided to change lanes, confident that there was no need for further mirror checks since nothing was behind me. Just as I started moving laterally, the car zoomed past me at 150 mph, and I barely avoided a collision. The Autobahn has no speed limit, so I was unprepared for a car approaching at such a high speed differential.

Lastly, the term "search" sometimes implies active information seeking. Cole and Hughes (1990) wrote an article entitled "Drivers Don't Search: They Just Notice," to highlight their observation that drivers spend an extended time monitoring the road but not looking for any specific information. People who perform such monitoring tasks generally exhibit "vigilance decrement" (Mackworth, 1948), where the ability to notice declines rapidly after a period as brief as 20–30 minutes. Late at night, when the down-phase in circadian rhythms[5] adds to the already monotonous nature of highway driving, vigilance decrement is likely. Experts evaluating the behavior of drivers who have been on the road for extended periods should remember that most studies collect data from highly aroused drivers who perform relatively brief tests during high points on their circadian cycles.

**2. Detection/Sensation/Visibility**

While searching, the viewer senses whether anything is there. Light rays from the scene strike the eye, initiating a chain of neural activity. If the activity level reaches a threshold point, then the viewer senses the object. In psychophysics, the scientific discipline that studies sensory thresholds, we say that the sensed object is "detected."

Detection is preattentive, occurring before the attentional filter operates on the input. Since people only consciously perceive objects that engage attention, the detection of an object does not ensure that the viewer should or will consciously perceive it. *Detection sets the bound of the possible but does not necessarily imply that conscious perception is likely.* If an object is below detection threshold, then it cannot be consciously perceived. If it is above threshold, it may or may not be seen. In fact, people *usually* fail to see the information that they detect.

If the sensory input has spatial structure, the eye next performs figure-ground segregation, a divide-and-conquer strategy that decomposes the image into pieces. The division of image chunks is initially based on raw sensory characteristics, color, brightness, and/or texture. The eye determines which chunks are foreground that should be considered for inspection and which are background that can be ignored. In general, the eye places chunks that are brighter and warmer in color (red, yellow, orange) and larger in the foreground. The viewer also selects, by means of stereopsis, disparity between retinal images in the two eyes that can determine relative depth.

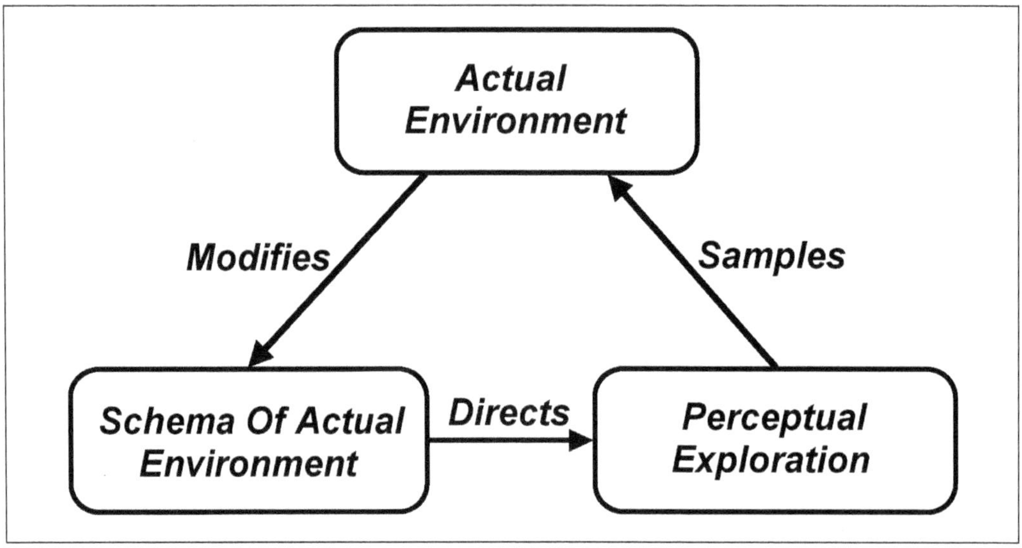


***Figure 1.4*** *Neisser's (1976) perceptual cycle.*

I have said that figure-ground segregation is a purely sensory process, but this is not entirely true. Later cognitive processes may refine the division based on knowledge and expectation. As with many visual processes, it is impossible to cleanly separate sensory from cognitive influences. Issues such as control of eye movements, attention and conspicuity, and figure-ground segregation invariably contain elements of both. The sensory influences usually operate first and faster, but not always.

Lastly, I should clarify some terminology that laypeople (and even some experts) often confuse. Some authors use "detection" to mean a stage of visual processing that includes conscious perception. This is an error that blurs the distinction between preattentive sensation and attentive perception. It further obscures the critical observation that a viewer may fail to see even the most highly detectable object for very good reasons. There is often a large gulf between sensing and conscious seeing.

Similar confusion surrounds the term "visible," which some also use to mean conscious perception as well as sensing. An object is visible if it exceeds detection threshold and can be sensed. In laboratory experiments where the viewer is on alert and knows exactly what the target looks like and when and where it will appear, the difference between sensation and perception may be small.[6] In the real world, however, the difference can be very large. Lastly, "visibility" is the degree to which the target exceeds detection threshold.

### 3. Attention and Conspicuity

The enormous amount of information pouring in through the senses is far too large to process. To avoid being overwhelmed with useless information, humans have evolved an attentional filter to block irrelevant input. Attention allows only important information to reach consciousness and to affect behavior. It allows us to focus our limited mental resources efficiently to the task at hand. Seeing then requires more than simply pointing the eyes in the right direction.

Attention's selection criteria are among the most important and intensively studied topics in visual science. It is also a critical topic in safety since incorrect (but not necessarily unreasonable) selection is a major cause of accidents. Attentional selection falls into two general categories: object and spatial. People may tune attention to see specific objects and/or specific locations in space.

There are a wide variety of circumstances where a person may fail to see an object because attention has filtered it away. One well-known phenomenon is "tunnel vision," or "perceptual narrowing,"[7] which is an exaggeration of the normal concentration of attention around the sightline. The viewer tightly focuses attention and shrinks the "useful field of view" so that objects in the visual periphery are unseen. Several factors promote perceptual narrowing, including stress, poor viewing conditions, expectation, aging, and alcohol and some drugs.

However, people can also fail to notice objects even when they fall on or near the sightline. The viewer is said to be "inattentionally blind." It cannot be stressed often enough that seeing is much more than mere detection of sensation. A person who does not see due to an attentional failure is just as blind, in a real sense, as a person who is blind due to an eye disease such as glaucoma.

Although the term "inattentional blindness" originates from a recent book of laboratory experiments (Mack and Rock, 1998), researchers have noted the phenomenon for many years. Gasson and Peters (1965), for example, performed a series of studies for the Royal Air Force to test the effects of a secondary task on visual field "shrinkage." They found that "*The target could be brought, on some occasions, into the fixation point, indicating 100 percent shrinkage.*" Later authors (Sabey and Staughton, 1975; Hills, 1980; Mai-Britt Herslund and Jørgensen, 2003; Brown, 2005) used the term "look but fail to see" error ('LBFS' error) to describe the common situation in which a person has an accident by simply failing to see the obvious.

Inattentional blindness can occur for several reasons (see Chapter 4). For now, it is important to remember that once the object is detected, attention must decide whether it should or should not be filtered. "Conspicuity" is the property that allows the object to break through the filter and enter consciousness. It refers to both the object's sensory properties and to the viewer's mental set.

In my experience, inattentional blindness is a far more common cause of accidents than lack of visibility. My initial forensic case, for example, involved a woman who drove a truck into the same gas station every workday for a year. The time was always early morning during twilight. To enter the gas station, she had to drive across a sidewalk that ran parallel to the street. As the truck edged past the sidewalk, she heard a thud. Looking back, she saw that she had struck a bicyclist who was lying injured on the ground. She claimed that she looked down the sidewalk as she entered the station and could only guess that there was insufficient light to see him.

A visibility analysis (Chapters 13 and 14) showed that seeing the bicyclist was well within human capability. She was inattentionally blind because of expectation. She had developed a script: pick up the truck, drive to the gas station, look down the sidewalk, see nothing, enter the gas station, fill the tank, etc. There were two sources of violated expectation. First, she entered the same gas station every workday for a year and had never seen anything on the sidewalk, so she had developed the expectation that no one would be there in the future. Second, pedestrians may be common on sidewalks but bicycles are not. Her attention was likely tuned, if at all, to look mainly for pedestrians. The bicyclist on the sidewalk was not part of the schema.

### 4. Recognition

If the viewer attends the sensation, the next step is recognition and identification—to determine what it is. Perception occurs when the viewer applies knowledge stored in long-term memory to organize and to interpret the sensation. For example, the blob of light down the road suddenly becomes a bicyclist, or the face suddenly becomes your cousin.

People are generally unaware that sensation and perception are distinct mental processes because the transition is usually quick and effortless. The sensation-perception distinction, however, is more obvious when the sensory input is ambiguous. Figure 1.5 demonstrates the gap between attending a sensation and recognition. At first glance, the image appears as a meaningless jumble of dots. Continue looking, however, and the visual system organizes the dots into the scene of a dog sniffing the ground. (The dog is outlined in endnote 8.) Sensation has engaged attention, but due to the high ambiguity, organization and recognition require time and effort.

For accident investigation and blame assignment, this example is a cautionary tale. Once you see the dog, it becomes obvious and you cannot lose the percept. Similarly, after the accident, the investigator already knows the correct interpretation, so it is obvious. It is easy to fall into the hindsight trap of ascribing post-accident knowledge to the actor before the accident. In reality, people acting before the accident had less knowledge, different goals, expectations, etc. Their interpretation may have been perfectly reasonable *given their context*. When the part of the context is a man-made product or environment, the fault may lie with the person who created the context rather than the person acting in it (Green, 2006).

The dog example may seem the exception. Perception normally operates much faster and with less effort. However, sensations at night in low illumination are frequently ambiguous. Is the blob a piece of litter or a pedestrian? Are those dots of light a vehicle nearby or just some traffic lights far away?

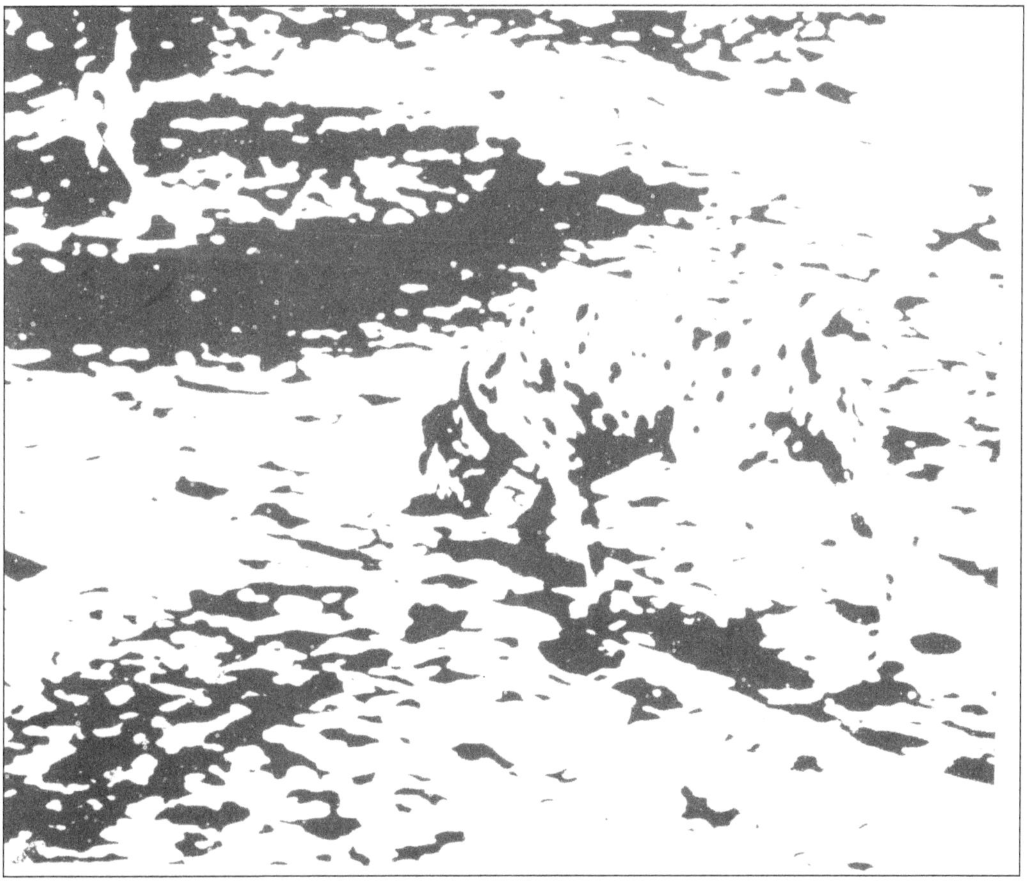

***Figure 1.5*** *The dots form a dog sniffing the ground.*

In good daylight there is usually little ambiguity, so the viewer need only draw on readily available memories. Even in these circumstances, however, knowledge guides interpretation. The two images in Figure 1.6 show bumps and dents. The two pictures are actually identical, except that the right hand one is inverted. The dots on the left appear as dents while the dots on the right appear as bumps. Why the change of interpretation? The answer lies in an environmental regularity that we have all learned—light usually comes from above. As a result, a brighter top indicates a bump while a brighter bottom suggests a dent. This is a more typical case where the viewer automatically uses implicit knowledge to perceive almost instantaneously. Another example is "aerial perspective," where objects that are fuzzy and bluish seem farther away. In this case, the environmental regularity is that light from more distant objects hits more air molecules, scatters and creates a fuzzy image. Since the atmosphere scatters short wavelength light more, the image is both fuzzy and blue.

In some cases, interpretation arises from strong innate perceptual tendencies and from context. People do not perceive objects in isolation but rather as being embedded in a scene context. For example, perception of even basic properties such as size depends greatly on context. Figure 1.7 shows two classic examples. In Figure 1.7A, the two middle circles are the same size, yet the circle surrounded by bigger circles appears smaller (Ebbinghaus illusion). In Figure 1.7B, the two dark lines are the same length, although the left one appears much smaller (Ponzo illusion). The effect occurs because the left line appears much closer due to the environmental regularity that parallel lines converge in the distance (linear perspective). If two objects create the same size retinal image but one is farther than the other, it must be larger. The mind uses apparent distance to judge apparent size, but also uses apparent size to judge apparent distance. One theory holds that child pedestrians are frequently struck by cars because drivers perceive them as being normal size people who have small retinal images because they are farther away. Conversely, drivers are less likely to rear-end large trucks, because they appear closer. In the Ebbinghaus illusion, the small dot in the center of large dots also looks further away because a small retinal image is a cue for greater distance.

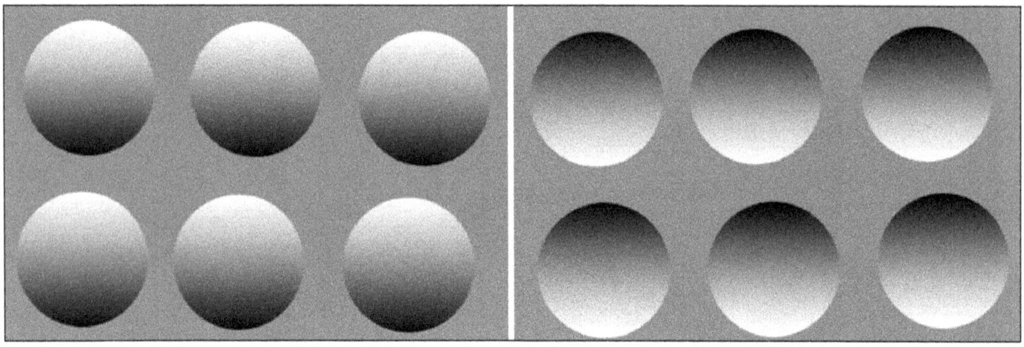

***Figure 1.6*** *Direction of light determines dot appearance.*

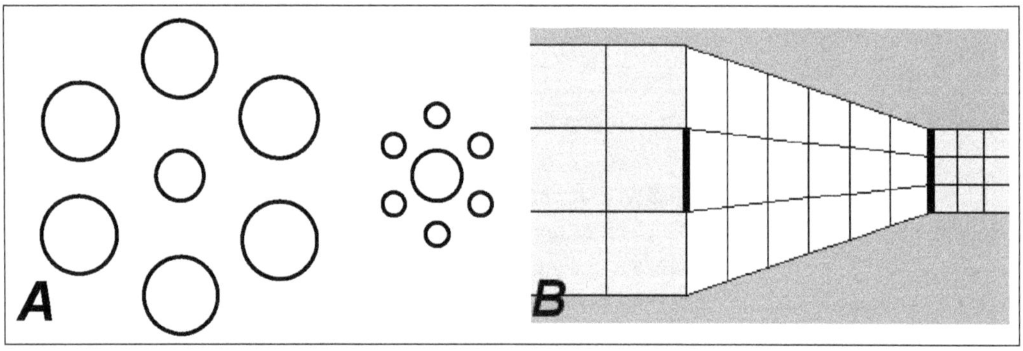


***Figure 1.7*** *Two illusions of size and context. A is the Ebbinghaus illusion and B is the Ponzo illusion.*

One final example shows how experience and learning cause perceptual changes. A classic research study (Chase and Simon, 1973) examined the differences between the perceptions of skilled and beginner chess players. Both groups briefly examined a series of board positions from real games. They recreated the position of the pieces on an empty chessboard. The chess experts recreated the piece locations with high accuracy, but the low skill beginners placed the pieces in the wrong locations. The difference wasn't simply due to expert chess players having superior memory. Further research had both groups examine chessboards with pieces placed at random positions. In the test, experts and beginners performed similarly.

This research is frequently cited because it demonstrates how perception is an active process in which viewers organize visual information into meaningful units. The expert chess players looked at the real board positions and instantly perceived, not a large number of individual pieces, but rather a few meaningful chunks. The beginners did not have the experience to perform the organization. When confronted with chess pieces placed randomly, the experts acted like the beginners because they could not project a meaningful organization on to the board. Similar effects occur in other activities, such as driving. Novice drivers are less able to anticipate collisions because they are inexperienced at perceiving the unfolding pattern of events to warn of upcoming danger. Jurors looking at pictures of an accident scene are unlikely to have the same perceptions as a person familiar with the location.

There are a few lessons in the examples shown in this section. The retinal image constrains scene interpretation but does not specify it. Much of what we see arises from our cognitive processes. This is exactly the point that Morris and Hampson were making. Further, these perceptions are "cognitively impenetrable" because we cannot introspect and change them and because they occur automatically and without control or awareness. They just happen and we have no choice, as Norretranders says. Cognitive impenetrability also gives us the illusion that we see the world directly and that nothing is really happening between the ears. It explains why most people never think about vision. Of course, this is usually a good thing. People would be overwhelmed and immobilized if normal perception required a series of conscious decisions. On the other hand, cognitive impenetrability leads to naïve realism, which can be a bad thing, especially in court.

### 5. Situation awareness

Situation awareness is most concisely defined as "the perception of elements in the environment within a volume of space and time, the comprehension of their meaning, and the projection of their status in the near future" (Endsley, 1995). It is the direction of consciousness to generate skilled performance in a given, unfolding situation (Smith and Hancock, 1995). The viewer may need to integrate several sources of perceptual information, draw on memory, and predict the immediate future—which then becomes one of the contextual factors in the person's decision making. This is the point at which the person decides whether there is a potential hazard and whether action will be required.

In a typical example, a person might have recognized the object on the road ahead as a pedestrian. Next, the driver must evaluate what the pedestrian is doing and how it relates to his current speed and heading and how it affects the current goal of driving the car to its destination. The meaning might be that the pedestrian is on a collision course with the car and that an accident will occur in the future. It might mean the pedestrian is moving away from the car and no action is required, so it is OK to look elsewhere for possible dangers. The driver bases his assessment on expectations created by past experience with pedestrian behavior as well as on psychophysical/perceptual judgments, usually of time, motion, and distance. How far is the pedestrian? How fast is she moving? How much time do I have? How often do pedestrians step into my path? If I steer what will happen? If I brake what will happen? Is it worse to steer into the oncoming lane or off the road into a ditch? A driver might be partly conscious of this thinking but much occurs outside of awareness.

### 6. Response Selection

Once a person decides that he must act, the next problem is choosing the proper response. In some cases, the choices are obvious. A driver facing a short time to avoid an accident can typically only brake or steer. Again, people apply their knowledge and experience. Moreover, people have built-in tendencies that limit control. Some factors operating here are automaticity, stimulus-response compatibility and affordance perception.

*Automaticity.* Learning can essentially expand attentional capacity. Extended practice allows people to perform tasks with minimal attentional supervision. For example, a person learning to use a device must initially attend in order to know where the hand and fingers go, read instruction or warnings, locate switches, etc. With extended practice, the response becomes automatic, meaning that the individual movements become linked in a chain. Once the viewer perceives the appropriate situation, he triggers the chain which then runs off of its own accord. In some cases, the behavior becomes open-loop and the need for external visual information is replaced by "muscle memory" as internal ("proprioceptive") feedback from each movement guides the next. The person seemingly performs the task without attention and can simultaneously carry on other activities, have a conversation, read, etc. Virtually all skilled performance, driving a car, operating machinery, etc., involves this replacement of conscious, attentive response with automatic behavior.

In driving, the most obvious example of automatic behavior is steering. People have little conscious awareness of how they manage to maintain lane position and to steer within the roadway. People behaving automatically generally cannot explain how they perform the behavior. If, for example, you asked a driver how he was maintaining lane position or knows how much to turn the wheel to steer a curve, he could not tell you. It has required extensive research (e.g., Land and Lee, 1994), for example, just to determine how people steer through curves because drivers don't know how they do it. In general, people who have become expert in routine tasks do not make conscious decisions: they simply do what works (Dreyfus and Dreyfus, 1986). Skilled behavior is fluid and unbroken by any conscious decision-making. In fact, one way to degrade expert behavior is to induce conscious deliberation.

Automatic behavior is usually beneficial because it partially circumvents attentional limitations and smoothes performance. In many cases, this offloading of conscious decision making to automaticity is a crucial part of skill development. Unfortunately, automaticity can also produce disastrous results. Since the task requires little attention, people then operate in open-loop mode or become blind to situational changes such as wear, equipment fault, warnings and other unexpected changes in the environment (e.g., Green, 2004). The collision of skilled, automatic behavior with unexpected circumstances is a major cause of accidents.

*Stimulus-Response Compatibility.* "Stimulus-response compatibility" refers to innate connections between vision and response selection. The tendency to move away from a threat is a good example. If a driver sees another car coming on a collision course from the left, the overwhelming predisposition is to steer rightward and away from the impending threat. The natural tendency to move away from objects heading toward us is good because the conscious analysis of a projectile's path could cause a fatal delay. However, it often causes the driver to steer into the path of the approaching vehicle. If the driver had time to calmly and rationally calculate the trajectory of the approaching vehicle, he would likely realize the safest strategy would be to steer toward the vehicle's current location or even straight ahead. (In fact, racecar drivers learn to steer straight toward a collision that occurs in front of them.) However, time pressure forces immediate response to threats, so the driver acts on hard-wired predisposition rather than deliberate calculation.

Another common scenario occurs when a driver goes into a sideways skid. If skidding left side forward, the overwhelming urge is to turn the wheel rightward to move away from the threat. This, of course, is opposite to the correct response, which is to turn the wheels leftward into the skid. People can overcome the incompatibility with training, but under stress may revert. In some cases, it is almost impossible to train out the incompatibility. Even with years of intense practice, very few highly trained baseball players can avoid bailing out when a curveball initially heads toward them.

Figure 1.8 shows another kind of compatibility called "mapping." The left side depicts the switch plate from my house's upper landing. One switch controls the upstairs overhead light, one the downstairs overhead light and the other the bathroom. In spite of living in the same house for 23 years, I frequently select the wrong switch. There is no compatibility in the design because mapping from perception->response->effect is arbitrary. The switches should be arranged to be compatible with their effect on various locations in the house. The right side shows how the switches should have been designed. The switch on the top should control the upstairs light, the switch on the bottom should control the downstairs light and the third switch is orthogonal because it controls the bathroom, not the hallway.

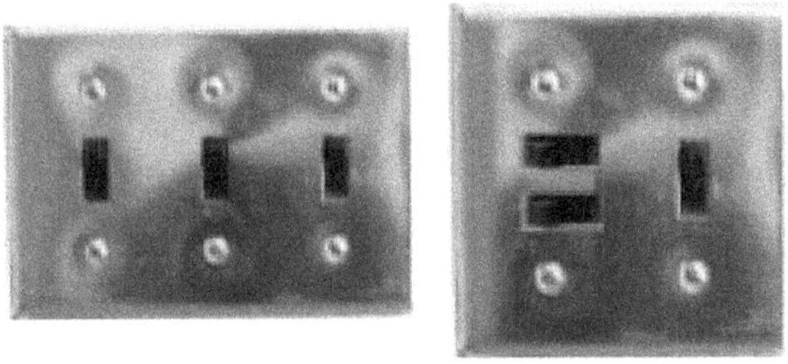

***Figure 1.8*** *Poor and good stimulus-response mappings.*

Despite knowing all this, I still sometimes curse myself for being stupid when hitting the wrong switch. Like most people, I automatically place causation on the event occurring just before the error—my behavior. Fault really belongs to the person who designed the switch. He should have known about mapping compatibility and that the design would cause frequent error. People are what they are and designers should be held responsible for taking likely human behavior into account. Of course the designers would accuse me of misuse, and say that I should have carefully inspected the switches and made a deliberate decision before every use (Green, 2006). However, there is no point in wishing that people would act in some perfect, idealized way that runs contrary to human nature.

I'm sure that most people reading the last two paragraphs are wondering why I never learned the switch positions. A similar question arises in many accident cases, where a person is injured because he failed to use information available from previous encounters with a product or environment. In one case, a man was injured leaving a building by a clear glass door with an unusual design. He had entered the building a few hours earlier through the same entrance. Why didn't he notice the odd design then?

The answer lies partly in the fact that the door appeared in a different context going in and going out and partly in the distinction between "knowledge in the world" and "knowledge in the head" (Norman, 1980). In order to behave adaptively, we have to know much about how the world works. Some of that knowledge is stored in memory and applied as needed. For example, doors are a means of moving from one bounded area to another. In our lifetimes, however, we pass through thousands of different doors. Each has a particular mode of operation. We could memorize the way every door works, so that next time we would know how it operates. That would require lots of memory. Instead, it is better if we learn a few general rules and let the door tell us which rule applies and how it operates—the required knowledge is in the world rather than in the head.

Objects often communicate their operation by their size, shape, color, location, etc. If a door has a handle, it should open toward us because handles are for grasping and for pulling. If the door opens outward, it should not have a handle because people will automatically try to pull it. Instead, it should only have a flat plate that permits pushing but not pulling. In sum, the door should be designed to tell the user what to do.

Getting back to the accident, the man failed to notice the door's operation on the way into the building because it was not important and slipped through short-term memory before consolidation. Further, he implicitly learned that the door would tell him how to get out. The door failed to give him the proper information and so he was injured. The accident did not occur because of the man's poor memory or "inattention," but rather because the door was improperly designed.

*Affordances*. The discussion of "knowledge in the world" naturally leads to the concept of "affordances" (Gibson, 1977), another class of "hard-wired" relationships between vision and responding. The actions that an object permits are one of its perceptual qualities, just as much as its size, shape and color. For example, a handle affords grasping. When a person sees a handle, he sees the grasping affordance just as much as he sees the shape, size, color, etc.

In a slightly broader meaning, an affordance is a set of environmental factors that define possible from impossible goal-oriented behavior. For example, a pedestrian reaches a curb and looks down the road to judge a gap. If the oncoming traffic is sufficiently distant, the road affords the opportunity for crossing safely. However, people of different walking speeds may perceive different affordances. A road that affords crossing for an athletic young person may not afford crossing for an older, slower person. Still, the idea is the same: to see something is to see what you can do with it.

Object affordances are partially a function of user goals. A hammer can afford driving nails or it can afford weighing papers down. Accidents frequently occur because a product signals unintentional affordances. When the user perceives and uses the affordance, it is sometimes inaccurately called "misuse" (Green, 20006). For example, step ladder manufacturers frequently put an extra step at the top of the ladder. The instructions tell the user not to use this rung, although it appears identical to the others. (Presumably it makes the ladder unstable or can't support sufficient weight.) However, the rung affords stepping and reaching higher. It is thoroughly predictable that many users will use this extra rung to achieve a goal.

Affordances may also cause road accidents. In one case, a driver who hit and killed a child had placed papers on the dashboard. The reflection on the windshield created glare and obscured vision. He should be held at fault for putting the papers on the dashboard—a conscious voluntary decision. However, the manufacturer is also to blame by making the dashboard a flat surface. When a person sees a flat horizontal surface, such as a tabletop or dashboard, he perceives the affordance of putting objects on it. The dashboard invited the behavior.

Lastly, the "population stereotype" is a concept that many confuse with the affordances. While affordances are innate perception-response connections, "population stereotypes" are learned perception-response conventions shared by most people within a culture. If a user wants to increase loudness on a new stereo, for example, should he turn the volume knob clockwise or counterclockwise? Most people would automatically turn it clockwise because they have internalized that norm. Any North American who has tried to cross the street in Britain knows our locally adaptive population stereotype of looking left as we step off the curb can be dangerous in a different culture.

### 7. Response

In the final stage, the person moves the muscles required to perform the response. In closed-loop behavior, this stage will circle back to sensation as the viewer assesses the effect of his action.

In open-loop behavior, the person ceases sensing the external world but may transfer control to proprioception.

Response intent, however, does not always translate to proper execution. People frequently make "slips," a type of error that occurs when the actual response is not the intended response. For example, one common type of slip is a capture error. If a person's phone number is 212-555-1212 and his dentist's number is 212-555-4343, he might intend to call his dentist and end up dialing his own number. The initial sequence is the same for both numbers, but the home number is dialed far more often. This habit captures the response and diverts the last 4 digits from 4343 to 1212. Similarly, a driver might take the same route every day from home to office. One day he decides to go to the supermarket, a less common destination that starts off in the same direction but requires an earlier turn down a different street. The driver starts thinking about what he will buy at the store and suddenly finds himself at the office. Despite the intent, the more familiar behavior has captured the less familiar.

Capture errors are more likely with automatic behavior, where a practice has turned a sequence of individual responses into what amounts to a single response, a phenomenon called "chaining." Once the sequence begins going down the practiced path, it simply continues under its own inertia. These chained responses might be conceived as a subroutine that the main processor sets off on its own or as a mental servant sent out to perform a specific task so that we can attend to something else.

Slips contrast with "mistakes," errors of intention or planning (e.g., Reason, 1990). For example, suppose the person drives to the wrong address because he has forgotten that his dentist has moved. The person drove to the intended destination, so there was no slip. Instead, the error occurred in the formation of the intent, so it arose from a different stage of behavior.

The "violation" is a third class of response. Both mistakes and slips are "honest errors" because the driver is not aware he is going to do anything wrong. Violations are like mistakes because they result from a conscious intent, but differ from mistakes because the person is aware that the behavior breaks some rule or guideline. A driver traveling 65 mph in a 55 mph zone is making a mistake if he believes the speed limit to be 65 mph, but making a violation if he knows that it is 55 mph. A driver who intends to slow to 55 mph but inadvertently presses the accelerator rather than the brake pedal has made a slip.

## 1.3 Example: The Underride Accident

The common accident scenario of a side underride demonstrates many aspects of the typical behavior sequence. A tractor-trailer blocks all lanes of a roadway at night, either while making a sharp turn or backing out of a driveway. A driver traveling 55 mph down the roadway goes under the trailer, shearing off the car's top, and is instantly killed.

When such cases occur, the defendant trucking company will often send an "expert" out to the accident scene. The expert will stand 1000 feet from the point of collision and then will say that the truck was visible at that distance. The implication is that the driver should have seen the trailer at a sufficient distance to permit braking and to avoid the accident.

While the observation is presumably true, it is also misleading. It disembodies vision from the driver's context. There may have been enough light (actually contrast) for the truck to produce a detectable sensation in the visual system. However, vision involves much more than mere activation of photoreceptors and reaching of sensory thresholds. The assessment of such accidents should start with a realistic appreciation of driver context:

> "Although motorway driving involves high speeds, it is relatively undemanding and unarousing most of the time. Due to advances in vehicle and highway design, together with the fact everyone around the driver is traveling in the same direction and at similar speed, little sensation of speed is obtained. Driving becomes largely a matter of monitoring one's lane position, maintaining a safe distance from the vehicle in front, and changing lanes to overtake slower vehicles if necessary. Other vehicles are generally behaving quite predictably and little attention has to be paid to them, other than cursorily registering their presence. Also drivers very rarely encounter stationary vehicles on such roads (at least not immediately in front of them), and so have no reason to look out for then. In terms of vigilance theory, the event which is to be detected occurs with a very low frequency amongst many other, fairly similar events (Langham, Hole, Edwards, and O'Neill, 2002, p. 179).

Given this starting point, what will happen when a driver approaches a trailer blocking the roadway? Drivers typically spend most of the time scanning the open road directly ahead (stage 1). He would probably be looking toward the end of his headlamp beam, about 300 feet ahead, because that's the most well-illuminated part of the roadway. Light reflected from the truck must provide enough contrast with the background to reach detection threshold (stage 2). If the truck has reflectors, then light from the reflectors must provide enough contrast with the trailer surface or other background.

Next, the truck must engage attention (stage 3). The attentional filter makes its selection of the relevant information based on many years of driving experience. However, most drivers have little or no experience of seeing an entire road blocked by a thin and white red line. It runs contrary to their expectations and is more difficult to perceive. The investigator who arrived after the accident knew exactly where to look and what he would find there, so the truck appeared obvious to him at 1000 feet. Moreover, the investigator had not been monitoring the road for extended periods, unaroused or experiencing vigilance decrement. Likewise, photographs and videotapes shown later to witnesses and jurors who know the case facts will similarly be misrepresentations of the driver's perceptions. (See Chapter 18.)

Attention can also be sometimes drawn by some physical scene attributes, especially size. As the driver approaches, the image of the truck grows on the retina, the headlamps throw more light to increase contrast and it eventually engages attention. The next stage is object recognition (stage 4); the driver must recognize the image as being a tractor-trailer across the road, and not mistake the trailer's flattop for the horizon. If the driver sees only the reflectors, he may be confused as to what they represent. The rarity of the event impairs and slows the recognition—it's not something that the driver has seen before. There are no salient depth cues, so distance can be difficult to judge. The driver frantically searches memory trying to organize and interpret the image in terms of previous visual experience. Once he recognizes the object, the driver must gain situation awareness (stage 5) and decide what to do (stage 6). The situation is that a collision is imminent. Unless he responds, he is going to drive into the trailer and be killed. While all this thinking occurs, his car is racing forward at 81 ft/sec (55 mph). By the time the driver appreciates the situation, he is very near the truck and there is no clear-cut response. Competition among response alternatives wages on because there is no time to brake and nowhere to steer. It is common for the collision to occur without the driver having made any response at all (stage 7 not completed).

## 1.4 Conclusion

This chapter has introduced vision and made several points. First, vision may seem simple, but it is highly complex. As a result, the subject is both difficult to understand and to explain. Judges and jurors probably are not even aware that there is anything to explain. At best, they might naively and implicitly assume the homunculus theory.

Second, vision is a much broader topic than just the study of the eye and of sensations such as contrast, brightness and color. Vision incorporates many aspects of cognition, including memory, attention, learning, and reasoning. We do not see in order to detect light and contrast, but rather to understand the world so we may act adaptively and intelligently. This is why much of this chapter on vision has wandered into human factors and cognitive psychology.

Third, like all other human behavior, vision is imbedded in a context that includes the past and future as well as the present. Human behavior occurs at a specific time in a specific context. This is one reason that government regulations, accident statistics and epidemiological data can be useful but are never definitive in defining accident causation. They are generalities that cannot take context into account, they may or may not apply to any particular situation, and do not address causation directly. It is folly to disembody action from context by relying on generalities. I stress this point because it so frequently occurs in assigning blame.

The discussion now turns to more specific issues in basic vision. The reader may be tempted to skip these chapters and proceed directly to the more obviously applied material toward the end of the book. I advise against this. In order to understand why vision may fail in some circumstance, it is necessary to understand how it operates normally. Moreover, much of the forensic application will only make sense in light of the underlying science. The discussion of basic vision highlights issues and problems faced by anyone wishing to perform a forensic vision analysis of any kind, whether it be road accidents, warnings, intellectual property or witness reliability. Lastly, if a person expects to pass Daubert as a scientific vision expert, then he should be able to demonstrate a deep knowledge of basic vision science, including both fundamental concepts and methodology.

The next two chapters provide a brief background on psychophysics, the scientific discipline that studies the senses and issues such as visibility. The ensuing chapter moves on to more cognitive issues of the attentional filter and conspicuity, the ability to penetrate the filter. Other cognitive issues, such as memory, learning and reasoning arise in later chapters, but will not be covered in the same detail.

## References


Bartlett, F. 1932. *Remembering*. Cambridge: Cambridge University Press.

Brown, I. 2005. *Review of the 'looked but failed to see' accident causation factor*. London: Department for Transportation. (Road safety research report. No. 60).

Chase, W. and H. Simon. 1973. The mind's eye in chess. In W. G. Chase (ed.), *Visual Information Processing*, 215–281. New York: Academic Press.

Cole, G. and P. Hughes. 1990. 'Drivers Don't Search: They Just Notice', In Brogan, D. (ed.), Visual Search Procedures, *1st International Conference on Visual Search*, University of Durham, September 1988, London: Taylor and Francis.

Dekker, S. 2002. *The Field Guide to Human Error Investigations*. Burlington, Vermont: Ashgate Publishing.

Dreyfus, H. L. and S. E. Dreyfus. 1986. *Mind over Machine: the power of human intuition and expertise in the era of the computer*. Oxford: Basil Blackwell.

Endsley, M. 1995. The out of loop performance problem, situation awareness and workload in a dynamic control task. *Human Factors*, 37, 381–394.

Gasson, A. and G. Peters. 1965. The effect of concentration upon the apparent size of the visual binocular field Part I. *The Optician:* London.

Gibson, J. J. 1977. The theory of affordances. In Perceiving, Acting, and Knowing, edited by R. E. Shaw and J. Bransford, 67-82. Hillsdale, NJ: Lawrence Erlbaum Associates.

Gibson, J. J., 1979. *Ecological Approach to Visual Perception*. Hillsdale: Lawrence Erlbaum Associates Publishers.

Green, M. 1992. Conceptions and Misconceptions of Design. In *Knowledge Aided Design*, edited by M. Green, 1–23. London: Academic Press.

Green, M. 2002. Inattentional Blindness. *Occupational Health & Safety Canada* Jan/Feb, 23–29.

Green, M. 2006. Human error vs. design error. *Trial* June, 231-233.

Hampson, P. and P. Morris. 1996. *Understanding Cognition*. Oxford: Blackwell.

Herslund, M-B. and N. Jørgensen. 2003. Looked-but-failed-to-see-errors in traffic. Accident Analysis and Prevention 35, 885-891.

Hills, B. 1980. Vision, visibility, and perception in driving. *Perception* 9, 183-216.

Holst, V. and K. Pezdek. 1992. Scripts for typical crimes and their effects on memory for eyewitness testimony. *Applied Cognitive Psychology* 6, 573-587.

Land, M. 1999. The roles of vision and eye movements in the control of activities of daily living. Perception 28, 1311-1328.

Land, M. 2006. Eye movements and the control of actions in everyday life. *Progress in Retinal Eye Research* 25, 296-324.

Land, M. and D. Lee. 1994. Where we look when we steer. *Nature* 369, 742-744.

Langham, M., G. Hole, J. Edwards, and C. O'Neil. 2002. An analysis of 'looked but failed to see' accidents involving parked police vehicles. *Ergonomics* 45, 167-85.

Lee, D. 2006. How movement is guided. http://www.perception-in-action.ed.ac.uk/PDF_s/Howmovementisguided.pdf. Downloaded 30 May 07.

Lunenfeld, H. and G. Alexander. 1990. *A Users' Guide to Positive Guidance. Washington D. C.: U. S. Department of Transportation* Federal Highway Administration, Office of Traffic Operations (Report No. FHWA-SA-90-017).

Macdonald, W. and E. Hoffmann. 1991. Drivers' awareness of traffic sign information. *Ergonomics* 34, 585–612.

Mack, A. and I. Rock. 1998. *Inattentional blindness.* Cambridge, Ma: MIT Press.

Mackworth, N. H. 1948. The breakdown of vigilance during prolonged visual search. *Quarterly Journal of Experimental Psychology* 1, 6-21.

Miller, G. 1956. The Magical Number Seven, Plus or Minus Two. *Psychological Review* 63, 81-97.

Neisser, U. 1976. *Cognition and Reality: Principles and Implications of Cognitive Psychology.* New York: W. H. Freeman.

Norretranders, T. 1998. *The User Illusion Cutting Consciousness Down to Size.* New. York: Viking.

Norman, D. A. 1980. *The Psychology of Everyday Things.* New York: Basic Books, Inc.

Posner, M. I. 1980. Orienting of attention. *Quarterly Journal of Experimental Psychology* 32, 3-25.

Reason, J. 1990. *Human Error.* Cambridge, UK: Cambridge University Press.

Sabey, B. and G. Staughton. 1975. Interacting roles of road environment, vehicle and road user in accidents. Paper presented to the 5th International Conference of the International Association for Accident and Traffic Medicine and the 3 rd International Conference on drug abuse of the International Council on alcohol and addiction, 1–5 September 1975, London.

Simon, H. A. 1956. Rational Choice and the Structure of the Environment. *Psychological Review 63, 129-138.*

Sivak, M. 2002. How common sense fails us on the road: Contribution of bounded rationality to the annual worldwide toll of one million traffic fatalities. *Transportation Research Part F* 5, 259-269.

Smallman, H. and M. St. John. 2005. Naïve realism: Misplaced faith in realistic displays. *Ergonomics in Design* 13, 6-13.

Smith, K. and P. Hancock. 1995. Situation awareness is adaptive, externally directed consciousness. Human Factors, 37, 137-148.

Summala, H., E. Pasanen, M. Räsänen, and J. Sievänen. 1996. *Accident Analysis and Prevention* 28, 147-153.

## Endnotes

1. Obviously, the question is still left as to how the homunculus sees the world. There would have to be a second homunculus inside the first and so on into infinite regress. There is also a homunculus theory of memory. Here, the little man just rewinds the videotape and views the screen again.

2. More correctly, it is "luminance" contrast. Brightness is the perceived amount of light. Luminance is the physical amount of light. They are often, but not always, related to one another. In psychophysics, it is essential to distinguish between physics and perception. See Chapter 2. Still, even experts sometimes use this shorthand.

3. Detection is only one of the three basic types of sensory judgment. The other two are discrimination and magnitude. See Chapter 2.

4. Technically, the eye is an outgrowth of the brain. Still, the metaphorical distinction between eye and brain is useful.

5. Circadian rhythms are normal 24-hour cycles of high and low arousal.

6. In some forced-choice psychophysical methods, for example, viewers detect objects yet never consciously see them. They believe that they are just guessing, but they are not.

7. The term "perceptual narrowing" is often used as a synonym for tunnel vision. In the original meaning (Estabrook, 1959), however, it is general restriction on the sources of information used in decision-making. He meant a cognitive as well as sensory narrowing.

8. The dog is outlined.

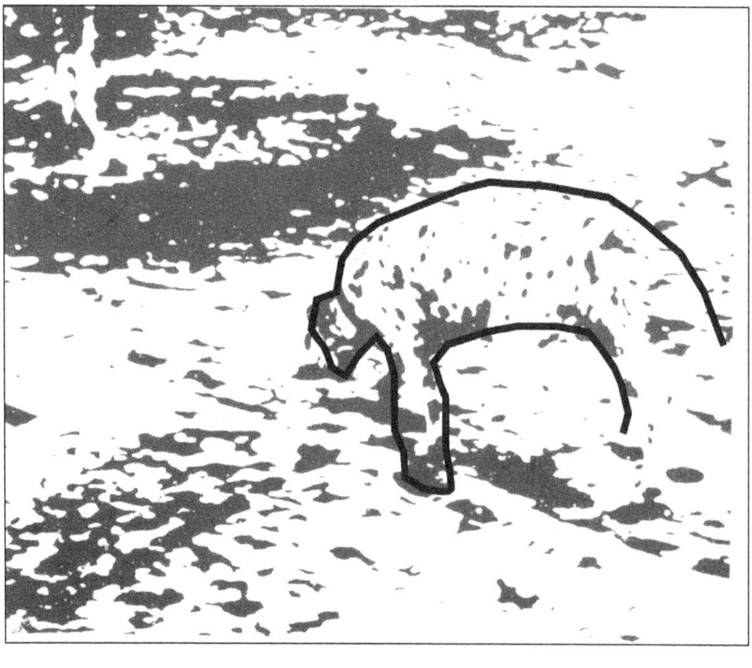

# Chapter 2

# Psychophysics

Marc Green, Ph.D.

*"We live on the leash of our senses."*
—Diane Ackerman

***Synopsis***



## 2.1 Introduction

The previous chapter noted that vision is sensation + perception. The scientific field that studies sensation is "psychophysics," a term that aptly describes its focus: the relationship between psychological and physical variables (psycho-physics). Despite this rather abstract definition, psychophysics is important as the bedrock science for any expert opinion concerning vision, audition, smell, taste, etc. Whether he knows it or not, anyone giving a scientific opinion on these issues is claming to be a psychophysics expert. Despite this, psychophysics remains largely anonymous, and few people are aware that the science even exists. In fact, I have never yet met an attorney who had heard the term "psychophysics."[1]

Most introductory perception texts begin with a chapter on psychophysics because it is the foundation of all behavioral research on vision. It is an essential science because the relationship between sensation/perception and the physical world is complex. For example, suppose someone illuminates a lamp, and light energy reaches a viewer's eye. The viewer experiences an increase in the sensation of brightness. The amount of light reaching the eye is a physical variable while apparent brightness is a psychological variable. Suppose we want to know the minimum amount of light needed to create an increase in apparent brightness. Suppose we want to know whether a fluorescent bulb would create a bigger brightness increase. Suppose we want to know how much brighter the room becomes when the lamp output is doubled. Physics alone cannot answer these questions. First, there is no simple one-to-one relationship between light intensity and brightness. Doubling intensity will not double brightness. Second, a meter can measure light intensity, but no meter can measure brightness. In fact, no meter can measure any sensation or perception—they are private, internal experiences. This is where psychophysics comes in. It provides practical methods and theoretical analyses for measuring these private experiences and for answering questions about the senses. The task of performing a visibility analysis, as described in Chapters 13 and 14, is a good example of psychophysics at work. Only psychophysical measurement and analysis can determine whether a given level of contrast would be detectable.

This chapter provides a general overview of psychophysical theory and practice. There are two vantage points for explaining psychophysics. The first is to treat psychophysics as a set of specialized fields, each devoted to a different sense modality: visual psychophysics (vision), auditory psychophysics (hearing), olfactory psychophysics (smelling), gustatory psychophysics (taste), etc. Each has its own scientific literature and specific knowledge base. A single legal case may require multiple psychophysics experts. For example, a railroad crossing accident may require a visual psychophysicist to evaluate train visibility while an auditory psychophysicist evaluates driver ability to hear the horn.

The second vantage point takes psychophysics as a single field. All psychophysicists share a common body of scientific knowledge, basic methodology and core set of assumptions, which were originally set out by Gustav Fechner who formally founded psychophysics in 1860 with *Elements of Psychophysics.*

While much of this book takes the first approach and discusses only visual psychophysics, this chapter will focus on the general psychophysical analyses and methods used by scientists in all sense modalities. These include concepts such as Weber's Law, Stevens' Law, Fechner's Law, the "classical psychophysics" methods and Signal Detection Theory. Still, the topic of this book is vision so the discussion leans heavily toward visual psychophysics.

## 2.2 Psychophysical Concepts

Despite the zen sounding name, psychophysics is about as hardcore as science gets. It is an experimental science that measures human response to changes in physical energy. A psychophysical study produces data usually depicted in a graph similar to Figure 2.1. The X-axis has a physical variable (phi: $\Phi$) such as light intensity, contrast, sound intensity, odor concentration, etc. while the Y-axis has a psychological variable (psi: $\Psi$) such as "percent detected," brightness, loudness, etc. The resulting relationship is a "psychometric function" (psycho=psychological and metric=measure) that maps the relationship between psychological and physical worlds.

The graph's exact form depends on the question being asked. Psychophysics has traditionally examined three fundamental sensory questions: detection, discrimination and magnitude (Table 2.1) Each question has forensic application. Detection is the most common issue in personal injury litigation. The question might be: whether the driver could detect the stopped truck (vision), whether the pedestrian could hear the approaching vehicle (audition) or whether the homeowner could smell the propane (olfaction). Discrimination plays a lesser role in personal injury cases, except in the ability of witnesses to make identifications among similar objects and colorsv. It is, however, important in intellectual property cases where trademark or tradedress confusion is at issue. Magnitude scaling is relevant when assessing both driver and witness accuracy about factors such as size, brightness, speed and distance.

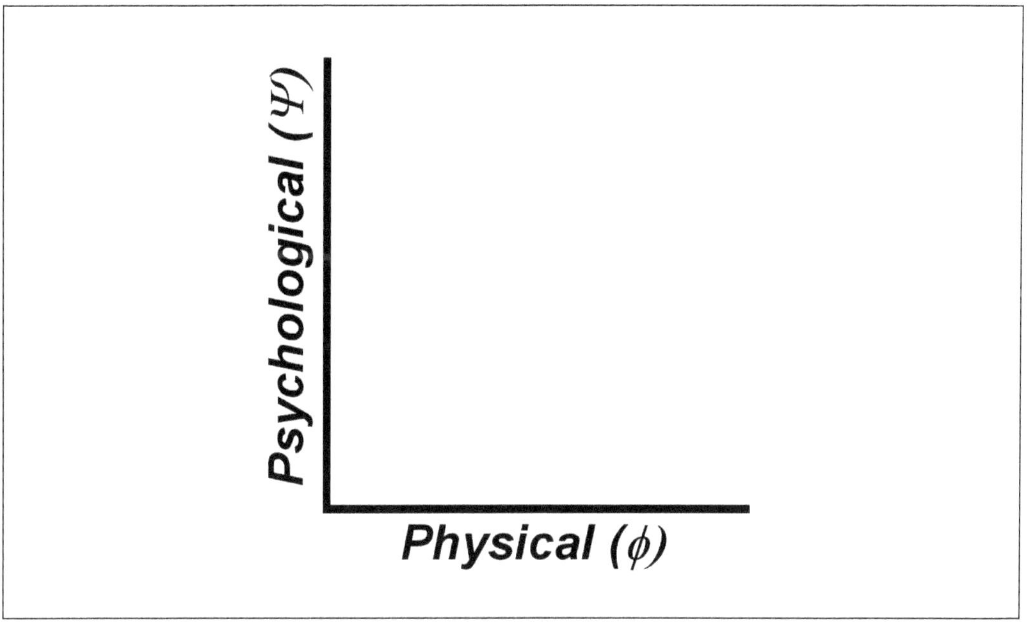


***Figure 2.1*** *Psychophysical data appear on a graph of Ψ vs. Φ.*

The psychophysics of detection and discrimination is the science of sensory "thresholds," the border between detecting/discriminating and not detecting/discriminating. For example, suppose the viewer's task is to detect a light. If the light is very dim, then he cannot detect it. The light is gradually made brighter and brighter. At some point, the viewer can see the light, so it has crossed from undetectable to detectable. This point is the detection threshold, and the light's intensity is its detection threshold value. Similarly, two colors may be indistinguishable. As one color is made increasingly different, it crosses the line from being the same to being different. This is the difference threshold. The concept of threshold, however, is far more complicated than these simple examples suggest. Threshold is not a fixed, unvarying point. Rather, it changes with conditions and testing methodology and can be affected by many factors. Anyone can compute threshold values or look them up in a table. The real expertise lies in interpreting and adjusting the thresholds given the context. The forensic visibility chapters will explain the complexities.

Magnitude scaling is a different task that examines "suprathreshold" (above threshold) information. A detection problem would determine threshold for the dimmest light that a person could detect. In contrast, a simple magnitude question would ask whether a light of 20 cd/m$^2$ appears twice as bright as a light of intensity 10 cd/m$^2$. Or whether a light of intensity 40 cd/m$^2$ would appear four times as bright as intensity 10 cd/m$^2$. In other words, how does the sensation of brightness (or loudness, weight, etc.) grow with the actual, physical energy? In most cases, the relationship is nonlinear and fits one of the basic psychophysical laws described below.

**Table 2.1**
**Psychophysical questions and examples**

| Judgment | Question | Example | Forensic Application |
|---|---|---|---|
| Detection | What is the smallest amount that is detectable? | What is the dimmest light that a viewer can detect? | Was the stopped truck visible to the driver? |
| Discrimination | What is the smallest difference that is discriminable? | What is the smallest difference between two shapes that a viewer can perceive? | Could the police officer distinguish between a gun and a wallet? |
| Magnitude Scaling | What is the relationship between sensation and physical magnitude? | If an object moves twice as fast, does it appear to move twice as fast? | How fast was the car traveling? |

## A. Classical Psychophysics

### 1. Sensory Thresholds

Thresholds define a boundary between detecting (discriminating) and not detecting (not discriminating). There are several ways to compute and to express thresholds, but the most common formulation starts:

$$I_o - I_B = \Delta I = JND$$

$I_o$ is object intensity and $I_B$ is background intensity. The formula takes the intensity of a just detectable intensity, $I_o$, subtracts the background intensity, $I_B$, to give the $\Delta I$, which is the change in intensity needed for detection. The $\Delta I$ can be greater than the background, an "increment threshold," or lower than the background, a "decrement threshold." In either case, it is a JND ("just noticeable difference") for that background. In vision, intensity will usually be measured in luminance (cd/m$^2$). $I_o$, $I_B$ and $\Delta I$ become $L_o$, $L_B$ and $\Delta L$.

The required $\Delta L$, however, changes with the background intensity. For example, a small increment that is visible on a dim background at night might be invisible on a higher background intensity in daylight. Rather than expressing threshold as $\Delta L$, normal practice makes threshold a ratio of $\Delta L$ to background:

$$k = \frac{L_o - L_B}{L_B} = \frac{\Delta L}{L_B}$$

k is the required percent change on the background. In many situations, the k remains constant as the background changes. For example, suppose detection requires an increase of 1 on a background of 10, so k=0.1. If k is constant, then $\Delta L$=5 when the background is 50 because 5/50= 0.1. This constant relationship is "Weber's Law" and k's value is the Weber fraction."[2] In vision, k is the contrast needed to detect the object. This same reasoning applies equally to all of the senses.

Weber's Law is by far the best-known psychophysical relationship, but several factors limit its applicability. It operates only over a limited range of background intensities. Figure 2.2 shows a "tvi" (threshold vs. intensity) curve and how $\Delta L$ changes as backgrounds become more intense. "Dark light" (internal neural activity that is spontaneously generated by the photoreceptors) is the limiting factor at very low luminances. The $\Delta I$ remains constant with rising $L_B$. As background intensity increases, the limiting factor becomes the quantal flux variability, which grows with intensity. Increment thresholds begin to rise, but not as fast as Weber's Law would predict.

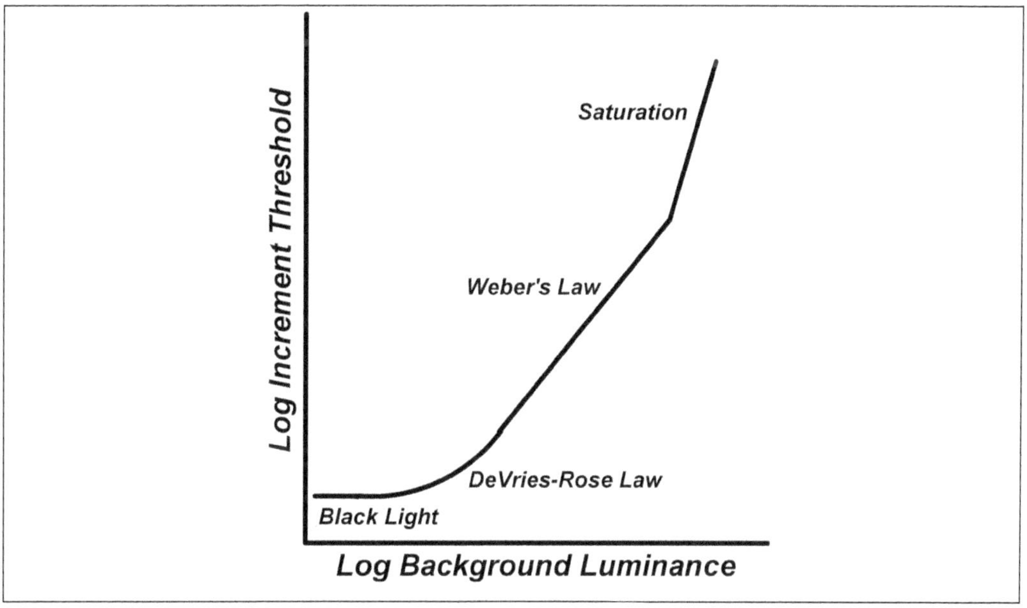


***Figure 2.2*** *Increment thresholds as a function of background for a large target.*

Much of the range approximates the DeVries-Rose Law, where thresholds increase with the square root of the background:

$$k = \frac{L_o - L_B}{\sqrt{L_B}} = \frac{\Delta L}{\sqrt{L_B}}$$

Then there is a large range where Weber's Law holds, at least in theory, and k no longer depends on background intensity. The transition point between DeVries-Rose and Weber's Laws occurs roughly at luminances where the sun is about 4°–8° above the horizon. In theory, variations in normal daylight luminance levels have no effect on contrast threshold.

However, Weber's Law has further limitations. The transition point from DeVries-Rose to Weber's Law is at higher luminance for smaller objects (e.g., van Nes, Koederink, Nas, and Bouman, 1967) and may never be reached for very fine detail. As a result, increased light levels continue to improve visibility in fine acuity tasks such as reading small print, so the tvi curve would look different. On the other hand, tasks such as seeing a large nearby vehicle are little affected by higher illumination once the sun is much above the horizon. Older people are an exception because their optics are opaque and reduce the amount of light entering the eye. Their thresholds become much more dependent on luminance level than those of younger people.

Increased luminance can also aid vision even when Weber's Law holds. Higher luminance creates a smaller pupil opening, which limits spherical aberration (effect of optical irregularities) and improves image quality. Small pupils also increase depth-of-field, so objects that are nearer or farther than the fixation point are sharper and more detectable.

Lastly, most psychophysicists speak of "sensitivity" rather that threshold. Sensitivity is simply the reciprocal of threshold:

$$\text{Sensitivity} = \frac{I_B}{\Delta I}$$

For example, if a viewer becomes better at detecting contrast, his threshold might fall from .02 down to .01, which equates to sensitivity improvement from 50 to 100. Many psychophysicists find sensitivity more intuitive because increasing numbers mean better performance.

### 2. Detection and Discrimination

Detection and discrimination both focus on threshold measurement. However, a new psychophysics, Signal Detection Theory, questions the classical notion of threshold and suggests that visibility and other elementary judgments depend on much more than just the senses. The ensuing sections first present the classical view and then the Signal Detection approach.

### 3. Psychophysical Methods And Interpretation of Thresholds

Psychophysical methodology is the set of procedures used to elicit sensory judgments. It may seem a boring and abstract topic,[3] but it has immense practical importance; different methodologies produce different results. In testimony on issues such as visibility, an expert may compare a driver's ability to detect an object on the road or other environment to the ability of research subjects to detect an object in the lab. Presumably, the subjects' research data are a standard against which to judge the driver. To make this comparison, the expert should consider any differences between the methodologies used to elicit the subject responses and the implicit methodology the driver was using. If the subject and driver judgments represent different methodologies, then some adjustment must be made.

This discussion is a window into a much larger and critical issue, namely "what is science?" and "who is a scientific expert?" *Science is not a collection of facts; it is the method used to collect the facts. Anyone who wishes to speak authoritatively about scientific data must be completely familiar with methodology. Otherwise, it is impossible to intelligently interpolate and extrapolate research data to real-world situations. The science is in the methodology even more than in the data.* (See the preface.)

Classical psychophysics has three basic methods for determining thresholds: "method-of-constant stimuli," "method-of-limits" and "method-of-adjustment." As already noted, each produces a different threshold and hence would produce a different visibility estimate.

Methods of limits and of constant stimuli use a "Yes-No" method to determine a "percent seen." Suppose we want to measure threshold for a light seen against a background. Both constant stimuli and limits methods consist of a series of trials where the investigator presents a light. The viewer then says, "yes I see it" or "no I don't see it" after each presentation. The process repeats for various light intensities, ranging from relatively low to relatively high.

The notion of threshold suggests that the result will appear as in Figure 2.3A, where percent seen ($\Psi$) is plotted against intensity ($\Phi$). At low intensities, the viewer always says "no" and at high intensities, the viewer always says "yes." In between, there is a specific intensity at which the viewer shifts from "no" to "yes."

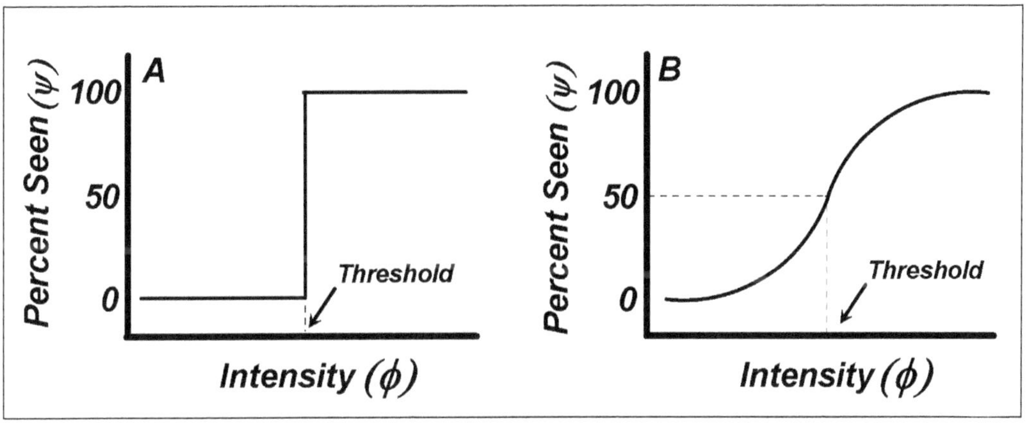


***Figure 2.3*** *The psychometric functions. A shows the theoretical function while B shows the function that is actually obtained, the ogive, a cumulative normal distribution.*

**Table 2.2**
**Typical method-of-limits data. Threshold on each run is halfway between the transition between yes and no**

| | | | | |
|---|---|---|---|---|
| 110 | | | | Y |
| 109 | | Y | | Y |
| 108 | | Y | | Y |
| 107 | | Y | | Y |
| 106 | | Y | Y | Y |
| 105 | Y | Y | N | Y |
| 104 | N | Y | N | Y |
| 103 | N | Y | N | N |
| 102 | N | N | N | |
| 101 | N | | N | |
| 100 | N | | N | |
| | ↑<br>104.5<br>ascend | ↓<br>102.5<br>descend | ↑<br>105.5<br>ascend | ↓<br>103.5<br>descend |

Real results do not look like those in Figure 2.3A but instead resemble those depicted in Figure 2.3B. As contrast grows, detection probability gradually increases from near 0 to near 100 percent[4] along a curve called an "ogive." There is no specific intensity that divides detecting and not detecting. Since detection is not all or none, threshold could be defined at any value, 25 percent, 50 percent, 75 percent, etc. The 50 percent point is convenient but is also somewhat arbitrary. As explained in Chapter 14, many practical applications use a 99 percent "yes" point.

Method-of-constant stimuli and method-of-limits differ in the order that the lights are presented. In the method-of-constant stimuli, the sequence is random. The next light might be either brighter or dimmer than the previous. The method-of-limits, in contrast, presents lights in one of two specific orders, ascending or descending series. In the ascending, the lights start below threshold and then increase step-by-step in intensity (hence the name "ascending"). The viewer starts by saying "no" repeatedly until eventually the light is bright enough to elicit a "yes" response. The descending series starts above threshold where the viewer is sure to say "yes" and then presents dimmer and dimmer lights until the viewer says "no."

Now, here's the rub; the three psychophysical methods produce differing estimates of the 50 percent threshold level. Ascending limits produces the highest threshold, descending limits the lowest threshold while constant stimuli thresholds lie in the middle. The ascending method creates a "no" bias that pushes up the threshold. Table 2.2 shows typical data. The viewer starts saying "no" at 100 and perseverates in saying "no" until he is absolutely sure that he sees the light at 105. The opposite occurs in descending limits, where the viewer perseverates with "yes," pushing the threshold down. Ascending limits almost invariably produce very high thresholds and descending limits very low ones.

In constant stimuli, the lights appear in random order, so there is no perseveration as the "yes" and "no" responses are intermixed. Most research studies would average the ascending and descending series in the hopes of canceling out the response bias and equaling constant stimuli thresholds.

The relevance of method becomes clear when considering that a driver who is heading toward a pedestrian on a dark road is essentially performing the method of ascending limits. He starts saying, "no, I don't see anything." As the vehicle moves forward, increasing amounts of headlamp illumination reach the pedestrian. Eventually, the pedestrian reflects enough light for the driver to make a "yes" response. In a court case, the driver's behavior might be evaluated by determining reasonable visibility based on laboratory data. If the laboratory data are derived from the method-of-constant stimuli, the threshold values will be too low because the driver was performing ascending method-of-limits, which produces higher thresholds.

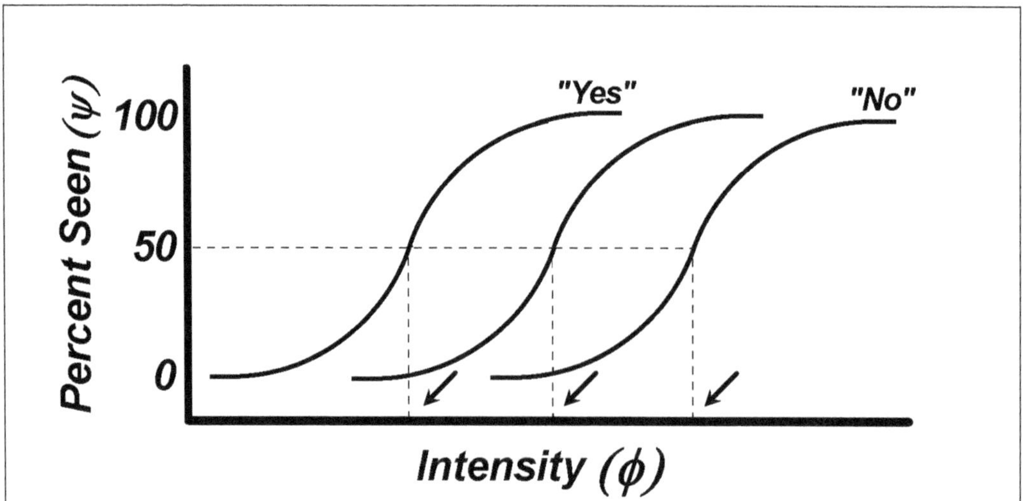


***Figure 2.4*** *Ogives shift with bias in "yes" and "no" responding.*

Both method-of-limits and method-of-constant stimuli are subject to a range of biases that can push the ogive one way or the other and change threshold. Figure 2.4 shows how changes in "response bias" affect threshold. If the viewer has a bias toward saying "no," then the ogive moves right and the threshold is higher. If the viewer is biased toward saying "yes," then the ogive moves leftward and the threshold is lower. In sum, cognitive decision-making factors confound attempts at determining a purely sensory threshold.

Many factors could cause the viewer to be biased toward "yes" or "no." For example, I have tested both children and elderly viewers and found that children have strong tendency to say "yes" while elderly viewers tend to say "No." On this basis alone, elderly viewers would then create higher thresholds. Viewers can change their tendency toward saying "yes" or "no" because of expectation or payoffs, as explained in the discussion of Signal Detection Theory in the next section.

The third classical technique is method-of-adjustment, which allows the viewer to control the intensity directly by turning a knob, pushing a button, etc. until it is just perceptible. The result is a single contrast threshold number rather than a function relating "percent seen" to contrast. However, method-of-adjustment thresholds are very high and would likely correspond to the 99+ percent point on the psychometric function, indicating certain detection. It is also subject to the same biases that afflict "Yes-No" methods.

The major alternative to the classical methods is "forced-choice." In the standard "Yes-No" method, the target appears at one location and the viewer's response is "Yes, I see it" or "No, I don't." In forced-choice, the target may appear at one of several different locations (spatial forced-forced) or at one of several different times (temporal forced-choice). The viewer responds with the correct location (or correct time). He cannot say "no" and is forced to choose even if he consciously sees nothing. For example, Blackwell (1946) had subjects view a small red dot and then presented a target at one of eight locations (the major compass points) on an imaginary circle that ran around the dot. The subjects scanned the display for 6 seconds and responded with the correct position of the target. This would be called an "eight-alternative spatial forced-choice" (8ASFC) method.

Forced-choice methods generally do not use the 50 percent detection level as the threshold because they must correct for guessing. Suppose, for example, that a visibility study used a two-alternative forced choice where the target appeared randomly in one of two locations. The subject could get 50 percent correct just by guessing, so the 50 percent level would be pure chance and indicate no detection. The usual solution is to split the difference between perfect performance and chance, and then add it to the guessing level. That is 100 percent – 50 percent= 50 percent. Half is 25 percent. Adding this to the guessing level of 50 percent gives 75 percent. In Blackwell's eight alternative method, guessing could get 12.5 percent (one in eight) correct. Splitting the difference gives (100 percent – 12.5 percent)/2=43.75. The threshold is then set to 12.5 percent + 43.75 percent= 56.25 percent.

Forced-choice methods produce data that are extremely stable and reliable, largely because there is no "Yes-No" decision, and hence none of the response biases that can affect classical methods. It is a purer measure of sensory ability because cognition plays a lesser role.

Forced-choice methods also generate lower thresholds than yes-no and adjustment methods. It is a very unnatural task because the viewer must pick one alternative even if it a guess. Subjects frequently complain that there is nothing to see, and the researcher must sternly insist that they pick an alternative. Amazingly, viewers perform well above chance even when they say that they consciously see nothing and are sure that they are guessing. In other words, they are somehow able to detect a target that they do not consciously see and that would have elicited a "no" response if it had been permitted. This further illustrates the gulf between sensing and perceiving.

The forced-choice method, however, has a downside. Real-world viewers make Yes-No rather than forced-choice decisions, so the task is somewhat artificial. The forced-choice threshold must be increased to reflect more realistic conditions. Blackwell (1959) estimated that forced-choice thresholds should be multiplied by 20 percent in order to equal "Yes-No" thresholds for the same conditions. In my experience, the difference is much greater.

This examination of methodology underscores the important point that thresholds are not fixed values. While the concept of threshold is useful, it is ultimately nothing more than an arbitrary point on a psychometric function. It provides a starting point, but every psychophysical expert knows that there is no absolute line between detecting and not detecting. As a result, interpreting the threshold number from an ogive is not straightforward. The ogive's position can shift left or right due to a large number of psychological factors. I have already described how the psychophysical method can elevate threshold by biasing the viewer to say "No." That would shift the ogive rightward so that threshold increases. Sensory threshold judgments depend partly on decision factors that are independent of intensity. In fact, there is an entire branch of psychophysics, 'Signal Detection Theory,' (D. Green and Swets, 1966) that is devoted to separating sensory from "nonsensory" or decision factors.

## B. Signal Detection Theory

Psychophysicists have long known that "Yes, I see it" and "No, I don't see it" judgments depend on more than just sensation. Figure 2.4 demonstrated how changes in response bias alter thresholds. "Signal Detection Theory" (D. M. Green and Swets, 1966) presents an alternative to classical psychophysics that explicitly separates sensation and response bias (cognition) in order to obtain more accurate assessments of sensitivity and detection. While classical psychophysics has only a single dependent variable ("percent seen," "detection probability," etc.), Signal Detection Theory (SDT) studies have two: sensitivity, $d'$, and bias, $\beta$. SDT also differs from classical psychophysics by replacing the concept of threshold with the concepts signal, noise, and uncertainty.

SDT's core is a simple notion: people decide whether to say "yes" or "no" for two distinctly different reasons. The first is "sensory" factors—signal strength. A viewer can more readily detect an intense light than a weak light and is accordingly more likely to say "yes." In some cases, the light might be so intense that it is very obvious and the viewer has little uncertainty that "yes" is the correct response. In other cases, the light might be weak, so the viewer is uncertain as to whether it actually appeared. SDT says that viewers resolve the uncertainty by establishing a criterion based on two "nonsensory" factors, probabilities and payoffs. I'll delay explaining the nature of this criterion until the next section. For now, the crucial point is that viewers can change criterion and likelihood of saying "yes" or "no," without affecting the measured sensitivity. SDT gives a pure measure of detection, uncontaminated by variations in response bias. This fixes a problem of classical psychophysics, where threshold and response bias vary together.

SDT may seem abstract and possess little obvious application. In its total glory, SDT and its more sophisticated offshoot "Ideal Observer Theory" (e.g., Green, Odom and Yates, 1995) are sophisticated mathematical models with many components. SDT's major scientific utility lies in its ability to determine the best possible detection performance in a given situation. However, it also is possible to strip the math from the model and to simply use SDT as a general viewpoint on perceptual decision-making under uncertainty. Here, it has important implications for viewer behavior, safety promotion, and juror attitudes toward defendants.

**1. Sensory Factors**

Before explaining SDT in detail, I'll start with a thought experiment that provides an intuitive grasp. Imagine looking at a uniform TV screen for a small blip to appear. If the blip is strong enough, it is readily detectable. Now imagine looking at a TV screen that is tuned to a channel with no station and that appears as a boiling array of dots. If a large blip appears, it is still detectable. If the blip is small, there is uncertainty because the apparent blip could be due to either a real blip or to an especially noisy bit of the background. SDT sees psychophysics as the second case. The same sensation is sometimes due to a real signal and sometimes due to noise.

There are several sources of noise. The first is "external noise" originating in the environment; in this case the boiling background of dots is noise.[5] The second is "internal noise" created by spontaneous activity in the nervous system. A full SDT model has even more noise sources, but the following discussion considers only internal noise in order to simplify the explanation. The main point is that detectability of a signal in noise (and all signals are in noise) is determined by the signal to noise ratio (SNR).

SDT originated as a means for analyzing a problem similar to this TV thought experiment, the detection of signals on radar screens. Radar operators are often faced with making decisions based on blips mixed with background noise. They would literally have to make decisions such as: is that fuzzy blip on the screen really an object and if it is, is it a flock of birds or a Russian ICBM headed for Washington? The flock of birds does not require a response while the Russian ICBM does. Similar problems are common. A driver must decide whether there is an object on the road ahead, a police officer must decide whether a suspect is holding a gun or an innocuous object like a wallet, a radiologist must decide whether the area on the X-ray is a tumor or just a random glitch, etc. Do I brake? Do I fire my weapon? Do I schedule surgery? How do people make such decisions when visual information is uncertain?

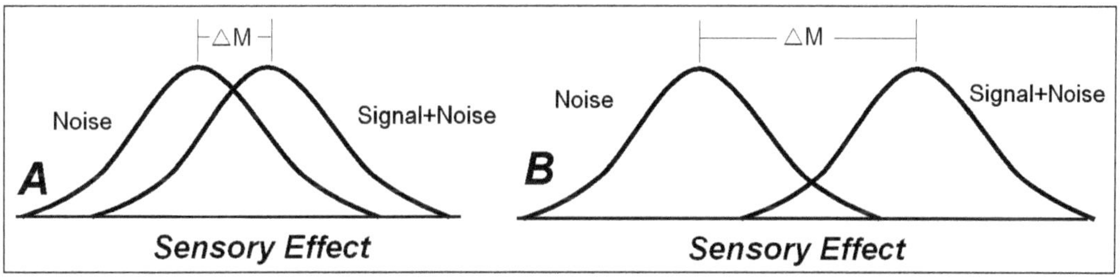


***Figure 2.5** Distributions of sensory effect for noise and for signal+noise. The vertical axis is probability. Figure A shows a relatively strong signal and Figure B shows a relatively weak one. The figures are slightly misleading because the distributions never touch the X axis—the probabilities never become 0 percent.*

Figure 2.5 diagrammatically shows how SDT views uncertainty and decision-making. Look at Figure 2.5A first. The distribution on the left is the noise; the likelihood of having a given noise level changes from moment to moment. For internal noise, imagine attaching a meter to the optic nerve and recording the activity level at each second in time. The momentary noise samples would be normally distributed with standard deviation $\sigma$. (Environmental noise, like the bubbling TV dots or even just the moment-to-moment quantal flux of ambient illumination would add to the internal background noise, pushing the distribution rightward.) The viewer, of course, has no direct access to the noise, but rather has an experience resulting from the "sensory effect" created by the noise. Small noise levels create small sensory effects and higher noise levels create greater sensory effects. Ultimately, the viewers must make their yes/no decisions based on magnitude of this sensory effect.

If the light turns on, it emits quanta that activate the eye and generate a signal up the optic nerve through the nervous system. This signal has a sensory effect, which adds to the sensory effect created by the noise alone. The result is the signal+noise distribution shifted to the right. It is also normal with variability of $\sigma$. The difference between the noise distribution and the signal+noise distributions is $\Delta M$. The amount of overlap between the distributions is *d'* ("d prime"):

$$d' = \frac{\Delta M}{\sigma}$$

The d' is a function of both separation and variability. In SDT terminology, these are "sensory factors" and are fixed properties of the situation that limit detectability. Further, d' is the measure of sensitivity, analogous to "percent seen" in classical psychophysics. The viewer cannot change d' by simply altering the preference for saying "yes" or "no."

The viewer faces a problem according to this model. He has no direct knowledge of whether the light flashed. All he knows is that he is experiencing a sensory effect. His task is to determine whether the sensory effect is due to the noise (so there is no signal and no light) or whether it was due to signal (there was a signal and a light). If the distributions overlap, then there will always be a sensory effect range where the viewer is uncertain. The sensory effect could be due to noise or it could be due to signal+noise. The viewer must make an educated guess.

Figure 2.5A shows two distributions with little overlap. There is only a small range of uncertainty; signal sensitivity should be good. Signals create sensory effects greater than all but a small percentage of noise distribution. In Figure 2.5B, the distributions overlap greatly. There is a large range of sensory effects that reasonably could have originated from signal or from noise. Sensitivity must be low. The important message from the figure is that as long as the distributions overlap to any degree, there will be a range of uncertainty and some errors are inevitable. Smaller signal strength means more overlap and more errors.

The viewer must decide whether to say "yes" or "no" when encountering a sensory effect in the uncertainty range. He knows that weak sensory effects are more probably from noise while high sensory effects are more probably from signal+noise. At some fixed sensory effect, he establishes a criterion, $\beta$ (Figure 2.6), a level where he considers the likelihood high enough that the sensory effect probably arose from signal+noise. He will say "no" whenever the sensory effect is lower than $\beta$, and "yes" whenever it is above.

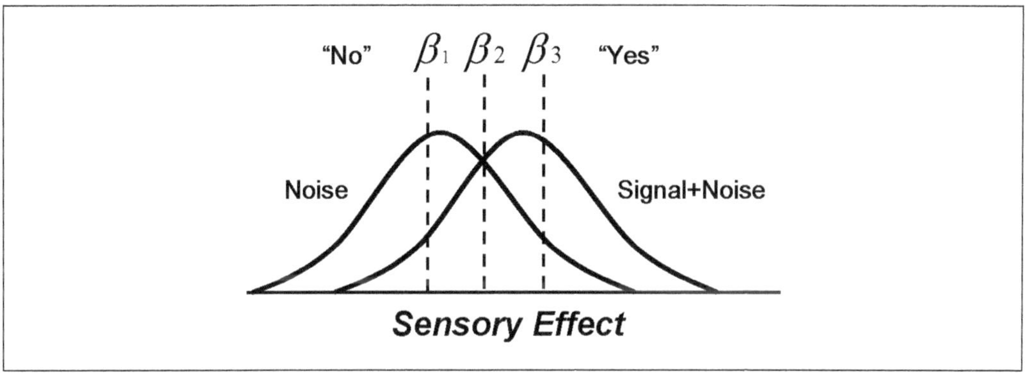


***Figure 2.6*** *Signal detection with three different criteria.*

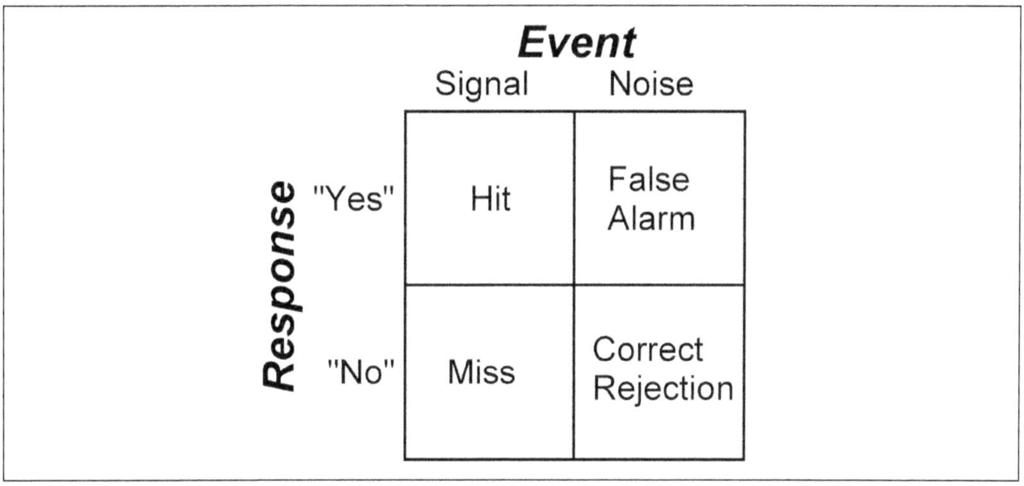


***Figure 2.7*** *SDT payoff matrix.*

The viewer's dilemma becomes clear when viewed as the decision matrix of Figure 2.7. There are two possible events, signal and signal+noise (or just signal for short) and two responses "yes" and "no," giving four outcomes. Two will be correct and two will be incorrect:

- Correct
  - "Hit:" The signal is present, and the observer says, "Yes."
  - "Correct Rejection" (CR): Only noise is present, and the observer says "No."
- Incorrect
  - "False Alarm" (FA): There was only noise, but the observer says, "Yes."
  - "Miss." The signal was present, but the observer says "No."

An actual SDT experiment might have a viewer watch the a screen in a series of trials. In a randomly selected number of the trials, the signal+noise appears. In the remainder, there is no signal and only noise ("catch trials"). The viewer says "yes" or "no" after each trial, generating hits, false alarms, correct rejections and misses. The sensitivity d' cannot be directly observed—the underlying distributions are unknown. However, d' can be inferred by calculating the following formula:

$$d' = z(pFA) - z(pH)$$

where z(pFA) is the z-score of the false alarm probability and z(pH) is the z-score of the hit probability. In practice, it is more common to simply consult a table containing d' for each possible combination of pFA and pH.[6]

The viewer can change his criterion and the proportion of error types, misses and false alarms without changing d'. Figure 2.6 shows the consequences of changing criterion. The criterion labeled $\beta_2$ is located at the intersection of the noise and signal+noise distribution. It is "unbiased," because the viewer will make equal numbers of miss and false alarm errors (assuming that signal and signal+noise occur equally often). This is obvious from looking at the figure: the area of the noise distribution falling on the "yes" side of the criterion (false alarms) is the same as the area of the signal+noise curves falling on the "no" side of the criterion (misses).

If the viewer adopts $\beta_1$, then the criterion is very low and he is biased toward saying "yes." The area of the noise distribution falling on the "yes" side of the criterion grows greatly while the area of the signal+noise curve falling on the "no" side of the criterion shrinks. The viewer will make many more false alarms than misses. The high criterion of $\beta_3$ has the opposite effect. The viewer is biased toward saying "no" so he makes many more misses than false alarms. None of this affects d!

The scheme shown in Figure 2.6 has other theoretical and applied consequences. First, hits and false alarms must vary together. Any criterion change that increases hits must also increase false alarms. Any criterion that increases correct rejections also increases misses. This is why sensitivity remains constant. Second, safety often requires use of a very low criterion, so false alarms greatly exceed misses. However, environmental circumstances often favor a high criterion and misses over false alarms. This creates safety problems and promotes accidents, as I discuss later.

**2. Nonsensory Factors**

So far, I have discussed how "sensory" factors of $\Delta M$ and $\sigma$ combine to determine sensitivity. I have also explained that observers can change their criteria, altering the relative likelihood of hits, false alarms, correct rejections and misses. I have further explained that criterion changes do not affect sensitivity. The next obvious issue is why a viewer would alter his criterion.

The answer lies in "nonsensory" factors, which fall into two categories: "probabilities" (the past) and "payoffs" (the future). Probability is the expected likelihood of an event. If a driver has traveled a rural road 1000 times and has never seen a pedestrian, then the *a priori* probability of encountering a pedestrian is low. The driver will then have a high criterion and will be biased toward saying "no." His errors will be misses rather than false alarms, and he will make many correct rejections rather than hits. That is, he will seldom deem the blip a pedestrian. If he were driving by an apartment complex where he had often seen children playing in the street, then his criterion would be low; he would be biased toward "yes" errors (false alarms) but would have a very high hit rate. Note that the term "biased" here is merely descriptive and is not pejorative. It simply says that the observer will tend toward one response more than another, a decision largely based on unconscious mental information-processing. In many cases, biased responding is proper strategy because it maximizes utility. In SDT the goal is to get the biggest utility, and not necessarily the highest percent correct. This is where payoffs become important.

The viewer must consider both benefits and costs of various outcomes. Here is an example of the payoffs for a driver on a dark road at night. He sees something up ahead:

- Hit: believes it is a pedestrian, and it is. He brakes, and the benefit is high—avoids running over pedestrian;
- CR: believes it isn't a pedestrian, and it isn't. He does not brake, and the benefit is low—he doesn't slow down unnecessarily;
- FA: believes that it is a pedestrian, and it isn't. He brakes and the cost is low—he slows unnecessarily; and
- Miss: believes that it isn't a pedestrian and it is. He fails to brake, and the cost is high(!)—he strikes the pedestrian.

### 3. Individual vs. Societal Perspective On Nonsensory Factors

In the pedestrian example, the payoffs obviously weigh heavily toward making false alarms rather than misses. However, the observer must also combine the *a priori* probabilities with the payoff matrix in order to set a criterion that optimizes utility. If the probability is very, very low, the bias might shift back toward misses. Accidents are generally rare, so the probabilities often favor a high criterion. Many everyday decisions require the same weighing of probabilities and payoffs. For example, people can almost always speed, tailgate, drive intoxicated, cross against the light, ignore product warnings, etc. without suffering ill consequences. People learn that the contingencies, the relationship between behavior and consequences, favor a high criterion in many tasks.

This creates a conflict between individual and societal perspectives on safety. Yes, leaving your seatbelt unbuckled increases injury risk. From the viewpoint of any particular individual, however, the likelihood is very low that he will have a crash where a buckled seatbelt prevents death. (Isn't that what airbags are for, anyway?) On the other hand, the societal perspective assumes a very high probability that the buckling of seatbelts will save the lives of some people at some time. The difference in perspective is obvious—individuals are concerned only with the probabilities facing themselves while society is summing outcomes across many individuals.

Individuals are likely to ask themselves whether they should care about the societal perspective. For example, airlines now tell passengers to keep their seatbelts buckled throughout the flight in order to prevent being thrown from their seats by a sudden air turbulence. Should I wear my seatbelt throughout an airline flight and suffer the cost of a false alarm (being uncomfortable in my seat, having to buckle and unbuckle when someone in my row wants to go to the lavatory, experiencing a feeling of being controlled, passively complying with the nanny state, etc.) when the likelihood of my encountering that turbulence is miniscule? Sure, the cost is low, but so is the probability. From the airline perspective, passengers' buckling of seatbelts has high utility by preventing injury and lawsuits. The probability multiplied by the number of passengers makes it highly likely that turbulence will occur on some of their many flights and that wearing the seatbelt will be a "hit" for a small number of passengers. Moreover, the airlines aren't the ones who pay the costs of the false alarm. For them, it's a pure gain. For individual passengers, the correct decision is not so obvious.

In many cases, society attempts to promote safety by persuading people to adopt a low criterion (many false alarms but very few misses) despite their personal experiences suggesting very low signal probability. This, of course, is why safety authorities attempt to inflate statistics on the role of alcohol in road accidents by every means possible. Safety authorities also attempt to maximize the perceived cost of a miss (e.g., pictures of diseased lungs on cigarette packages) and to minimize the cost of the false alarm. Experience shows that this strategy has, at best, mixed success against peoples' personal experiences. This is why hazards should be designed out if possible and why reliance on warnings or other forms of persuasion is unreliable or worse. It also explains why overwarning is bad—it increases the *a priori* probability that warnings are just noise. Lastly, it explains why enforcement and high penalty are often the best strategy; it changes the contingencies by adding to the real cost of a miss.

In court, jurors tend to take the societal perspective. They will likely care more about payoffs than about probabilities. After all, they are looking at an accident probability of 1 so there is no uncertainty. Since the jurors do not have the driver's perspective prior to the accident, they cannot see the *a priori* probabilities in the same way. Jurors unconsciously fail to consider that the defendant had to deal with the uncertainty of what *might* happen rather than the certainty of what *did* happen. This is one core factor contributing to hindsight bias.

## 4. SDT Applications

SDT applies widely because people frequently must make decisions under uncertainty. I have already described a road accident scenario, and there are other examples: drivers approaching rail crossings (Raslear, 1995), the effectiveness of retroreflective material (Multer, Conti, and Sheridan, 2001) and response to warning systems (Parasuraman, Hancock, and Olofinboba, 1997), etc. Even the response biases and accuracies of jury verdicts are amenable to SDT analysis (Arkes and Mellers, 2002).

SDT is especially useful in low light situations because visual information is often uncertain. One scenario occurs when a police officer must decide whether to fire at a suspect . A police officer sees an object in a suspect's hand and fires, only to discover that it was a wallet (Green, 2005). These incidents usually occur at night (Aveni, 2003), when visibility is low and uncertainty great. The problem is difficult, because there is little time and because the object is small and moving in dim light. The nonsensory factors, however, play an equally important role in the decision on whether or not to shoot.

The officer must consider the payoff consequences of each response. Of course, the officer will attempt to be correct, but, since the situation is uncertain, he must also consider the consequences of an error. If he makes a correct "yes" response he may save his own life while a correct "no" response leaves the situation as status quo. There are two types of error possible. If he makes a false alarm (says gun when there is no gun), he shoots an unarmed and possibly innocent suspect, may face legal action, etc. If he makes a miss (does not shoot when there is a gun), he and/or a fellow officer or bystander may end up wounded or even dead.

The officers have no way to assign objective values to the outcomes of the "yes" and "no" responses. Is it worse to shoot an unarmed suspect than to have a fellow officer shot? Is there any worse outcome than being shot and killed? Expectations (probabilities) also add to the likelihood of a "yes" if the officer is in a part of town regarded as dangerous, has just come from pre-patrol briefing where he is told that a dangerous person is on the loose or if the suspect resembles a known dangerous person.

The same analysis can explain why motorcycle accidents are common. Drivers are far more likely to detect a car, which has a high probability, than a motorcycle, which is relatively rare (e.g., Hole and Tyrrell, 1995). Further, the consequences of colliding with a car are high, creating a "yes" bias, but are relatively low for colliding with a motorcycle. Both probability and payoff bias the decision toward "yes" for the car and "no" for the motorcycle. The driver is likely not consciously biasing his response, but rather simply responding to his implicit understanding of the way the world works.

To conclude, SDT is instructive because it highlights an important point made in Chapter 1: vision is more than just the eye, and visibility analysis requires examination of cognitive factors. However, SDT treats nonsensory factors in a very crude and global way. It does not attempt to examine specific cognitive processes, such as attention, memory and learning, the mechanisms by which nonsensory factors operate. While providing a good framework, SDT may require more detailed elaboration. People do not base their decisions solely or even primarily on simple statistics. Rather, they tend to think causally, so their knowledge, schemata and mental models qualitatively govern decision-making. Chapter 4 picks up this thread and discusses nonsensory factors in detail.

## 2.3 Magnitude Scaling

Magnitude scaling is the area of psychophysics that measures the relationship between perceived intensity and physical magnitude. It is a common task. Any person making a judgment such as the brightness of the light, the speed of the car, the distance of the train, the vividness of a color, the loudness of the sound, the strength of the smell, etc., is judging magnitude.

In a typical research study, the viewer might see a series of lights. After the first, he gives a number indicating the light's brightness. The viewer then sees another light of greater or lesser intensity and again gives a number that reflects the apparent brightness. The process iterates until there is a function that relates apparent brightness to actual intensity (Figure 2.8).[7]

There are both scientific and practical reasons for performing such a study. The scientific reason is to understand how the senses transform physical energy into sensation. In practical application, magnitude scaling provides a scientific means for evaluating and interpreting some witness statements. Suppose that a witness testifies about the speed of a car. He didn't have a radar gun and can only judge what his senses have presented to him. His judgment's accuracy then depends on the degree of correspondence between perceived speed and the actual, physical speed. In a sense, the witness is acting as a speed meter, but the "calibration" between perceived speed and physical speed must be known in order to evaluate accuracy of his response. This calibration cannot be performed with any physical instrument; while a meter can measure actual speed, no meter can measure perceived speed, brightness or any other percept.[8] Psychophysics is the only tool for performing the calibration.

Magnitude scaling calibrates the human meter against the physical world. It provides a way to evaluate the human ability to act as a light meter, loudness meter, speed meter, distance meter, time meter (clock), etc. As I will explain, magnitude scaling reveals that the human meter often is inaccurate in highly predictable ways.

Magnitude scaling[9] typically creates results similar to those shown in Figure 2.8. The relationship between perceived brightness and physical intensity is nonlinear and "compressive." At low levels, perceived brightness increases relatively quickly, but at higher levels, perceived brightness grows very slowly. Curves for most other sensory judgments exhibit this same compressive function, although there are a few exceptions. Some curves are linear (length) while a very few are "expansive" (shock), with perceived sensation growing faster than physical energy.

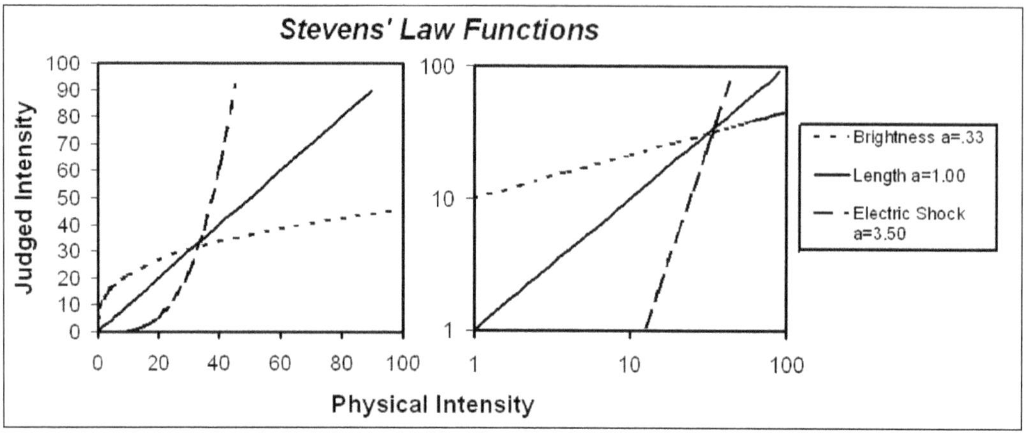


***Figure 2.8*** *Stevens' Law on linear and log-log coordinates. K=1 for length, K=10 for brightness, and K= .00015 for shock.*

Psychometric functions for magnitude usually follow Stevens' Law:

$$\psi = k\Phi^a$$

The $\Psi$ (psi for psychological) is perceived intensity, $\Phi$ (for physical) is intensity, *a* is the exponent and k is a scaling factor. When Stevens' Law applies, plotting the data on log-log axes produces straight lines (Figure 2.8), and the equation's exponent is the slope of the line. Exponents and slopes less than one are compressive, greater than one are expansive. Exponents of 1 are linear. The closer the exponent is to 1, the more "veridical" (truthful) the viewer's judgment. A doubling of the physical quantity produces a doubling of the percept. A witness making a sensory judgment for a variable with a slope of one will be more accurate. On the other hand, a witness, making a judgment on a sensory dimension with a slope much above or below 1 will make predictable errors.

In some cases, psychometric functions are a better fit to Fechner's Law:

$$\psi = k\log(\Phi)$$

which produces a straight line on log-linear axes. Fechner's Law follows directly from Weber's Law, as it is merely the result of summing $\Delta I$'s. In English, the difference between the laws is: Stevens' Law says that equal ratios of energy produce equal ratios of sensation. Fechner's Law says that equal ratios of energy produce equal *intervals* of sensation. However, the two laws fit many compressive functions equally well.

Let's put Stevens' Law to work. Suppose that a witness testifies to the speed of a vehicle. How are people calibrated for speed perception, and what types of errors are they likely to make? Rachlin (1966) found that perceived speed gave an exponent of .8, which is compressive like brightness. At low speeds, the function increases rapidly but at high speeds it flattens off. This suggests that people will overestimate low speeds and underestimate high speeds. Hills (1980) confirmed this prediction in a study where viewers judged the speed of passing vehicles. Viewers overestimated speeds below about 45 mph and underestimated higher speeds.

**Table 2.3**
**Typical exponents, a, for Stevens' Law**

| Dimension | Exponent |
|---|---|
| Brightness (5° target) | .33 |
| Brightness (point source) | .5 |
| Visual length | 1 |
| Heaviness | 1.45 |
| Smell (Heptane) | 0.6 |
| Loudness | 0.67 |
| Electric shock | 3.5 |
| Taste (salt) | 1.4 |

Like detection and discrimination, however, nonsensory factors affect judgment. People do not typically think numerically. They see a car and may think "fast," "slow," "very fast," etc. They judge distance as "near," "far," "very far," "extremely far," etc. When asked to provide a numerical estimate, they must translate a remembered image or general impression into a number. The assignment of a number to a percept or to a memory has several known quirks.

One is "regression error." People tend to avoid using extremes of a scale. For example, if asked to rate something on a scale of 1 to 10, people tend to avoid using the 1 and the 10. This also promotes the overestimation of low values and underestimation of high values, since it pushes up the low end and pushes down the high end. Sometimes the scale is merely implied.[10] For example, people know that vehicles have a practical range of 0-100 mph. They are unlikely to use the extremes in speed estimation. If the car is on a city street, however, they are likely to adjust the scale's top downward, since cars do not normally travel 100 mph on city streets.

On the other hand, people may use "magic numbers." If you want someone to wait a short while, you say, "I'll be back in 5 minutes." The number "5" is not meant literally, but rather simply expresses that the duration will be short. No one ever says, "I'll be back in 3 minutes" or "I'll be back in 7 minutes." Similarly, a witness might say that a very fast car was going 100 mph. One-hundred may be a magic number, which simply means that it was going very, very fast. I have heard a witness state that a car was moving 1 mph, a value that cannot be taken too seriously. He probably meant that the car was moving very slowly.[11]

Witness answers are also highly sensitive to "frame effects," the specific way that a question frames the issue. Advertisers, for example, typically describe products as "99 percent fat free" rather than "1 percent fat." A marketing study had found people judged the "99 percent fat free product" as being healthier. In one well-known study (Loftus and Palmer, 1974), viewers saw a film clip of an accident and then answered the question, "How fast were the cars going when they *X* into each other." The *X* was a different verb for different viewers. The resulting speed estimates were higher for verbs such as smashed and collided than for verbs such as contacted.

In some cases, there are nonsensory factors specific to the type of judgment. Speed judgments are especially sensitive to the contextual factors discussed in the previous chapter. For example, people believe that sports cars are fast, teenagers are wild and that loud engines are working harder, all cognitive factors indicating greater speed and biasing sensory judgments upward. Speed judgments are also sensitive to background. Objects appear to move faster on a patterned than on a uniform background. Apparent speed also increases when the background is moving in the opposite direction. As a result, a car will appear to move faster when seen against traffic going in the opposite direction. Briefer motions appear faster than longer motions. Sudden motions seem faster than predictable motions. I could belabor the point that should be obvious by now; evaluating witness judgments of even seemingly simple percepts, such as speed, is highly complex due to the myriad of variables at work.

## 2.4 Conclusion

This chapter has outlined the scientific field of psychophysics and explained its focus on human abilities to detect, to discriminate and to judge magnitude. Psychophysics provides the scientific bases for any forensic analysis of issues such as visibility and judgments of speed, distance, time, color and other percepts. However, psychophysics is the starting and not the end point for expert opinion sensory judgments. As Signal Detection Theory highlights, human judgments are always affected by nonsensory cognitive factors that are described in Chapter 4.

## References


Adrian, W., 1989. Visibility of Targets. *Lighting Research Technology,* 21, 181-188.

Arkes, H. and B. Mellers. 2002. Do Juries Meet Our Expectations? *Law And Human Behavior* 26, 625-639.

Aveni, T. 2003. Police Marksmanship Under Fire: Paradox And Promise. *Law & Order* August.

Blackwell, H. R. 1946. Contrast thresholds of the human eye. *Journal of the Optical Society of America* 36, 624-643.

Blackwell, H. R. 1959. Development and use of a quantitative method for specification of interior illumination levels on the basis of performance data. *Illuminating Engineering 54*, 317-353.

Blackwell, O. and H. R. Blackwell. 1971. Visual performance data for 156 normal observers of various ages. *Illuminating Engineering*, October, 3-13.

Gescheider, G. 1997. *Psychophysics: The Fundamentals, 3rd ed* Matawan, NJ: Lawrence Erlbaum Associates.

Green, D. M. and J. A. Swets. (1966) *Signal Detection Theory and Psychophysics*. New York: Wiley.

Green, M. 2005. 'Is It A Gun? Or Is It A Wallet?' Perceptual Factors In Police Shootings of Unarmed Suspects," *Police Marksman*, July/August, 52-54.

Green, M., J. V. Odom, and T. Yates. 1995. Measuring situational awareness with the "Ideal Observer." *Proceedings of the International Conference on Experimental Analysis and Measurement of Situation Awareness*, Embry-Riddle Aeronautical University Press, FL.

Hills, B. L. 1980. Vision, Visibility, and Perception in Driving. *Perception*. 9. 183-216.

Hole, G. J. and L. Tyrrell. 1995. The influence of perceptual "set" on the detection of motorcyclists using daytime headlights. *Ergonomics* 38, 1326-1341.

Loftus, E. F. and J. C. Palmer. 1974. Reconstruction of automobile destruction: An example of the interaction between language and memory. *Journal of Verbal Learning and Verbal Behaviour* 13, 585 –589.

Multer, J., J. Conti, and T. Sheridan. 2001. Recognition of rail car retroreflective patterns for improving nighttime conspicuity. John A. Volpe National Transportation Systems Center Report DOT/FRA/ORD-00/07.

Parasuraman, R., P. A. Hancock, and O. Olofinboba. 1997. Alarm effectiveness in driver-centered collision warning systems. *Ergonomics, 39*, 390–399.

Rachlin, H. 1966. Scaling, subject velocity, distance and duration. *Perception & Psychophysics*, 1, 77-82.

Raslear, T. 1995. Driver behavior at rail-highway grade crossings: A Signal Detection Theory Analysis," In: *Safety of Highway-Railroad Grade Crossings, Research Needs Workshop, Volume II-- Appendices,* A. A. Caroll and J. L. Helser (eds.). Report No. DOT/FRA/ORD/14.2, DOT-VNTSC-FRA-95-12.2, pp. F9-F56. U.S. Department of Transportation, Washington, D.C.

Roper, V. and E. Howard. 1938. Seeing with motor car headlamps. *Transactions of the Illuminating. Engineering Society* 33, 417–438.

## Endnotes

1. A note on terminology. Psychologists sometimes call the field "sensory psychology." When speaking of visual psychophysics, ophthalmologists and especially optometrists may refer to it as "physiological optics." Lastly, some restrict the term "vision" to mean "visual psychophysics" only and treat perception as cognition.

2. "Weber" is pronounced "Vayber." Hence, it is "Vayber's Law." Germans invented psychophysics, so names are always pronounced in German.

3. William James, the father of experimental psychology, was no fan of psychophysical methods. He once famously observed that "Psychophysics proves that you can't bore a German."

4. The curves never actually reach either 0 percent at the bottom or 100 percent at the top.

5. A note for the more mathematically inclined reader: In SDT, the "Ideal Observer" has a mental template of the signal. He performs a cross-correlation between this template and the stimulus in order to determine whether it is a signal. Any variation or uncertainty in signal size, shape, location, time, etc. constitutes noise that spoils the cross-correlation and lowers detectabilty.

6. There is no need to worry about correct rejections and misses because hits and false alarms specify their probabilities. Suppose there were 200 trials, half signal and half noise. Assume that 65 were hits (p(H)=.65) and 20 false were alarms (p(FA)=.2). There must have been 35

misses (p(M)=.35) because p(H) + p(M) must equal 1. More generally, p(M)= 1-p(H). Similarly p(CR)=1-p(FA).

7. Sensory magnitude is only one of many types of scaling. "Hedonic scaling" measures continua such as goodness, preference or virtually any property that a subject can identify. I know a psychophysicist who worked for a food company and measured the "Italianness" of spaghetti sauces containing different amounts of basil and oregano. "Multidimensional scaling," as the name implies, measures several different dimensions at the same time. It is useful when the dimensions are not known in advance, but can be inferred from the data. For example, it might be used to determine the ways in which different products or political candidates differ from one another.

8. Magnitude scaling deals with direct sensory judgments. There is a small but separable field called "memory psychophysics," which specifically examines how sensory judgments change with memory. For now, I'll ignore the distinction between perception and memory as they have much in common.

9. There is a wide variety of methodologies for performing magnitude scaling. Most fall into one of two categories: ratio scaling or interval scaling. See Gescheider (1997) for a good introduction.

10. Most magnitude scaling methods reduce or eliminate regression errors by allowing subjects to use any number they please. The best example is "free-modulus magnitude estimation."

11. I have it on authority from a biblical scholar friend that 40 is a very popular magic number in the bible. Many quantities are 40 or multiples of 40, which may represent the span of one generation.

# Chapter 3

# Physics, Physiology, Psychology

Marc Green, Ph.D.

*"What error drives our eyes and ears amiss?*
*Until I know this sure uncertainty,*
*I'll entertain the offer'd fallacy"*
—Shakespeare

***Synopsis***

## 3.1 Introduction

Shakespeare may have been referring to the fallacy of naïve realism, the persistent belief that we see the world as it really is. In reality, we perceive an array of electrical signals created by physiological mechanisms in the eye and brain in response to a retinal image. This chapter provides general background on this process by outlining vision's three supporting disciplines: physics, physiology and psychology. Physics includes both light and optics while physiology includes the operation of the eye and the higher visual pathways. Psychologically, vision begins with the sensation of brightness and of color.

The ensuing discussion is a whirlwind tour through foundational areas of visual science. It is meant to achieve three goals. First, it provides some background needed in later, more applied chapters. Most notably, chapters on various forensic analyses use and extend some of the concepts described below. Second, the discussion alerts the reader to the breadth of knowledge required to be a genuine expert in vision. This plus the previous psychophysics chapter is a mini introductory perception course. I emphasize the "mini" because it contains far less than students completing an introductory perception class should know. Third, the discussion is a springboard for readers who wish to learn more. Each section is only a peek through the keyhole into a much bigger world. I admit to freely using much technical terminology, but there is a reason. For many, research these days often amounts to typing words into an internet search engine. Such searches are far more productive with the right key terms. The ancient Chinese likely did little googling, but they did have a proverb saying, "The first step towards wisdom is calling things by their right names."

## 3.2 Physics

### A. Light

Light is radiant energy capable of producing visual sensations of brightness and color. It is not the only form of energy that can create visual sensations. For example, visual sensation also may result from mechanical (pushing on the eyeball or hitting the head, as Helmholtz's unfortunate assistant learned) or electrical (phosphenes) energy. However, light is the "adequate stimulus for vision," meaning that it is the form of energy to which the eye is most attuned.

#### 1. Quantum and Wave Theories of Light

Scientists conceptualize light in two ways. "Quantum theory" views light as a collection of particles, "quanta" or "photons," traveling in straight lines through a medium. Quantal speed depends on the density of the medium, but is about 299,792,458 feet per second in a vacuum. Most fundamentally, a light has two properties, quantity and quality. Quanta vary in energy, so total amount of light energy (quantity) is equal to the number of quanta multiplied by the energy of each. For quanta of a given energy, intensity is the number of quanta. Light consisting of high energy quanta would typically have a quality called violet color. Quanta of decreasing energy move up the rainbow to green, yellow, orange and finally to red.

"Wave theory" views light as a vibration or wave in the electromagnetic spectrum. It quantifies intensity by amplitude, the distance between wave peak and trough. Quality is related to wavelength, distance between wave peaks measured in nanometers (nm), 1 millionth of a meter.[1] Short wavelength lights typically appear violet or blue while long wavelength lights typically appear red. The eye responds to a limited range of wave frequencies, the "visible spectrum." In normal cases, this extends from roughly 370 to 730 nm. Frequencies below 370 are ultraviolet, while frequencies beyond 730 nm. are infrared.[2]

Visual science uses both sets of concepts. Scientists usually express the amount of light in quantal language, especially when discussing low intensities. Light output might be expressed as quantal flux, number of quanta per second. The eye's response to light might be described by "quantal catch," the number of quanta activating photoreceptors. A classic experiment (Hecht, Schlaer and Pirenne, 1942) showed that rods can respond to a single quantum and that a viewer can detect as few as 5-14 absorbed quanta.

In contrast, research on light quality, color vision, usually employs wave theory. Color scientists physically specify lights by their "spectral composition," the amount and distribution of their constituent wavelengths. A light may be monochromatic, consisting of a single wavelength, or polychromatic, consisting of many. Among polychromatic lights, those with only a small range of wavelengths are "narrowband" and those with a large range are "wide band." Generally speaking, the wider the band the less pure ("saturated") the color will appear. A light with roughly equal amounts of all wavelengths appears white—at least in theory.

## 2. Light Measurement, Quantities and Units

There are two separate, but related worlds of light measurement. Radiometry measures the light's radiant energy while photometry measures the effect of light on the human eye. The two systems create a mind-numbing array of measurement units, a confusion further complicated by parallel sets of English and SI (metric) units. Below, I briefly describe the measures in SI units.

Radiometric theory starts with a hypothetical entity called a point source, an infinitesimally small light emitter. A point source's fundamental property is total energy output. A point source continually emits quanta, so that energy output is a function of the number of quanta, the energy of each and the period of time over which the energy is summed. The standard measure is called "radiant flux," which is expressed in joules per second (in units called Watts).

**Table 3.1**
**Radiometric and photometric quantities and units**

| Pictorial Representation | Radiometric Quantities | Photometric Quantities |
|---|---|---|
| 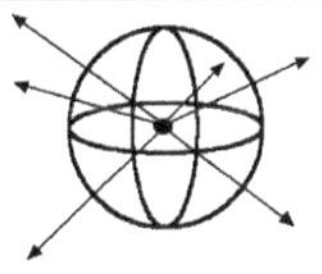 | radiant flux (Watts) | luminous flux (lumen, lm) |
| 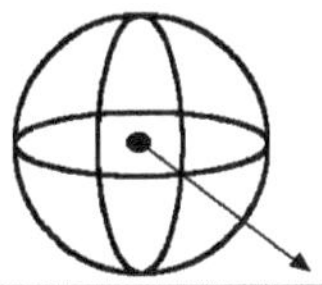 | radiant intensity (W/sr) | luminous intensity (lm/sr = "candela," "cd") |
| 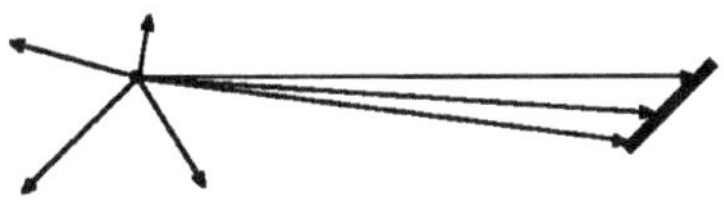 | Irradiance (W/m$^2$) | Illuminance (lm/m$^2$ = "lux," "lx") |
| 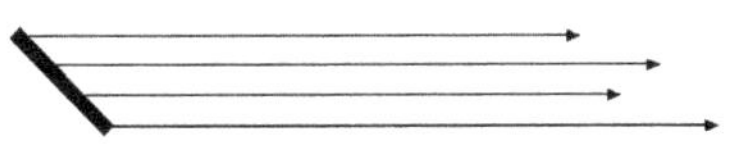 | radiance (W· m$^{-2}$· sr$^{1}$) | Luminance (lm/m$^2$ sr = "nits," "cd/m$^2$") |

The total radiant flux could be measured by enclosing the point source in a sphere and measuring all light that falls on the sphere's inner surface. The amount of energy emitted by the source direction within a given solid angle is the radiant intensity (W/sr).

Two interesting changes occur as the sphere becomes bigger. First the sphere's surface area increases. Since the amount of light is constant, less must fall on any given area inside the sphere. The sphere's surface area grows as the square of its radius, which is the distance of the sphere from the light source. This gives rise to the "inverse square law": the amount of light falling on a given area of surface decreases with the square of the source distance.

Second, each section of its surface more and more approximates a flat plane, such as a road or a street sign. The same logic used in measuring light on a sphere's inner surface applies to measuring real-world surfaces, as long as the distance between source and surface is sufficiently large. The amount of energy falling on a specific area of surface is called "irradiance" and is measured in watts per square meter ($W/m^2$) or centimeters ($W/cm^2$).

Point sources are only imaginary concepts that do not actually exist. In the real world, light originates from "extended sources," which can be treated as arrays of point sources. However, there is minimal error in treating an extended source as a point source if the distance from source to surface is sufficiently large relative to the source size.

Finally, "radiance" is the amount of light that the source throws in a given direction, as defined by solid angle, or steradian (in units of $W/cm^2/sr$). Radiance has the nice property that it is independent of distance, so long as the source is uniform and extended. The inverse square law is still in effect, but increasing amounts of the extended source fall within the measuring angle. The summation of light from a larger area exactly offsets the loss due to the increasing distance.

Visual scientists seldom use radiometric measures. Humans are not equally sensitive to radiant energy of all wavelengths. For example, suppose there were two light sources emitting the same amount of energy. One produced 570 nm light (appearing yellow) and the other 660 nm light (appearing red). The yellow one would appear brighter because humans are more sensitive to 570 nm. than 660 nm light.

If the goal is to determine the effect of light on vision, photometric units replace radiometric units. Photometric units are simply the radiometric units weighed by the eye's response at each wavelength. Each radiometric unit has a corresponding photometric unit. Radiant flux becomes "luminous flux," which is expressed in "lumens." Radiant intensity becomes luminous intensity, which is expressed in "candela." Irradiance becomes "illuminance," measured in lumens per square meter (lux). Illuminance is still commonly expressed in the English unit of foot-candles (ft-c), lumens per square foot, which converts to lux as 1 ft-c to 10.76 lux.[3] Lastly, radiance becomes "luminance," measured in candelas per meter squared ($cd/m^2$), units occasionally called "nits." The foot-lambert (= 3.43 $cd/m^2$) is a common older unit of luminance.

Finally, some vision work uses "retinal illuminance," the amount of light actually falling on the retina. Pupils change size with light level, so dilations and contractions alter retinal illuminance. The unit "trolands " is the product of luminance (in $cd/m^2$) × pupil area (in $mm^2$). Do not confuse trolands with "illuminance at the eye," referring to light at the cornea and not including a correction for pupil size.

### 3. Light and Vision: Mueller's "Law Of Specific Nerve Energies."

The fundamental law of all sensory science is Mueller's "law of specific nerve energies." Visual experience is determined by the part of the brain that is activated. If a hit on the head activated the same brain cells as the sight of your cat, you'd see your cat when you were hit on the head. If the nerves from the ear were somehow attached to your visual cortex, you would see a flash every time the telephone range. Sensation and perception are all in your head. This is the fundamental message that all people interested in visual science should firmly appreciate. Naïve realism makes us think otherwise, but that is just as well.

Having briefly discussed the physics of light, this is a place to talk about the relationships between light's physical properties and vision. These relationships are beyond complex. We live blithely in our day-to-day naïve realism because our visual systems have many tricks to disguise the complexities in order to give us the illusion of a stable world.

Be warned, however, that commonsense intuitions about the relationship between light and vision are almost invariably wrong. For example, an object's brightness is *not* determined by the intensity of the light that it sends to the eye. An object's color is *not* determined by wavelength of the light that it sends to the eye. Neither brightness nor color is a fixed property of any object.

## B. Optics

Optics is the science that studies the behavior of light. Light moving from one medium to another can be reflected, absorbed or transmitted.[4] If the light is transmitted, it may refract (bend), depending on the speed difference with which it passes through the media. Light may exhibit all three behaviors when striking a single surface. Lastly, the amount of light exhibiting each of these behaviors may depend on wavelength.

### 1. Reflectance

Light entering the eye may originate from a light source such as the sun or a lamp. More commonly, viewers see light that has been reflected off a surface. The reflected light's intensity and wavelength depend on properties of both the incident light and the reflective surface.

Incident light may vary in both intensity and spectral composition. Surface properties include reflectance and texture. Different surfaces reflect different percentages of the incident light. A piece of coal might reflect 5 percent while a sheet of paper might reflect 90 percent. Surfaces also vary in their reflectivity for different wavelengths. A surface illuminated with white light appears blue, for example, if it reflects short wavelength light and absorbs middle and long wavelengths. Similarly, a surface that appears white or gray reflects all wavelengths about equally.

The same surface illuminated with colored light will appear different. A surface that reflects short wavelength light appears blue in white or blue light because it reflects the wavelengths contained in the incident beam. It appears black, however, when illuminated with narrowband yellow light. There are no short wavelengths in the incident beam reflected back to the eye. The surface absorbs the long wavelength yellow light, so none reflects to the eye.

Surfaces also vary in texture, which determines the direction of reflected light leaving the surface. Textures fall into four categories: specular (mirror), spread, diffuse and retroreflective. Chapter 13 discusses surface texture in the context of practical light measurement issues.

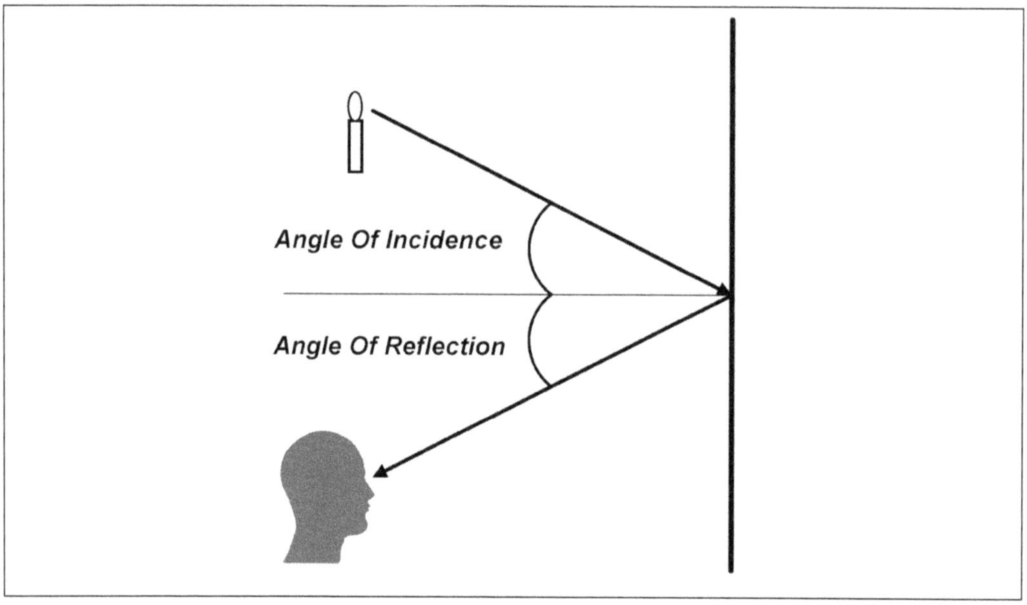


***Figure 3.1*** *Angle of incidence equals angle of reflection.*

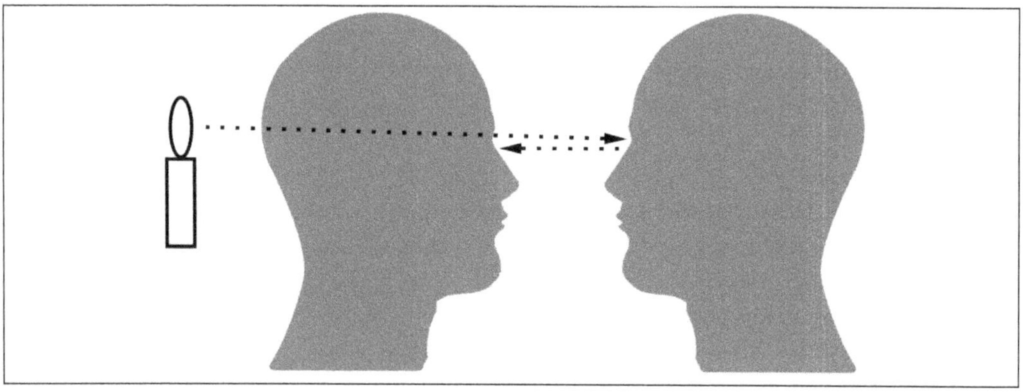

***Figure 3.2*** *Light rays from another person's eye would have to originate from behind the viewer's head.*

Specular surfaces are the simplest, because they follow the rule: "angle of reflection equals angle of incidence" (Figure 3.1). Incident rays strike the surface and reflect the same angle relative to the surface normal (the line perpendicular to the surface). Conversely, the eye sees only the image of objects whose rays strike the surface at the same angle as the viewing angle. This fact explains the great mystery of vision: why can people look out through their eyes, but no one can look in? That is, if you try to see into another person's pupil, there is only black. Obviously, the eye transmits light, otherwise you could not look out.

The answer lies in the rule about reflectance angle. As Figure 3.2 shows, rays from the other person's eye reflected to your eye would have to originate from a point behind your head. Since your head blocks the rays, there is no reflected light and everyone else's pupils appear black. Optometrists and ophthalmologists circumvent this problem with an "ophthalmoscope"[5] that the viewer holds up to the patient's eye. The ophthalmoscope contains a light that enters into the patient's eye at just the right angle to reflect rays back to the viewer's eye.

### 2. Transmission

Transparent surfaces transmit some of the incident light and reflect or absorb the rest. Transmission is characterized by two variables: density and wavelength selectivity. Density refers to the overall amount of light that the surface blocks. "Neutral density filters" affect all wavelengths equally, so they change brightness but not color.[6] Wavelength selective filters transmit some wavelengths better than others, so they alter both color and brightness. For example, if a transparent surface appears green, it is transmitting "green" middle wavelengths and blocking short and long wavelengths (red, yellow, blue and violet). Another way to think about filters is in terms of complementary colors. If the filter is yellow, then it is blocking blue. The eye contains several yellow filters, as explained below.

If the incident light is colored rather than white, a filter may produce different results. For example, a filter that looks blue in white light will appear black or very dark in yellow light. Blue filters pass blue light and block longer wavelengths.

An example of wavelength-selective filtering occurs when roadway sources emit very narrow spectra. For example, low pressure sodium lamps are a very narrowband yellow, which would poorly penetrate blue-tinted windshields. As a result, a blue-tinted windshield that would have 85 percent transmittance for white light would have a much lower transmittance for low pressure sodium street lighting.

### 3. Refraction

Light normally travels in a straight line at a fixed speed, which depends on medium density. When light moves from one medium to another of different density, it changes speed and bends or "refracts." A "lens" refracts light to produce the image of an object at some distance. The image is a 2-dimensional projection for a 3-dimensional object. In vision, the object is distal, and the retinal image is proximal, so viewers only "see" images but never objects. Since the image is all the nervous system has to work with, it is the starting point of all visual analyses. A sharp reader might ask, "How do we see a 3-D world using 2-D images? Where does the extra dimension come from?" The mind/brain somehow manufactures it.

Figure 3.3 shows a lens forming an image. Incident rays bend upon both entry and exit from the lens. If the lens is sufficiently thin, this double bending can be ignored. The image formed by the lens is upside down.

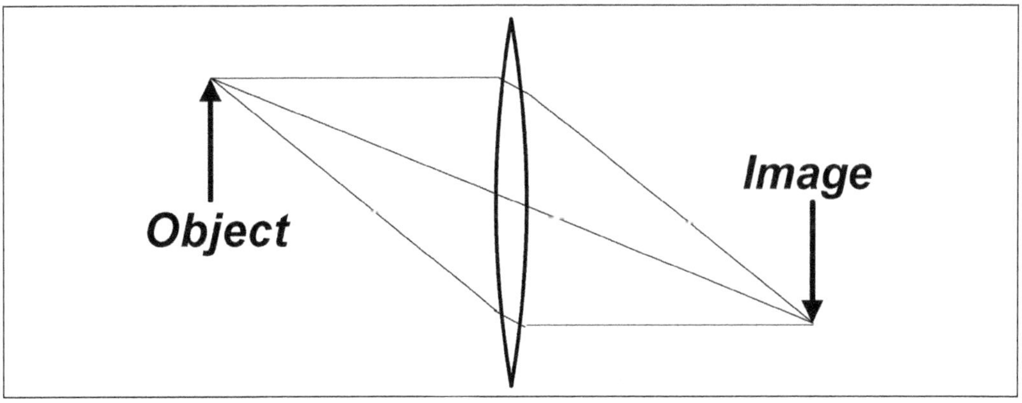


***Figure 3.3*** *Schematic of lens performing refraction.*

Now, imagine a distant point sending light rays to a lens. The rays are nearly parallel, and the lens converges them back to an image of the point (Figure 3.4). The distance between the lens and the focal point is the lens's "focal length." Figure 3.4B shows a lens that bends the light more sharply and has a shorter focal length. The second lens has more refractive power because it has a shorter focal length. The unit of lens power is the "diopter," 1/focal length measured in meters.

The lenses shown in the Figures 3.4A and 3.4B are converging (also called positive, convex or +) lenses since they cause the incident parallel rays to meet. Figure 3.4C shows a diverging (negative or -) lens that causes incident rays to spread apart. These "coke bottle" lenses have negative power because their focal point is in front of the lens rather than behind. They are useful in subtracting optical power from an overly powerful optical system, such as the myopic eye. In Figure 3.4, placing a negative lens in front of either lens A or B would move the focal point rightward.

If the lens is not ground perfectly, it may not be able to focus all incoming parallel rays to the same point, and some part of the image will invariably be out of focus. The two major types of optical error are spherical and cylindrical. If the curvature error is symmetrical over the surface, the result is a "spherical aberration." Different parts of a scene focus sharply at different distances, and it is impossible to sharply focus the entire scene. One way to limit spherical aberration is to use a small aperture so that light rays must pass through a relatively limited area of the lens.[7] If the lens has different focal lengths along different radial axes, then the error is cylindrical and the result is astigmatism. Lines of different orientation focus at different lengths.

## 3.3 Physiology

### A. Eye Anatomy and Optics

The eye consists of muscular, optical and neural components. Muscles aim the eyes at an object; optics sharply focus the image; the retina transforms the image into a neural code.

To some extent, the optical components resemble a camera; they refract incoming rays in order to sharply focus an image on its "film." However, this eye-camera analogy breaks down quickly. The eye's method of creating a sharp image differs from the technique used in cameras. More importantly, the eye's retina is not a passive recorder of light like film but is the first step in an active series of image processing operations. There are many other differences, such as dynamic range, gamma and temporal integration, but I'll save these issues for Chapter 18.

Figure 3.5 shows a schematic eyeball and the major components. Light first strikes the cornea, passes through the pupil, hits the crystalline lens and then reaches the retina. The pupil diameter, and hence the amount of light entering the eye, varies with conditions. Pupil size grows to admit more light in dimmer conditions. However, the pupil also shrinks when people feel anxious or threatened and grows when people feel aroused. If you are playing Hold 'Em poker and your opponent's pupils pop open, fold immediately.

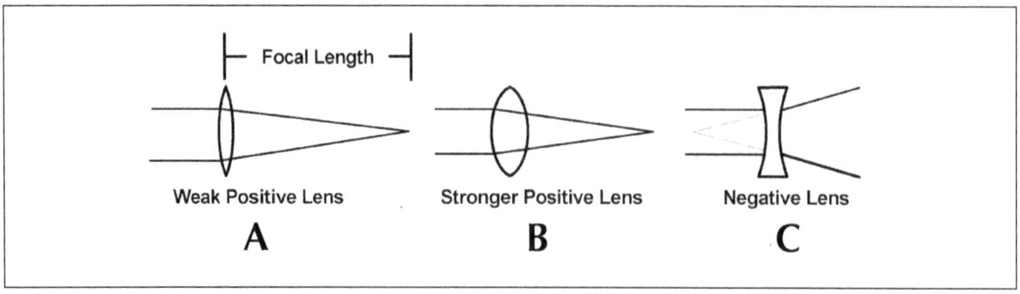


***Figure 3.4*** *Example lenses.*

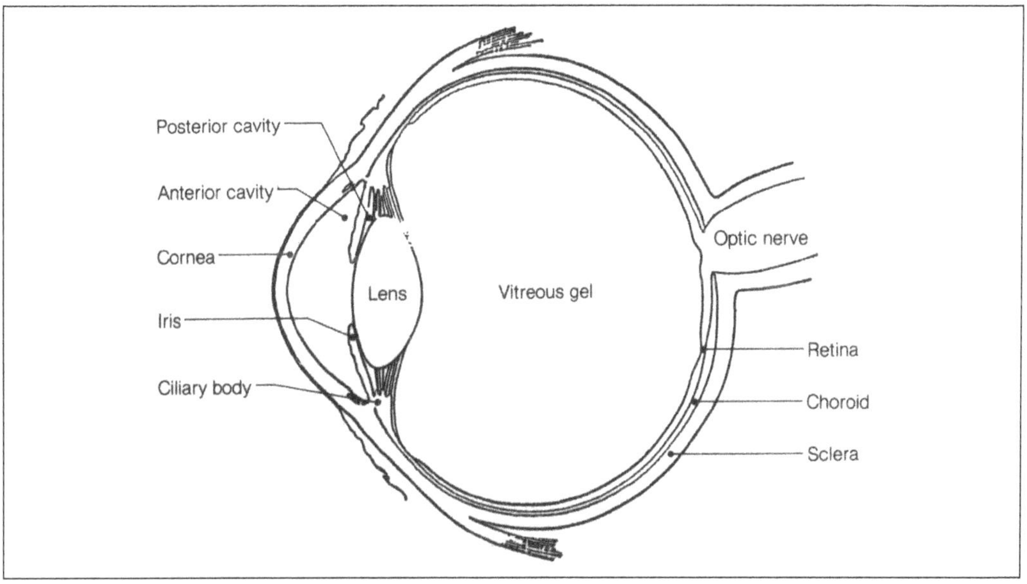


***Figure 3.5*** *Eye schematic.*

The pupil has other functions besides light regulation. Normal pupil diameter varies from 2–8 mm, resulting in a 16:1 range[8] in light admittance. Since people can see over a light intensity range of several million to one, the pupil's effect is really very small. Perhaps the pupil's main function is control of image quality. As noted, smaller apertures reduce spherical aberration and expand depth-of-field.

The cornea and the lens both refract light. The cornea is the eye's principal optical component with a power of about 40 diopters. It performs most of the focusing but has fixed optical power and cannot adjust for distance. The lens is weaker at 20 diopters when relaxed but has a variable power of about 8 diopters. It can "accommodate," changing thickness to sharply image objects at a wide range of distances. From age 16 onward, however, ability to thicken the lens declines and viewers have increasing difficulty in accommodating nearby objects. By age 40 most people become "presbyopic" and need reading glasses. The lens and cornea are both tinted yellow, which filters blue light. This is advantageous because the atmosphere scatters blue light, making objects slightly fuzzy. The yellow tint removes the bluish fuzz and sharpens the retinal image. However, aging increases the yellow density to the point where it impairs vision.

Optically, eyes fall into three classes depending on their ability to create sharp images through accommodation (Figure 3.6). In the "emmetropic" eye, the length of the eye matches the optical power so incoming rays focus sharply on the retina. As a result, an emmetropic viewer can see sharply without the aid of optical correction. However, aging emmetropes will eventually become presbyopic and need reading glasses. The "myopic" eye has too much optic power for the eye length. The focal point is in front of the retina, so images are blurred rather than sharp. To see sharply, the myope must move the focal point back to the retina by means of negative correction. Lastly, the hyperope (or hypermetrope) has too little optical power, so the focal point falls behind the retina, again blurring the retinal image. The solution is positive correction.

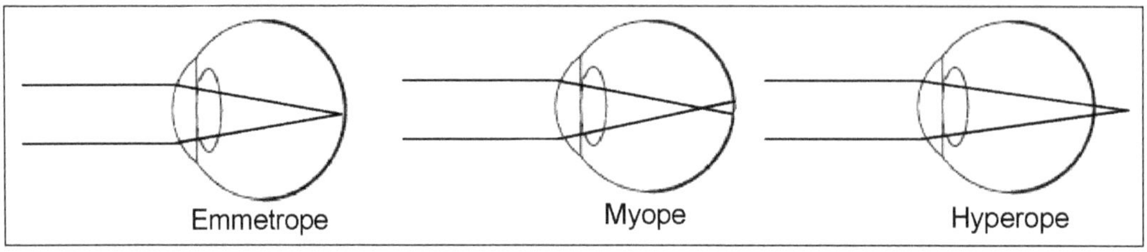


***Figure 3.6*** *Three optical classes of viewer.*

## B. Eye Muscles

The eye has two primary sets of muscles. The ciliary muscles alter lens shape in order to accommodate to objects of different distances. When ciliary muscles are at rest, the lens is accommodated to a distance of about 1.52 diopters or 66 centimeters. Individuals, however, vary greatly.

The oculomotor muscles control eye movements, changes of eye orientation within the socket. Eye movements fall into several categories, including saccades, smooth pursuit, vergence and nystagmus. I have already discussed saccades, the sharp, ballistic jumps from one fixation point to another. The eyes may also perform smooth pursuit, the tracking of an object as it moves across the visual field. Viewers cannot perform smooth pursuit without a specific target to track. The eye also performs vergence movements, an inward turning of the eyes toward the target. Most viewers have two laterally offset eyes, yet see the world as a single image. In order to accomplish this feat, each eye must point at the object and fuse left and right eye images. As objects come nearer, the eyes must verge at a sharper angle in order to maintain fixation. If you hold a finger up close to your face, notice that the background becomes a double image because the eyes are not verged for that distance. Vergence is discussed more below in connection with stereopsis. Nystagmus is an involuntary movement in which the eyes move in one direction and then snap back to the other. For example, a viewer standing in front of a train moving rightward automatically tracks the train rightward (slow phase). When the eyes reach the limit of their rightward motion, they suddenly snap back leftward (fast phase) and then begin another rightward motion. The eyes then continue the fast-slow cycle while the train passes. Nystagmus can also be a congenital condition that occurs in the absence of a driving visual stimulus. Finally, some people under the influence of alcohol and drugs also exhibit nystagmus, so police use it as a sobriety test.

## C. The Retina

### 1. Rods and Cones

Ultimately the light rays strike the retina, a neural layer containing photoreceptors. Each photoreceptor contains molecules of photopigment that can convert light energy into a neural signal.[9] The light strikes the molecule causing it to isomerize (change shape) and to release energy. This is also called "bleaching" because the photopigment turns clear. The photopigment temporarily stays in the bleached state before regenerating and again becoming available to catch quanta. Even without being struck by a quantum, however, photopigment molecules spontaneously bleach to create a "dark light" that is indistinguishable from real light. As a result, it is literally impossible to be in the dark. In fact, people in the dark don't see black, they see "eigenlicht," an "intrinsic light" of gray. More importantly, dark light limits detection at very low light levels.

Photoreceptors fall into two classes, rods and cones, which further subdivides into three classes based on wavelength preference of their photopigment: short-wavelength ("blue"), middle-wavelength ("green") and long wavelength. Rods come in only one variety.

The rods and cones constitute the retina's "photoreceptor mosaic." Cone photoreceptors are packed closely together in the retina's center. The central fovea has no rods and few, if any, short-wavelength cones. This is the area of highest visual resolution. As distance from the fovea increases, the cone mosaic becomes sparser and more irregular, and virtually all visual functions decline. Viewers usually attempt to see with the fovea—that is, they move their eyes so that the object of interest forms its image on the fovea.

Rods have a different retinal distribution and are most concentrated about 20° from the fovea. Visual function peaks at about 10° from the fovea, but for targets of any significant size, sensitivity varies little over the central 20–40° of the visual field—except for a dip right at the fovea where no rods exist.

## 2. Visual Angles

Object size affects visibility and many other visual functions, so visual science requires a metric that specifies the size of viewed objects. However, specifying size in simple measurements such as feet or meters will not work. People directly perceive only the images that an object projects onto the retina and not the objects themselves. Retinal image size, however, changes with object distance. Any useful measure must scale physical size by distance. The "visual angle" is an angular dimension of an object at the eye and is a good metric for retinal image size. As shown in Figure 3.7, a larger distant object and a smaller near object can create the same size retinal image and are theoretically equally detectable.[10]

Visual angle, $\theta$, may be computed several ways. The most accurate is:

$$\theta = 2 * \arctan\left(\frac{\text{size}}{2 * \text{distance}}\right)$$

Unless the angle is large, however, most psychophysicists simply calculate visual angle as:

$$\theta = \arctan\left(\frac{\text{size}}{\text{distance}}\right)$$

For small angles, such as those in looming detection (see Chapter 16), a simpler formula is applicable:

$$\theta = \left(\frac{\text{size}}{\text{distance}}\right)$$

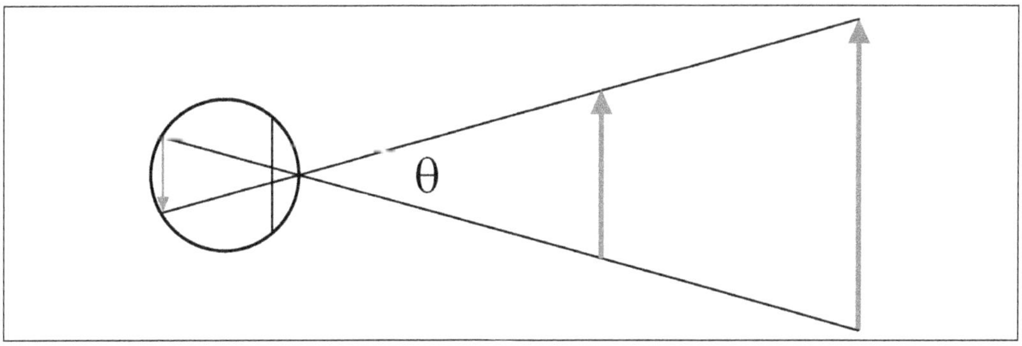


***Figure 3.7*** *Visual angle of an object's image projected on to the retina.*

**Table 3.2**
**Some typical visual angles**

| Visual Angles Of Common Objects | |
|---|---|
| Quarter held at arm's length | ~2.5 degrees |
| Thumbnail at arm's length | 1.5-2 degrees |
| Diameter of the fovea | ~1 degree |
| Diameter of the sun and moon from Earth | 30 minarc |
| Tractor-Trailer rear (8′ wide) at 1 mile | 5.2 minarc |
| Headlamp (5.25′ diameter) at 1500 ft. | 1 minarc |
| Strip of reflective tape (3″) at 850 ft. | 1 minarc |

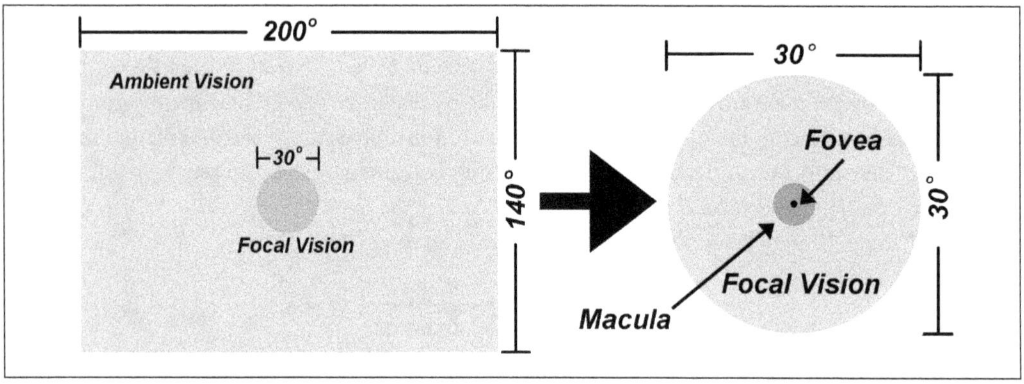


***Figure 3.8*** *Schematic representation of the visual field. This is a rough approximation, as the visual field is not literally rectangular.*

The visual angle is expressed in degrees, minutes (arcmin or minarc) or seconds (arcsec or secarc). In rare cases, such as angular velocity (Chapter 16), the unit of convenience is the radian. Lastly, visual angle can be converted to actual retina image size, where 1° = 288 μm.

Figure 3.7 highlights an interesting point. If large distant objects and nearby small objects can create the same retinal image size, then how does the viewer know which he is seeing? This is seemingly no problem in most cases; a pedestrian down the block makes a tiny retinal image, yet the viewer perceives him as normal size and not as a tiny person. Somehow, the brain creates a "size-distance constancy" by taking distance into account when judging size. This is another reflection of the fundamental problems inherent in creating a 3-D world from a 2-D image. By now, it should be increasingly clear why this book started with the sentence, "*Vision is the most complex task that humans perform.*" There is more proof below.

### 3. Visual Fields

The retina is not uniform, so visual function varies with location in the visual field. Figure 3.8 shows that the entire field subsumes a visual angle of roughly 200° by 140°.[11] Most of the field is used for ambient vision ('Where am I?') with the center 30° devoted more to focal vision ('What is it?').

The visual field has four functional divisions: 1) center-surround, 2) left-right, 3) up-down and 4) nasal-temporal (toward-away from the nose). All four have known effects on vision, but center-surround is certainly the most powerful.

Working from the center out, the fovea is about 1-1.5° in diameter and is the area of sharpest vision. Roughly speaking, the fovea covers the area defined by the thumbnail held at arm's length. The fovea's center is pure cone with no rods. A line extending from the fovea's center out through the pupil's center is called the "optical axis."

The "macula lutea," ("yellow spot") is a yellow area surrounding the fovea. It has a diameter of about 4–10° and maintains relatively good resolution. The area immediately around the fovea is also sometimes called the "parafovea." Finally, the central 30° area is focal vision, Roughly speaking, it is the area that viewers use when normally searching the world and viewing scenes.

The fovea and even the macula cover only a small portion of the visual field, so the eyes move frequently in a series of saccades to inspect scenes. Each movement stops briefly, bringing both the fovea and attentional focus to bear on some target for the brief dwell time. Since saccades are seldom more than 15°, focal vision is the area over which a viewer can make a single saccade bring the target to the fovea.

The area further out in the visual field is the far periphery. Photoreceptor spacing increases and spherical aberration becomes significant. Visual functions such as contrast sensitivity, acuity and motion detection fall dramatically. Viewers also suffer a loss of color vision as the number of cones decreases. The viewer first loses reds and greens and then blues and yellows. This color loss can cause accidents, as drivers can misidentify the color of red signals viewed in the far periphery as being yellow (Sivak, Flannagan, Miyokawa, Traube, 1999). Peripheral vision is also poorer because viewers focus attention around the fovea. Moreover, situational factors, such as traveling at high speed, suppress peripheral detection. Lastly, each eye has a blind spot about 20° from the fovea where the optic nerve leaves the eyeball and there are no photoreceptors. Disease can create other blind spots called "scotomas."

The area outside of focal vision is sometimes termed "ambient vision." While viewers use focal vision search to perceive objects in the environment, they use ambient vision for spatial orientation. Drivers and pedestrians unconsciously monitor their peripheral visual fields for information to guide their heading and direction as they move forward. A little introspection will reveal we have no idea how we manage to keep our car on the road or walk down the sidewalk without going off into the street. Like so many visual functions, we simply take the maintenance of heading and direction for granted without realizing that it is a difficult feat. The attempt to maintain heading when not looking in the direction of travel, for example, may cause the "moth-effect" (Green, 2006).

Ambient vision may use "optic flow." Gibson (1958) noted that the visual scene changes in predictable ways as people move through the world. Figure 3.9 shows the changes for a person traveling forward in a straight line. Points in the visual field stream outward to form the "flow field." The field's central point, where the viewer looks, is the "focus of expansion" (FOE). Points farther from the FOE stream outward with increasing speed. Points on the outer limit are constantly leaving the flow while new points are born at the FOE. The faster the person moves forward, the faster the points stream. If the viewer alters heading, relative direction and speed of the points change. Drivers and pedestrians can use these changes for steering in order to maintain their heading and direction. On straight roads, it is also possible to maintain a straight heading by simply steering toward the FOE, which is the only station at any point in the visual field. Optic flow is a central concept in most theories of driving and walking through the environment.

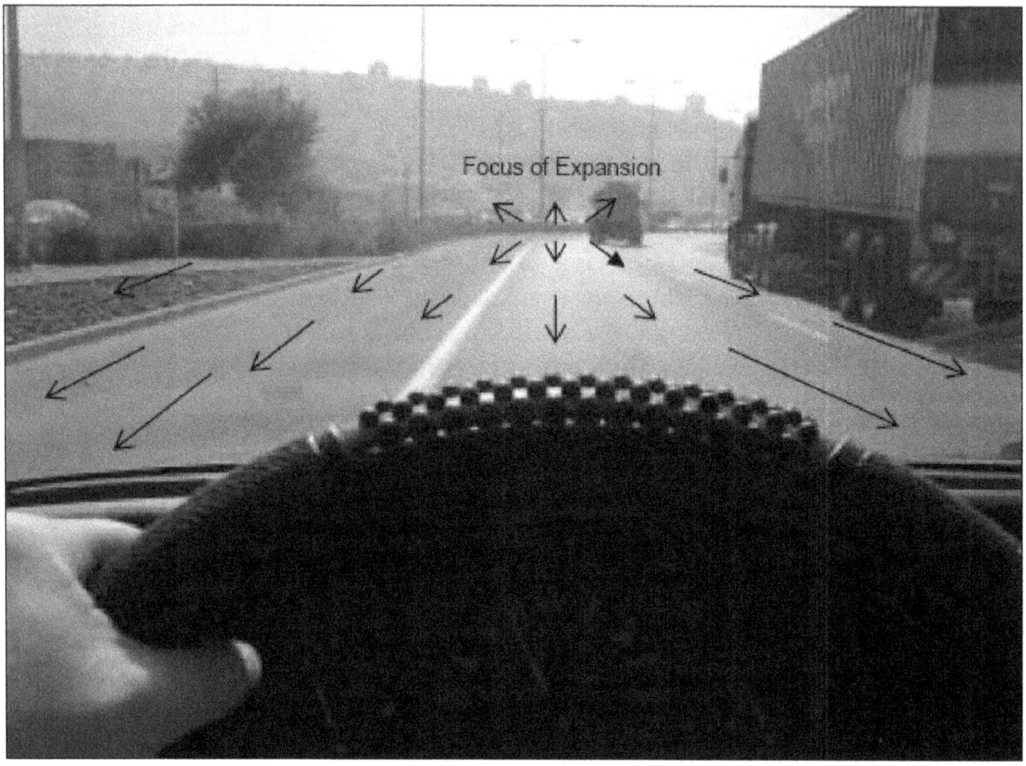


***Figure 3.9*** *Example of optic flow field, showing movement of points in space. Arrow orientation indicates direction and length speed. Reprinted with permission of Zhonghai Li.*

Ambient vision is very robust, operating relatively well even in dim light, even as focal vision sharply declines. The "selective degradation" hypothesis (Leibowitz and Owens, 1977) suggests that many accidents occur because drivers fail to understand the different effect of dimming focal and ambient vision. As light dims, drivers then have no problem steering and maintaining lane position, so they grossly underestimate their loss of contrast sensitivity and ability to detect obstacles on the road ahead. They drive too fast for conditions and do not have enough time/distance for braking and steering should an obstacle appear.

*Binocular and Monocular Fields*. Figure 3.8 showed the "achromatic binocular visual field," the area covered when both eyes are operating. Normal viewers use the two eyes together and don't notice that each eye covers only part of the visual field. The one-eyed "monocular" visual field is about 160–170° field, although it declines with age. The two monocular fields overlap in the central 120°, but the extreme peripheral 30–40° is covered only by the eye on the same, ipsilateral side. If a viewer cannot use an eye, he loses that 30–40°. For example, a person without use of the right eye would not see the leftmost 30–40° of the visual field. Some one-eyed viewers, however, maintain a slight head turn to compensate. A left-eyed viewer looking straight ahead, for example, might turn the head slightly to the right in order to cover some of the lost 30–40°. Of course, the total field is still 160–170°, so the area gained to the left is offset by an area lost on the right. Monocular viewers, however, tend to compensate for visual field loss by frequent head turns that sweep the eyes through the entire scene (Westlake, 2001). Lastly, everyone's nose blocks some of the area on each eye's opposite, contralateral side. There is also a smaller "chromatic binocular field," of about 110°

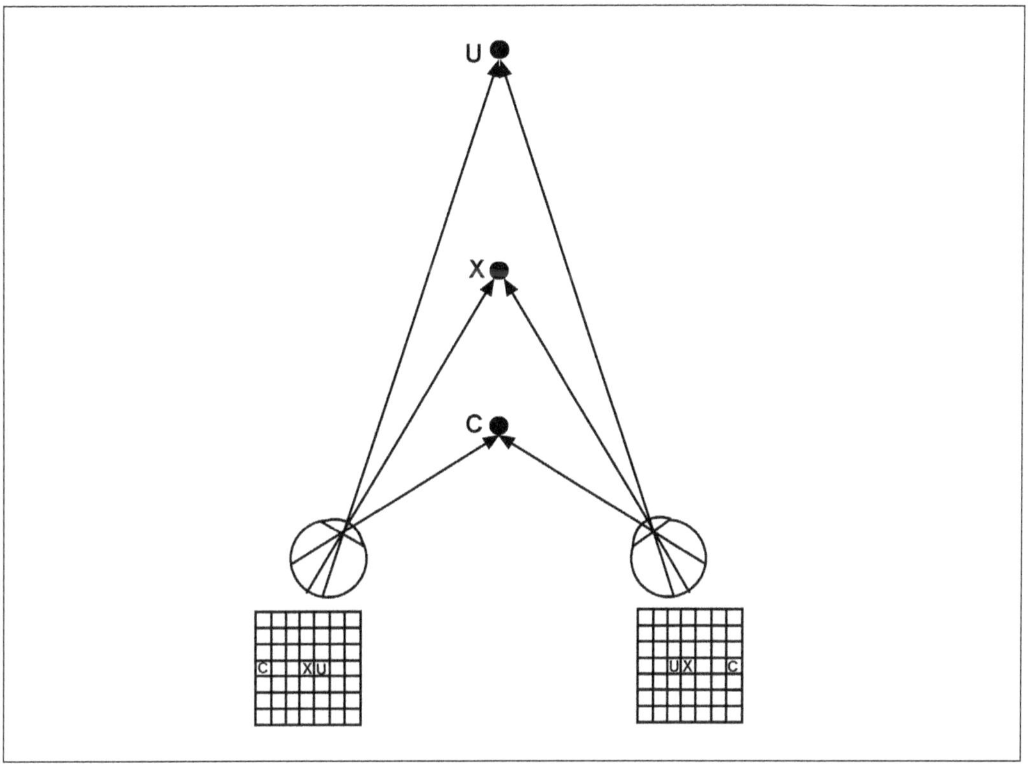


***Figure 3.10*** *Schematic diagram of stereopsis. X marks fixation and the corresponding retinal points. Point U lies farther and point C nearer.*

width and 90° height in which viewers can see chromatic color. The limits of the field are difficult to specify, however, because color vision declines gradually at the extremes. The blue-yellow field is somewhat larger than the red-green field.

*Stereopsis.* Binocular vision also permits stereoscopic depth perception. The retina in each eye is something like a map with a set of coordinates (Figure 3.10). A normal viewer typically points the two eyes at the same fixation point in 3-D space, which then registers at the same coordinate on each map. In technical jargon, points falling on the same retinal coordinates in each eye are "corresponding." Further, the fixated point is fused, so the viewer sees only a single image although he is really looking at separate left and right eye images.

Since the eyes are laterally offset from one another, however, each eye has a slightly different view of 3-D space and registers all non-fixated points at noncorresponding locations on the two retinal maps. Viewers can still fuse these noncorresponding points into a single image, but they will have "disparity" since they do not fall on the same coordinate in each eye. Viewers use the disparity information to create stereoscopic depth, the sensation seen when looking through 3-D glasses. Ability to detect small disparity differences, "stereoacuity," is one of vision's keenest abilities.

Figure 3.10 illustrates disparity and stereopsis. The fixated point "X" falls at the same coordinate in each eye and has 0 disparity. The distant point, U, and the nearer point, C, create images at noncorresponding points. The lateral shift in non-corresponding points creates two types of disparity that signal depth. Point C is in "crossed disparity," where the image points are too far to the left in the left eye and too far to the right in the right eye. This pattern of disparity signals that the point is closer than fixation. Conversely point U is in "uncrossed disparity," which occurs when the image point is too far to the right in the left eye and too far to the left in the right eye. This disparity signals an object beyond fixation. Suppose that the viewer shifts fixation to point C. Then both X and U will be beyond fixation in uncrossed disparity. This does not change apparent depth of the points. Stereopsis codes only *relative* depth rather than absolute depth, so that changing the fixation point does not cause objects to suddenly jump around.

If the disparity grows sufficiently, however, viewers can no longer fuse the left and right eye images, resulting in "diplopia" or double vision. Various impairments of the eyes and eye muscles as well as drugs and alcohol can also cause diplopia. Further, stereopsis has a range limited to about 1200 ft. At greater distances, the disparity is so low that it falls below stereoacuity and is not detected.

Finally, most nonexperts harbor misconceptions about stereopsis, and its role in spatial vision. First, many sources incorrectly say that a person who has lost an eye has lost depth perception. This is obviously untrue. Try closing one eye, and you see that depth still exists. Depth perception can use a wide variety of monocular cues: linear perspective, height in the visual field, aerial perspective, motion parallax, interposition, size, brightness, and others.

Stereoacuity's advantage is that it is much finer than other depth cues, as a simple demonstration shows. Close one eye and hold both hands out near arm's length with the index finger raised. Move the index fingers to the same distance from the face. Now open the other eye. Chances are that the fingers are not at the same distance. Without stereopsis, the ability to see the small depth difference is lost.

Second, many people mistakenly believe that stereopsis is a distance cue. Stereopsis says little or nothing about *absolute* distance, except perhaps for objects within a few feet of the face. As explained above, stereopsis signals only *relative depth*, whether one point in space is relatively nearer or farther than another. Viewers use this information to decompose scenes into different surfaces and to perceive object shape. They also use stereopsis to judge whether an object is moving closer or further away. (See Chapter 16.) They do not use stereopsis to judge distance.

## D. Visual Modes

Humans are able to see over a light intensity range of several million to one. In order to achieve this extraordinary feat while maintaining good contrast sensitivity, the eye adjusts to the prevailing conditions and changes its mode of operation as light levels vary. These modes are called "photopic," "mesopic" and "scotopic" vision. Figure 3.11 shows typical situations where the eye would be in each operating mode.

Photopic vision occurs at higher light levels where cone receptors in the center of the visual field dominate vision. Photopic vision also exhibits 1) low light sensitivity, 2) high acuity and 3) color vision. Scotopic vision occurs at very low light levels where rod receptors outside the central field dominate vision. Scotopic vision also exhibits 1) high light sensitivity, 2) poor acuity and 3) lack of color vision. Mesopic mode is mixed, with both cones and rods active.

The visual mode switch also affects spectral sensitivity, the ability to detect lights of a given wavelength. As noted above, photometric units are radiometric measurements that have been weighted by human eye sensitivity. There are two standard weighting functions or "luminous efficiency curves," $V_\lambda$ for photopic and $V'_\lambda$ for scotopic conditions (Figure 3.12). The scotopic curve and peak efficiency shift down the spectrum to shorter wavelengths in dim light. The change in viewing spectral sensitivities is called the "Purkinje shift." During photopic vision, viewers are most sensitive to light that appears greenish-yellow. In scotopic vision, viewers are most sensitive to light which would appear greenish-blue during the day. Viewers also lose most long wavelength (red) sensitivity.

It is common to read that "blue is the most visible color at night." Figure 3.12 shows this statement to be incorrect.[12] Scotopic vision shifts sensitivity to lower wavelengths, but the peak is in the bluish-green and not in blue. Moreover, a viewer using scotopic vision cannot see color. The correct statement is, "the brightest wavelength in scotopic vision would produce a color appearing blue-green if it had had enough intensity to stimulate cones." This may seem nitpicking, but the original statement is quantitatively wrong and confuses physics and perception.

The shift from scotopic to photopic is much more than just changing from cones to rods. The shift involves a complete rewiring of the retina due to a delicate balancing act between the contradictory demands of light sensitivity on the one hand and contrast sensitivity on the other. During the day, the eye is optimized for seeing contrast. The photoreceptors connect to ganglion cells, which essentially throw light away by creating inhibitory, edge-sharpening responses that decrease neural activity in response to light (e.g., Green, 1984). The effect is similar to the edge-sharpening function on a computer graphics program. Blurred images become clearer and more distinct.

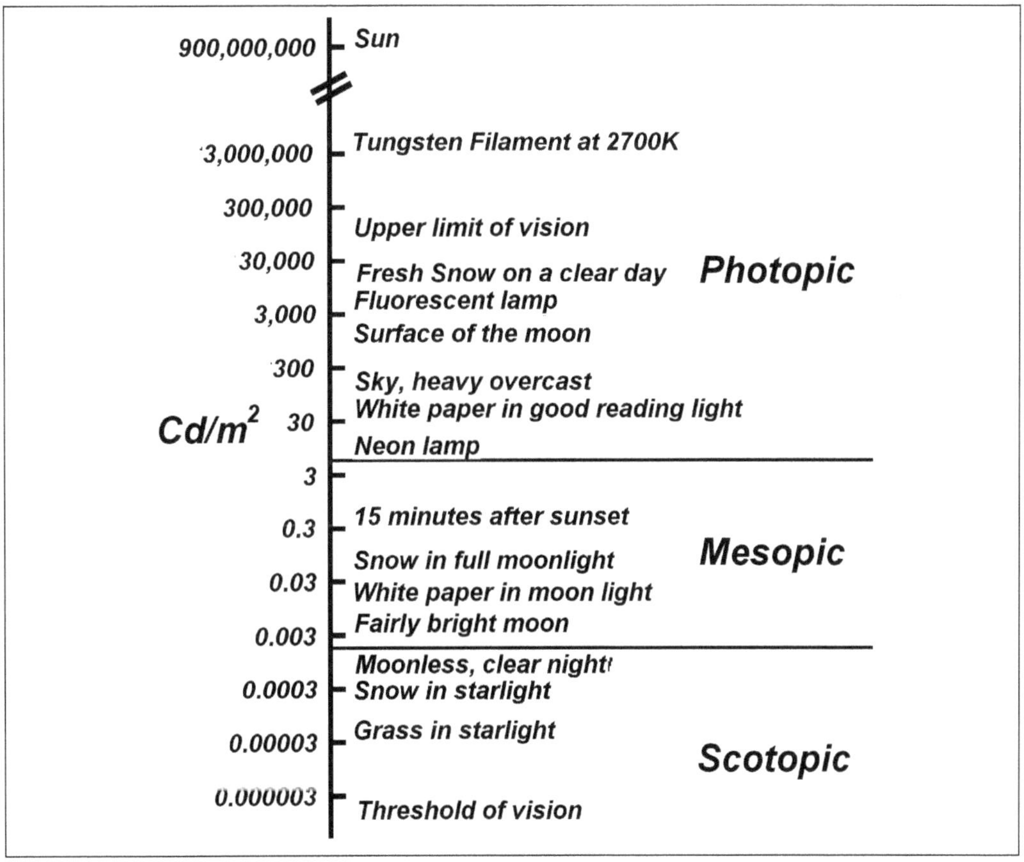


***Figure 3.11*** *Light levels which produce photopic, mesopic and scotopic vision.*

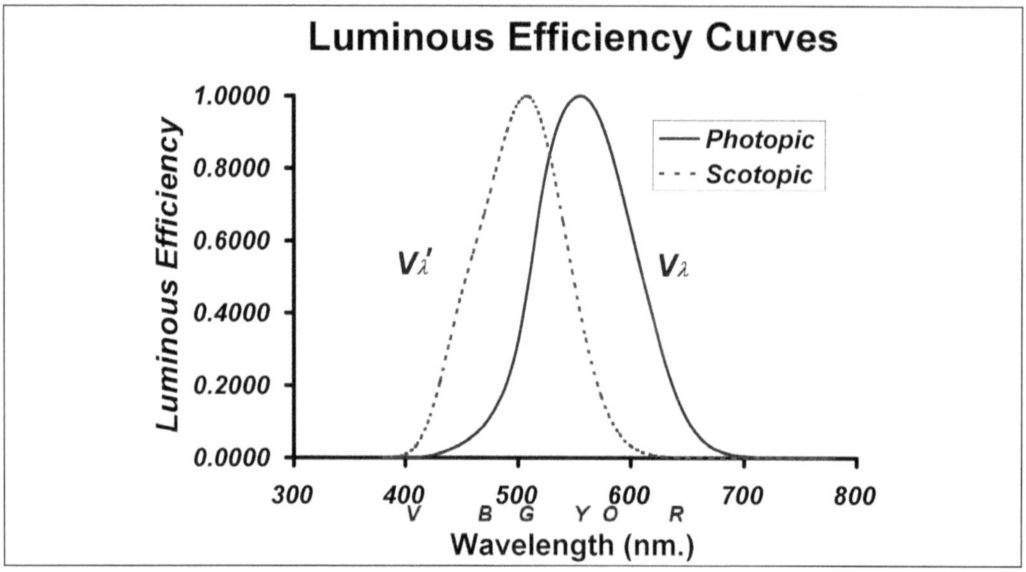


***Figure 3.12*** *Photopic and scotopic luminous efficiency curves. R=red, O=orange, Y=yellow, G=green, B=blue and V=violet.*

As illumination declines, the visual system starts conserving light in order to gain sensitivity. Photopic inhibitory responses weaken, and eventually stop. Eventually, inhibition is replaced by convergence, where the many photoreceptor outputs pool together to increase sensitivity but also further reduce resolution. In very dim light, the visual system switches to scotopic rod vision to conserve light and reduce contrast sensitivity even more.

Light sensitivity also improves in dimmer light because more photopigment is available. A bleached photopigment molecule is unable to respond again for a period of time. During daylight, the large number of quanta striking the eye means that much of the photopigment is bleached. At night, most of the photopigment is unbleached and ready to respond to the next quantum.

Mesopic wavelength sensitivity lies between the photopic and scotopic and does not have a standard spectral response curve. Mesopic vision is also more complex because it is a transition range that mixes cones and rods, each having a different spectral sensitivity and retinal distribution. The high mesopic level covers luminances where the cones are still operating relatively well. Vision is still best in central vision and the viewer can perceive color. At the bottom of the mesopic range, the cones have almost ceased to function and rods dominate. Sensitivity is almost constant throughout the visual field and there is no color vision. In between, there is a highly mixed mode where central vision remains photopic but where the periphery is a rod-cone mix. In sum, there is no easy way to characterize mesopic vision. This is highly unfortunate, because many, if not most, nighttime road accidents occur in mesopic conditions. Although people often equate cones with daylight vision and rods with night vision, this is an error. Urban environments, even at night, have enough sufficient ambient light to maintain mesopic adaptation. Even a full moon in a rural road can maintain a mesopic state.

## E. Higher Visual Pathways

The rods and cones are only the first stage of the visual pathway. They connect to a network of other retinal neurons, the most important being ganglion cells whose axons form the optic nerve that transmits information to higher visual areas. The point where the optic nerve leaves the retina has no photoreceptors and forms a blind spot in the visual field.

The first stop in the primary visual pathway[13] is the "lateral geniculate nucleus," where input from the two eyes combines. The next is "primary visual cortex"[14] where basic processing occurs. From there, information divides into dorsal (location, attention) and ventral (perception, identification) pathways. The ventral system further divides into an array of area specialized for various attributes, such as color.

A detailed account of this physiology is beyond the scope of this book and is probably unnecessary, anyway. However, there is one physiological distinction worth remembering. The primary pathway contains two streams: "transient" or "magnocellular" and "sustained" or "parvocellular," which have different functions.[15] Much like rods and cones, they are complementary and permit vision over a much larger range of conditions than would be possible with a single processing stream.

The transient/parvocellular pathway is specialized for detecting motion and temporal change. It likely directs orienting and attention. The other pathway ("sustained" or "parvocellular") is less sensitive to motion and flicker but is specialized for detecting fine shape and color. This division of labor is necessary because it is impossible to have a single pathway specialized for both temporal and spatial vision (Green, 1984).

This distinction also has an important practical consequence. Objects will be more conspicuous if they activate the transient/parvocellular pathway, which responds best to large size and to rapid flicker and motion. Small stationary or slow-moving objects stimulate only the parvocellular system and will be less conspicuous. Very roughly speaking, the systems divide at about 10 minarc in size and at about 4 Hz in time. I shall return to this topic in Chapter 4 when discussing conspicuity.

## 3.4 Brightness

The two fundamental sensations are brightness[16] and color. Brightness is the perceived quantity of light while color is the perceived quality. Both are psychological experiences manufactured by the mind/brain. They do not exist in the real world and are not fixed properties of objects. No meter can directly measure them, and they are only very roughly related to measurable physical properties of light, intensity and wavelength. Still, an astonishing number of sources will say that illumination or luminance is a measure of brightness or refer to red light rather than light that appears red. These are errors at the most fundamental level of visual science; they confound psychological and physical variables.

The ensuing discussion very briefly covers some basics about brightness and color. I begin with brightness, which is a function of several variables, most notably relative reflectance and adaptation level.

### A. Brightness and Reflectance

Most people would say that an object appears bright because it sends more light to the eye. For example, a sheet of white paper is brighter than a lump of coal because it reflects more quanta. This explanation sounds plausible, but it is incorrect and simply represents naïve realism at work.

Earlier, I gave an explanation of how surfaces produce varying brightness by reflecting varying amounts of incident light. A simple experiment demonstrates that this story is simplistic and that light intensity and brightness are not closely related. I could take a light meter and measure the luminance of white paper inside a building and then measure the luminance of coal in the sunlight. The readings would show that the coal actually had the higher luminance. According to the naïve view, the coal should appear brighter, but obviously it does not.

A more sophisticated reader might suggest that brightness is not due to amount of light *per se* but rather to the reflectance of the object. That is, white paper is brighter because it has higher reflectance. This too sounds plausible, but it is also incorrect, or at least incomplete.

Brightness is really related to *relative* reflectance. The eye judges brightness by comparing the amount of light coming from the object and from the background. Further, the eye apparently assumes that the amount of incident light on the object and background is the same, so that it is judging the relative reflectance of the object and background. Paper only appears white because it has higher reflectance than the backgrounds against which it is commonly viewed. Similarly, coal only appears black because it reflects a smaller percentage of light than any other common background. I routinely demonstrate this point to perception students with the "Gelb effect,"[17] which turns a piece of black paper to white by putting it on a background of essentially 0 reflectance.

The dependence of brightness on relative reflectance further demonstrates a fundamental visual principle. The eye does not care much about absolute properties of light; the eye is a difference detector that is tuned to see *relationships* between objects and backgrounds. If real estate is "location, location, location" then vision is "contrast, contrast, contrast."

This may seem an unnecessarily complicated way of designing a visual system, but it has great advantages. By operating on relative rather than absolute light levels, the eye keeps the perceptual world stable and maintains visual constancy across large changes in illumination level and wavelength. Suppose that brightness really were a function of object luminance. The same piece of paper that appears white in daylight would fade to gray and to black as the light level fell. The same piece of coal that looked black in a dimly lit mine would turn white when taken out in the daylight. Instead, the eye maintains "brightness constancy," and white objects are always white and black objects are always black. "Color constancy" works on the same principle, so objects keep their apparent color over wide ranges in illumination. The eye "discounts the illuminant," a principle that Edwin Land used to create Retinex color theory and to develop Polaroid cameras. However, both brightness and color constancy have limits and fail under extreme conditions.

## B. Adaptation

Brightness also changes with adaptation level. After walking into a theater during the day, everything appears dark. Eventually the scene becomes brighter as the eye adapts. Conversely, walking out of the theater creates a temporary period of dazzling brightness. Here is more proof that brightness is a function of the eye and not of the light and that brightness is not a property of objects in the world.

Adaptive changes fall into four categories. The eye can dark adapt, going from bright to dark environment, or light adapt, going from dark to light. Each of these comes in two varieties, slow and transient phase. Most people are familiar with the slower phase process that takes about 45 minutes to complete but there is also a transient adaptation effect that has a time scale of seconds.

The classic slow phase dark adaptation curve (Figure 3.13) shows the sensitivity change as a function of time. For a viewer using photopic vision when the lights dim, the initial dark adaptation occurs within the cones, by convergence and loss of inhibition. As time proceeds, the cone sensitivity increases but then levels off. Simultaneously, the rods also adapt. At higher light levels they are inactive and cones determine threshold. As time passes, they increase sensitivity. Roughly 5–7 minutes into adaptation, the photopic and scotopic curves cross (the "rod-cone break") and the scotopic system becomes the more sensitive. Depending on the initial adaptation level, complete dark adaptation may require 30–45 minutes.

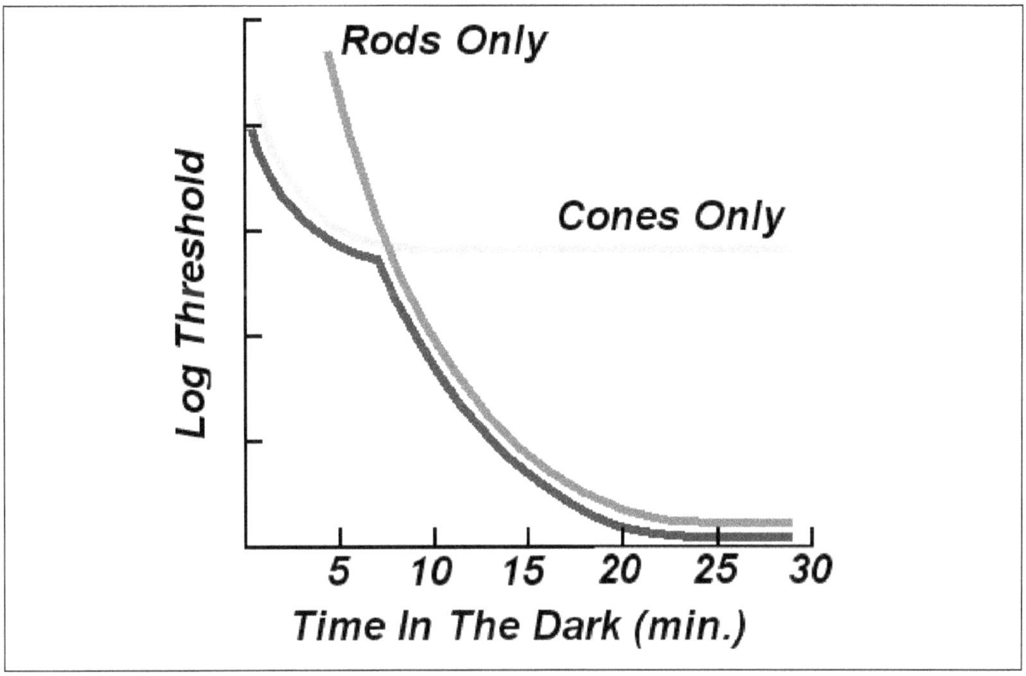


***Figure 3.13*** *Rod and cone activity during dark adaptation.*

However, this classic rod-cone break only occurs for large targets that stimulate both foveal cones and peripheral rods. Small, foveal targets do not activate rods, so their dark adaptation curve follows the cone curve and exhibits no break.

It is overly simplistic, however, to say that the eye has shifted from cones to rods. Rods set the lower sensitivity bound, but the cones do not simply disappear and still respond to a sufficiently intense light. For example, a driver on a very dark rural road may be in scotopic mode, but he could still see the color of a sufficiently intense warning light. If a viewer sees color, he must be using cones. If a viewer sees a blue light at night, you can be sure that the choice of blue was suboptimal for visibility since cones prefer yellow-green.

The exact timing of dark adaptation depends on two factors: 1) the higher the initial adaptation level, the longer the adaptation time and 2) the lower the final resting light level, the longer the adaptation time. For example, a person going into a movie theater during the day will take longer to adapt than a person going into the theater at night.

Viewers also experience light adaptation[18] effects when switching from dark to light. It is not a mirror image of dark adaptation. The viewer sees a dazzling glare, which temporarily impairs vision. Light adaptation also occurs far more rapidly. The major effect is complete in about a minute, although complete adaptation may take a few minutes longer. Again, the size and duration of the effect is greater when the light transition is greater.

Transient light and dark adaptation occur much faster than the normal adaptation effects described above. The classic source paper is Crawford (1947), research designed to determine how light adaptation would affect a driver entering and leaving a tunnel. Crawford investigated this problem by measuring sensitivity to an object presented at various times just before, during and after a "conditioning flash." There was a large spike in thresholds for a brief period when a light went on (light adaptation). More surprising, there was also a large spike in threshold just after the light went off (dark adaptation). These sharp, brief threshold spikes are called "transient adaptation" (also called "Crawford masking" or "masking by light," e.g., Green, 1984) because they occur on a short time scale, lasting about a second or less in most cases. The effect means that light flashes, such as from a gun, strobe or oncoming car headlamp, will impair vision greatly for a brief period.

## 3.5 Color

Color vision is an especially large and complex topic. No brief overview can even scratch the surface without being highly selective and without oversimplifying many issues. Even defining color is a surprisingly difficult problem. The naïve answer is that color is a property of light. We see red light, blue light, green light, etc. In reality, color is a psychological experience that the mind/brain creates in response to light. A meter can measure a light's spectral composition, but no meter can measure color, and there is no such thing as a "red light," etc. There is only light which appears red. More precisely, there is only light which creates an experience that you or I label with the designation "red." Of course, I have no idea if your experience of "red" is the same as mine.

In visual science, color's precise definition is "any aspect of visual sensation that is not due to spatial or temporal attributes of a light." This definition isn't very satisfying or informative because it says what color is not rather than what it is. That's the problem—color simply is. Color is a cognitively impenetrable experience, and people cannot easily introspect and describe it in words.

Experts more commonly avoid a direct definition and simply say that color is a psychological experience having three components: quality, quantity and purity (Figure 3.14). **See Appendix A (on supplementary CD-ROM to this book) for Figures 3.14 through 3.17.**

- Hue: quality of the experience (red, green, blue, etc.).
- Brightness: quantity of the experience or the amount of light apparently coming from an object.
- Saturation: purity of the experience.

Two lights which differ on one or more of these three dimensions differ in color. Note that brightness is technically a dimension of color. Even experts, however, will often use the term "color" to refer to variations in hue and saturation alone and treat brightness as a different sensation. In common use, however, the term "color," may refer to any combination of hue, saturation and brightness. For example, "color" may mean differences in hue (red vs. green), saturation (red vs. pink) or brightness (electric blue vs. navy blue).

### A. Basic Color Vision

#### 1. Wavelength and Color

Many sources will present a table resembling Table 3.3, purporting to show the relationship between color and wavelength. As already explained, however, color is neither a property of light nor of objects. Moreover, the relationship between color and wavelength is very rough. So what is Table 3.3 really saying?

The answer lies in the distinction between aperture color and surface color. Aperture color is about lights and wavelength. It is typically studied by scientists examining the most basic aspects of color vision in the laboratory. Test subjects view small, disembodied patches of color, which they usually see on a black backdrop with no other images visible. Aperture color is good for isolating the effects of wavelength on color vision, and for explaining color matching and discrimination, the effect of light on cones, etc. However, aperture color is an artificial world that is purposely designed to eliminate many of the variables operating in the normal world. It is not very good at predicting color appearance under more natural viewing conditions.

The world of surface color reflects normal viewing conditions. Viewers normally see colors as belonging to the surface of objects that are embedded in a scene and viewed under illumination. Here, backgrounds, adaptation, expectation, and other objects in a scene can greatly influence perceived color. In fact, colors which appear identical in aperture viewing can look very different in a real scene and colors which look different in aperture color can appear identical in a real scene. In surface color, wavelength becomes only one of many factors which determine apparent color.

Table 3.3 describes the relationship between color and wavelength, but only for aperture color. The statement, "A light of 555 nm will appear green" is from the aperture color viewpoint. In surface color, it may or may not be true. Unfortunately for beginners, most experts confusingly move back between the two worlds when speaking of color. It is easier to describe color vision from a more simplistic aperture vantage point. Below, for example, I make many aperture color statements. It may cause confusion, but it is unavoidable.

**Table 3.3**
**Colors with "corresponding" wavelength ranges**

| Color | Wavelength (nm.) |
|---|---|
| Red | 780–622 |
| Orange | 622–597 |
| Yellow | 597–577 |
| Green | 577–492 |
| Blue | 492–455 |
| Violet | 455–390 |

## 2. Classification of Lights and Colors

Visual scientists classify lights and colors in many different ways. Each classification reveals a distinction that is important for understanding color vision.

- Chromatic vs. Achromatic colors: Achromatic colors are the neutrals, black, grays, whites. Chromatic colors are everything else, reds, greens, blues, etc. Despite common belief, black is not the absence of light. Like red, green or blue, it is a visual experience created by the mind/brain. I've already mentioned that people in the dark see eigenlicht, an intrinsic gray. You need contrast to see black.
- Spectral vs. extraspectral hues: Spectral hues, red, green, blue, orange, etc., exist in the visible spectrum. Extraspectral hues do not exist in the spectrum and can only be created by combining spectral lights. For example, there is no spectral purple, but it can be created by mixing red and blue.
- Unique (unitary) vs. Non-unique (intermediary) hues: Most light appears as a combination of colors. For example, if you look closely at red on a computer monitor, there is a trace of yellow in the red color. A unique hue is one which has no trace of another color—a

red which contains neither yellow nor blue. Similarly, there is a unique yellow, unique green and unique blue. This concept is important when considering color categories.

- Warm and cool colors: Red, orange and yellow are warm colors while green, blue and violet are cold. Warm colors produce the feeling of closeness while cool colors produce the feeling of distance. Most notably, objects that are blue-violet and fuzzy appear much further than they actually are ("aerial perspective").
- Complementary and noncomplementary hues: complementary hues are those which lie directly opposite each other in color space and which have the highest chromatic contrast. When mixed, they cancel each other's chromaticity and produce neutral color, i.e., green-magenta and blue-yellow/orange. Noncomplementary colors are everything else.
- Monochromatic and polychromatic lights: Monochromatic lights consist of a single wavelength and have the highest saturation. Polychromatic lights have more than one wavelength and usually have reduced saturation. A light's constituent wavelengths are its "spectral composition."
- Metamaric and nonmetamaric lights: Metamers are lights that are physically different (have different spectral compositions) but appear identical.

### 3. Basic Color Theory

Color is a private experience, so the only way to study color is to ask viewers to perform some task requiring color judgments. No single theory is able to explain the results of all tasks. There are two principle color theories: Trichromatic Theory and Opponent Process Theory. They were competitors for many years, but color scientists now consider them complementary. Each is good at explaining some aspects of color vision but relatively poor at explaining others. Together, the two theories can account for the way people perform most color vision tasks. The most common tasks include:

- Discrimination: determining whether two colors are the same or different;
- Matching: combining two or more colors to match a sample color;
- Mixing: combining two or more colors to create a specific color appearance;
- Naming: using a word to designate a color. E.g., "The apple is red";
- Memory: identifying or naming a previously seen color.

Trichromatic Theory can explain color discrimination, matching and mixing and can further predict errors made by color deficient viewers. The theory originated in 1801 when Thomas Young found that viewers could match any color sample with three primaries.[19] Young concluded that the eye must have three different color elements. These elements have proven to be the three cone types, each containing a different photopigment. The cone types are normally classified as "long wavelength," (L) "middle wavelength" (M) and "short wavelength" (S). Experts often use short-hand and refer to them as red, green and blue cones.

When light strikes the eye, photopigment molecules may absorb quanta and release energy. The L, M and S cones each contain a pigment with a different spectral sensitivity. Once the photopigment absorbs a quantum, however, it cannot know the wavelength of the incident light (the "principle of univariance"). As a consequence, lights can contain very different wavelengths yet appear identical. The only requirement is that they activate L, M and S cones in the same ratio. For example, a viewer can match a monochromatic yellow light with red and green lights. Yellow stimulates both L and M cones, so a red light that stimulates R cones and green light that stimulates M cones can add to match yellow.[20] This dependence of color vision on cone activation rather than directly on wavelength is crucial for understanding many color phenomena.

Trichromatic theory is very good at explaining tasks that require judgments of same-different, but it doesn't do so well explaining tasks involving color appearance—whether lights were red, blue, pink, etc. Trichromatic Theory has other obvious problems. For example, it posits three basic elements. Perceptually, however, there are four primaries: red, green, blue and yellow. Further, the cancellation of color possible with complementary hues suggests that some color pairs are somehow antagonistic.

Opponent Process Theory (Figure 3.15) better explains color appearance and the malleability of color under different circumstances. It posits three color elements, but they consist of color pairs, red-green (R-G), blue-yellow (B-Y) and black-white (B-W). The B-Y and R-G units are the "chromatic system," which provides the four perceptual primaries. The B-W pair is the "achromatic system"—without hue. Actually, B-W is something of a misnomer, since it is the brightness channel.

Opponent-Process Theory says that color appearance depends on the amount and polarity of each process. The red and green are antagonists, so you can only see one or the other at a time. Obviously, you could have red and green lights next to each other. It's just that they cannot appear at exactly the same spatial location at exactly the same time. For example, Opponent Process correctly predicts there can be no such color as reddish green or greenish red. It isn't even possible to imagine such a color. In contrast, purple is red + blue. Opponent Process Theory explains purple by saying that the red part of the R-G pair and blue part of the B-Y pair dominate. The B-W channel determines the purple's brightness. Opponent process theory also readily explains cancellation by complementary colors, the existence of four perceptual primaries, and color aftereffects.

Although long-time antagonists, the discovery of opponent-process neurons in the visual system has created a color vision model that sees the two theories as complementary. As shown in Figure 3.15, the three cone classes send their outputs to the three opponent processes. The R-G system pits red against green cones while the B-Y system adds red and green cones to form Y and blue cones to form antagonistic B. The B-W brightness system adds input from all three cones types, although blue cones are relatively unimportant in brightness perception. When trying to make sense of color vision, it helps to keep this figure in mind.

### 4. The Number of Discriminable Colors

Color discrimination is that task of determining whether two colors are the same or different. The number of discriminable colors varies greatly with circumstances. The most precise method for testing color discrimination places colors side-by-side and asks a viewer whether they appear the same or different. The number of colors is too great for an actual experiment, so several scientists have made rough estimates based on theory. The most common estimate (e.g., Halsey and Chapanis, 1951) is that under optimal conditions, there are about one million distinguishable colors—combinations of hue, saturation and brightness.[21] Other estimates, however, put the number as high as 7 million. In less optimized conditions, the number of discriminable colors is far smaller. As spatial or temporal separation increases, discrimination declines very rapidly. Color discrimination is also worse for small sizes and for brief viewing times. Lastly, discrimination is not uniform through the color gamut; viewers discriminate shades of yellow far better than shades of blue.

### 5. The Number of Color Categories

Viewers have a strong tendency to perceptually group similar colors into a limited number of categories. When people perceive and remember colors, they tend to rely heavily on these color categories. They name colors by category and readily confuse colors within a category.

One fundamental property of color is that it is both continuous and categorical. It is continuous because one color gradually shades into another. For example, going from yellow to green, there is pure yellow, various shades of green-yellow, then yellowish green and then finally green. Color is also categorical because yellow and green are different percepts at some fundamental level. Berlin and Kay (1969) performed a very famous study which concluded that color has eleven basic color categories that fall into three classes:

- achromatic: black, gray, white
- primary: red, green, blue, yellow
- secondary: brown, orange, purple, pink

Later work suggests that Berlin and Kay is not the last word on color categories, but there is little doubt that viewers classify the many thousands of discriminable colors onto a much smaller number of color categories. As a result, *the same category name will apply to the many distinguishable colors.* For example, a viewer may term both a fire engine and a person's hair as "red," although they are highly distinct colors. Knowing the category is often good enough. People use color in a very contextual way. By saying that a person's hair is "red," the person is making a statement about color relative to all other colors possible for the domain—in this case hair color. "Red" has a different meaning in this context than in a fire-engine context.

Categories are not uniform. Some colors are "good" examples of a category while others lie at the border of categories and have uncertain membership. Imagine starting with unique green, a green so perfect that it apparently contains no trace of yellow or of blue. It would be the best member of the green category. Now start gradually adding more and more blue. The color turns bluish-green and becomes a poorer member of the category green. At some point, the color crosses a mental border and becomes greenish-blue. It ceases to be a member of the green category and becomes blue, albeit a poor blue category member.

These categories are important in both color appearance and in witness descriptions of color. People are good at distinguishing between color categories, but readily confuse colors within a category. People typically remember colors as closer to the central category than they actually were. If the person categorizes the blue-green color as green, then he will later remember the color as greener than it actually was. If categorized as blue, he will remember it as bluer than it actually was. In many cases, people are not recalling an actual color but rather the color category name by which they coded the perception. Lastly, bright colors are usually remembered as brighter than the original and dark colors as darker.

Color memory is also a function of expectation, belief and social convention. For example, people call both apples and tomatoes red. If you go to a supermarket, however, it is clear that tomatoes are frequently more orange. Color memory is even more malleable when the object in question does not have a strong innate connection to color. For example, people might readily remember that a lemon was yellow because lemons are always yellow. However, they are more likely to err in remembering the color of a shirt or vehicle because there is no strong innate connection between object and color. Of course, if the person remembered that the vehicle were a sports car, then there might be a bias toward remembering a bright color. Overall, color memory is astoundingly poor. We seldom notice this because color memory errors usually have little consequence.

### 6. Color Appearance Changes Readily

Like brightness, people mistakenly believe that color is a fixed property of an object. Also like brightness, perceived color is dependent on background as well as object. Both shade and even category membership can change drastically with viewing conditions, most notably with lighting and background.

Figure 3.16 demonstrates the effects of background on color perception. It may be difficult to believe, but the "H" in the left and right pictures is exactly the same color. The color appears uniform on the neutral background. However, the color of the left and right halves changes dramatically when shown in different colored backgrounds. The color category of the "H" is also uncertain. In the right panel, I would call the left part of the "H" orange and the right "red," although someone else might call the right part "purple or even "brown." Factors such as object size, lighting conditions and adaptation (what was viewed before looking at the colors) also affect judgments.

This effect, "simultaneous color contrast," induces an approximately complementary color; a red background makes objects appear greener, a blue background makes them appear yellower, etc. Marketers frequently use simultaneous contrast to enhance appeal. Meat looks redder when viewed on a leafy green background. Paint sales have long manipulated color appearance by altering background. My father was the manager of a paint department and intuitively understood simultaneous color contrast. If a customer said that a yellow paint sample was too orangey, he would retire to the back and pretend to get a new sample. Instead, he returned with the same sample, but held it on a red sheet of paper. The red paper induced green into the sample. The induced green cancelled some of the red in the sample and made it appear less orange.

Other factors affecting color appearance include wavelength of the incident light, size, brightness and any degree of color deficiency (see below). In addition, high color contrast, e.g., red on a green background (a red stop sign against a hedge), also makes larger objects more detectable and conspicuous.

Apparent color also changes with other factors. "Chromatic adaptation" resembles light adaptation, except that it is wavelength specific. That is, looking at a strong red light will selectively adapt the L cones. Subsequently viewed yellow light will then appear greener. Color also varies with drastic changes in wavelength of the incident light. The eye's ability to discount the illuminant and to maintain color constancy has limits. Under very narrowband lights, colors can change drastically. Lastly, small objects lose color. If it is bright, it will become whiter and less saturated. If it is dark, it will become black.

## B. Color Deficiency

The term "colorblindness" is too vague to be useful, and the common statement that 8 percent of the population is colorblind is grossly misleading. There are seven types of color deficiency due to cone abnormalities. The term "color deficient" is more accurate because only a minority of people with abnormal color vision are literally colorblind. In addition, the elderly see colors differently, but their abnormal color vision is not due to cone activity and is not color deficiency in the usual sense of the term.

People with normal color vision are called "trichromats" because they require three primaries to match any arbitrary sample. The trichromatic eye has the full complement of three cone types,

S, M and L, each responding to a limited wavelength range. The major color deficiencies are abnormalities in the way cone pigment is distributed in the cones. In all, there are three deficit major classes.

### 1. Anomalous Trichromats

A subpopulation of trichromats requires three primaries to match a sample but makes abnormal matches. They use more of one primary than would be expected by a viewer with normal color vision. This suggests that they have all three cone types but that one cone type is rarer, has a reduced amount of pigment, or has a pigment tuned to an unusual wavelength.

These "anomalous trichromats" fall into three groups, based on the primary that they overuse:[22] Deuteranomalous (weak green) viewers far outnumber the protoanomalous (weak red), and male anomalous trichromats far outnumber females. People with a congenitally weak "blue" cone response, anomalous tritanopes, are virtually nonexistent. However, some eye diseases, such as glaucoma, attack blue cones creating "acquired" tritananomalous conditions. The loss of blue cones is usually greatest in the periphery.

Anomalous trichromats can see all hue categories, so they are not literally colorblind. However, they may have difficulty in discriminating colors which a normal would easily distinguish. Anomalous trichromats, however, are a very heterogeneous group. Some are only slightly different from normal trichromats, some are almost dichromats and others fall somewhere in between.

### 2. Dichromats

Dichromats, as the name implies, require only two primaries to match any sample. These people are presumably missing one of the three cones types. Unlike color anomalous individuals, dichromats are true color blinds in the sense that there are some hues which they cannot perceive. Protanopes and deuteranopes are red-green color blind and see only yellows and blues. The tritanope is analogously blue-yellow color blind. However, there is evidence that at least some dichromats use rods to compensate for the lack of the third cone. Studies find that these dichromats can often discriminate colors along the red-green axis of color space. Note that only 2 percent of males, 1 percent of the population, are dichromats and truly color blind in any sense.

### 3. Monochromats

Monochromats can match any light with a single primary. They generally have no cones and make all matches using rods. With only a single receptor type, they can have no color vision and are truly color blind because they distinguish only brightness levels. They are very rare, 1 in 10,000,000.

### 4. Color Deficient Perception

Some theorists like to say things such as "a color which would look deep red to a normal, looks dark yellow or brown to a dichromat." This is speaking very loosely because it assumes a commonality of perceptual experience. Of course, it is impossible to know what color blind, or any other, people experience. Given this caveat, here is common lore.

Dichromats have a spectral point called the "neutral point" where the light appears achromatic. The point is about the same for both common classes, 495 nm for protanopes and 500 nm for deuteranopes, wavelengths which would appear slightly bluish green to a normal (assuming aperture color).

All wavelengths below the neutral point appear blue while those at longer wavelengths appear yellow. In the first few nm away from the neutral point, apparent saturation increases rapidly, so dichromats can easily discriminate colors. The rest of the blues then appear similar as do the rest of the yellows and only discrimination of brightness is possible. Toward very long wavelengths, protanopes experience lights as becoming darker, so a very red apple, as already mentioned, might look dark yellow or brown. Likewise, tritanopes would have trouble discriminating hues located above or below their neutral points. Purples would also be difficult to discriminate since they differ in their blue content.

Dichromatic confusions are readily explainable by cone activation. Protanopes, who are missing "red" cones, cannot distinguish lights which produce equal ratios of activity in the "green" and "blue" cones. Similarly, a deuteranope, who is missing "green" cones, cannot distinguish lights that produce identical activity ratio between the "red" and "blue" cones. Experts often plot these as "confusion lines" on a CIE diagram, a standard method of depicting color space.

**Table 3.4**
**Percentage of anomalous trichromats, by cone type**

| Type | Cone | Male% | Female% |
|---|---|---|---|
| Protoanomalous | "red" | 1.0 | .02 |
| Deuteranomalous | "green" | 4.9 | .38 |
| Tritananomalous | "blue" | ~0 | ~0 |

**Table 3.5**
**Percentage of dichromats, by cone type**

| Type | Cone | Male% | Female% |
|---|---|---|---|
| protanope | "red" | 1.0 | .02 |
| deuteranope | "green" | 1.1 | .01 |
| tritanope | "blue" | .002 | .002 |

In addition to cone abnormalities, optical yellowing produces color perception changes in the elderly. Since yellow filters blue, older people see blue as relatively darker and yellow as relatively brighter. Colors, however, do not shift much. That is, oranges may look more yellow, but the effect is surprisingly small, probably due to color constancy.

### 5. Color Deficiency and Road Accidents

Some believe that color deficiency increases road accident risk. In Australia, for example, protanopes cannot hold a commercial driver's license because of their presumed difficulty in seeing red traffic signals. Research apparently supports this policy, as color deficient reaction time to red and yellow lights are as much as 85 percent longer than for color normals (Atchison, Pedersen, Dain and Wood, 2003). Protans are also less able to detect red signals (Cole, 2002), which have only about 25 percent of the luminous intensity as for normals (Dain and King-Smith, 1981).

Given these considerations, you might expect to find intersections littered with twisted wrecks once driven by color deficients. Research on accidents rates, however, does not fully support this prediction. One study (Verreist, Neubauer, Marre, and Uvijls, 1980) found increased risk for a small sample of color deficients while another (Norman, 1960) found no effect. The discrepancy between the proven performance loss of color deficients and accident rates has two possible explanations. One is that color-deficients avoid nighttime driving, which would lower their accident rates (Tagarelli, Piro, Tagarelli, Lantieri, Risso and Olivieri, 2004). Alternately, color-deficient drivers may take advantage of "redundancy coding." Traffic signals are red, yellow and green, but they are also coded top, middle and bottom. That is, they are redundantly coded by color and by position. A person with weak color vision could simply use the position cue rather than the color. Road signing is frequently coded redundantly. Stop signs are redundantly coded with color and shape, for example. Redundant codes, however, can also cause accidents if the two perceptual dimensions are not perfectly correlated. People come to rely on the more salient one to the exclusion of others. This can cause a person to choose the wrong dimension for decision-making (Green, 2004).

### C. Color and Brightness

Color can play an important role in visibility. The eye detects contrast borders created by differences in object and background. Like brightness, color differences produce detectable contrast. However, color contrast is less significant for detection in central vision. Compared to brightness contrast, it has only about 15–20 percent of the acuity and only about 20 percent of the perceived contrast (Kaiser, Herzberg and Boynton, 1971) obtained with achromatic intensity. Viewers cannot see color contrast when the object is very small. For example, NTSC TV signals don't even bother coding color for fine details because they are invisible and just consume bandwidth.

The situation changes in the peripheral vision. Brightness contrast declines with eccentricity. There, only large objects are detectable, so color contrast may become more visible. For example, look at a traffic sign in peripheral vision. At some point, the sign color is more detectable than the print on the sign.

Even in central vision, however, brightness and color are connected. Different colors have different brightnesses and produce different brightness contrasts. The highest possible brightness contrast occurs with the achromatic black and white, the darkest and brightest colors. Chromatic colors are neither as bright as white nor as dark as black, so they create lower brightness and lower contrast.

Figure 3.11 depicts the photopic luminosity curve which shows how brightness varies with wavelength. Colors in the middle of the spectrum (yellow and green) are bright while colors at the extremes of the spectrum (blue, violet and red) are dim. From the luminosity curve, it is obvious that yellow on blue (or blue on yellow) would create high brightness contrast and promote visibility. On the other hand, yellow on green or blue on red would have small brightness differences and hence poor visibility.

While color may play a secondary role in visibility, it can be important in promoting conspicuity. Yellow-Black is an especially good color combination because it promotes both good visibility and good conspicuity. Conspicuity is a separate, although slightly related, visual function from visibility. I take up this topic in the next chapter.

## 3.6 Conclusion

This chapter has been a mini-perception course that discussed some basic principles in physics, physiology and psychology. An expert needs knowledge of all three fields because vision is the physiological conversion of light energy into psychological experience. Vision, however, is more than the sum of these parts. Expertise in vision begins by shedding naïve realism and by accepting that the world we see is a creation by the mind/brain. The physical world of meter measurements is a highly chaotic and unstable place. Our visual systems have evolved some magic that takes the flat 2-D image of this world and give us a three-dimensional perceptual world. This a world of stability and constancy. It is a world where white objects remain white even in dim light and do not fade to gray. It is a world where objects maintain their size despite variation in distance and visual angle. It is a world where upside down retinal images appears right side up. And it is a world where the series of snapshots created by eye movements is sewn together without any noticeable discontinuity. Yes, vision is the most complex task that humans perform.

## References


Atchison, D. A., C. A. Pedersen, S. J. Dain, and J. M. Wood. Traffic signal color recognition is a problem for both protan and deutan color-vision deficients. *Human Factors* 2003 Vol. 45 (3), 495-503.

Berlin, B. and P. Kay. 1969. *Basic Color Terms: Their Universality and Evolution.* Berkeley: University Press.

Cole, B. 2002. Protan colour vision deficiency and road accidents. *Clinical & Experimental Optometry: Journal Of The Australian Optometrical Association* 85, 246-53.

Cole, B. L. and J. D. Maddocks. 1997. Defective colour vision is a risk factor in driving In: Cavonius, C. R. (ed.) Colour Vision Deficiencies XIII Kluwer Academic.

Crawford, B. 1947. Visual adaptation in relation to brief conditioning stimuli, *Proceedings of the Royal Society of London* B 134, 283-302.

Dain, S. and P. King-Smith. 1981. Visual thresholds for dichromats and normals: The importance of postreceptoral processes. Vision research 21, 573-580.

Gibson, J. J. 1958. Visually controlled locomotion and visual orientation in animals. *British Journal of Psychology* 49, 182-194.

Green, M. 1984. Masking by Light and the Sustained-Transient Dichotomy. *Perception and Psychophysics* 34, 617–635.

Green, M. 2004. Nursing Error and Human Nature, *Journal of Nursing Law*, 9, 37-44.

Green, M. 2006. Is the moth-effect real? *Accident Reconstruction* May/June, 18-19.

Halsey, R. and A. Chapanis. 1951. On the number of absolutely identifiable spectral hues. *Journal of the Optical Society of America*, 41, 1057-1058.

Hecht, S., S. Schlaer, and M. H. Pirenne. 1942. Energy, quanta and vision. *Journal of the Optical Society of America*, 38, 196-208.

Kaiser, P., P. Herzberg, and R. Boynton. 1971. Chromatic border distinctiveness and its relation to saturation. *Vision Research* 11, 953-968.

Leibowitz, H. and F. Owens. 1977. Nighttime driving accidents and selective visual degradation, Science 197, 422-424.

Li, Z. 2006. *An Empirical Investigation of the Effect of Manipulating Optical Looming Cues On Braking Behaviour In A Simulated Automobile Driving Task.* Ph.D. dissertation, University of Toronto.

Norman, L. 1960. Medical aspects of road safety. Lancet 1, 1039-1094.

Sivak, M., M. Flannagan, T. Miyokawa, and E. Traube. 1999. Color identification in the visual periphery: consequences for color coding of vehicle signals. University of Michigan Transportation Research Institute.

Tagarelli, A., A. Piro, G. Tagarelli, P. B. Lantieri, D. Risso, and R. Olivieri. 2004. Colour blindness in everyday life and car driving. *Acta Ophthalmologica Scandanavia* 82, 436-442.

Verreist, G., O. Neubauer, Marre, and M. Uvijls. 1980. New investigations into the relationship between congenital colour vision defects and road safety. In Verreist, G. (ed.) Colour Vision Deficiencies. Bristol: Adam hilger, 331-342.

Westlake, W. 2001. Is a one eyed racing driver safe to compete? Formula one (eye) or two? *British Journal of Ophthalmology* 85, 619-624.

## Endnotes

1. In special cases, the variable "wave number" replaces wavelength.

2. Light also has two other properties, polarization and coherence, that are less relevant for vision.

3. One meter is 3.28 feet. A square foot is 1 × 1 = 1. A square meter is 3.28 feet × 3.28 feet = 10.76 feet.

4. For simplification, I'll ignore internal reflection.

5. Hermann Helmholtz, the first visual expert, also invented the ophthalmoscope.

6. Brightness changes by themselves can change color, e.g., the Bezold-Brucke effect, where colors become yellower and bluer at higher intensities.

7. If you lose your reading glasses, just poke a hole in paper with a pencil and look through the tiny aperture. You can see clearly at any distance.

8. Area is equal to pi × $r^2$. For a diameter of 8, the radius is 4 and the area is pi × 16. For a diameter of 2, the radius is 1 and the area is pi × 1. This gives the 16:1 ratio.

9. The retina also contains layers of ganglion and bipolar cells. Ganglion cells are particularly important because they receive output of many photoreceptors to form "receptive fields." If this were a straightforward scientific text, there would be extensive discussion of receptive fields, one key concept in visual science.

10. Note that the arrow's image inverts when focused on the retina. We actually see the world upside down. This seems a major philosophical problem for some people, but it isn't. The sense of upright and inverted, like everything, is a perceptual creation of our brains. Up and down are arbitrary conventions.

11. No, this is not a mistake. The cornea extends slightly in front of the eye, so the visual field is bigger than 180°, and viewers can image objects slightly behind.

12. The fixed relationship between wavelength and color is an aperture vision concept and is not generally true.

13. This is only the primary pathway. There are many other secondary paths.

14. Primary visual cortex is located in the occipital lobe at the very back of the head where it is protected. In contrast, the "thinking" area for higher cognitive areas is located in the exposed frontal cortex. Evolution has apparently concluded that seeing is more important than thinking.

15. Strictly speaking the transient/sustained and magnocellular/parvocelluar distinctions are not equivalent. Their predictions for psychophysics and perception, however, are the same.

16. Many people confuse brightness with "lightness," which is a different concept. For simplicity here, I ignore the distinction. For a fuller explanation, see "The Basic Color & Design SB FAQ" http://visualexpert.com/FAQ/Part1/cfaqPart1.html.

17. It's a simple trick. Hang the piece of black paper in a doorway and turn the lights off. Then project a light that just illuminates the paper. There is essentially no background, so the black paper becomes silvery white.

18. Some people use the term "light adaptation" to mean "dark adaptation," i.e., any adaptation change due to light. This can obviously become very confusing.

19. This isn't literally true. Sometimes the viewer must use negative light—add color to the sample to make a match.

20. This is a gross oversimplification, however, because the spectral sensitivities of L and M cones overlap greatly.

21. This has always sounded suspiciously like one of those "magic numbers" described in the previous chapter.

22. The listed percentages of color deficient classes in the population varies somewhat from source to source.

# Chapter 4

# Attention and Conspicuity

Marc Green, Ph.D.

*"Only those items which I notice shape my mind—without selective interest, experience is utter chaos."*

—William James (1890)

***Synopsis***



## 4.1 Introduction

There is more to vision than meets the eye. Sensing is only the first step in seeing because cognitive processes must interpret the sensations and bring them into consciousness. Attention mediates this transition by filtering sensory input and by allowing the viewer to focus mental resources on the relevant information. The viewer is effectively blind to the lost information.

A viewer's failure to see can be due to either psychophysics (visibility) or cognition (attention). If sensory analysis reveals that information was below detection threshold, then there is no need to proceed further. If the information exceeded sensory threshold, then the next step is to examine cognitive explanations.

Psychophysics and visibility factors play a role in some failures to see, but more accidents probably have their origins in cognitive processes. The usual culprit is attention. Selective attention filters away most of the information bombarding the senses. It may seem that evolution has taken a wrong turn by allowing people to filter away potentially important information. As the quote by William James suggests, however, filtering is necessary. The senses receive far more input than the brain can process. If we did not have attention, it would be impossible to focus on a task or set of tasks. Everything would have equal importance, and we would not be able to separate the relevant from the irrelevant. We simply could not function.

Attention, however, is an imperfect mechanism. Sometimes there is more relevant information than a person can handle, so the filter must make a choice. Sometimes the attentional filter chooses incorrectly, blocking critical information. This does not necessarily mean that the person acted badly, even if hindsight makes it appear that way. The important questions are whether the person 1) made a conscious decision that led to lower attentional capacity and 2) allocated attention in a reasonable manner given the context and what was possible at the time. The answer to these questions lies in the normal operation of attention.

This chapter discusses the filtering process as well as conspicuity and the variables that determine attentional capture. It also discusses the role of attentional failure in road, medical and other accidents. Lastly, it highlights the importance of understanding attention and inattention in blame assignment.

## 4.2 Laws Of Attention

There is much to say about attention, but a relatively short list of basic properties captures the key elements. (Adapted from Reason and Mycielska, 1982):

- *Attention is a limited resource.* People have a fixed amount that must be allocated according to need. Attention is like a bucket of water. People draw upon it as needed but every dipper full, and every teaspoon full, leaves less for other purposes. However, the total attentional capacity can vary in different circumstances. First, each sense modality has some separate attentional resource. An auditory task interferes less with a visual task than would a second visual task. It is much easier to monitor the road ahead while talking on a cell phone than when looking at the navigation system. However, attention to one modality can impair attention to another (Sinnett, Costa, and Soto-Faraco, 2006). Second, overall capacity varies. People who are fatigued, bored, older or under the influence of alcohol or drugs may exhibit low arousal and have less attentional capacity. Even "normal" people suffer from the "vigilance decrement," the lowering of attentional capacity after 20–30 minutes of monitoring the same situation, and from the effects of circadian rhythms, 24 hour cycles of biological arousal. Conversely, humans have evolved some adaptive mechanisms to simulate an expanded attentional capacity. Examples include automaticity, heuristics and biases (see below).
- *Attention is selective.* People attend to some things to the exclusion of others. Attention is always divided, however, as people are invariably performing multiple tasks simultaneously. The manner in which people voluntarily and involuntarily allocate attention is the main focus of this chapter.

- *Consciousness requires attention.* Viewers only consciously perceive an object that has engaged attention. This is true as a general statement, but always remember that attention is not an all-or-none phenomenon. It is possible to be aware at different levels. In the cocktail party, for example, people may be dimly aware of the vague background buzz or may not be aware at all.
- *Attention does not require consciousness.* People are only partially conscious of their attentional allocation. Some attention may be allocated without awareness to a task that is using capacity. This occurs in behaviors that have become automatic through overlearning, the practicing of a skill well past the point of mastery. Much of normal driving occurs automatically and outside of awareness. Drivers have little or no conscious awareness of steering, using the foot pedals, etc. This can go so far as the common phenomenon of "highway hypnosis," where a motorist travels for an extended period with no conscious awareness or memory of having driven the car.
- *All tasks require some degree of attention, although the required amount may be small.* It is not surprising that operating the in-car navigation device or reading a billboard can distract a driver and cause an accident. Research (Stutts, Reinfurt, Staplin, and Rodgman, 2001) suggests that a task as apparently undemanding as listening to the radio can also cause distraction and increase accident likelihood. Even the most seemingly effortless tasks, like walking, consume and require attention. For example, distraction is a major cause of accidents during stair descent (Templer, 1992).
- *All tasks have an optimal level of attention.* Novel and complex tasks may suffer from lack of attention while highly overlearned and automatic tasks may suffer from too much attention. Every golfer, for example, knows the ploy of disrupting an opponent by commenting, "That's a wonderful pause you have at the top of your back swing." For more analysis on this topic, see the authoritative source, *The Theory and Practice of Gamesmanship: The Art of Winning Games Without Actually Cheating*, Potter (1948).

Lastly, while most models treat attention as a filter, it also operates as a mask. Attentional tuning is not just deciding what to focus upon but is also sometimes deciding what to block out. Most people have had the experience of trying to block out noise, music, etc. while attempting to concentrate on a visual or mental task. For example, novice drivers frequently prefer to avoid conversation while driving. Both physiological and behavioral evidence (e.g., Green and Odom, 1991) further suggest that even within vision, people organize the percepts by actively suppressing unwanted information.

## 4.3 Types of Attention

Selective attention can operate in different ways depending on two factors: source of control and filtering criteria. Source of control refers to the mechanism that directs attention toward an object. James (1890) distinguished between "active" (endogenous) control, originating from higher mental processes, and "passive" (exogenous) control, automatic attraction by something in the visual field. For example, a driver can decide to scan the road looking for a specific house number (endogenous) or simply have attention attracted by an overhead flashing signal light (exogenous). Both endogenous and exogenous attention are under control of attention set, a preexisting bias toward noticing specific information.

The filtering criteria determine which sensory information is fully processed. Viewers may filter based on two criteria: spatial location and object properties. In spatial attention, the viewer tunes attention to different areas of 3-D space. For example, road signs are on the right side of the road, so drivers will be less likely to notice signs located on the left side. Spatial tuning can also be near or far.

Viewers also control spatial attention through gaze direction; they can only notice objects located in the field of view. Even then, a viewer will most likely notice targets falling on or near the sightline. Viewers prefer having the attended target's image fall on the fovea for maximum visual sharpness. Peripheral objects trigger saccades that bring the object to the fovea. Knowing where to look is just as important as knowing what to look for. In general, people look where they expect to find relevant information.

Object attention directs focus toward items with a specific attribute. One set of attributes is sensory qualities such as shape, color, movement, etc. A second set of attributes is properties such as meaning and task relevance. In Chapter 1, I described, for example, how my attention was drawn to the letter string "Pitt" in newspapers.

The viewer's spatial and object tuning at a given moment form an "attentional set", which is a function of expectations and goals. As explained in Chapter 1, people are not blank slates. The viewer enters the situation and senses cues that evoke schemata telling him what to expect and what to do. The viewer's goals then determine the spatial and object tuning of attention. Lastly, general search strategies, such as "cue generalization," may affect filter tuning.

## A. Source of Control

Control sources are either endogenous or exogenous. Originally, endogenous control equated to a conscious direction of attention and exogenous control equated to an involuntary, externally driven direction of attention (Posner, 1980). Trick, Enns, Mills, and Vavrik (2004), however, suggest further subdividing control strategies by the automatic-controlled distinction (Schneider and Schiffrin, 1977). Behavior in automatic mode seems to occur with little or no attention or conscious direction. In contrast, controlled behavior requires effort and occurs under top-down supervision.

**Table 4.1**
**Types of attentional control**

| | **Endogenous** | **Exogenous** |
|---|---|---|
| Automatic | Habit | Reflexive |
| Controlled | Deliberation | Exploration |

Table 4.1 shows the four resulting control strategies. Deliberate and reflexive are the two extremes. In deliberate control, viewers consciously choose to scan a scene. Top-down influences both initiate and control the eyes. A driver looking for a parking place, for example, looks along the street in order to find an opening. Another example occurs when a driver looks at the cell-phone keypad in order to punch in a number. In contrast, reflexive mode prevails when attention seems automatically drawn to an object in the visual field. Neither the initiation nor the direction of the attentional control is voluntary. A driver might notice the oil light on the instrument panel illuminate or the flashing light of an emergency vehicle by the roadside. It will be clear later, however, that even apparent reflexive control depends on attentional set.

"Habit" is a form of control that is endogenous, yet not conscious or deliberate. In highly practiced tasks, the viewer controls attention top-down but has no awareness. For example, drivers reaching a curve unconsciously direct attention to the key steering cue, the curb tangent point (Land and Lee, 1994; Land, 2006). The driver has initiated the eye movement based on expectation of the needed information rather than by reflexive attraction. On the other hand, the control is not deliberate because he made no conscious decision. One reason that novice drivers have more accidents is presumably that they have not developed the proper habits and have not learned to reduce the attentional load by making driving largely automatic. On the other hand, driving habits can cause accidents when people are not in their normal situation—as any North American who has driven in Britain can tell you.

"Exploration" occurs when a viewer with spare attentional capacity samples the scene and when goals and expectations are not well-defined. The internal control initiates the eye movement and stops only when an object of interest falls on the fovea. Unlike deliberation, the viewer is not consciously moving the eyes. Unlike reflexive eye movements, the eyes do not feel drawn to the target. Unlike habit, the control is not based on highly overlearned experiences. However the line between habit and exploration is blurred. Even in exploration, drivers do not search randomly. Drivers are often in exploratory mode unless their attention is required for a specific task, such as car following or inspecting an intersection for traffic controls.

Of the four control strategies, only deliberation is completely under conscious control. Automatic behaviors (habit and reflexive control) occur without conscious volition. Exploration is also mostly controlled by unconscious processes. As a result, telling drivers to "look where you are going" and "to pay attention" will usually have little effect. Such instructions have a significant effect only on conscious driver behaviors.

## B. Filtering Criteria

The viewer has two ways to select sensory input. Spatial filtering restricts input to a limited area in three-dimensional space. Object filtering restricts input based on object properties, which further subdivide into sensory and cognitive.

### 1. Spatial Attention

A popular spatial metaphor conceptualizes attention as a spotlight that emanates from the eyes and "illuminates" part of the visual field where we look. The spotlight is centered at the fovea, surrounds the line-of-sight and generally moves with the eyes. Viewers can notice information falling within the beam while anything outside goes unnoticed. In order to inspect the entire scene, the viewer must move the fovea in a series of saccades, jumping the beam from place to place.

Like a real beam, intensity is stronger in the center and weaker in the periphery, so viewers notice objects along the sightline more readily. Moreover, the beam can be wide and weak or narrow and intense. Since attention is a fixed resource, a wide and weak beam allows the viewer to attend large parts of the visual field without close scrutiny or concentration. The beam is unitary and may not be subdivided into pieces, so a viewer can attend only one area of space at a time. To attend a larger area, the viewer must widen, and weaken, the beam.

When the beam is very narrow and intense, then the probability of noticing objects in the peripheral field becomes small. Obviously, intense narrowing of attention is a recipe for disaster when unexpected events occur. In one classic airline crash, the crew of a jumbo jet became so engrossed in fixating a blinking light on the instrument panel that they failed to notice what was happening in their peripheral vision—the ground approaching through the windshield.

The spotlight metaphor is incomplete because spatial attention is three-dimensional. That is, people direct attention not just up, down, left, right but also near and far. If two objects align at different distances near the sightline, the viewer might not see both. In one common accident scenario, for example, a driver pulls out while looking down the road for oncoming traffic and is completely oblivious to the pedestrian walking right in front of his car.

The three-dimensional nature of attention complicates application of any technology that requires people to look through a transparent surface, such as an automobile windshield or "heads up displays" (HUD). HUD's are presumed beneficial because the driver need not take the eyes off the road in order to view the instrument panel. If a driver focuses on the HUD, however, he may fail to notice objects on the roadway ahead. In aviation, where HUD's are more common, there are cases of a pilot viewing his HUD and failing to see a jumbo jet crossing right in front of him. The Mandelbaum effect and vergence error may be part of the problem. However, much of the impairment is purely cognitive. As Figure 4.1 demonstrates, it is very difficult to read the numbers while looking down the road or vice versa. The problem cannot lie in accommodation or vergence.

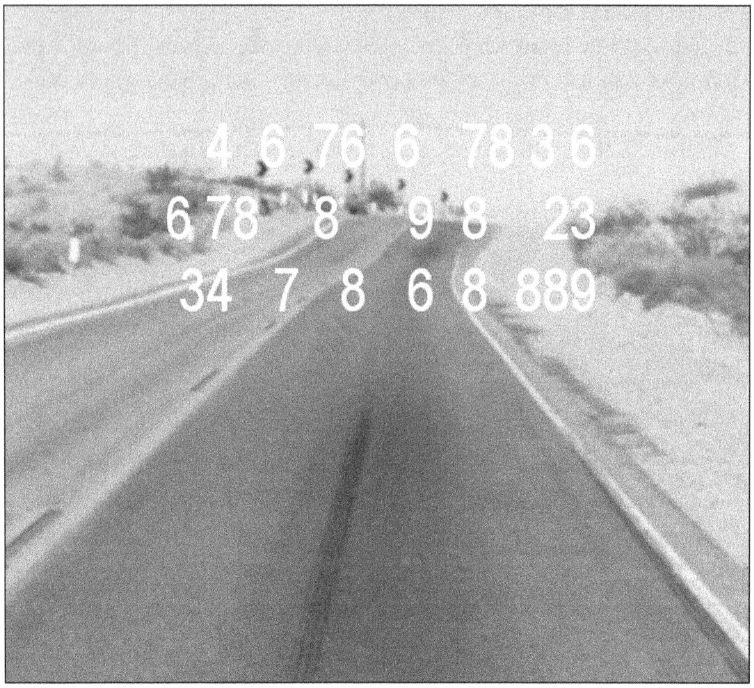


***Figure 4.1*** *Simultaneous focusing near and far is difficult.*

**2. Object Attention**

Viewers can also tune attention based on sensory or semantic object properties. Sensory properties include color, shape, motion, etc. Semantic properties include meaning and task relevancy. Sometimes, high familiarity is sufficient.

Recall from Figure 1.3 in Chapter 1 that sensory information must pass the attentional filter in order to reach short-term memory and to be perceived. The figure had two attentional filters, one labeled "early selection" and the other "late selection." Most older models of attention posited early selection, placing the filter between sensory and short-term memory. If this were the actual location, then attentional filtering could only be based on sensory properties because the input has not yet been interpreted. The late selection placement puts filtering after the input has been at least partly interpreted. Attention can then select input based on meaning as well as on sensory characteristics. The cocktail party phenomenon demonstrates that the early selection model is untenable because attention allows your name through the filter.

## 4.4 Conspicuity

Conspicuity is the likelihood that a viewer will notice and perceive visible information. Even experts often confuse the concepts of visibility and conspicuity, but they are distinctly different mental processes and should be treated separately. Visibility refers only to whether the viewer can detect a sensation. It does not specify whether the viewer will likely notice the sensation.

Visibility and conspicuity overlap somewhat. All things being equal, a viewer will more likely notice objects of greater visibility. However, viewers *usually* fail to notice objects even if they are highly visible. I can't make this point too strongly: *there is much more to seeing than the mere registration of a visible retinal image*. The best way to conceptualize visibility is that once an object reaches detection threshold, contrast is just one of many factors that determines conspicuity. (If it is below threshold, of course, the viewer cannot notice the object.)

The classic view of conspicuity usually assumes an "early detection" model of information processing, stressing sensory factors and largely ignoring attentional set. This is obvious from most conspicuity definitions, which follow Engel (1976): "the ability of an object to attract attention and to be easily located" or "the property of an object that makes it stand out from the background." Hills (1980) even mistakenly incorporates visibility into the definition by saying, "It can be defined partly as the extent to which the object is above the just visible limit." Such definitions are misleading because they imply that 1) the "early selection" model holds and filtering is purely sensory, 2) conspicuity is an object property and 3) viewer variables are irrelevant. All three assumptions are incorrect.

Early selection and tuning for sensory quality occurs frequently in everyday life, although such tuning is perhaps most evident when it fails. When I go to the mall with my wife, for example, we sometimes separate to do errands and agree to meet later. One time, I walked right by her without noticing. The explanation lay in the coat that she was wearing that day. I had remembered the wrong color. I had unconsciously thought that she was wearing her pink coat, but she was wearing her blue one. My attentional filter was tuned to notice pink, so blue was meaningless for the current task and did not register. This tuning to pink was unconscious and made without deliberate direction. I was not aware of it until after I had realized my mistake.

It might be asked why I didn't simply look for my wife's face, a much more accurate strategy. The answer is highly instructive in understanding how attention works. Face perception is effortful and requires detection of high-resolution detail. In facial attention, I would have to foveate all likely candidates to find her. Color perception is much easier because it requires only detection of a low-resolution blob, so there is little effort. Color perception does not require foveal vision, so my attentional spotlight was widened to include the low-resolution periphery. I could then search most of the visual world in a single glance and did not need to move my eyes from face to face. Lastly, color forms distinct categories that are readily discriminable. It differs from quantitative continua, such as brightness, where there are no clear categorical boundaries.

I had performed "cue generalization," a phenomenon where a viewer switches from a cue requiring effort and close inspection to one that is easy and effortless. This most often happens when attention switches from reading, a highly effortful, focal task and high-resolution cognitive process, to simpler color, shape or location. *People invariably attempt to reduce mental effort and complexity in familiar tasks*. People seldom attempt to optimize outcomes in any task. Rather, they "satisfice," meaning that they settle on a heuristic strategy which is good enough to achieve reasonable, if not perfect, results.

A recent study (Most and Astur, 2007) experimentally demonstrates the mall phenomenon and suggests that it applies on the roadway. Viewers operating a driving simulator looked for either a blue or yellow sign at an intersection. A blue or yellow motorcycle suddenly veered into their paths. When the motorcycle color matched the sign color, accident probability was far lower than when the sign and motorcycle had different colors. Like the mall visit shows, people can set attention for some object attribute and will be less likely to notice objects that do not match.

However, the ability of even sensory variables to attract attention depends on attentional set. Triesch, Ballard, Hayhoe, and Sullivan (2003) provide a particularly compelling demonstration of attentional set in an article aptly entitled, *What You See Is What You Need.* Viewers performed different tasks manipulating objects in a virtual world while the experimenters monitored their eye movements. The objects could suddenly change size or color during the task. The viewers failed to notice the change unless it was task relevant. If the task did not require color judgments, for example, the subjects didn't notice color changes. Most amazingly, the attentional failure could occur even when the viewers were looking directly at the object during the change.

Further, there have been some notable failures of introspectively eye-catching conspicuity aids. British authorities found that drivers frequently rear-ended stopped police cars. To reduce accidents, authorities painted the rear of police cars with presumably conspicuous patterns such as the one shown Figure 4.2.[1] Despite the bright new pattern, accident rates actually increased. **See Appendix A (on supplementary CD-ROM to this book) for Figure 4.2.**

Others have adopted the "late selection" model, which assumes that the factors responsible for conspicuity can be either sensory or cognitive. Cole and Hughes (1984) concluded that "conspicuity cannot be regarded simply as an object attribute; whether an object attracts attention must be strongly dependent on the state of attention of the observer." In short, conspicuity is a joint function of both viewer and object. The next section discusses both sensory and cognitive conspicuity.

## A. Sensory Conspicuity

Some sensory signals seemingly have an innate ability to attract attention, even without attentional tuning. A note of caution is necessary, however, because introspection is not a reliable method for determining attentional attractors. Many people, for example, assume that motion and flicker are highly conspicuous. Everyone has had the experience of having attention drawn to a flashing target seen out the corner of the eye. This observation is a biased sample, however, because viewers are *unaware* of the times that they failed to see movement. We know about the times a particular cue works but not about the times that it fails. Moreover, introspection does not reveal whether there are specific conditions that determine a cue's conspicuity. The only way to evaluate conspicuity is through research.

Not surprisingly, sensory conspicuity has been the focus of intense study because of the obvious safety implications. Unfortunately, most "conspicuity" studies have limited application. First, most measured visibility rather than conspicuity. To the extent that attentional attraction increases with visibility, these studies are relevant to conspicuity. However, visibility is not conspicuity. Second, conspicuity is important to draw viewer attention to the unexpected, but virtually all studies employed subjects who were seeking expected, specific objects. They are relevant to search conspicuity but not necessarily to attention conspicuity. Schieber, Larsen, Jurgensen, Werner, and Heimstra (2001) nicely illustrate the conspicuity difference between active search and just noticing the unexpected. The study tested the ability of fluorescent colored objects to attract viewer attention. When viewers expected to see a fluorescent color, it greatly improved search time. When the fluorescent color was unexpected, however, it had little effect. This research used an "inattentional blindness" paradigm, which can test for conspicuity of truly unexpected objects. It is a major advance in conspicuity research and is described more fully later.

There are many potential sensory conspicuity cues, including size and contrast, but the two most commonly used cues are color and "temporal transients," flicker and motion. Each is a very large topic on its own, so the following is just a very brief overview.

### 1. Color

Color is a popular means of enhancing conspicuity. Road signs, product warnings, worker clothing, advertising, etc. all rely heavily on color to attract viewer attention. As with everything perceptual, however, color conspicuity depends on context and attentional set.

Several factors contribute to color conspicuity. Some colors apparently have a better innate ability to attract attention, but even these colors are ineffective without color contrast. As in brightness contrast, a color will not be highly visible or conspicuous unless it stands out from the background. A red STOP sign against green trees, for example, has very high contrast since red-green are complementary colors. A green sign against the same trees will be less conspicuous even at the same brightness contrast. Cluttered backgrounds and scotopic light levels also decrease color conspicuity. Lastly, color conspicuity depends on viewing factors such as object size and visual field location.

For many years, safety experts had errantly assumed that red is the most conspicuous color. Red is only a modestly bright color during the day and a dark color at night. In dim light, the viewer is adapted to mesopic or scotopic vision, where rods are predominating in the peripheral field. Since rods don't see long wavelengths ("red") well, a viewer would not readily notice a red object.[2]

Recent research in commercial and safety fields has converged on the same conclusion: the most conspicuous colors are yellow and yellow-green, sometimes called "lime yellow." Here are just a few examples:

- Lime yellow fire engines have fewer accidents than red ones. The lime yellow engines are more conspicuous to motorists. (Solomon and King, 1995)
- Lime yellow is the most detectable color for forestry worker clothing. (Isler, Kirk, Bradford, and Parker, 1997)
- A large-scale study asked over 12,000 people to rate the "visibility" of a mannequin dressed in a variety of colors. Yellow was the clear winner. It also was chosen by 97 percent of 119 color deficient observers. (Minnesota Department of Transportation)

Lime yellow is likely so conspicuous because it is the brightest chromatic color.[3] As Figure 3.12 showed, it is the color at the peak of the luminous efficiency curve. Yellow is also relatively rare, so it contrasts well with backgrounds, especially a complementary blue sky. Moreover, warm colors, such as yellow, appear nearer. When the eye first views a scene, the initial "figure-ground segregation" decomposes the image into foreground objects that are worth inspection and attention and background that is irrelevant. Areas perceived as closer are more likely seen as foreground and attended. Since warm colors, such as yellow, are seen as nearer, they are more readily perceived as foreground and more likely to attract attention. Lastly, some have even suggested that yellow is an attention-grabber because of its associations with sun, happiness, etc., but research support is weak.

Yellow combined with black creates the perfect mix of good visibility and good conspicuity. Visibility requires high brightness contrast. White is the brightest color, so it provides optimal brightness contrast with a dark color such as black. However, white is achromatic and has little innate conspicuity. Yellow is the brightest chromatic color, so it gives good brightness contrast with black while simultaneously providing chromatic conspicuity.[4]

Orange, however, might be more conspicuous if the object is small and/or viewed in the periphery.[5] Under these conditions, colors lose their apparent saturation. Yellow is a low saturation color to start, so it fades toward a less conspicuous white. Similarly, objects viewed in the far periphery begin to lose chromaticity and yellow fades. Orange is generally the second best choice for color conspicuity. It is also more saturated and holds its chromaticity and conspicuity better and is likely a better choice under these adverse conditions. Amber, although a bit darker, is another alternative since it mixes yellow and orange. In sum, the most conspicuous color changes somewhat with circumstances.

Lastly, the myth that blue is the most conspicuous (or most visible) color at night persists despite clear psychophysical evidence to the contrary. Chapter 3 discussed the common misunderstanding of the "Purkinje Shift," the change in spectral sensitivity as light level falls from photopic (cones) to scotopic (rods) levels. Optimal sensitivity changes to shorter wavelengths in scotopic vision, but this is sometimes incorrectly stated as saying that optimal sensitivity changes to blue. In reality, it shifts *toward* blue, and is better described as a change from yellow-green to blue-green. Even this is a misstatement because a viewer cannot see hue in scotopic vision. The correct statement is: "the most visible scotopic wavelength would appear blue-green if seen in photopic vision."

Applicability of the Purkinje shift is further debatable because ambient roadway lighting is not scotopic but rather mesopic. Cones still operate and predominate in foveal vision. The rod periphery likes shorter wavelengths, but cones are still active down to very low mesopic levels. The whole issue is probably irrelevant anyway, since warning lights are usually bright enough to activate cones regardless of ambient light level. If a viewer sees a light, such as the gumball machine on an emergency vehicle, and can judge that it is blue, then he is obviously using cone vision. A green, yellow, amber and possibly orange light would have been brighter and more conspicuous than blue.

Red is about the only color possibly less visible/conspicuous than blue at night, and even then only in scotopic vision or in low mesopic vision with peripheral stimulation. However, absolute intensity is still an important factor. Warning lights create colors by using housing covers that selectively transmit different amounts of various wavelengths. By one account (Tijerina, 2003), yellow housings transmit 60 percent of the light, red housings 25 percent and blue housings only 15 percent. As a result, blue warning lights will have the lowest intensity. I say more about the effectiveness of blue flashing lights below.

### 2. Flicker and Motion

Temporal transients, flicker and motion, are the other main conspicuity cue. Many warnings, railroad crossing lights, overhead flashing beacons, and emergency vehicles use flashing lights on the presumption that they create a significant increase in conspicuity.

The early research literature supported the notion that temporal change is highly conspicuous (Yantis and Jonides, 1990) and not easily suppressed during active search, but others (e.g., Mack and Rock, 1998; Pashler and Harris, 2001) found that motion and flicker are not magically powerful attention grabbers. Moreover, the conspicuity of temporal transients likely depends on several variables:

*Modulation amplitude.* The magnitude of change between on and off phases is "modulation" or "temporal contrast." All things being equal, lights having greater modulation are more detectable and likely more conspicuous. Modulation amplitude is a function of several factors, including age of the bulb and dirt on the housing. It can also be affected by modulation rate and sunlight reflecting off the housing. Lastly, it is not necessarily desirable to make the flashes as high amplitude and bright as possible. Very intense flashes may produce glare or mask pedestrians standing near the light.

*Modulation rate.* The number of flashes per second is "modulation rate" or "flicker rate" and is expressed in units of Hertz (Hz) or cycles per second (cps). The temporal modulation transfer function (TMTF) is the psychophysical relationship between sinusoidal modulation rate and detection threshold. The TMTF peaks at middle frequencies, meaning that there is an optimal frequency and flash duration. The optimal rate/duration will appear brighter than shorter or longer flashes and will even appear brighter than a steady light of the same luminance (the "Broca Sulzer effect," [e.g., Green and Corwin, 1978]). In laboratory studies, the optimal modulation rate is about 3–5 Hz, although it varies with intensity. In the world-at-large, several factors push the optimal rate lower. First, lower intensity light produces lower optimal flicker rate because of greater temporal summation. Second, some lights have bulbs that require heating and cooling to turn on and off. If flicker rate is too high, the bulbs don't completely cool down and turn off before the next cycle, reducing modulation amplitude. Despite their lower visibility and conspicuity, however, faster modulation rates may have advantages because they can signal greater urgency (ICE Ergonomics, 2002) and presumably induce faster response.

*Modulation waveform.* The same flicker rate can be presented in a variety of waveforms (e.g., sharp vs. gradual on and offsets) and different duty-cycles (the relative amount of time on and off in the cycle). If total energy remains constant, short flashes will almost certainly be more conspicuous. If the off-phase is too long, however, the viewer may miss the flash. In addition, flicker is more conspicuous with a sharp on/offset. Strobe lights, with their sharp on/offsets will likely be slightly more conspicuous than rotating beacons, which produce a more gradual light on and offset. However, strobe lights are likely more difficult to spatially localize.

*Beam pattern.* Signal lamps send out a directional beam pattern that is strongest in the center and weaker with distance from the primary axis. Some beams are broad while others are narrow, requiring the viewer's eye to be precisely located for high conspicuity. Railroad crossing signals are a good example. They use batteries, so lamp power consumption is low, and bulbs have less intensity than normal traffic signals. The low-wattage bulb is then covered with a red glass roundel, which filters and reduces light by as much as 80–90 percent. In order to compensate for the weak output, reflectors mounted behind the bulbs concentrate light into a narrow beam of about 30° width. However, most energy is concentrated near the primary axis. One study (Andrews, 1987) found that intensity could drop by more than half at only 3° off axis—about twice the width of the thumb seen at arm's distance. To ensure that drivers' eyes intersect the beam, railroad signal flashers aim down the roadway several hundred feet in advance of the crossing. In one accident, the driver turned off a side road 75 feet before the crossing, so his eye never intersected the beam. Moreover, he was in a truck, putting his eye above beam height.

*Color.* I have already discussed the misconception that blue is the most visible color at night and have noted that any light perceived as colored must be stimulating cones. Of course, blue may be a good choice for other reasons. People readily attach meanings to each of the other primary colors: green means "go" and "safety," red means "stop, and yellow means "caution." Among primaries, only blue does not start with connotations which might cause viewer misinterpretation. Moreover, blue signals are likely less common than those of other primaries. Lastly, Berkhout (1979) concluded that drivers perceive blue as advancing and red as receding. Blue signals presumably increase safety because drivers perceive them as approaching. However, Tijerina (2003) noted that Berkhout's results did not clearly support the advancing blue hypothesis. Moreover, Berkhout was careful to note that his results were limited. He made all measurements with a completely black background containing no other objects to act as reference points. Berkhout (1979) also found that direct judgments of speed and direction were superior for single red over blue lights. Further, Berkhout (1979), and most similar research, is difficult to evaluate because they confound brightness, hue and saturation and because they provide no photometric or colorimetric data—chromatic color is less important with low saturation. It is quite possible, for example, that his results were due to brightness differences in the lights and not to chromatic differences. Lastly, blue lights might actually be the worst choice because aerial perspective makes blue objects appear the farthest away. At this point, the issue is far from settled.

*Sunlight.* Flickering lights will be less conspicuous in daylight. Sunlight reflects off the lamp housing and masks the flickering by lowering apparent modulation (Green, 2002). The worst situation occurs when the light originates from behind the viewer, and direct rays reflect off of the light housing to produce glare. Hoods, such as those on railroad signals prevent direct glare from sunlight, but are less effective at lower sun altitudes. By one reckoning (Cox, 1971), a railroad signal covered by a 9-inch hood would have the most glare when the sun is within 15° of the horizon and behind the driver.

*Background.* I once read a deposition of a highway patrol officer who said that he always turned on his steady headlamps rather than flashers at an accident scene—steady lights stood out much better against the emergency vehicle lights that were flickering all around him. He knew what research has shown: a flickering light is less conspicuous when the background also contains flicker (e.g., Nikolic, Orr, and Sarter, 2001). Crawford (1963), for example, found faster reaction time to flashing lights, but only when the background contained steady lights. The presence of even one flashing light in the background reversed the relationship, and viewers responded faster to a steady light. Like everything else, flickering lights are highly detectable only when they contrast with the background. In one accident, for example, a driver approached an intersection with a flashing yellow overhead signal. With this in the visual field, he missed the rotating amber beacon of unexpected construction machinery stopped on the road. The situation would have been worse in the rain, where raindrops on the windshield and the wipers create more temporal transients. Even in dry weather, a driver's own movement through the visual field causes motion and changes in the optic flow field, so there is almost always some motion in the scene.

*Size.* Large flickering lights have much better conspicuity than small ones. The visual system has two mechanisms for detecting motion/flicker: the "sustained" and "transient"[6] systems (e.g., Green,

1984). Objects activating the transient system are more effective in drawing attention. The transient system likes objects at least 10–15 minarc in size. Any flickering light below this size will not be as effective for conspicuity and orienting. For example, a 6-inch diameter flickering light seen at 300 feet would subtend only 5.7 minarc at the eye and fail to strongly activate the transient system. The needed size likely increases in peripheral vision due to cortical magnification (e.g., Rovamo, Virsu, and Näsänen, 1978). See Chapter 14.

*Visual Field Location.* Many falsely believe that the visual periphery is specialized for seeing motion and flicker. Research clearly shows that the opposite is true. Makela, Rovamo and Whitaker (1994), for example, found that peripheral flicker thresholds were almost invariably much higher. A 3 Hz flashing target, for example, was about 8–15 times more detectable in the fovea than at 20° in the periphery. The foveal advantage grew when light size decreased. Green (1983) further found that motion detection falls rapidly and perceived motion stops if the object is only a few degrees from the sightline.

*Number of "Stations."* Many conspicuity aids attempt to create apparent motion by using alternately flickering lights. Railroad signals, for example, use two "stations," that is, two lights that flicker on and off alternately and appear to move back and forth.[7] The use of two stations is a poor method for creating motion because 1) it requires almost perfect timing of the lights, as expressed in Korte's (1915) Three Laws of Motion and 2) the lights frequently appear as two independent flickering lights rather than as one moving light. Three stations far more reliably produce motion (Green, 1989). Lastly, motion that goes from the periphery toward the central field is slightly more effective and produces faster reaction times than motion that starts in the center and goes toward the periphery.

### 3. Humans

Recent evident suggests that the human form has an innate ability to draw attention. Several studies (e.g., Ro, Russell, and N. Lavie, 2001) show that the human face has strong innate conspicuity. Another study's (Downing, Bray, Rogers, and Childs, 2004) conclusion is stated in its title *Bodies Capture Attention When Nothing Is Expected.* Other evidence from biological motion, discussed in Chapter 15, further suggests that humans are innately recognizable as well as innately conspicuous.

## B. Cognitive Conspicuity

The variables that create cognitive conspicuity are more difficult to define. People may learn that some information has general relevance, promoting its conspicuity. The cocktail party, for example, suggests that self-references create conspicuity. I have explained how I am often drawn to words containing the letter string "Pitt." Spammers frequently capitalize on self-reference by sending attention-grabbing emails that use the recipient's name in the subject. For example, my former email address was *vexpert@visualexpert.com*, and I received many spam messages with the subject lines like "Vexpert, your credit has been approved."[8] Lastly, overlearning and high familiarity alone are sometimes sufficient to promote attentional "pop out," at least in deliberate searching (Wang, Cavanagh and Green, 1994).

Meaningfulness can be task dependent and based on highly symbolic reasoning. One day, I went to the nearby mega-hardware store to buy a new BBQ. I got five feet in the door, suddenly looked up at the ceiling and saw the black, round surveillance camera spheres depicted in Figure 4.3. I'd been in that store dozens of times and never previously noticed the spheres. Why did I notice them this time? I entered the store looking to buy a BBQ. A very common type of BBQ is the kettle (Figure 4.3) which closely resembles the black sphere hanging from the ceiling.

The explanation for the attentional control may seem obvious: it was primed for black spheres. However, that can't be the explanation. I had gone to the hardware store to buy a stainless steel gas BBQ, which looks nothing like a round black sphere. The connection was purely semantic. I was looking for a BBQ, so my attention was tuned for any object fitting the concept. Research (Koivisto and Revonsuo 2007) has demonstrated this effect experimentally.

The BBQ example shows attention tuned by a goal. In other cases, viewer attention is tuned by expectation. Information learned through experience does not exist in memory as random, isolated bits. Instead, people create organized knowledge structures called "schemata" and "scripts." Chapter 1 described schemata (Bartlett, 1932) as mental models of an object or environment. Shinoda, Hayhoe, and Shrivastava (2001) showed the power of driving schemata by pitting bottom-up, sensory conspicuity against attentional set created by driver expectation. Viewers drove a virtual world where STOP signs could suddenly appear either at intersections or unexpected midblock locations. Under normal driving, viewers detected almost all the STOP signs located at intersections but only a third of the STOP signs located midblock. Midblock stop signs violate normal driving schemata.

Expectation is a leading cause of accidents. Motorcycle accidents are a case in point. For many years, authorities attributed the high rate of motorcycle accidents to low sensory conspicuity because their small size limited visibility. Safety experts strongly encouraged the use of bright clothing, reflective materials, headlamps, etc. However, accidents still occurred when the motorcycles should, in theory, have been highly visible. Several authors (Hills, 1980; Wulf, Hancock and M. Rahimi. 1989; Hole and Tyrrell, 1995) have concluded that drivers fail to see motorcycles, at least in part, because they are relatively uncommon, unexpected events. Statistics on pedestrian accidents show the same trend; cars hit fewer pedestrians where they are expected—in a crosswalk. Instead, the majority of accidents occur when pedestrians cross at unexpected locations in the middle of a block (See Chapter 15).

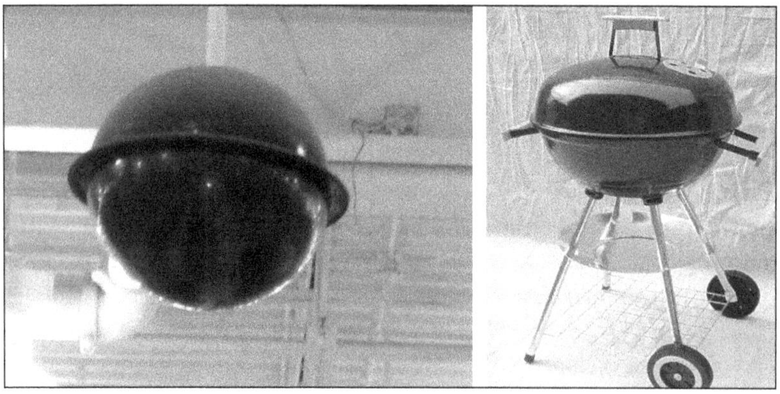

***Figure 4.3*** *Surveillance system (left) and BBQ (right).*

Lastly, attentional set also affects where we look in the first place. If a viewer has learned that a spatial area is not relevant, then he will not look in that direction. A common accident scenario is a driver coming to an intersection intending to turn right. Drivers have learned that the only threat are cars approaching from the left. There is no need to check right, so they do not see pedestrians and bicycles approaching from the right. Conversely, pedestrians may also put themselves in harm's way because of violated expectation. In one accident, a car struck a newly arrived Pakistani student as he stepped off a curb. Pakistan uses the British drive-on-the-left rule, so the student had looked right instead of left as he entered the roadway.[9] The control of eye movements is discussed further in a later section.

## 4.5 What Is Inattention?

The topic of inattention deserves some attention. Failure to notice information frequently leads to accusations of faulty behavior. In the usual case, the plaintiff blames the defendant for "inattention" (or for its alter ego, "improper lookout"). The term "inattention" is loaded because it has two subtly different meanings that laypeople (and some "experts") readily confuse.

First, inattention can be a mere restatement of events. Suppose that a driver fails to see a pedestrian and strikes him with his vehicle. Inevitably, someone will blame the driver for being "inattentive." Here's the logic used to reach this conclusion:

Question: Why did the driver fail to see the pedestrian?
Answer: Because the driver was inattentive.
Question: How do we know that the driver was inattentive?
Answer: Because the driver failed to see the pedestrian.

This is circular reasoning called a tautology in deductive logic. It cannot be refuted because it uses "inattention" as a simple restatement of what happened. We already knew that the driver failed to see the pedestrian. In this sense, the concept of "inattention" is merely a shorthand label and adds nothing to an understanding of events. This is the sense with which I use the term in several articles (e.g., Green, 2002).

Second, "inattention" can be a type of a mental aberration (for lack of a better word). This second meaning refers to blameworthy behavior. The driver not only failed to notice the pedestrian, but he did so because he had some mental aberration that put him outside the realm of reasonable behavior. Here, "inattention" is more than description. It is a cause.

This is a different meaning from the first. People can fail to notice but still be acting reasonably and without mental aberration. That is, if the driver says that he didn't see the pedestrian before hitting him, then he obviously was "inattentive" in the first sense, but not necessarily in the second. Humans have constraints on their behavior. Just as the human body's physical construction limits the weight that can be lifted, the mind's construction limits our ability to attend. Moreover, remember that "inattention" is not an aberration but rather the norm. As frequently stated above, the senses receive far more information than our minds could possibly handle, so we are all inattentive to most of the world at any moment. People need good reason to direct attention to some place or to some object.

The question that an expert must answer is whether the causes of this failure to see ("inattention" in the first sense) can be explained by the normal workings of human vision given the context. If so, the driver acted normally, and the accident was not caused by mental aberration ("inattention" in the second sense). A person can act reasonably and intelligently and still have an accident because the circumstances violate expectation or have some other peculiarity.

Now, suppose that after looking at the facts, I cannot explain the driver's behavior in terms of the normal limitations/predispositions imposed by the human mind. I would conclude that the driver had not acted reasonably. At that point, I might be tempted to say that the driver caused the accident through "inattention." Here, I would be using "inattention" as a shorthand for saying that I cannot find any "normal" reason for the failure to see. Of course, there are some cases in which the inattention's cause is obvious. The driver, for example, may have been dialing a cell phone or looking at the screen of a navigation system. In this case, it is better to simply attribute causation to the misbehavior rather than to invoke inattention.

However, I try to avoid using "attention" in the second sense because it is so easily confused with the first. An attorney might ask me whether the driver was inattentive. If he failed to see the pedestrian, then I would have to answer "yes," at least in the first sense. But I might have concluded that the answer is no in the second. If the attorney wants to lay blame at the driver's feet, he will take the opportunity to use the second interpretation of my answer.

These sentiments are not new. Davis (1959) noted that a typical accident inquiry report

> attributes error to such things as 'lack of attention,' 'inattention,' 'failure of judgment,' or 'fatigue.' Explanations in terms such as these are, however, unsatisfactory because either they do no more than give a name to what has obviously occurred, or they suggest a cause without giving any insight into the way in which it might have operated to produce the accident in question. (p. 24)

Davis is saying that inattention is not an explanation but rather something to be explained. Fortunately, recent scientific research has provided great insight into how attention normally operates and how and why it fails.

## 4.6 Causes Of Attentional "Failure"

### A. Insufficient Capacity

To a first approximation, attention is a fixed pool of mental resource that people draw upon as needed to perform tasks. The pool can become taxed for several reasons. One is a general capacity shrinkage that reduces the total amount of attention available. For example, fatigued drivers have less overall attentional capacity. A second reason is that attention divides among concurrent tasks. The more attention paid to one task, the less available for other. A driver tuning his car radio, for example, has less attention available for noticing pedestrians. When the total attentional demand exceeds the supply, there is insufficient capacity for carrying out all tasks. However, people adapt and learn to perform tasks automatically, so that they consume minimal attention. However, this means that the person is less likely to notice new information should novel factors arise.

#### 1. Total Capacity: Too Much and Too Little

The general pool of attentional resource can change with circumstances. The most common examples include fatigue, alcohol and some drugs. Further, arousal level and attentional capacity level vary in 24-hour cycles called "circadian rhythms." Lastly, attentional capacity generally declines with age.

However, too much capacity can be as big a problem as too little capacity. Different tasks have different optimal attention levels and, somewhat intuitively, too much capacity also promotes accidents. While safety experts have traditionally focused on attentional overload, attentional underload is becoming a more common problem. The major culprits are computers and other technological advances that have automated an increasing number of job functions. In theory, human error should decline because important tasks are transferred from the fallible human to the reliable machine. However, automation often decreases rather than increases safety because humans go into a state of low arousal.

Automation causes the human to switch roles from operating to merely monitoring the equipment. They soon exhibit vigilance decrements and begin to lose attention. In England, for example, there have been major train collisions that occurred when the crew simply failed to see a plainly visible signal. This type of accident occurs so often that it has its own name, SPAD, for Signal Passed At Danger. Accident inquiries usually attribute SPAD's to low arousal caused by boredom, sometimes abetted by fatigue. The infrequency of the signals and the monotonous clickety-clack of the tracks lowered arousal and reduced attention. Similar accidents occur in aviation. A Continental flight barely avoided disaster when it plunged 12,000 feet due to wing icing. Prior to the incident, the captain was sitting with his foot up on the console and failed to notice what was happening. With autopilot, it is often "set it and forget it." Thanks to automation, viewers often become so dependent on technology that they quit using their own senses.

Perceived risk is another important variable in the control of attentional arousal and capacity. People are more likely to notice warnings, for example, when they believe that a situation contains risk. This produces a classic catch-22 because people notice warnings most when they already perceive risk and notice warnings least when the risk is hidden and unanticipated—the very time that the warnings are most needed.

Perceived risk also has a major effect on attention and arousal during driving. When Sweden switched from driving-on-the-left side of the road to driving-on-the-right, authorities predicted a huge increase in accident rate. Instead, accident rates *fell*. Drivers appreciated the increased risk and became extremely attentive and cautious. Unfortunately Swedish drivers adapted within a few years and accident rates returned to previous levels.

The Swedish drivers demonstrated the human tendency to adapt behavior to degree of perceived risk. Wilde (1982) introduced the concept of "risk homeostasis," the notion that people are willing to accept a given level of risk to perform a given task. If perceived risk increases, they act more cautiously to bring the risk level back to the homeostasis point. If some technological innovation reduces perceived risk, then they act less cautiously. Similarly, Gibson and Crooks (1938) suggested that drivers create a "safe field of travel," an area surrounding the car that provides an acceptable level of response time to the sudden appearance of an obstacle. They further suggested that improved technology such as better brakes will have no effect on driving safety. The driver perceives a narrower safe field of travel and allows the same relative margin for error.

Some research supports the risk compensation view. Studies have shown that drivers in vehicles with anti-lock brakes driver faster (e.g., Aschenbrenner and Biehl, 1994) and take more risks (Biehl and Aschenbrenner and Wurm, 1987). Wilde's original notion suggested than any gains in safety will be exactly offset by an increase in risky behavior. While there is little evidence of such a perfect tradeoff, it is true that people often change their behavior in response to lower and higher perceived risk.

Lastly, the safety benefits of automation are often consumed in the name of efficiency. Autopilots should make flying safer by automating functions, leaving pilots free to attend other tasks. The airlines, however, soon started using autopilots as a means for reducing safety margins, such as the time between takeoffs and landings on the same runway. Now, pilots have even less room for error than before automation. Of course, the autopilot also means that the human pilots have one more instrument to monitor and one more piece of equipment that can go wrong.

**2. Automaticity**

Learning can in a sense expand attentional capacity. As already described, developing expectations help by removing the need to waste attention on the irrelevant. People know exactly what they need and where to look. With extended experience, people learn to perform some tasks with minimal attentional drain. For example, an operator learning to use a device must initially attend in order to know where the hand and fingers go, read instruction or warnings, locate switches, etc. With extended practice, the response becomes automatic, meaning that the individual movements become linked in a chain, which once started, seems to run off of its own accord. In the extreme, "muscle memory" (internal "proprioceptive") feedback from each movement guides the next and no external visual information is used. The user seemingly performs the task without attention and can simultaneously carry on other activities. For example, a pianist learning a new piece of music must concentrate on the keys while playing. After extensive practice, the pianist simply runs off the piece automatically and has enough spare attention to simultaneously hold a conversation or watch TV. If stopped in the middle of the chain, the pianist might even have to go back to the beginning and start over. Virtually all skilled performance involves this replacement of conscious, attentive response with automatic behavior.

Automatic behavior is usually beneficial because it circumvents attentional limitations and improves performance, but it can also produce disastrous results. Since attention is no longer required, people then become inattentionally blind to situational changes such as wear, equipment fault and warnings. An American hand surgeon who has treated hundreds of shop-related injuries from power tools confirms that accidents most often occur when an experienced person is performing a highly repetitive task. He further notes that frequently accidents occur when an unexpected event occurs, probably because it interrupts the response chain at a critical point.

Automaticity also helps explain why people frequently fail to see warnings when they learn that they are not task-relevant. Experienced people soon learn the 'contingencies,' the relationship among information, behavior and outcome in a specific situation. When information has no link to the outcome, it is task-irrelevant and often tuned out. The most experienced and skilled practitioners are the most likely to tune out information; they have successfully performed a task repeatedly, have learned the contingencies well and have the most efficient performance. For example, diving team members are the least likely to notice 'no diving' signs (e.g., Goldhaber and deTurck, 1988). They also have the strongest sense of control and perceive the least risk (Green, 2004b).

A similar situation occurs when an operator is highly practiced with one machine, but then must use a similar but slightly different device. The operator continues to rely on muscle memory and fails to notice differences in the new situation because of inattentional blindness. One employee operating a press brake, for example, lost fingers from both hands using a new, unguarded press. His usual machine had a guard, but he failed to notice the difference.

As the Laws of Attention noted, however, all behavior consumes some attention. Land (1999) found that even during automatic behavior, viewers were unconsciously monitoring the environment and engaging in closed-loop behavior to some degree. (Recall that in the cocktail party phenomenon, you must be monitoring the background at some level in order to recognize your name.) Land concluded that the difference between controlled and automatic behavior does not equate to the distinction between open and closed loop behavior. Rather, the distinction is whether the control occurs under conscious supervision.

The dichotomy between controlled and automatic behavior is one of the most central concepts in information processing and attention. It is also an important consideration in forensic analysis. Did the person make a conscious decision (mistake) that led to the accident or was his behavior controlled by automatic processes over which he had no volition? If automatic, were the controlling expectations and goals reasonable?

### 3. Divided Attention and Driver Distraction

Since it is a limited resource, attention to one task may interfere with performance in another. The use of cell phones and other in-car technology has become a focus of study in the field of "dual task performance," the ability of one task to impair the performance of another. Concern about distracted drivers is nothing new. As early as 1906, highway authorities denounced a new technology that would increase accident rates by hypnotizing and distracting drivers from the road. Despite the protests, the new technology, called "windshield wipers," became a standard automobile feature in 1913. A similar concern over driver distraction arose in 1923 when the Springfield Sedan introduced car radios. Some, however, disputed the distracting effects of radios. Nicholas Trott, for example, wrote in the 1930 Farmer's Almanac that "the sound of Rudy Vallee's voice would be less disturbing than backseat conversation." Again, technology triumphed over caution and radios became standard within a few years. Except for some mild concern about CB radios in the '60s, the issue of driver distraction from in-car technology lay dormant for 70 years until the dramatic spread of cell phone-wielding drivers has reawakened fears that new technology will distract drivers and cause an increase in accident rates.

There are two main classes of distracting in-car technology that are becoming commonplace. One "enhances" performance of driving tasks. Some cars already have navigation systems that give routing information and infrared vision systems that provide the ability to see better at night and in fog. Before long, cars will come equipped with "head's up displays" (HUD's) to project the instrument panel onto the windshield. In theory, drivers will no longer have to look down and away from the road to read their speed, gas tank contents, etc. Lastly, car manufacturers are beginning to supply devices that give auditory warnings of everything from impending collision and straying from the lane to driver drowsiness.

The other class of technology involves nondriving tasks. Most focus on telematics, the ability to communicate with the outside world while in the car. Radios and cell phones are the best-known examples, but others include internet access, text messaging, and wireless fax. Increased sophistication and reduced cost of wireless technology is a principle factor driving telematics, but social factors are also important The growth of cities and skyrocketing of house prices has driven workers into the distant suburbs where they face longer commutes on increasingly congested roads. Telematics affords a means to turn unproductive commuting time into productive work. The car becomes a portable branch office.

Even this list of potential in-car technologies is merely the skin on the pudding. Several companies are already marketing systems that turn the car into a virtual computer network with the ability to install "plug and play" devices from third party vendors. The number of potential in-car devices will then be limitless and will likely include functions that are beyond current imagination. Judging by the operation of the computer industry, many will be developed by small companies with neither the resources nor interest for proper human factors testing or for assessing the potential for driver distraction. Authorities in the future will have little ability to control the scope and the amount of distraction caused by in-car electronics.

The assessment of risks posed by new in-car technology has become a cottage industry, so even a brief discussion of the research would fill several volumes. Suffice to say, most studies conclude that cell phones and other in-car technology impair driver performance and cause accidents. The level of risk, however, is still unclear and fundamental issues, such as whether hands-free sets are safer, are still unresolved.

Unfortunately, social-political overtones cloud the issues, especially with cell-phone use. The actual risk posed by cell phones is difficult to assess because it is a classic example of advocacy driven research—authorities and organizations like MADD, insurance and other safety groups *want* to find evidence for ill effects of cell phones. University and other researchers know that they have to find such effects in order to receive grants. No one gets grant funding renewal by finding negative effects. Further, cookbook science runs rampant because the advocates are interested in snappy slogans that support their agenda and not in what the actual data say. Unfortunately, the will to believe is the enemy of rational thought.

The "will to believe" is common in research on cell phone distraction. One recurring assertion is a prototypical example: the assertion that cell phone use is equivalent to drunk driving. The notion goes back to Redelmeier and Tibshirani (1997), which identified 699 drivers who had been using cell phones at the time of crashes. They examined the drivers' cell phone records for both the day of the crash and the preceding day to determine whether accidents correlated with phone use more than would be expected by chance. Redelmeier and Tibshirani concluded that cell phone use could increase likelihood of accidents by as much as a factor of 4, equivalent to that of drunk drivers. However, the study was a classic case of sampling bias. Samples should be selected at random from the population which they purport to represent. The study only examined drivers who had accidents—possibly a population of bad drivers. The study also included other sources of sampling bias: subjects self-selected whether to participate in the research, and the study included only relatively minor, noninjury accidents.

More recently, Strayer, Drews and Couch (2003) resurrected the claim that cell phone users were as impaired as drunk drivers. It is worth examining this paper because it nicely demonstrates the problem with cookbook science and highlights the necessity of looking at actual data before accepting second-hand conclusions. The abstract's conclusion says that "the impairments associated with using a cell phone while driving can be as profound as those associated with driving while drunk." Strayer stated in a later press release that "We found that people are as impaired when they drive and talk on a cell phone as they are when they drive intoxicated at the legal blood-alcohol limit of 0.08 percent" (What's New At the U, 2007). In fact, his actual data tell an entirely different story. Cell-phone using drivers performed worse than the control subjects, sober drivers who had no cell phone, on tests such as reaction time and number of accidents but not on other tests, such as following distance and braking force. Drunk drivers performed as well as controls on reaction time, traveling speed and number of accidents, but followed closer necessitating harder braking and causing Strayer, Drews and Couch (2003) to label them as more aggressive drivers. The important point, however, is that cell-phone drivers behaved nothing like drunk drivers. The two groups showed *qualitatively* different patterns of behavior. Anyone merely reading the article abstract or, worse, the public relations release, would be getting an entire false impression of what the data actually show.

Examination of the study's data raises another important issue about statistical versus practical significance. Strayer, Drews and Couch (2003) called the drunk drivers more aggressive because they followed more closely, 26.0 m compared to 27.4 m for control drivers. This is a difference of 5 percent! Perhaps the difference would be greater in the real world, but who knows? The important point is that statistically significant does not necessarily mean practically significant.

The political/social bias in interpreting cell phone studies becomes even more obvious when looking at the relative effects of various driver distractions. Stutts, Reinfurt, Staplin, and Rodgman (2001) found that other distractions, such as listening to the radio and in-car eating, produce about as much distraction as cell-phone use, yet no one is claiming that radio users are equivalent to drunk drivers or that R.I.D.E programs should stop vehicles to see if anyone has been eating. Stutts, Reinfurt, Staplin, and Rodgman (2001) also found that sources of distraction outside the car create *far* more distraction than cell phones, but this result receives very little attention. Few people are calling for a ban on billboards or store signs. There is little doubt that the political and funding climate biases research and interpretations of cell phone risk.

This is not to say that cell phone use while driving entails no risk, but the general equation of cell phones to drunk drivers is going far beyond the data. In fact, the causal relationship between cell phone use and accidents is difficult to assess (Hancock, 1999; Green, 2001). The effect of cell phones, or any other potential distractor, is highly contextual. A second task interferes with the first only when it taxes capacity or when it causes cross-task interference. Drivers on an open road in good visibility and light traffic have spare capacity, so talking on a cell phone may not impair driving performance significantly. The same cell phone conversation on a rainy night in heavy traffic or on a winding road or by an older person, conversely, may absorb attention needed for driving. All tasks use some capacity and can tip the balance from safe to risky behavior. As always, context is critical.

While on the subject, what about real drunk drivers? NHTSA defines an accident as "alcohol-related" if either the driver or a pedestrian has a BAC of .01, far below the legal limit. As a result, it includes accidents where the driver might not have been drinking at all or had a minimal BAC. It also includes accidents where the driver in question did not cause the accident. NHTSA further uses a model to estimate BAC incidence for cases where actual BAC was unknown because the driver was never tested, so it is including hypothetical data. As far as I know, there is no such model for any other accident risk factors. NHTSA's analysis of 2005 alcohol-related accidents (National Highway Transportation Safety Administration, 2006) concluded that legally impaired drivers caused only 59 percent of "alcohol-related" accidents, however, and this percentage includes both the hypothetical analysis and cases where the impaired driver may not have been at fault. Obviously, NHTSA's "alcohol-related" accident data overestimate the causative relationship between drinking and driving. Yet many sources with an agenda equate this "alcohol-related" accident rate as drunken driver accident rate because they want the rates to appear as high as possible.

The point here is not that alcohol, cell phones and other in-car technology have no role in accident causation. Rather, the point is Judkins' Law. Accepting second hand conclusions, especially in hot button social/political issues, can lead to mere parroting of faulty conclusions. Any assessment of risk level and of remedial measures should be founded in close examination of the actual data. Lastly, as forensic scientists, we are concerned with causal factors in specific cases and not with general risk factors. General statements like "cell phone users are equivalent to drunks" are essentially useless and misleading. The real question is how independent variables such as alcohol, cell phone use, etc. affect specific behaviors, such as reaction time, visual fields, attentional arousal, etc. in a specific situation.

## B. Attentional Set

Psychologists have discovered many examples of how attentional set creates blindness, including change blindness (Simons and Levin, 2003), repetition blindness. (Kanwisher, 1987), inattentional blindness (Mack and Rock, 1998), attentional blink (Shapiro, 1994), perceptual narrowing

(Easterbrook, 1959), and automatic behavior (Schneider and Shiffrin, 1977). The ensuing section describes some of these phenomena and explains their roles in accidents.

### 1. Perceptual Narrowing and Tunnel Vision

A viewer intently focusing attention at the fixation point is less likely to notice objects in the visual periphery. This phenomenon goes under many names, including "perceptual narrowing," "tunnel vision" and "coning of vision." The central area that has attentional capacity is the "useful field of view" or "functional field of view."

Several factors may cause tunnel vision. One is deep concentration on a difficult task, such as tracking of a target that has poor visibility due to small size, low contrast, cluttered background, etc. A driver fixating on a car directly ahead in the fog at night, for example, is far less likely to notice a pedestrian stepping off the sidewalk than he would on a bright, sunny day. In one accident, a driver who had become lost and anxious focused very narrowly on a freeway entrance ramp in the distance. She failed to notice a "STOP Ahead" sign, three sets of rumble strips, and a STOP sign before driving into an intersection and colliding with a crossing vehicle. Some attribute the presumed increased accident rate of older drivers to a reduced useful field of view. (See Chapter 9.)

Novices frequently exhibit narrowing because they are struggling with a task that experienced people simplified by offloading mental processing on to automatic behavior. For example, Underwood, Chapman, Bowden, and Crundall (2002) found that novice drivers spent more time focused on the road ahead, presumably because they had not fully automated steering and had limited capacity available. Similar effects occur in other fields, such as aviation (Williams, 1995).

Drivers who are fatigued or under the influence of drugs or alcohol attempt to compensate by concentrating their diminished attentional capacity around the sightline. Such drivers may show surprisingly little impairment in detection and response of targets located directly in the sightline but major impairments for objects in the peripheral field. Further, drivers under stress, in a hurry or highly goal directed also exhibit perceptual narrowing. Environment stressors, such as heat and loud noise, can also create narrowing.

### 2. Change Blindness

Change blindness is the failure to notice scene alterations. I have already described the Triesch, Ballard, Hayhoe, and Sullivan (2003) experiment where people failed to see a color change, even when looking directly at the object. The underlying message is that people don't see what they don't attend to, and they don't attend to what is irrelevant.

A series of experiments using the "change blindness paradigm" has led to the same conclusion. A viewer watches two pictures alternate every few seconds, with a very brief flash of white screen occurring during the picture switch. The pictures are identical, except for a major detail, and the viewer's task is to identify the difference between the two pictures. In one popular example, one picture shows a large jet plane and the other shows the identical image with one of the plane's engines air-brushed out. The engine is not a tiny detail in the corner but rather a sizeable part of the central image. Remarkably, very few viewers detect the difference between pictures. The same effect occurs in the real world. One demonstration involved a change at a fast food restaurant. The customers came to the front of the line and ordered. The cashier rang up the order and then pretended to bend down behind the counter to pick up something on the floor. In reality, he had moved aside and a different cashier popped back up to continue the food purchase. Very few customers noticed the change of cashier.

Several researchers have suggested that change blindness might cause road accidents. A driver looks right and sees a clear road (picture 1). He then checks left (picture 2) and looks back right (picture 1). The saccadic suppression[10] during the eye movement is equivalent to the white flash. A new vehicle may have appeared, but the driver doesn't see it because of change blindness.

Velichkovsky, Dornhoefer, Kopf, and Helmert (2002) found some evidence for driver impairment due to change blindness, but the results were mixed. Caird, Edwards, Creaser and Horrey (2005) found that young and middle-aged drivers detected only about 75 percent of traffic scene changes, such as "taxi incurring from left." Older drivers were about 20 percent worse. They also found that size or contrast had no reliable effect on perception, reinforcing the importance of distinguishing between visibility and conspicuity factors. Overall the results suggest that change blindness can afflict real drivers and cause accidents, but the effects are smaller than those found in the laboratory with less meaningful images. However, these studies used objects in their normal locations. When objects are at unexpected locations, even highly relevant information may go unnoticed (Shinoda, Hayhoe, and Shrivastava, 2001).

### 3. Inattentional Blindness

Until the last ten years, very little was known about viewer ability to detect unexpected objects. I've already noted that most applied conspicuity studies are really visibility studies. Until recently, most laboratory conspicuity studies examined "search conspicuity," where the viewer actively searched for a specific target. There was little known about just noticing, "attention conspicuity," although the phenomenon of "look but failed to see" accidents had been appreciated for many years (e.g., Sabey and Staughton, 1975).

Mack and Rock (1998) initiated research interest in conspicuity of truly unexpected objects with their 1998 book, *Inattentional Blindness*, which described experiments testing viewer awareness and attention. The results were absolutely startling; viewers missed a large proportion of clearly visible objects presented in the center of the visual field. Subsequent research has confirmed and extended Mack and Rock's work for a wide variety of situations and found even more surprising failures to see the obvious.

Mack and Rock used brief flashed images, but research also demonstrates "sustained" inattentional blindness (e.g., Neisser, 1979; Most, Scholl, Clifford, and Simons, 2005), where viewers watch film clips and fail to see highly salient objects that are present in the scene for several seconds. Similar effects are readily apparent in the real world. In one demonstration,[11] for example, a driver counted the number of two-door cars as she drove up to an intersection. She stopped for a light and continued counting. While waiting, a man in a gorilla suit walked right in front of her car. She and about half of the other test participants failed to notice the "gorilla." It is not unusual for inattentional blindness studies to find that 50 percent or more of viewers fail to see the "obvious." When giving talks, I routinely show a movie where only 5-10 percent of the audience sees a person located directly in the middle of the scene. When I tell the audience what to look for and replay the clip, they are invariably astounded to have missed something so obvious.

Inattentional blindness likely plays a role in many accidents (Green, 2002). Recall from Chapter 1 the example of the woman who failed to see the bicyclist because she had spent a year entering the gas station without ever seeing anyone on the sidewalk. Her failure to see the bicyclist was due to expectation and confirmation bias. She had developed a script: pick up the truck, drive to the gas station, look down the sidewalk, see nothing, enter the gas station, fill the tank. On the day of the accident, there were two sources of violated expectation. First, she entered the same gas station every workday for a year and had never seen anything on the sidewalk, so she had developed the expectation that no one would be there. Second, pedestrians may be common on sidewalks but bicycles are not. Her attention was likely tuned, if at all, to look mainly for pedestrians. The bicyclist on the sidewalk was not part of the schema.

The human tendency toward *confirmation bias* strengthens expectancy effects. People who hold a belief or expectation tend to seek evidence that confirms and ignore or avoid evidence which refutes. For example, people who favor one political candidate will listen to her speeches but immediately turn off the TV if someone starts extolling the virtues of the opponent. The same effect occurs unconsciously. The driver looked down the sidewalk for confirmation of what she already knew.

There are some truly extraordinary cases of confirmation bias leading to accident. In one that killed 500 people, a train collided with another when seven highly trained and experienced crew members failed to notice that they pulled out of the station going in the wrong direction. Even though familiar with the station and the surrounding area, they proceeded for several minutes before running into another train on the track.

Inattentional blindness and confirmation bias also commonly generate medication errors. In one case, a highly experienced hospital nurse selected a bottle of Lasix from a cart full of medications. She checked the bottle three times before injecting the patient, who subsequently died. She had actually injected the patient with a different drug, KCL. The vial was correctly labeled, so why the error? The Lasix bottle was always in a specific location on the cart. The nurse had learned that she could select by cart location and that reading the label was superfluous, that is, she cue generalized. Like the driver who became inattentionally blind to the bicyclist, she simply failed to detect the violated expectation.

The general lesson to be learned is that people are adaptive. They learn to change behavior, tune attention, etc. based on circumstances. Accidents frequently occur when usually adaptive, intelligent and unconscious behavior meets unexpected and unusual circumstances. Ironically, highly skilled and highly practiced experts are *more* likely to commit inattentional blindness accidents than are beginners. They have had more chance to develop expectations and to have the expectations repeatedly reinforced by experience. Recall that the Swedish drivers who effectively became beginners when required to drive "on the wrong side of the road" had fewer accidents.

Inattentional blindness accidents are especially likely when expectation and distraction combine. In one famous accident, Cmdr. Scott D. Waddle of the submarine USS Greeneville surfaced his boat, overturning a Japanese fishing trawler and killing 9 people. With visiting dignitaries onboard, the sonar operator told Cmdr. Waddle that there were no blips on the screen. Cmdr. Waddle had learned through long experience that a clear sonar screen meant no ships in the area. When he subsequently scanned the ocean through the periscope prior to surfacing, he did not expect to see the 500-ton trawler. Moreover, the visitors and their care doubtless occupied his attention, further reducing likelihood of seeing the boat. Lastly, Cmdr. Waddle likely was suffering from confirmation bias. He doubtless peered through the periscope, unconsciously looking for evidence to confirm the sonar reading.

Expectation and confirmation bias can also cause viewers to see things that aren't actually there. The nurse who mistakenly selected KCL checked the label three times before injecting the patient. Each time she saw what she expected—"Lasix." In another accident, a pharmacist filling in for an absent colleague on a pediatric care unit made an error which led to an overdose and death. She consulted a medical reference and misread the dosage, mentally adding an extra 0. Moreover, she consulted a second reference and made exactly the same error. The explanation lay in her expectation and attentional set. She had no previous pediatric experience and normally dealt with adult size doses. When she consulted a pediatric reference, she "saw" dosages consistent with adults and not with babies. When she checked a second reference, expectation and confirmation bias again supplied the extra 0.

Inattentional blindness is far less intuitive than tunnel vision and far more difficult to explain in court. Even under normal circumstances, everyone is less able to notice objects in the peripheral field. Central vision has both better resolution and the focus of attention. Tunnel vision is merely an accentuated version of normal visual tendencies. The failure to see objects at or near the sightline, in contrast, is almost incomprehensible to most people. This is why demonstrations of the phenomenon are often both necessary and effective.

In sum, inattentional blindness is so powerful because it highlights the fallacy of naïve realism and the notion that vision is complete. It shows that there is much more to seeing than registering a retinal image. It underscores the fact that visibility and conspicuity are vastly different functions. Lastly, it shows that many people accused of inattention are doing no more than acting adaptively and skillfully.

### 4. Eye Movements and Attention

Research into eye-movements and attention have dramatically demonstrated the role of experience, expectation and goals in attentional failures. This set of studies measured eye-movements of people involved in a variety of common tasks. Like inattentional blindness, it has boomed in the past ten years, mostly due to development of light-weight portable eye-tracking systems that viewers can wear while going about everyday activities. The results of these studies have revealed how people normally direct attention in routine tasks and have been almost as surprising as those from the inattentional blindness research.

Yarbus (1967) was perhaps the earliest to demonstrate how viewer goals direct eye movements and attention. He measured eye movements of viewers who examined the painting of a family. Viewers tended to look at the parts of the painting that held the most important information, which in turn was a function of their task. In free viewing, the viewers looked at eyes and lips. When asked to remember the clothes worn by the family, however, the viewers instead fixated various pierces of clothing. When asked to perform other tasks, the eye movements and attention again changed pattern. Yarbus' study had important implications—people look and direct attention to where they expect to find the important information for the particular task. If the task changes, then eye movements and attentional allocation change, even with the same scene.

More recent research (reviewed in Land, 2006) shows that eye movements operate on a "just in time basis," with viewers transferring fixation to the relevant information about .6–.8 seconds before it is needed. This is the endogenous-automatic "habit" control of attention shown in Table 4.1. Land further concluded that people seldom notice task irrelevant objects: "the eyes are driven by top-down information from the script of the activity rather than by the intrinsic salience of objects in the scene." In other words, "sensory conspicuity" is not very important when people are engaged in a specific task.

The forensic importance of this research is enormous. When people are performing a task, the standard conspicuity aids, such as color, contrast and flashing, have little effect. It explains why people quickly tune out warnings of all kinds and why warnings are so generally ineffective (e.g., Ayres, Wood, Schmidt, Young, and Murray, 1998; Green, 2004).

## 4.7 Conclusion

This chapter has outlined basic attentional mechanisms and explained why "attentional failures" occur. Beyond the basic science, the discussion has underscored five general messages.

1. Visibility and conspicuity are different mental processes. A large number of cognitive processes determine whether a particular viewer will "see" a particular object. Visibility is a factor in attention and conspicuity, but it is only one of many. Attentional set is generally far more important, as shown by studies where viewers fail to see highly visible objects directly in the sightline. This issue arises again later, especially in Chapter 18 which explains why pictures introduced as evidence of what a viewer would have seen are almost invariably misleading.
2. Labeling a person "inattentive" explains nothing. Inattention is not an explanation but rather something to be explained.
3. Attending is the exception and "attentional failure" the rule. Accidents frequently occur because attention filters away critical information. The filter allows only a small subset of impinging sensory information into consciousness, so we are oblivious to almost everything. This is not intuitive for several reasons. Naïve realism leads us to believe that seeing is complete. We are not aware when we are not aware. Moreover, we all have largely similar interactions with the world and hence have similar expectations and goals. As a result, we all generally learn to attend to similar information in a given situation. All experienced drivers expect traffic signals, pedestrians, signs, etc. at various times and places on the road. This gives the illusion that attending to the right information is innate and that attentional failure is likely due to a mental failing. In fact, each situation has its own peculiarities and each person a set of idiosyncratic experiences, expectations and goals which may affect attentional allocation in a specific context.
4. People are far too often blamed for "inattention" when they are merely behaving intelligently and adaptively but have met unusual circumstances. This is not to say that all attentional failures are excusable, but rather that the reason for the "inattention" should be closely examined before assigning blame (Green, 2006). In some jurisdictions, the law says the viewer should see whatever there is to see. This presumption is both unscientific and simply unreasonable.
5. Could does not imply should. Detection and perception are related somewhat because, all things being equal, higher contrast is more conspicuous. Of course, all things are seldom equal, as the inattentional blindness and other research show and as the common underride scenario discussed in Chapter 1 demonstrates. The driver *could have* seen the trailer at a sufficient distance to permit braking and to avoid the accident. The unstated assertion is that the driver *should have* seen the trailer and avoided it. *Could*, however, does not necessarily imply *should*. As many inattentional blindness, change blindness and eye-movement studies have shown, moreover, size, contrast and other sensory conspicuity cues often have little effect. In any event, "should" is not a scientific concept, and a scientific analysis carries no value judgment or moral imperative.

There is often great misunderstanding about what a scientific analysis of cognition represents. It does not read the minds of individuals. It says what a "normal person" would be expected to achieve in a given situation, within the bounds of variability. To draw a simple analogy, I frequently cross a busy intersection when the facing light turns green and the "Walk" sign is illuminated. I trust that drivers will stop for the red light and allow me to cross safely. I don't know the exact thoughts of each driver, but then I don't have to know. I have knowledge of "normal" human behavior for the population as a whole in that situation.[12] In this case, my knowledge arises from direct experience and vicarious observation. In a scientific analysis, the knowledge of normal arises from controlled research.

To sum up, whether a viewer's behavior were reasonable depends on the entire process of seeing that includes visibility, attention, expectation, and goals—the viewer's entire mindset (Dekker, 2002). Vision isn't just about the eyes, it's about much of psychology as well. As Kay (1971) said, "We shall understand accidents when we understand human nature."

## References

Andrews, W. 1987. Improving the visibility of railroad-highway grade crossing signals. *Public Roads* 51, 25-35.

Aschenbrenner, K. M. and B. Biehl. 1994. Empirical studies regarding risk compensation processes in relation to anti-lock braking systems. In R.Trimpop, G.Wilde (Eds) *Challenges to Accident Prevention: The issue of risk compensation behaviour*. Groningen: Styx Publications.

Ayres, T., C. Wood, R. Schmidt, D. Young, and J. Murray. 1998. Effectiveness of Warning Labels and Signs: An Update on Compliance Research. *Proceedings of Ergon* 98.

Berkhout, J. 1977. Information content at night of roof mounted emergency vehicle lights. Final Report. Contract DOT DS 50121. Department of Transportation, Office of University Research.

Berkhout, J. 1979. Information transfer characteristics of moving light signals. Human Factors 21, 445-455.

Biehl, B., M. Aschenbrenner, and G. Wurm. 1987. Einfluss der Risikokompensation auf die Wirkung von Verkehrssicherheitsmassnahmen am Beispiel ABS. Unfall-und Sicherheitsforschung Strassenverkehr, No. 63, Symposion Unfallforschung '87.

Caird, J., C. Edwards, J. Creaser, and W. Horrey. 2005. Older driver failures of attention at intersections: Using change blindness methods to assess turn decision accuracy. *Human Factors, 47*(2), 235-249.

Cole, G. L. and P. Hughes. 1984. A field trial of attention and search conspicuity. *Human Factors* 26, 299-313.

Cox, J. 1971. The viewing of railroad flashing light signals. In *Perception And Application of Flashing Lights*, 189-207. London: Hilger.

Crawford, A. 1963. The perception of light signals: The effect of mixing steady and flashing irrelevant lights. *Ergonomics* 6, 287-294.

Davis, D. 1959. Human Errors and Transport Accidents, Ergonomics 2, 24-33.

Dekker, S. 2002. *The Field Guide to Human Error Investigations*. Burlington, Vermont: Ashgate Publishing.

Downing, P., D. Bray, J. Rogers, and C. Childs. 2004. Bodies capture attention when nothing is expected. *Cognition* 93, B27-B38.

Easterbrook, J. A. 1959. The effect of emotion on cue utilization and the organization of behavior. *Psychological Review* 66, 183-201.

Engle, F. 1976. *Visual Conspicuity As An External Determiner of Eye Movements And Selective Attention*. Eindhoven: Technische Hogeschool.

Gale, G. 1979. *Theory of Science*. Toronto: McGraw-Hill.

Gibson, J. J. and L. Crooks. 1938. A theoretical field analysis of automobile-driving. American Journal of psychology, 51, 453-471.

Goldhaber, G., and M. deTurck. 1988. Effectiveness of warning signs: Gender and familiarity effects. *Journal of Product Safety* 11, 271-284.

Green, M. 1983. Contrast detection and direction discrimination of drifting gratings. *Vision Research* 23, 281-289.

Green, M. 1984. Masking by Light and the Sustained-Transient Dichotomy. *Perception and Psychophysics* 34, 617-635.

Green, M. 2001. Do Cell phones Pose An Unacceptable Risk? A Complete Look at the Adequacy of the Evidence, *Risk Management* Nov, 40-48.

Green, M. 2002. Inattentional Blindness. *Occupational Health & Safety Canada* Jan/Feb, 23–29.

Green, M. 2004. Why warnings fail. *Occupational Health and Safety* Feb, 20-24.

Green, M. 2006. Human error vs. design error, *Trial* June, 60-65.

Green, M. and J. V. Odom. 2001. Occlusion, segmentation and the aperture problem. Association for Research in Vision and Ophthalmology Meeting, Sarasota, Florida.

Hancock, P. 1999. The driving question. *Transportation Human Factors* 1, 47-55.

ICE Ergonomics, 2002. Motor vehicle conspicuity: — Warning beacons. Loughborough University: Leicestershire, UK. http://www.unece.org/trans/main/wp29/wp29wgs/wp29gre/greinfdoc/48inf02.pdf. Downloaded 1 June 06.

James, W. 1890. *Principles of Psychology*. New York: Henry Holt.

Johnsson, G. 1973. Visual perception of biological motion and a model for its analysis. *Perception and Psychophysics*, 14, 201-211.

Kanwisher, N. G. 1987. Repetition blindness: Type recognition without token individuation. Cognition, 27, 117-143.

Kay, H. 1971. Accidents: Some facts and theories. In P. Warr ed *Psychology at Work,* 121-145. Baltimore: Penguin.

Koivisto, M., J. Hyönä, and A. Revonsuo. 2004. The effects of eye movements, spatial attention and stimulus features on inattentional blindness. *Vision Research* 44, 3211-3221.

Koivisto, M. and A. Revonsuo. 2007. How Meaning Shapes Seeing. *Psychological Science* 18, 845-849.

Korte, A. 1915. Kinematoskopische untersuchungen [Kinematoscopic investigations]. *Zeitschrift für Psychologie 72,* 194–296.

Land, M. 1999. The roles of vision and eye movements in the control of activities of daily living. Perception 28, 1311-1328.

Land, M. 2006. Eye movements and the control of actions in everyday life. *Progress in Retinal and Eye Research* 25, 296-324.

Makela, P., J. Rovamo, and D. Whitaker. 1994. Effects of Luminance and External Temporal Noise on Flicker Sensitivity as a Function of Stimulus Size at Various Eccentricities. *Vision Research* 34, 1981-1991.

Mandelbaum, J. 1960. An accommodation phenomenon, *Archives of Ophthalmology*, 73, 923-926.

Most, S., B. Scholl, E. Clifford, and D. Simons. 2005. What you see is what you set: Sustained inattentional blindness and the capture of awareness. *Psychological Review 112(1)*, 217–242.

Most, S. and R. Astur. 2007. Feature-based attentional set as a cause of traffic accidents. *Visual Cognition* 15, 125-132.

National Highway Transportation Safety Administration. 2006. Traffic Accident Facts. Washington, D. C.: National Highway Transportation Safety Administration.

Neisser, U. 1979. The control of information pickup in selective looking. In A. D. Pick (ed.), *Perception and its development: A tribute to Eleanor J. Gibson,* 201-219. Hillsdale, NJ: Lawrence Erlbaum.

Nikolic, M. I., J. Orr, and N. Sarter. 2001. Why onsets don't always capture attention: The importance of context in display design. *Proceedings of the 11th International Symposium on Aviation Psychology.* Columbus, Ohio, March.

Posner, M. I. 1980. Orienting of attention. *Quarterly Journal of Experimental Psychology* 32, 3-25.

Potter, S. 1948. *The Theory and Practice of Gamesmanship: The Art of Winning Games Without Actually Cheating*. London: Henry Holt.

Previc, F. 1998. The Neuropsychology of 3-D space. *Psychological Bulletin* 124, 123-164.

Reason, J. and K. Mycielska. 1982. *Absent-minded?: The Psychology of Mental Lapses and Everyday Errors*. Englewood Cliffs, NJ: Prentice Hall, Inc.

Redelmeier, D. A. and R. J. Tibshirani. 1997. "Association between Mobileular-Telephone Calls and Motor Vehicle Collisions." *New England Journal of Medicine 336,* 453-458.

Ro, T., C. Russell, and N. Lavie. 2001. Changing faces: a detection advantage in the flicker paradigm. *Psychological Science* 12, 94–99.

Sabey, B. and G. Staughton. 1975. Interacting roles of road environment, vehicle and road user in accidents. Paper presented to the *5th International Conference of the International Association for Accident and Traffic Medicine and the 3rd International Conference on drug abuse of the International Council on alcohol and addiction*, 1–5 September 1975, London.

Schieber, F., J. Larsen, J. Jurgensen, K. Werner, and G. Heimstra. 2001. Fluorescent colored highway signs don't 'grab' attention; They 'guide' it Proceedings of the Human Factors and Ergonomics Society, 1622-1626.

Shapiro, K. 1994. The *attentional blink:* The brain's 'eyeblink.' *Current Directions in Psychological Science* 3 86-89.

Shinoda, H., M. Hayhoe, and A. Shrivastava. 2001. What controls attention in natural environments? *Vision Research* 41, 25-26.

Simons, D. J. and D. T. Levin. 2003. What makes change blindness interesting? In D.E. Irwin and B.H. Ross (eds.), The psychology of learning and motivation, Vol. 42 (pp. 295-322). San Diego, CA: Academic Press.

Sinnett, S., A. Costa, and S. Soto-Faraco. 2006. Manipulating inattentional blindness within. and across sensory modalities. *Quarterly Journal of Experimental Psychology*, 59, 1425-1442.

Solomon, S. S. 1990. Lime-yellow color as related to reduction of serious fire apparatus accidents: The case for visibility in emergency vehicle accident avoidance. *Journal of the American Optometric Association* 61, 827-831.

Strayer, D., F. Drews, and D. Crouch. 2003. Fatal Distraction? A Comparison of the Cell-phone Driver and the Drunk Driver. Proceedings of the Second International Driving symposium on Human Factors in Driver Assessment, Training and Vehicle Design.

Stutts, J., W. Reinfurt, L. Staplin, and E. Rodgman. 2001. *The Role Of Driver Distraction In Traffic Crashes*. New York: AAA Foundation for Traffic Safety.

Tejerina, L. 2003. Committee report: conspicuity enhancement for police interceptor rear-end crash mitigation. https://www.fleet.ford.com/showroom/CVPI/pdfs/CVPI_Conspicuity_Report.pdf. Downloaded 1 Nov 06.

Templer, J. 1992. *The Staircase. Studies of Hazards, Falls And Safer Design.* Cambridge, Ma.: MIT Press.

Trick, L. M., J. T. Enns, J. Mills, and J. Vavrik. 2004. Paying attention behind the wheel: A framework for studying the role of selective attention in driving. *Theoretical Issues in Ergonomic Science* 5, 385-424.

Triesch, J., D. Ballard, M. Hayhoe, and B. Sullivan. 2003. What you see is what you need. *Journal of Vision 3,* 86-94.

Underwood, G., P. Chapman, K. Bowden, and D. Crundall. 2002. Visual search while driving: Skill and awareness during inspection of the scene. Transportation Research Part F: Traffic Psychology and Behaviour 5: 87–97.

Velichkovsky, B. M., S. M. Dornhoefer, M. Kopf, J. Helmert, and M. Joos. 2002. Change detection and occlusion modes in road-traffic scenarios. Transportation Research Part F: Traffic Psychology & Behaviour, 5, 99-109.

White, W. T. and J. Toomath. 1980. Motorcycle exposure to risk of accident, *Proceedings international conference on motorcycle safety*, Washington, DC, May Vol. 4, 1613-1638.

Wilde, G. J. S. 1988. Risk homeostasis theory and traffic accidents: Propositions, deductions and discussion of dissension in recent reactions. *Ergonomics 31*, 441-468.

Williams, L. 1995. Peripheral target recognition and visual field narrowing in aviators and nonaviators. *International Journal of Aviation Psychology* 5, 215-232.

Wulf, G., P. Hancock and M. Rahimi. 1989. Motorcycle Conspicuity—An Evaluation And Synthesis of Influential Factors, *Journal Of Safety Research* 20, 153-176.

Yarbus, A. L. 1967. Eye movements during perception of complex objects, *in* L. A. Riggs ed., *Eye Movements and Vision*, 171-196. New York: Plenum Press.

## Endnotes

1. The Ontario Provincial police have recently reverted to "Panda Cars," cruisers painted white and black. In terms of conspicuity, this is a very foolish decision.

2. Note that having STOP signs as white on red, however, is a good idea. At night, the red becomes dark, creating good brightness contrast with the white lettering.

3. Recall that colors fall into two categories. Achromatics are white, gray and black while chromatics are everything else, i.e., red, green, yellow, blue, etc.

4. Road signs showing diagonal stripes of alternating yellow and black optimize both color and shape conspicuity. Diagonal lines are more conspicuous than verticals or horizontals.

5. In the very far periphery, red fades before yellow, so there is little difference between yellow and orange (which is red+yellow).

6. The sustained-transient dichotomy has been replaced by the parvocellular-magnocelluar dichotomy. They are not identical but are functionally very similar.

7. People frequently, and incorrectly, call this "phi motion." In fact, this is "beta motion." Phi motion is a quite different phenomenon of "disembodied" motion.

8. In fact, anyone wishing to learn about conspicuity would do well to study spammer techniques and the variety of trick banners that appear on the internet.

9. Such accidents are so common among tourists in Britain that "Look Right" is stenciled on the ground at crosswalks. Ireland uses "Stay Left" signs along the roadway to warn continental and North American drivers.

10. Saccadic suppression is a mechanism that blots out vision during an eye movement. It is the reason that the world does not appear to smear when the eyes move.

11. The test was performed during a segment on CTV television, Canada.

12. Certainly, I may supplement my knowledge by perception. If a car is approaching the intersection at a high speed, I may conclude that he will not stop. This still requires no mind reading.

# Chapter 5

# Systemic Diseases and Highway Safety

Leslie Weintraub, O.D.

***Synopsis***



## 5.1 Metabolic Diseases

Metabolic disorders refer to dysfunctions of the endocrine glands. The endocrine glands work with the nervous system, to maintain homeostasis, or a balanced internal environment. Endocrine glands produce hormones, which regulate metabolic activities such as growth, utilization of nutrients by cells, salt and water balance, blood homeostasis and metabolic rate.

If the endocrine glands are not functioning properly, debilitating symptoms may occur. For example, a generalized lack of strength, muscle weakness, spasm or tetany, sudden episodes of vertigo, or unconsciousness. Motor vehicle operation should be restricted until the particular metabolic disease has been treated sufficiently to prevent these dangerous symptoms.

### A. Diabetes mellitus

Diabetes, or the inability of the body to metabolize sugars, is very common. According to the Centers for Disease Control and Prevention 2002 National Health Survey, 6.3 percent of the U.S. population, or 18.2 million people, have diabetes. This survey also shows that the chances of developing diabetes increases with age. Non-insulin dependent, or NIDDM, is more common in the elderly than is insulin dependent, or IDDM.

Persons with NIDDM may experience hyperglycemia, or abnormally high levels of blood sugar. This will impair alertness, usually very gradually. Therefore, it does not inhibit one's safe driving ability, as long as they are properly counseled and monitored.

Persons with IDDM, and possibly those treated with oral hypoglycemic drugs such as diabeta, glipizide, glyburide, and starlix may experience hypoglycemia. Hypoglycemia, or abnormally low levels of blood sugar, can occur rapidly and without warning. Faintness or unconsciousness may result. For this reason, it is imperative for IDDM persons to self-monitor their blood-sugar levels. Only then can they ascertain their ability to drive safely. In fact, the U.S. Department of Transportation recommends a "restricted license" for persons subject to "stress hypoglycemia."

After reviewing several studies of driving records from the 1960s and 1970s, Janke, Peck, and Dreyer (1978), concluded that diabetes causes some increased driving risk. Both Janke et al., and Waller (1973), agree that the major cause of peril associated with diabetic drivers is most likely their susceptibility to hypoglycemic attacks. Table 5.1 shows a compilation of recent studies evaluating accidents or traffic violations of diabetic drivers (Janke, 1994). The results are mixed, but clearly show some increased risk associated with diabetes.

Diabetes may affect vision, and is one of the leading causes of blindness in our country. Eye disturbances associated with diabetic retinopathy, are discussed in Chapter 7.

## B. Thyroid disease

The thyroid gland, located in the neck, just anterior to the trachea, secretes two thyroid hormones. The two principal actions of the thyroid hormones, T3 and T4, are to stimulate metabolic rate and to promote growth.

Excessive amounts of thyroid hormone, or hyperthyroidism, causes an increase in metabolic rate, weight loss, and goiter. Symptoms of hyperthyroidism that may cause danger while driving include nervous excitability, tremors, breathlessness upon exertion, and a rapid heart rate.

Subnormal amounts of thyroid, or hypothyroidism, cause a decrease in metabolic rate, body temperature, pulse rate, respiration and mental capacity. Symptoms of hypothyroidism that may cause danger while driving, include physical and mental sluggishness, fatigue, and poor muscle tone.

Severe hyperthyroid or hypothyroid persons should not drive a motor vehicle at all. However, if well diagnosed and treated, persons affected with these disorders are able to safely drive motor vehicles.

## C. Hyperparathyroidism and hypoparathyroidism

Disorders of the parathyroid glands, which surround the lateral lobes of the thyroid gland, may cause abnormally high, or abnormally low blood and bone calcium levels. Normal levels of calcium are essential for normal nerve and muscle function, bone metabolism, cell membrane permeability, and blood clotting.

If calcium levels in the blood are extremely low, as may occur with hypoparathyroidism, nerve fibers become more excitable. Twitching and muscle spasms may ensue. Neuromuscular excitability, cramps, spasms and tetany, are all contraindications for driving.

If calcium levels in the blood are extremely high, as may occur with hyperparathyroidism, muscular weakness and hypotonia may ensue. Since so much calcium is removed from the bones in this case, they are weakened and easily fractured. Muscular weakness, loss of muscle tone and brittle bones, may prevent safe driving. If calcium levels are stable, with or without treatment, persons affected with hyperparathyroidism or hypoparathyroidism should be able to drive safely.

**Recent Studies Evaluating Accident or Violation Experience of Diabetic Drivers (Adapted from La Porte et al., 1991)**

| Study | N | Time | Type of Dbx | Accidents | | Violations | | Units | Comments |
|---|---|---|---|---|---|---|---|---|---|
| | | | | Dbx | Ctl | Dbx | Ctl | | |
| DeKlerk & Armstrong (1983) | 8623 | 9 years | Both | 72 | 73 | - | - | hospital admissions for road trauma | Hospital-recorded accidents. Does not consider driving exposure. Diabetic males had more hospital admissions than expected. |
| Songer et al. (1988) | 127 | 1 year | IDDM | 14.2 | 7.1 | - | - | per 100 drivers | Self-reported accidents. Small sample size for 1-year time. |
| | 121 | 1 year | IDDM | 10.4 | 3.9 | - | - | per 100 drivers/per million miles | Adjusted for driving exposure. |
| Eadington & Frier (1989) | 166 | 8 years | IDDM | 5.4 | 10.0 | - | - | per million miles | Self-reported accidents. Control was not age- or sex-matched. |
| Stevens et al. (1989) | 354 | 5 years | ITDM | 7.9 | 7.8 | - | - | per 1.5 million kilometers | Self-reported accidents. Adjusted for driving exposure. |
| | | | | 7.1 | 7.1 | - | - | per 100 drivers/year | |
| Chantelau et al. (1990) | 241 | 2 years | ITDM | - | - | 11% | 16% | % | Comparison group not matched on age, sex or driving exposure. |

N Sample size
Dbx Diabetics
Ctl Comparison group
IDDM Insulin-dependent diabetes mellitus
ITDM Insulin-treated diabetes mellitus
Both ITDM and non-insulin treated diabetics

res rpts/age related disability

### D. Posterior pituitary insufficiency

The posterior lobe of the pituitary gland, releases oxytocin and antidiuretic hormones (ADH). ADH increases water reabsorption from the kidney, to conserve the body's water. Persons with insufficient pituitary function may experience enormous fluid loss. Hypoglycemic episodes, as do occur in hyperinsulin states, may ensue. This causes faintness and unconsciousness, which clearly make it unsafe to drive. Proper therapy, however, should prevent this from occurring.

### E. Anterior pituitary insufficiency

The anterior lobe or the pituitary gland, releases six hormones, including the growth hormone, prolactin and several tropic hormones. Growth hormone has several actions that may directly or indirectly raise blood-sugar levels. Insufficiency may cause abnormally low carbohydrate levels and hypoglycemic events. This may impair alertness, making those persons unsafe drivers.

### F. Pituitary tumor

Tumors of the pituitary gland may cause visual field loss. The pituitary gland sits at the base of the cerebellum, just under the intersection of the optic tracts. The classic visual field loss, in this case, is a bitemporal hemianopsia. This is the loss of both temporal fields of vision. Loss of peripheral vision can prove to be hazardous for a motor vehicle driver. Loss of peripheral vision results in a slower reaction time to objects appearing from the sides, which is the scenario for most motor vehicle accidents.

Visual fields may or may not return after treatment of a pituitary tumour. Visual field examinations are recommended every 6–12 months after treatment.

### G. Adrenal cortical hypersecretion (Cushing's disease), and hypo-secretion (Addison's disease)

The two adrenal glands, located on top of the kidneys, contain an inner medulla and an outer cortex. The adrenal cortex secretes corticosteroids. The corticosteroids help regulate water and electrolyte balance in body fluids, normal cell metabolism, blood glucose levels, and secondary male sex characteristics.

Hyperfunction of the adrenal cortex (Cushing's disease) causes excessive water and sodium retention, with consequential high blood pressure and potassium loss. When associated with muscular weakness and osteoporosis, it inhibits safe driving ability.

Hypofunction of the adrenal cortex (Addison's disease) causes excessive sodium and water loss. This is associated with muscle weakness, asthenia, low blood pressure, and possible hypoglycemia and syncope. These symptoms contraindicate driving.

### H. Hyperfunction of the adrenal medulla

The adrenal medulla releases epinephrine and norepinephrine into the blood. This produces the "fight or flight" reaction during stressful situations. Epinephrine and norepinephrine increase heart rate, blood pressure, blood glucose, and blood oxygen. If hyperfunction of the adrenal medulla causes headaches, dizziness, weakness, blurred vision, a rapid pulse rate and increased blood pressure, driving a motor vehicle is clearly contraindicated.

## 5.2 Cardiovascular Disease

Symptoms of cardiovascular disease that would inhibit safe driving ability, are loss of consciousness, severe chest pain, and symptoms such as dizziness or blurred vision. Some heart conditions may also cause insufficient oxygenation of the brain. Lack of oxygen to the brain may impair mentation, or even cause sudden death behind the wheel. Cardiac deaths average about 4.6 per 1,000 man years, and 1.3 per 1,000 woman years in those aged 35–64 year of age (Shephard, 1987, cited in Janke, 1994). However, there is a 10 to 11 fold increase in the risk of cardiac deaths, in the age group of 60–64, as compared to the age group of 40–44.

A review of the more recent studies concerning the traffic accident risk of cardiovascular patients concluded that none of the well controlled studies have demonstrated a consistent increase in risk associated with cardiovascular disease (Potvin, Guibert, and Loiselle, 1993). Similarly, a review of studies done before 1978, concluded that the majority of cardiovascular patients pose no threat behind the wheel (Janke, Peck, and Dreyer, 1978). The researchers noted, however, that cardiovascular patients tend to reduce the amount of time they spend driving alone and driving in heavy traffic. This self restriction may account for the favorable results. Also, the researchers noted that the studies concerning cardiovascular patients and driving are full of methodological problems.

Although no definitive study has shown an increased private car crash risk associated with cardiovascular disease, persons afflicted with heart disease are usually restricted from obtaining a commercial drivers license. This is reasonable since commercial drivers, unlike private passenger car drivers, frequently need to drive long hours under adverse weather and lighting conditions. If a crash occurs, these large commercial vehicles can cause major damages and traffic congestion.

## A. Congestive heart failure

If the heart fails to pump the blood throughout the body efficiently, blood backs up into the lungs, liver, and veins. The causes congestion of fluid in the lungs, legs, liver, and possibly other parts of the body. Persons affected with congestive heart failure will have difficulty breathing, and may be driving hazards. In 1993, Wielgosz and Asad found that the prevalence of congestive heart failure increases with age: 3 percent in those aged 45–64, 6 percent in those aged 65 and above, and 10 percent in those aged 75 and above (cited in Janke, 1994).

According to the American Medical Association (AMA), persons with congestive heart failure should not drive commercial or passenger transport vehicles, even if their condition is stable. Driving a private motor vehicle is considered safe, as long as their condition is stable.

## B. Arrhythmias

Abnormal functioning of the ventricles, which pump blood out to the body, are very serious conditions that may cause sudden death. Rapid ventricular contractions tend to reduce cardiac output and may lead to heart failure. Therefore, any disorder of cardiac rhythm that causes very rapid ventricular contractions would contraindicate driving. For example, ventricular arrhythmias or atrioventricular blocks, associated with faintness or unconsciousness, contraindicate driving. The types of heart disease most frequently associated with ventricular tachycardia or ventricular fibrillation, are coronary artery disease (70 percent), dilated cardiomyopathy (7 percent), hypertensive heart disease (3 percent), and valvular disease (2 percent) (Larson, Stupey, et al., 1994).

Atrial rhythm disturbances, such as premature beats, or brief dysrhythmias, usually do not disturb safe driving ability. Atrial fibrillations or flutter, however, should be controlled by medication or a pacemaker, in order for the person to safely drive a private motor vehicle. The AMA advises that these persons should not drive a commercial or multi-passenger vehicle. Pacemakers usually alleviate disabling symptoms of cardiovascular disease, by maintaining proper cardiac rhythm.

Thus, if a pacemaker has been implanted, the person should not be at risk to drive a private motor vehicle.

### C. Angina pectoris (cardiac pain)

Persons with coronary artery disease, that experience angina at random times, are advised against driving, by doctors. This is because the resulting pain in the chest, arm or jaws can be so severe, it incapacitates the driver temporarily. Nitroglycerin dilates the coronary arteries, and usually alleviates cardiac pain.

Persons with coronary artery disease, whom experience angina only with moderate exertion, are advised by doctors against operating a commercial or multi-passenger vehicle. (No Class I or Class II licensing.)

### D. Hypertension

Although hypertension normally does not preclude driving, some symptoms of hypertension may. Complications of hypertension that may contraindicate driving are: frequent and severe headaches, heart failure, weakness, mental disturbances, dizziness, retinal hemorrhages, and cerebral vascular hemorrhages. The potential for syncope caused by severe hypertension has also been mentioned as a great hazard to driving (Balkanyi, 1971).

Hypertension has been associated with an increased driving hazard. In a 1970 study, randomly selected groups of drivers with arteriosclerosis, hypertension, rheumatic heart disease, and other heart diseases, were compared to groups of drivers with the same age, sex, and city of residence, without medical conditions. The arteriosclerotic and hypertensive groups were found to have significantly higher accident rates than those of the comparison groups. The rates for the other cardiovascular disease groups, however, were not significantly different from those of the comparison groups. Violation rates for all groups were comparable (Crancer and O'Neal, 1970).

Hypertensive drugs may also cause side effects that contraindicate driving. These side effects include depressed reflexes, somnolence, syncope, and others. See Chapter 8 for more detail. Complications of hypertension, and antihypertensive drugs, should be evaluated in order to determine safe driving ability.

The AMA recommends that persons with:

Class I licenses have blood pressure $< 180 / < 105$.
Class II licenses have blood pressure $< 200 / < 115$.

### E. Hypotension

Unless accompanied by syncope (faintness), hypotension does not preclude driving a motor vehicle.

## 5.3 Cerebrovascular Attacks (CVA)

Cerebrovascular accidents refer to those conditions where there is an interruption of blood supply to the brain. Eighty percent of CVA's, or strokes, are ischemic, or due to lack of blood supply to the brain. They are caused by an embolus or thrombus. Twenty percent of strokes are hemorrhagic, or due to leakage of blood outside the normal vessels. They can be caused by a ruptured aneurysm or hemorrhage from an arteriovenous malformation. It is estimated that each year 500,000 Americans have a stroke. Strokes are the third leading cause of death in the United States, and an estimated 2 million people are stroke survivors.

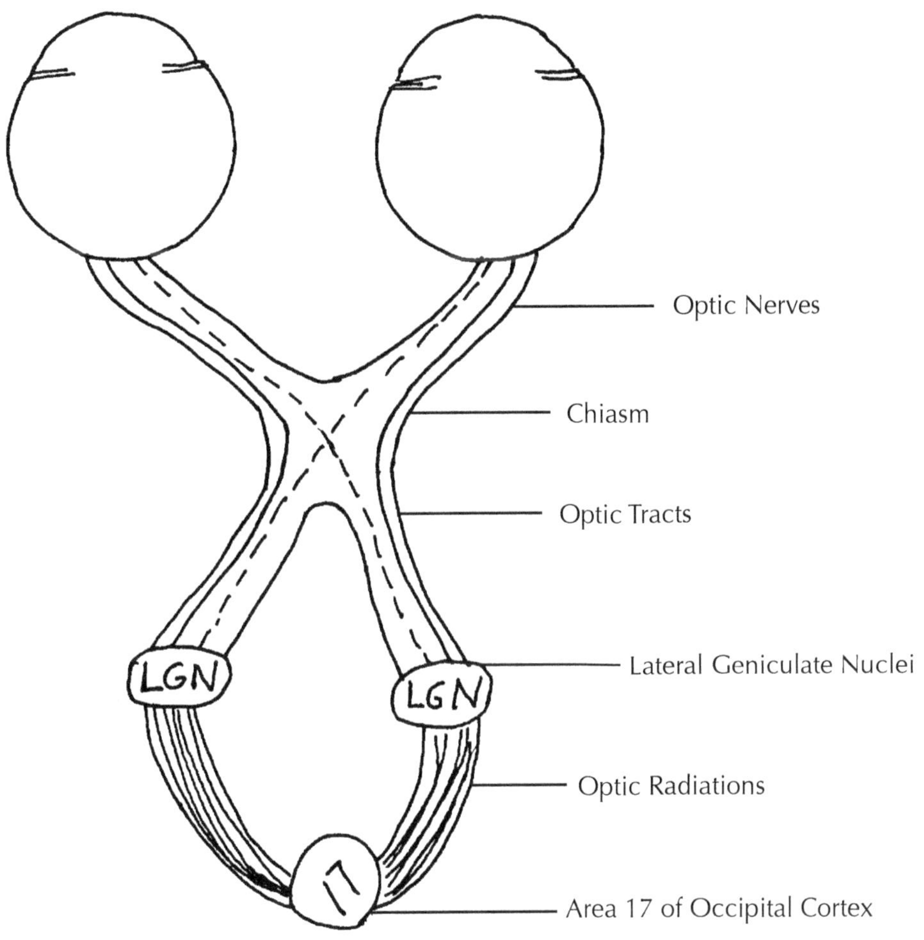


***Figure 5.1*** *Visual pathway.*

Brain tissue dies when it is deprived of adequate blood supply. Resulting disabilities that may increase crash risk include motor, sensory and behavioral changes, and visual and spatial deficits. Visual and spatial problems caused by stroke include visual neglect, and impairments in visual attention, oculomotor skills and visual fields. Up to 76 percent of stroke patients admitted to hospitals have visual and spatial deficits, which are a major cause of traffic accidents (Hills, 1980). In a 1983 study, stroke patients who had been cleared by hospitals to resume driving showed compromised driving skills and poor awareness of other vehicles. For example, these patients had difficulty entering and leaving the highway, driving in roundabouts, and performing two tasks at once in an emergency situation (Wilson and Smith, 1983).

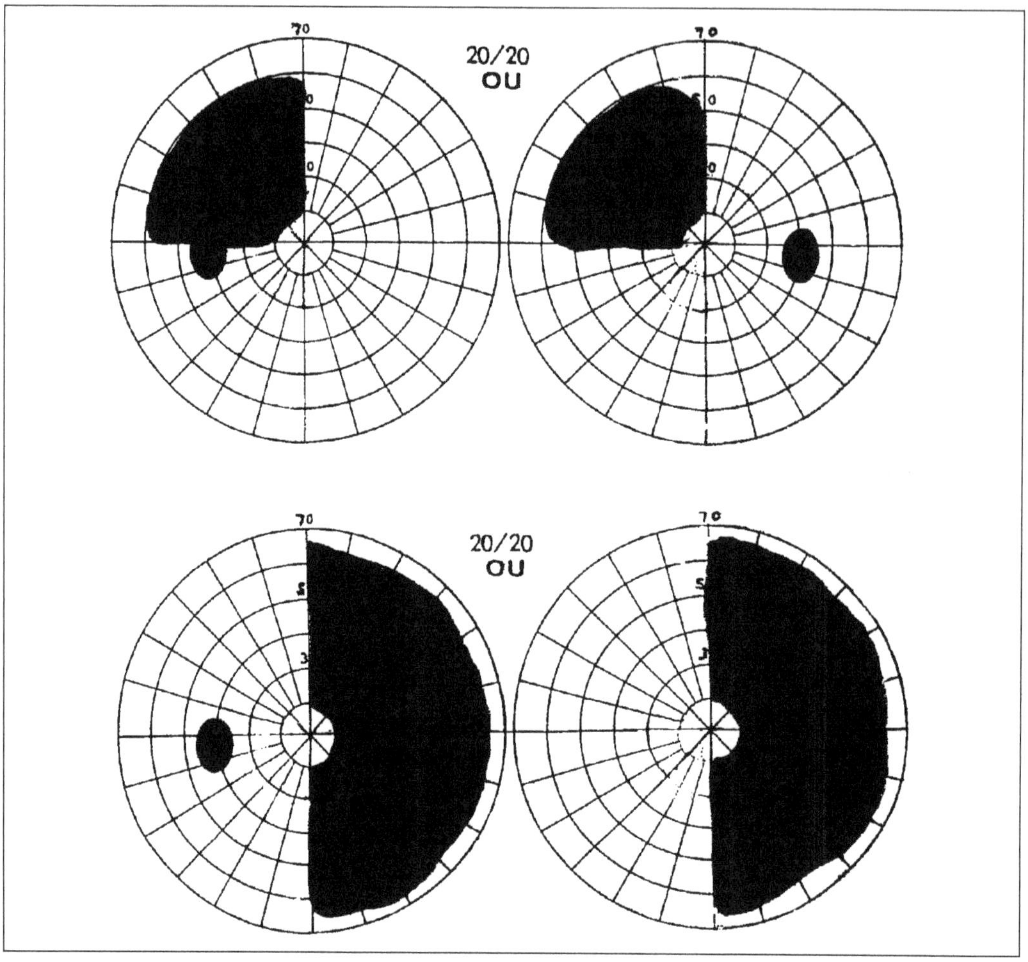


***Figure 5.2*** *Examples of post-CVA visual fields with resulting post-chiasmal lesions: left superior quadriceps (top), and right hemianopias (bottom). Both with 20/20 visiion. Notice how they respect the mid-line.*

Strokes may cause lesions of the nerves and pathways that control eye movements. Our extraocular muscles, which control eye movements, are innervated by cranial nerves (CN) located in the brain stem. They are the Oculomotor (CN III), Trochlear (CN IV), and Abducens (CN VI). Damage to them will most likely cause double vision, or oscillopsia (the sensation that objects are moving or oscillating).

Depending upon where the lesion is in the visual pathway, damage from stroke can affect one eye, or more commonly, one field of vision. Prechiasmal lesions will affect one eye, while postchiasmal lesions will cause hemianopias, or blindness in one-half of the visual field. In a study of over 100 hemianopias by Trobe et al., 89 percent were found to be caused by strokes (cited in *Clinical Ophthalmology*). Hemianopias or quadranopias may be extremely hazardous when driving. Objects or cars coming from the side can go completely unnoticed. See Figures 5.1 and 5.2.

Since the right cerebral hemisphere is dominant in visual and spatial abilities, while the left is dominant in language, we could assume that those persons suffering from right cerebral strokes would have more difficulty driving. In fact, this has been shown in a group of fifty post-CVA patients who underwent driver retraining: 74 percent of the patients with left CVA's passed the driving test, while 52 percent of the patients with right CVA's passed (Quigley and De Lisa, 1983).

If no new stroke occurs, deficits are stable within six to twelve months after the CVA. If antihypertensives are used to prevent future strokes, individuals can have visual impairments, drowsiness, light-headedness, and impaired attention in some (Toole, 1984). Stroke patients should be followed at least every six months with a visual field test, until stable, and counseled about their disabilities.

## References

Balkanyi, A., "Various causes of disturbance in consciousness important for traffic medicine," *Praxis*, 60(17), 532-534, 1971.

Benzodiazepine/driving collaborative group, "Are benzodiazepines a risk factor for road accidents?", *Drug and Alcohol Dependence*, 33, 19-22, 1993.

Bell, Emslie-Smith, Paterson, *Textbook of Physiology*, Churchill Livingstone, London and New York, 10th Edition, 1980.

Crancer, A. and O'neall, P., "A record analysis of Washington drivers with license restrictions for heart disease", *Northwest Medicine*, 69, 409-416, 1970.

Doege and Engelberg, editors, *Medical conditions affecting drivers*, American Medical Association, Chicago, 1986.

Hedden and Raffle, *Medical aspect of fitness to drive: A guide for medical practitioners*, Medical Association of South Africa, 1990.

Hu, P.S., Young, J.R., and Lu, A., *Highway crash rates and age-related driver limitations: Literature review*, Oakridge National Laboratory, Oakridge, Tennessee, 1993.

Janke, Mary, "Age-related disabilities that may impair driving and their assessment," California Department of Motor Vehicles, 1994.

Janke, M., Peck, R.C., and Dreyer, D.R., "Medically impaired drivers: An evaluation of California policy", California Department of Motor Vehicles, Sacramento, 1978.

Larsen, G.C., Stupey, M.R., Walence, C.G., et al., "Recurrent cardiac events in survivors of ventricular fibrillation or tachycardia", *Journal of the American Medical Association*, 271, 1335-1339, 1994.

*Physicians Guide for Determining Driver Limitation*, American Medical Association, Chicago, 1968.

Potvin, L., Guibert, R., and Loiselle, J., "Cardiovascular disease and traffic accidents: Weighing the evidence", *Journal of Safety Research*, 24, 233-241, 1993.

Reuben, D.B., Silliman, R.A., and Traines, M., "The aging driver: Medicine, policy, and ethics", *Journal of the American Geriatric Society*, 36, 1135-1142, 1988.

Solomon and Davis, *Human Anatomy and Physiology*, Saunders College Publishing, Philadelphia, N.Y., 1983.

Stewart, Moore, Marks, et al., "Driving cessation and accidents in the elderly: An analysis of symptoms, diseases, cognitive dysfunction and medications," Dept. of Pharmacy Practice and Department of Statistics, University of Florida, Gainsville, Fla., 1993.

Waller, Julian, *Medical Impairment to Driving*, Thomas Pub., Springfield, Ill., 1973.

www.cdc.gov/diabetes/pubs/estimates.htm. Natural Diabetes Fact Sheet, 2008.

# Chapter 6

# Vision Tests

Merrill J. Allen, O.D., Ph.D.

***Synopsis***



## 6.1 Introduction

The complete optometric examination will be outlined, and those areas of particular concern in vision tests for drivers will be discussed in detail. It is assumed that the reader of this chapter has a basic proficiency in making the tests so that the remarks can be directed to refinements in clinical testing and special precautions that may not be generally understood. This chapter is not directed toward the needs of the license bureau tester or legislator, although certain portions could be of general informational value. The visual and ocular examination (the "21 point" examination) is outlined as follows:

A. Case history:
  1. Chief complaint of patient
  2. Nature of work, lighting, distances, etc. associated with patient's activities
  3. Patient's statement of symptoms or history of ocular and systemic disease
  4. Medications, internal and external, currently being taken by patient
  5. Extent of use of alcohol and tobacco by the patient
  6. Patient's exposure to chemicals, both at home and work
  7. Scintillating scotoma, migraine and other headaches

B. Preliminary examination: A search for pathology or abnormality
  1. Visual acuity tests at distance and near, old RX
  2. Motility of the eyes
  3. Visual fields test of peripheral vision
  4. Pupil dynamics and the condition of the iris
  5. Lids and corneal health
  6. Lens and vitreous clarity
  7. Fundus study, inspection of retina and blood vessels
  8. Intraocular pressure measurements
  9. Photo myoclonic, photo convulsive, and photo phobic tendencies

C. Refraction
  1. Objective tests for lens prescription
  2. Subjective tests for lens prescription

D. Five fundamental variables of ocular muscle coordination
  1. Distance phoria (position of the eyes relaxed)
  2. Positive fusional convergence
  3. Negative fusional convergence
  4. Amplitude of accommodation
  5. A.C.A. (accommodative convergence divided by accommodation) ratio

E. Special tests
  1. Aniseikonia (difference in size of right and left eye images)
  2. Color vision
  3. Stereopsis
  4. Night visual performance
  5. Visual fields
  6. Reaction time
  7. Glaucoma (field defects, abnormal intraocular pressure)

## 6.2 Case History

If given the opportunity, the patient will tell what his major symptoms are and what he wants done. Through careful sympathetic questioning, most of the information needed about health, medication, diet, and intoxicants becomes readily available. Specific questions about driving should be asked, including what make and model automobile, the color of the hood and dash-panel top, and the location of chromium surfaces that can reflect the sky. Ask about seeing double at night, such as occurs by double reflection within the windshield. Ask if he wears sunglasses to drive; if so, take a look at them. They should not be clip-over glasses and should not be green or made of wavy glass or plastic. Ideally, they should be gray polarizing with prescription incorporated, with large lenses that tend to "wrap around" and with thin frames and high temples.

Ask if he wears night-driving glasses of any kind; if so, inspect them. They should not be tinted any color including yellow, except for the lightest shades of cosmetic pink. Green sunglasses, tinted windshields, and Thermanon all absorb red excessively and are not recommended for any driving day or night.

Does the patient have trouble seeing street signs at night; seeing against headlight glare; seeing with normal amounts of light in the home, in the yard at night, and so forth? Problems here can indicate increasing ocular scatter, as in a beginning cataract; the steamy cornea of glaucoma; increased light absorption; or pinhole pupils, all of which reduce the light available on the retina; or they may indicate a systemic problem which interferes with retinal metabolism, such as a vitamin deficiency or the presence of toxic agents harmful to the retina or neural pathways. Common toxic agents, carbon monoxide and alcohol, interfere with dark adaptation, accommodation, and fusion. Chronic alcoholism or inadequate diet may cause nutritional deficiencies.

Drugs of interest to inquire about are those that cause pupil constriction and accommodative activity (parasympathomimetic), paralysis of accommodation and dilation of the pupil (parasympatholytic), or dilation of the pupil alone (sympathomimetic). The *Physicians' Desk Reference* or equivalent will provide needed information on the effects of a particular drug the patient is using. The *Merck Manual* will provide information on what drugs are commonly used for what diseases. This will assist whenever the patient is unaware of what medication he is taking but knows the name of his disease.

Information on smoking is of two-fold interest. If the patient is a smoker of cigarettes about which he/she has repeatedly been warned, you know he/she has little regard for self or safety, and is also apt to be a less safe driver because of attitude (Adams and Williams). The second reason for interest in smoking is that tobacco smoke contains carbon monoxide. The street and highway atmospheres have significant levels of carbon monoxide as well. The adverse effects of carbon monoxide are exaggerated by altitude and alcohol, and consist of anoxia at the tissue level. Anoxia causes "red-out" and, finally, "black-out," just as positive g-forces cause these same symptoms in an aircraft pilot. Focusing ability is impaired, esophoria occurs, fusional amplitudes fall, and 0.50 to 1.50 diopters of accommodative myopia may occur. Asthenopia, diplopia, blurring, headache, and drowsiness can all result from smoking, or smoking combined with high levels of atmospheric carbon monoxide. In addition, the dark adaptation ability is impaired and the recovery from bright headlights will be delayed. These all produce a longer response time to driving hazards.

The need to know about environmental intoxicants is of importance for similar reasons. Many people do not realize that lead absorbed from food, drink, and from air amounts to 30 micrograms a day in the city for an average nonsmoker and 40 for a smoker. This can lead to symptoms of lead poisoning. Similarly paint solvents, gasoline, carbon tetrachloride, and many other chemical vapors common around the house and job can be detrimental to health. Hair sprays, hair dyes, perfumes, toothpaste, and other "harmless" items can cause trouble for some people. Symptoms often mimic eye disorders or cause eye changes.

Two classical examples are naphthalene (moth balls) and insecticides. Ingestion or long exposure to the vapors can cause cataract and accommodative spasms as well as wide systemic problems. Moth crystals, toilet and room deodorizers, isopropyl alcohol, insecticides, and cleaning solvents are common in many homes, with little thought being given to their hazardous nature. There are many other cataractogenic and systematically toxic chemicals that a workman may encounter on his job or to which a do-it-yourself artist may expose himself. They are all the more hazardous in spray form. Some researchers (Clark, 1993b) argue that toxic agents around the home and job can cause cancer, diabetes, AIDS, etc., by stimulating the growth of intestinal parasites (e.g., fluke worms, etc.) normally present in the body. Supposedly these parasites then invade the thymus gland causing AIDS, the pancreas then causing diabetes, the liver causing cancer, etc. Perhaps other conditions, like migraine headaches, can have a similar etiology.

The use of atropine and related drugs is common. Atropine and alkaloids are poisons that have some medicinal value. They have a parasympatholytic action, their effects are cumulative, and they require about two weeks to wear off. These alkaloids are available without a prescription in cold remedies (such as Contac), laxatives (Alophen Pills), rectal suppositories (Wyanoids), and asthma powders (Asthamador), among others. They and related compounds are regularly and freely prescribed for intestinal, digestive, and ulcer symptoms and to dry up mucous secretions. The effect of small doses over prolonged periods of time by self-medication or by prescription will most assuredly be worse than the illness it was intended to treat.

Typical symptoms are blurring of vision because of enlarged pupils and a paralysis of accommodation, dryness of the eyes, and asthenopia (visual discomfort) due to a higher than normal A.C.A. (convergence caused by focusing the eyes) ratio. Vague symptoms of eye distress, pain, and headache may be due to atropine-caused elevated intraocular pressure. Certainly, it is well known that atropine is a provocative test for glaucoma, yet apparently it is little realized that atropine anywhere in the body affects the eyes if ingested long enough. One interesting clue to atropine poisoning is male impotence!

Extensive use of alcohol is harmful to the liver, which is the important reservoir of vitamin A needed by the eyes. Tobacco-alcohol amblyopia appears to be due almost entirely to vitamin deficiencies. Night blindness and dry skin (xerophthalmia) with eventual corneal opacification, is the result of prolonged vitamin A deficiency. The effects of alcohol in some ways resemble carbon monoxide poisoning. The ability of alcohol to remove social inhibitions also seems to parallel losses of inhibitory behavior of visual pathways. Border contrasts, successive contrasts, and hence acuity and threshold visibilities are degraded. The increased reaction times and general disorientation of the "drunk," especially at night, make him, as statistics have shown, a poor risk on the highway, either as a driver or a pedestrian.

A record of a person's visual symptoms without pertinent questions about poisons, drugs, intoxicants, and nutrients is apt to prove misleading when one attempts to determine whether or not spectacles will relieve the symptoms.

Scintillating scotomas and migraine headaches have been the subjects of many papers and studies. Generally they are considered to be of little importance, and treatment is often only symptomatic. On the assumption that these phenomena are the result of vascular disturbances, the author has found experimental evidence that chewing niacin, vitamin $B_3$ in a 50 to 100 mg. dose at the first, prodromal visual symptom, will, in a high percentage of cases, halt the development of the scintillating scotoma and avert the headache that normally follows the visual disturbances. Recent medical evidence indicates that natural and induced migraine attacks can be aborted by increasing the level of serotonin in the system. During the height of the untreated scintillation phenomena, the retina has very poor sensitivity in the portions of the visual field affected, and may become completely blind for a short time. Since the scintillation effect usually starts as a small area in the periphery and grows over a ten or fifteen minute period to include a major portion of the field, often sparing the fovea, the patient has adequate warning of the impending headache. *Please note that niacin will cause a facial reddening, skin itching and a feeling of fever which lasts about 20 minutes and is a normal and harmless response to niacin.*

If relief medication is not at hand, the driver with a scintillating scotoma should not continue driving until after the scotomas have entirely disappeared. Even then, the migraine headache that usually follows would probably make driving unwise. A person with a history of migraine or scintillating scotoma should be studied carefully to determine whether a refractive error, aniseikonia, muscle imbalance or incoordination, or environmental chemicals could be contributing factors. Since many migraine patients have all but given up hope of obtaining relief from their malady, they may not know that relief can sometimes be dramatic. They should be referred, when indicated, for further medical consideration and treatment.

## 6.3 Preliminary Examinations

### A. Visual acuity

This portion of the optometric examination is a search for pathology and for hereditary, traumatic, or functional anomalies. The first test is visual acuity. While there are many factors that affect visual acuity, the test does give an indication of the general visual efficiency of the person at the test distance and for the test illumination.

A valuable aid to visual acuity testing would be an acuity chart with luminance variable from 150 down to 0.5 apparent foot candles. The Night Vision Performance Tester (Allen and Lyle, 1963) provides a suitably wide range of luminances, in addition to providing low contrast visual acuity targets which simplify the assessment of reductions in visual performance due to refractive error, abnormal pupil size, ocular scatter, and absorption in the ocular media.

It is certain that an acuity of 20/40 at high luminances will deteriorate, perhaps to less than 20/200, at night roadway luminances (Allen and Lyle, 1963; Richards, May 1966). Adjustment of luminance on a specific target, from too low upward until the target is just readable, provides a sensitive test for evaluating the effects of small lens-power changes or small changes in cataract density. Note: The Night Vision Performance Test was never marketed. Several other tests involving low contrast letters are available (see Chapter 12).

### B. Ocular motility

Ocular motility needs to be tested in all quadrants of the fixation field to determine whether a paresis or paralysis exists. Equally important is to watch the eyes track a moving target. Eye movement records may be taken with the Ober 2:Visagraph from Taylor and Associates, 200-2 East Second Street, Huntington Station, NY, 11746. A special pair of spectacles comfortably and quickly monitors eye movements while the patient watches a moving object, reads, etc., and it provides a computer print out for the record. A significant percentage of people are visually poorly coordinated. The result of general or ocular incoordination is easy disorientation, frequent errors of judgment, and ease of confusion, none of which is desirable while climbing stairs, walking across a street, or driving an automobile.

The value of testing for gross visual incoordination is that something can and should be done for it. The beauty of using an eye movement recording device is that the improvement in coordination can be shown to the patient, who will probably also have noticed a favorable difference in visual comfort and confidence. Gross motor coordination tests also give information about the visuomotor coordination and should be included whenever case history, examination results, or recent accident experience indicates a need. High degrees of esophoria or exophoria at distance are unusual. They should not be accepted as unchangeable. They should not be allowed to go untreated when the patient is likely to drive at night. Prism correction may work, provided ghost images from lens internal reflections do not negate their benefit. I do not recommend the use of prisms. Visual training is the best and can modify phorias favorably. When combined with spectacles (if needed), visual training can make a comfortable and safer nighttime driver.

If paresis (partial paralysis) is present, much improvement or even complete compensation can be achieved with visual therapy. If a paralysis exists, often enough rehabilitation work can be done to provide comfortable binocular vision in at least a portion of the visual field. An eye that has had muscle surgery will almost always show abnormalities of coordination and of muscle fields. Such eyes have been injured, and visual rehabilitation is needed just as surely as it is needed after facial and ocular injuries in an automobile crash. Such people should be studied carefully to see if it is safe or can be made safe for them to operate a motor vehicle at night. *Vision training is the ultimate therapy.*

## C. Visual fields

A number of authors have shown that glaucoma symptoms will appear in the central visual fields (tangent screen test) virtually every time there is a peripheral field restriction; hence, peripheral fields would not seem to be more valuable than central fields for glaucoma study. For this reason, it is desirable that a multiple-pattern visual field screening device be used on every patient regardless of age. The confrontation test is crude but often quite adequate to pick up extreme peripheral field lesions.

For drivers, the horizontal limits to the visual field should be tested on a perimeter or a screening device similar to those used in some driver licensing bureaus and driver training schools. Any loss in visual fields to less than 180 degrees is abnormal and is cause for suspicion of pathology. The driving limitation in some states of not less than 140 degrees of horizontal visual field is purely an arbitrary cutoff point for driver testing. A person with only 140 degrees of visual field has some kind of abnormality which may be in the retina, central neurology, or optics of the eye (usually lenticular). It may also be due to the field limitations due to high power lenses or even standard spectacles!

Since peripheral vision is essential to safe driving, any field anomaly should be evaluated as to its possible effects on driving. Even a reduction in the color fields for red and amber may be sufficient grounds for restricting driving. Fields are of little value unless taken through an adequate correction lens. The newer testing machines make testing and recording of visual field defects both easy and fast and are highly recommended.

## D. Pupil dynamics

The pupil can be a useful source of information to the examiner. A large pupil will provide higher retinal illuminations, and the pupils of younger people open wide at night. Since the pupil musculature is both sympathetically and parasympathetically innervated, it can show the systemic effects of sympathomimetic and parasympathomimetic agents. It also mirrors the effects of emotions, accommodation, convergence, light, mental activity, glaucoma, iritis, and neurological lesions. It even appears that abnormal binocular vision may cause an abnormal pupil size of one or both pupils.

An anisocoria which produces a two-to-one difference in image intensity between the two eyes will cause significant visual space perception anomalies (Lit, 1966). Greater differences can occur as, for example, in the early stages of monocular cataract formation with increased light absorption in the lens in one eye. Patients with image intensity differences between the two eyes will be confused by rapidly moving objects in the field of view. This is called the *Pulfrich stereo phenomenon.*

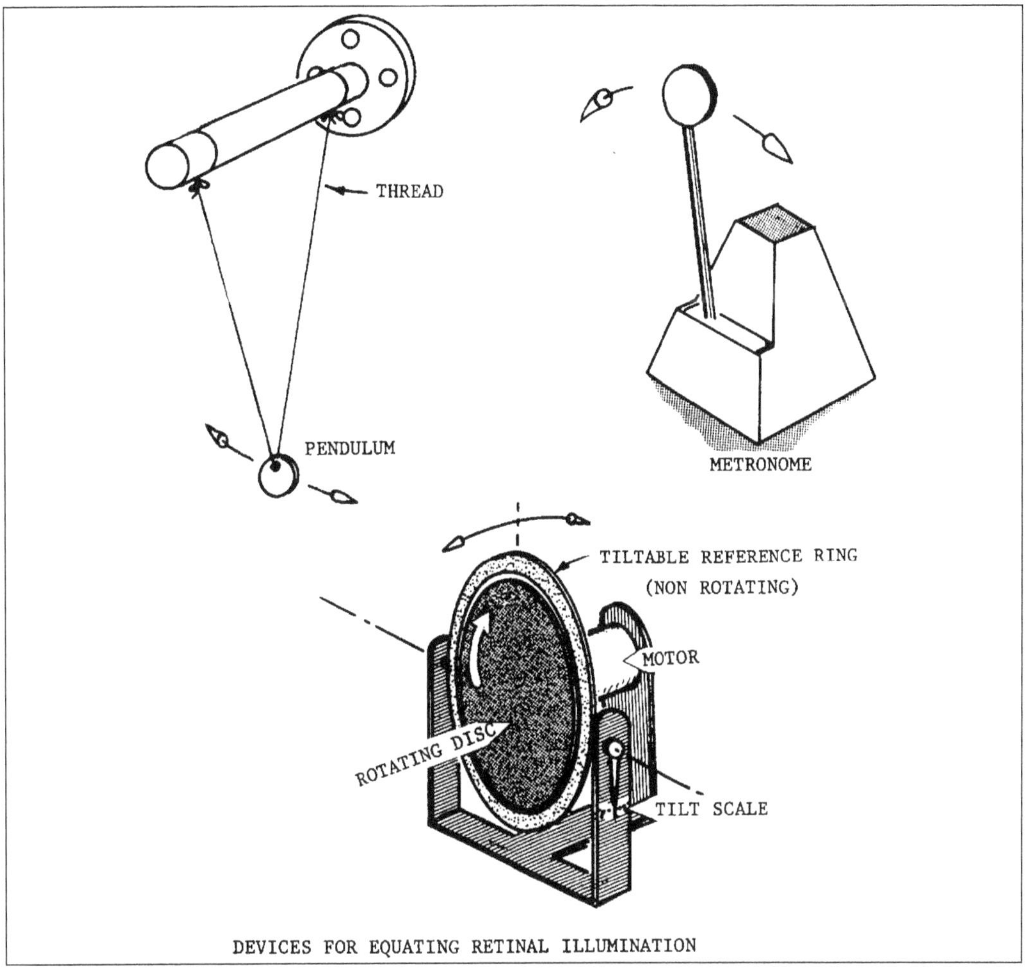


***Figure 6.1*** *Three methods for demonstrating the Pulfrich stereo effect. All involve a moving target and a difference in luminance levels at the two retinas, as by a filter before one eye.*

## E. Equating retinal illumination

Measurements of pupil size may not reveal the existence of a Pulfrich stereo anomaly because light loss may be due to absorption in the lens, to different focal lengths of each eye, to the presence of a neurological anomaly, or even to a blurred uniocular image which then behaves like a reduced intensity image. When any doubt exists, it is wise to test for the anomaly. Testing, of course, is unnecessary if the patient does not have good binocular vision with stereopsis.

Figure 6.1 shows a white pendulum which will move in a plane and be seen correctly by the normal patient. It will be seen to move in an ellipse by the person with unequal optical image intensities, with a lowered monocular border gradient due to ametropia or ocular scatter, or even with a difference in image size.

Figure 6.1 also shows the use of a metronome for testing the relative luminances of the retinas of the two eyes. A larger excursion can be obtained by casting a shadow of the moving disc on a translucent screen or on a large projection screen. The third device, a tiltable ring, rotating disc apparatus, offers a precise means of measuring the Pulfrich stereo phenomenon (Walker, 1968) or of balancing the two eyes with lenses or filters to eliminate the tilt of the moving disc.

## F. Lids and cornea

Lids, cilia, and the palpebral conjunctiva should be healthy and in normal relationship to the eyes. Evidences of chronic or acute inflammation should be treated or referred. Corneal hazing, epithelial edema, or purulent material in the tear fluid, are all contributory to increased ocular scatter and to poor night vision. In addition, such inflammation of the lids and conjunctiva may be symptomatic of vitamin A deficiency, which is important in nighttime vision. The cilia in an older person may turn in toward the cornea and account for photophobic symptoms, tearing, and asthenopia. The cilia may be absent, or not dense and dark enough to form a sun shade to help reduce sky glare, thus contributing to photophobia. On the other hand, the lids may droop so low that the cilia split the pupil into multiple pinholes, thus causing all manner of weird symptoms.

There is some evidence that eyelash cosmetics flake off and enter the eye, causing corneal abrasions similar to those from wearing contact lenses, thus producing photophobic symptoms. Hair sprays can also be a problem, especially for contact lens wearers. Exposure to ultraviolet light, as in snow fields, at high altitudes, in welding, over the water, in the laboratory, or under a sun lamp, may cause a painful burn of the corneal epithelium which, when severe, is called snow blindness. An ultraviolet burn is characterized by extreme photophobia. Iritis and uveitis are also characterized by photophobic symptoms. The post surgical cataract patient with an ultra violet absorbing artificial lens implant, is not likely to suffer excessively from photophobia. Cataract surgery requiring strong spectacle lenses, will cause photophobia because of the increased ocular transmission, and an increase in the effective aperture size of the eye due to the strong spectacle lenses.

## G. Lens and vitreous

The lens and vitreous contribute much of interest to the patient's symptoms. Excessive scattering and losses in transmission are usually lenticular in origin. Sometimes the cornea or vitreous or even the retina itself may be implicated in the intraocular scatter of light. The healthy cornea seems never to cloud up (Allen and Vos, 1967) even up to age eighty. Corneal clouding is usually indicative of glaucoma, vitamin deficiency, or interstitial keratitis.

The lens, on the other hand, shows progressive deterioration of optical clarity beginning in children. Vitamin C, the B vitamins, zinc, and antioxidants, along with good nutrition, offer hope of delaying or reversing the aging of the crystalline lens. Some encouraging results have been observed in improving ocular transmission and reducing lens opacity in selected cases using proteolytic enzymes. Since excessive amounts of proteolytic enzymes may have some hazard, studies should proceed cautiously.

The vitreous remains clear, unless uveitis or retinitis exists. Vitreous floaters, however, accompany liquefaction of the vitreous and are generally thought to be untreatable. Three points of interest are (1) the floaters are more conspicuous when a small pupil exists, (2) the floaters may pose less of a problem or disappear altogether after the patient improves nutrition and health, and (3) quick and large eye movements can often displace a large floater away from the fovea. Liquefaction of the vitreous is frequently found among those being treated for glaucoma with a miotic drug, such as pilocarpine. Iris nodules and other adverse symptoms may also appear in addition to the severe impairment of night vision by direct effects upon retinal sensitivity and by the extreme reduction of retinal illumination due to a small pupil.

## H. Fundus study

The fundus, the vascular and neural tissue lining the inside of the eye, offers clues to retinal health as well as neurological and systemic health. Retinopathies or other evidences of active ocular pathology usually must be referred for medical attention. Visual symptoms would be reduced acuity, reduced contrast sensitivity, excessive vitreous floaters, poor night vision, distorted retinal images, and so on. Patients with evidences of untreated hypertension, arterio or athero sclerosis, or diabetes should be referred for medical attention. A driver's license should not be permitted until cleared by a physician who is cognizant of the hazards of modern day driving and the probable risk involved of a cardiac crisis occurring during driving. Patients showing physical signs of liability to episodes that could render them incapable of operating a motor vehicle should be told of the seriousness of attempting to drive. Notification should be sent to the driver licensing agency if the physical or ocular conditions noted seem to contraindicate safe driving. Recent research (Michael and Allen 1994; Allen and Lowry 1998; Allen, Jarding and Zehner 1998) shows that nutrition and electrical stimulation of the eye can slow or reverse the symptoms of macular degeneration and even retinitis pigmentosa.

## I. Intraocular pressure

Intraocular pressure must be measured on all patients where symptoms or signs of glaucoma exist and on all patients forty years of age or older. Early glaucoma is not a basis for restricting driving day or night, provided the patient is not being treated with pilocarpine or some other miotic. However, when visual fields fall below 60 degrees to either side of the line of sight, the person usually should not be allowed to drive. Acute attacks of glaucoma (high pressure in the eye) cause increased ocular scatter similar to that seen through a lycopodium powdered plate[1] and will definitely be a hazard to attempted night or even daytime driving. In addition, the headache and nausea that often accompany acute glaucoma attacks would probably discourage a person from continuing to drive. Nutrition and general health should be evaluated.

## J. Photo convulsive behavior

High intensity light flashing at 15 to 18 cycles per second produce widespread abnormal central nervous system responses in a few especially sensitive people (Allen and Courtney, 1967). It is believed that one out of about 250 epileptic patients will have a tendency to grandmal or petitmal epilepsy when exposed to a strong natural photic environment such as picket fences, dashed highway stripes, or tree shadows, viewed while riding in an automobile or while walking. Helicopters at slow blade speeds may be a hazard to the pilot with photo convulsive sensitivity. Usually the person has no noticeable warning, loses consciousness and falls. The attack may last from a few minutes to twenty minutes or longer.

If the case history reveals any unexplained episodes of unconsciousness or other suspicious signs, patients who drive or whose occupations are potentially hazardous to themselves or others should be tested (Bickford 1948). A bright light viewed through a sectored disc chopping the light about 18 times per second should induce symptoms of an attack. Prodromal signs are a twitching of the eyelids and an interference in speech. In stroboscopic light, the lid twitching might be noted only by palpation. It may take less than ten seconds to induce an attack. Ask the patient to count as long as he can while he faces the flickering light. If he falters he may be nearing unconsciousness. The Translid Binocular Interaction Trainer which provides stimulation rates alternately to the eyes at 7 to 9 cycles per second is too slow and is not intense enough to produce seizures.

For therapy, treatments may be given consisting of a flashing light into both eyes while monitoring brain waves. Upon the first signs of epileptiform brain waves, the flashing light is turned off. When the brain rhythms have returned to normal, the flashing stimulus is again applied. Tolerance to flashing lights is thus built up in a few training periods. Without electroencephalograph equipment, the same effects could probably be obtained by a cautious treatment program starting with one to five seconds of low intensity light stimulation at 15 to 18 cycles per second followed by 30 to 60 seconds of no stimulation. An increase should be made in the length of time of stimulation or in the intensity of the flashing light at each succeeding visit. When the patient can withstand several minutes of high-intensity flickering light, he/she is probably beginning to be safe for driving.

There is also some evidence that red-free (green) light will not cause photo convulsions. There are cases in the literature of epileptics, uncontrolled by drugs, becoming symptom free after wearing red free filter glasses. The use of such green lenses should be tried. The hazard, of course, is the insensitivity to red signal lights while wearing green lenses. *No one should wear green colored glasses while driving.*

## 6.4 Refraction

### A. Objective tests

Retinoscopy with the patient looking at a distant wall chart, still is the foundation in refraction, even though a number of objective, automatic machines are available. The problem with these objective tests is the phenomenon called "awareness of nearness." The patient looks into a "box" which tends to induce accommodation (the near reflex) and is expected to relax the focus of the eyes. The usual error of these devices is too much minus lens power. Excess minus causes the further development of myopia.

For improved reflex brightness and a larger patient pupil, a blue free (yellow) filter (such as Corning's 3-67, glass no. 3482) could be placed over the retinoscope source. The older patient with excessive ocular scattering of blue light will be easier to scope with the yellow filter. There should be less than a quarter diopter difference between the scope findings with and without the filter.

A second item of importance to accurate retinoscopy is a spectacle made especially for the older optometrist to wear during retinoscopy. This spectacle should contain in the upper portion of the lens the examiner's distance prescription increased by the value of the usual retinoscopy working distance. A bifocal near add will be needed for writing. Such a bifocal prescription provides an unobstructed view of the phoropter and an in-focus view of the patient's pupil through the upper portion of the spectacle lens. The examiner must focus on the reflex in the plane of the patient's pupil for accurate retinoscopy. This retinoscopy spectacle will improve accuracy, and make the reflex easier to see.

If the pupil size is small, retinoscopy cannot be done accurately at the usual distance. By scoping at 33 or 25 cm. and by wearing the correct retinoscopy lenses as a fit-over to allow a clear view of the patient's pupil, the difficulties of scoping a small pupil may be circumvented. However, since ophthalmoscopy also is difficult with a small pupil, it is wise in such cases to dilate the pupils, using one or two drops of 10 percent ophthalmic Neosynephrine in each eye. Dilation should begin to occur within twenty minutes and be complete in thirty minutes. The effects should wear off in two to four hours. Visual fields should be taken as well as ophthalmoscopy and retinoscopy while the pupils are dilated. This will give a truer measure of field defects and, hence, of retinal health. However, for a driver's visual field test, the pupils should be at their normal size.

Another objective test, keratometry, can reveal evidences of elevated intraocular pressure because the cornea becomes irregular or bumpy at elevated pressures. This will cause the mires to look distorted or irregular and may cause corneal power readings to be different from time to time. A hazy corneal stroma or an irregular corneal surface precludes good visual acuity and suggests glaucoma.

## B. Subjective tests

### 1. Monocular

A patient with a small pupil cannot easily make the clarity judgments asked of him because of the large depth of focus and because of a reduced light level at the retina. Dilation of the pupil with 10 percent neosynephrine is helpful just as it is in retinoscopy. Raising light levels on the test screen and on the walls of the refracting room will also help. The refraction might be done with a cardboard letter test chart illuminated by about 250 watts of reflector flood lighting instead of the regular projector test chart. It should be apparent to doctor and patient that night driving should be avoided.

The generally useful red green test requires some care. The filters are subject to fading, which reduces the sensitivity of the test. In addition many filters, even when new, are not properly balanced both as to wavelength and total transmission. If the filters are a bright blue green and a bright orange red of equal brightness, you can be assured of good performance on the test. The red should actually appear brighter to a normal person, so that it will help the protanopic and protanomalous color defectives who are much less sensitive to red light. *High test chart brightness* will reduce the adverse effects of protanopia, and of the small pupils and greater media absorption in the older patient.

For the red green test, the projector's aluminized screen must appear dark when the projector is off, though the room should have 2 to 15 foot candles of illumination on the walls. The aluminized screen should be adjusted to reflect directly toward the patient. The projector lenses and targets should be clean and aligned to provide a high screen illumination. A higher wattage bulb in the projector will be beneficial. Caution: Some projectors cannot keep a high wattage bulb cool, and the optics may be damaged by heat. A change from 50 to 100 watts is a safe change and will give more than a two fold increase in screen luminance. Higher screen luminances as seen by the patient will speed up a subjective refraction and make it more accurate.

The fan dial test for astigmatism should be conducted under the right amount of blur, that is, the least amount to ensure control of the test. If a three line pattern and progressively more blur is used, the patient may first see three out of focus lines, then two clear lines, then multiple clear fine lines, and finally only a uniform gray area (see Figure 6.2).

Hence, upon asking which lines are clearest, one must also *ask how many lines the patient sees*. It is possible for the patient to pick out as clearest a pattern of two lines 90 degrees away, instead of correctly choosing the less blurred three line pattern which does not appear to be as clear. If a single line pattern is used in the sun burst or clock dial, then often two clear lines are seen instead of a blurred single line.

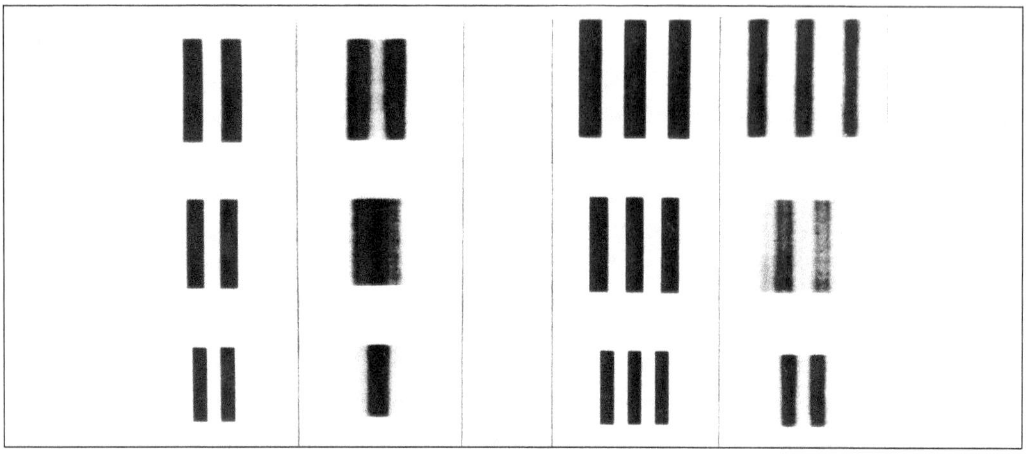

***Figure 6.2*** *One test for astigmatism uses a clock dial pattern of three lines at each hour position. The effect of blur on two and three line targets is shown. Constant blur with different line spacings, as shown, is like the effect of different amounts of blur on fixed line spacing, such as used in the astigmatic dial test. More intricate patterns can occur in a person's eye because the blur circle image for a point object is more complex than the image from a camera lens. A blurred image of three lines could look like a clear image of two lines.*

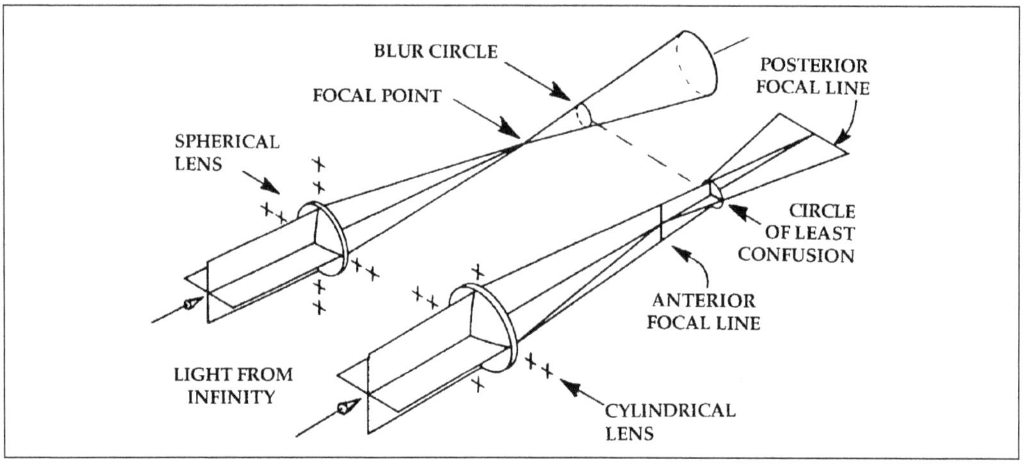


***Figure 6.3*** *The diagram on the left represents the focusing of a bundle of light rays by a spherical lens. If the rays intercept a surface such as the retina at the position labeled "blur circle", the light will be distributed in the circular area shown. In the diagram on the right the bundle of light rays is refracted by a cylindrical lens to produce an astigmatic focus. There is a position between the two focal lines which is called the "circle of least confusion" and resembles the spherical blur circle in the left diagram. The crossed cylinder test, properly applied, alternately increases and reduces the distance between the two focal lines and thus makes the circle of least confusion larger or smaller. This gives the patient an easy choice of which position of the crossed cylinder gives the clearest focus (smallest blur circle). People with astigmatism see things blurred but not slanted, as popularly depicted. The slant or distortion occurs when spectacles are used to correct the astigmatism. Contact lenses produce virtually no distortion.*

Similarly, locating the middle of the astigmatic interval upon the retina (see Figure 6.3) is critical to the success of the Jackson cross cylinder test. The standard procedure is to add +0.25 diopter of plus sphere for every –0.50 diopter of cylinder to keep the proper condition of "no blur." Similarly, if the patient keeps rejecting minus cylinder, add an 0.25 diopter of plus sphere and retest. If he keeps asking for more minus cylinder, give an 0.25 diopter of minus sphere and retest. Usually, this is enough to reverse the patient's pattern of answers and to bring them back into agreement with the objectively determined cylinder.

**2. Binocular**

The blur balance test is acceptable if the patient has good acuity in each eye, has equal pupil sizes and is binocular. If acuities are not the same, then a balance by blurring should not be used. The red green test chart used binocularly with vertical dissociation is a good test. If acuities are too poor for this test (20/40 or poorer), the retinoscope finding or the monocular subjective maximum plus sphere should be used to establish the balance.

The Turville infinity balance test is excellent as a means of determining the subjective and for checking aniseikonia, vertical phoria, and lateral phoria tendencies. In this test, an occluder about the width of the patient's interpupillary distance is placed halfway between the test chart screen and the patient. This gives the patient a view of the right half of the test chart by the right eye and the left half by the left eye. Polarizing techniques are available and the principles of testing are much the same. Though polarizing techniques simplify alignment, a serious light loss occurs which interferes with its use for older patients unless luminances are increased per the discussion in the section on Monocular Subjective Tests.

An effective "binocular" test may be performed with both eyes open, but with one blurred by about +1.00 diopter. The best subjective refraction of the clearer eye is determined; then the one diopter blur is moved from one eye to the other, and the best refraction of the second eye is determined

## 6.5 Five Fundamental Variables of Ocular Muscle Coordination

### A. Distance phoria

The phoria at distance is the position of rest of the lines of sight of the two eyes in the absence of fusional and accommodative innervation. The classical distance phoria provides the starting point in building and understanding the relationship between accommodation and convergence. Using the phoria as a starting position, the amount of fusional innervation needed for a given target will be proportional to the amount and direction of the distance phoria from ortho (eyes approximately parallel). The distance phoria, in turn, is somewhat affected by the direction, duration, and amount of fusional innervation as well as by classical considerations such as orbital fat, extraocular muscle size and strength, check ligaments, orbital shape, and compensatory tonicity innervation as from reading a book or driving a car before the test.

The distance phoria test involves zero stimulus to accommodation and to fusion. If a large distance phoria exists, or an intermittent tropia is present, the patient should be warned of the hazards in driving late at night where the conditions may approach a phoria test, that is, no stimulus to fusion. In many squinters, it is typical that the ability to maintain single vision depends upon keeping their eyes at their normal squint angle. Night driving removes many of the important visual orientation clues, and, hence, a squinter cannot be relied upon to remain fully compensated at night or in fog. A person who has crossed or out-turning eyes needs to have at least some vision training.

For exotropia and esotropia the cause usually is esophoria due to uncorrected hyperopia or to a high A.C.A. ratio. Thus the exotrope needs a plus RX for near, *usually with dramatic therapeutic success*, while the esotrope will require antisuppression and eye-straightening vision training, again with sensational normalcy resulting (see Figure 6.4).

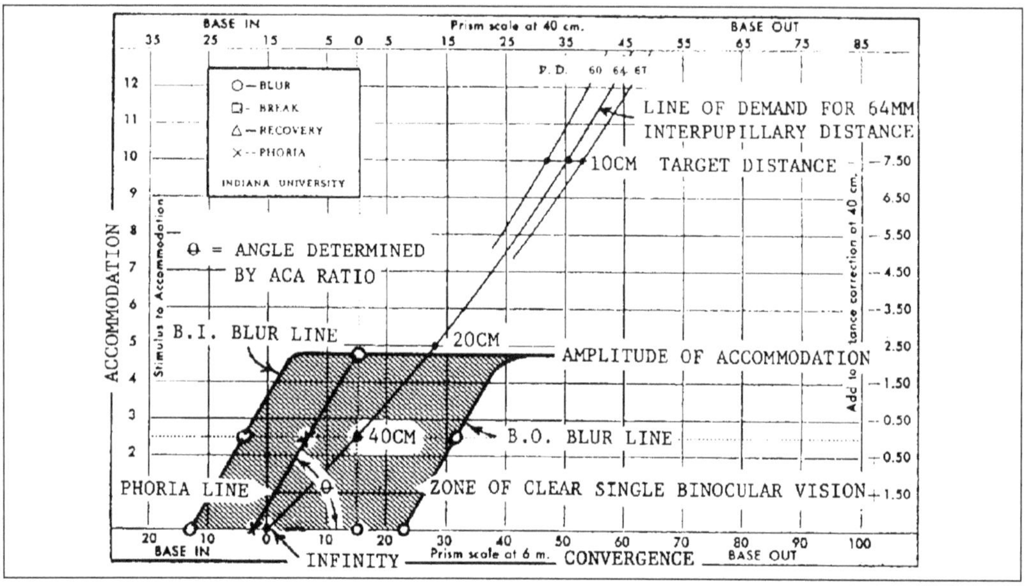


***Figure 6.4** The zone of clear single binocular vision is indicated by the cross hatched area. The hypothetical patient whose data are diagrammed here has a 2 exophoria, a base out blur of 23 prism diopters, and a base in blur of 13 prism diopters all at distance (infinity). At 40 centimeters, he has 8 exophoria, a base out blur of 16 prism diopters, a base in blur of 19 prism diopters, a plus lens to blur of +2.50 diopters, and a minus lens to blur of –2.25 diopters. The amplitude of accommodation is 4.75 diopters, and the A.C.A. ratio is about 3.33. The line of demand is curved because accommodation and convergence are not measured from a common point.*

## B. Positive fusional convergence

The ability to increase convergence from the phoria position without increasing accommodation is called positive fusional convergence. It is needed to align the eyes when an exophoria (out-turning tendency) exists. It appears to be impossible to induce fusional convergence by any means other than with a binocular fusional stimulus. It is a relatively slow posture adjustment, which is easier to induce gradually with variable power prisms than to induce suddenly with a quick change in prism. With the lids closed, the eyes tend to revert to the phoria position. Upon opening the eyes, a double image is seen until a fusional movement has occurred. Recovery findings in the blur, break and recovery prism tests, give some idea of the ability to recover fusion. For example, a high exophoria and a low positive fusional amplitude, as measured with the base out prism-to-blur test, indicates a need for a spectacle prescription, and/or visual therapy, and advice to avoid night driving until the condition is corrected.

## C. Negative fusional convergence

The ability to decrease convergence from the phoria position without a change in accommodation is called negative fusional convergence. Negative fusional convergence is the opposite of positive fusional convergence, and becomes important in visual analysis when an esophoria (tendency to turn inward) exists. A weak negative fusional convergence ability or a high esophoria or both indicates a susceptibility to seeing double under adverse conditions, because most adverse conditions, such as blur, fog, darkness, fatigue, or alcohol, tend to increase the esophoria. Visual therapy and abstinence from night driving are indicated.

## D. Amplitude of accommodation

The accommodative amplitude is an indication of the flexibility of seeing clearly at all distances. The amplitude is determined by how close an object can be and still be seen clearly. The lower the amplitude, the longer it takes to change accommodation and the more difficult it is to see objects nearby, such as the instrument panel. In some ways a reduced amplitude is favorable for driving, because it precludes the effects of accommodative spasms (night myopia), which may occur in an empty field, at low levels of illumination, after drinking alcohol, and after exposure to hypoxia or to carbon monoxide. Multifocals for dash panel and map reading are essential for safe driving when a low amplitude is present. They make an older driver able to read the dash panel quicker than a younger driver not wearing bifocals.

## E. A.C.A. ratio

The A.C.A. (accommodative convergence divided by accommodation) ratio is the amount of convergence change induced by a one-diopter change of accommodation. We know a great deal about the A.C.A. ratio, but we do not know how to make permanent changes in it. Pathological or pharmaceutical attacks on the accommodative mechanism can cause the A.C.A. ratio to rise. Similarly, impairments of the convergence mechanism will cause it to fall. Many factors are contributory, such as the strength and attachment of the medial recti muscles, the ciliary muscle size, the zonular fiber strength and arrangement, and the age of the lens in the eye. Even so, the A.C.A. ratio is surprisingly constant for a given individual year after year. (It does slowly increase with age because the lens in the eye grows larger and is less flexible).

Whatever the causative factors, an A.C.A. ratio outside the limits of four to six prism diopters of convergence per each diopter of accommodation is abnormal, and can contribute to discomfort in reading and driving, to learning disabilities, to myopia, and may even contribute to diplopia and crossed eyes under certain conditions. If the abnormal A.C.A. is of a transient nature, as for example resulting from atropine in medications for colds or ulcers, it is only necessary to wait a few weeks after cessation of medication for it to return to normal. If the abnormal A.C.A. ratio is a "natural" condition for the patient, appropriate lenses should be provided which may include a bifocal.

If a hazard of diplopia due to crossed eyes exists under low levels of illumination, visual therapy should be given to ensure that diplopia will not occur. Such therapy would include stress prisms or lenses, large excursion rotations, and eye-hand coordination training using a rotating pegboard and a training occluder (Oppenheimer, 1968) (see Figure 6.5). Stress prisms would be base in for a high A.C.A. ratio and base out for a low A.C.A. ratio. Stress lenses would be minus for a high A.C.A. ratio; but for an A.C.A. ratio of less than 3:1, stress lenses are of little value.

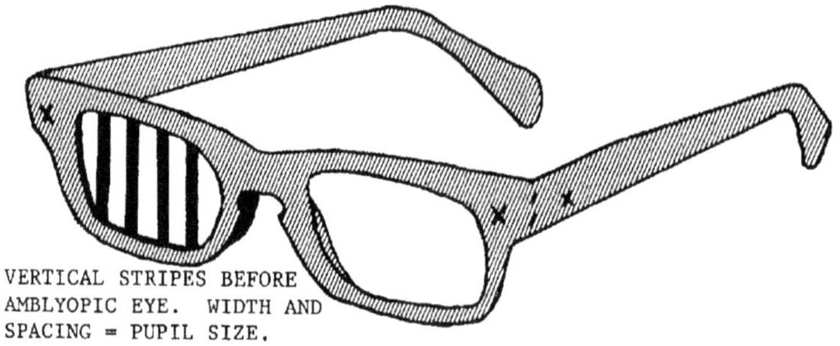


***Figure 6.5*** *Vertical stripes applied to a spectacle lens provide a unique stimulus to an amblyopic eye or a means of increasing binocular interaction. No serious interference with the field of view occurs when such a partial occluder is worn in contrast with complete uniocular occlusion. (Adapted from Oppenheimer, 1968.)*

A "new" and little understood concept is to use the patient's own tonicity reflexes to straighten the eyes as if surgery had been done. Once the eyes are straight (behind occluders), antisuppression and fusional training will permit normal binocularity to take over.

Eye straightening should be done as the first step in vision therapy before amblyopia or antisuppression treatment is given. By putting on increasing amounts of prism in the direction you want the eyes to go, and by letting the person interact with the environment for a few days or weeks, the eyes will adapt to the prisms. When the eyes are physically straight, put on binasal occluders for regular wear while you do the antisuppression and fusion training. You will have straightened the patient's eyes naturally without drugs or surgery. When fusion is reactivated by antisuppression treatment (the TBI), just remove the binasals.

## 6.6 Special Tests

### A. Aniseikonia

Aniseikonia is a perceived difference in the image sizes of the two eyes. It can be meridional, or overall, and can be a serious problem in spatial orientation. Aniseikonia is usually considered to be induced by spectacle differences, or differences in the lengths of the two eyes. However, photoreceptor distribution and cortical representations from the two eyes are equally important factors in aniseikonia. Indeed, like refractive errors and phorias, the wonder is that there are so few people with a significant amount of aniseikonia (5 percent or more). People adapt to their environment. Adaptation to a new pair of glasses is usually strangely distressing for a few minutes, hours, or days, but within two weeks it is usually complete. If a person has an appreciable natural aniseikonia, it is possible that binocular abilities have never been fully developed and that a program of building normal binocular function will permit a successful adaptation to the aniseikonia. Heavy emphasis should be placed on the maintenance of binocular vision while the patient does spatial orientation training, such as baseball, table tennis, or inserting golf tees in a rotating pegboard disc, etc.

In any event, aniseikonic spatial distortions, like chromeostereopsis errors, usually show up only when normal perspective clues are missing or are unreliable. This occurs in the leaf room[2] or behind the wheel of an automobile late at night, when other automobiles are seldom encountered, and when fatigue has reduced the driver's compensating ability. The symptoms of aniseikonia then will be illusions of going up or down hills, or being on a roadway that slopes to the right or left, or a combination of these effects. A sudden loss of normal perspective and overlay spatial clues could create a dangerous illusion for the aniseikonic patient when driving; this could result in disorientation, confusion, and perhaps an accident.

Aniseikonia is suspected when refractive and muscle balance corrections have been supplied and headaches or asthenopia persist. Further evidence is supplied if monocular occlusion for a few days eliminates the symptoms. The aniseikonia would then have to be differentiated from cyclophoria, lateral phoria, or vertical phoria anomalies, which can cause the same symptom complex.

It is never safe to rely upon assumptions about aniseikonia based upon refractive considerations alone, except where a person of known good binocularity has been comfortable and we are contemplating a change in base curves or thickness, as in safety glasses, or strong lenses after old fashioned cataract surgery. Then, we can use the present base curves, thicknesses, prescription powers, and vertex distances to determine intelligently these variables in the new prescription. Otherwise, the only safe procedure is to measure the amount of aniseikonia with an Eikonometer through the new prescription and to redesign one or both lenses as needed to bring the Eikonometer reading to zero.

Eikonometry can only be done if normal binocular vision with stereopsis is present. Binocular anomalies of suppression, anomalous correspondence, amblyopia, and strabismus can result from aniseikonia. But, persons with such anomalies cannot be tested with an Eikonometer because they do not have stereopsis. A technique based upon afterimages has been recommended by William Ludlam, O.D., Ph.D., Pacific University, College of Optometry. Have the person view a pair of parallel, lighted showcase lamps on a wall to induce an after image in the nonamblyopic eye. Turn off the lights. Occlude the after image eye and have the patient walk toward or away from the wall until the afterimages appears to be the same size as the unlighted bulbs. The ratio of the distance used to induce the afterimage, to the distance needed to make the second eye image the same size as the afterimage in the first eye, is the measure of aniseikonia in the meridian at right angles to the bulbs. At 10 feet, a one-foot difference between the viewing distances of the two eyes gives a 10 percent size difference; hence distances must be carefully measured and the test repeated on several different office visits if any question of accuracy exists.

The formula for computing the magnification ($M$) of a spectacle lens is as follows: $M$ = shape magnification × power magnification

$$M = \left\{ \frac{1}{1 - \frac{t}{n} F_1} \right\} \times \left\{ \frac{1}{1 - aF_v'} \right\}$$

where $F_1$ = Front surface power

$t$ = Center thickness of the lens

$a$ = Distance of entrance pupil from back vertex of lens

$F'_v$ = Back vertex power of the lens

$n$ = Refractive Index.

The ratio of the magnification of each spectacle lens should be the same as the aniseikonia ratio to be corrected, but opposite in sign; that is, the larger imaged eye would need the smaller spectacle magnification.

## B. Color vision

Dalton in 1798 wrote about his own color vision defect as follows:

> I found that persons in general distinguish six kinds of colour in the solar image, namely red, orange, yellow, green, blue, and purple. Newton, indeed, divides the purple into indigo and violet; but the difference between him and others is merely nominal. To me it is quite otherwise. I see only two, or at most three distinctions. These I should call yellow and blue, or yellow, blue and purple. My yellow comprehends the red, orange, yellow and green of others; my blue and purple coincide with theirs (Judd, 1943).

This lucid description of a visual problem clearly indicates the futility of designing a traffic-control signal system, based entirely on color. About 10 percent of the male population has a permanent color vision defect of some sort. One out of fifty can't see red light. It looks black! Very few females have any color blind problems. Acquired color vision defects from injury, disease and age also occur.

Color defective people tend to confuse red, green, and yellow signals, and the color vision defect may be slight or severe. Some tests for diagnosing the several types of color vision defects follow.

The anomaloscope is an instrument for mixing red and green to match yellow. The yellow is adjustable in brightness. An extra amount of red in the match indicates protanopia; of green, deuteranopia; and the ability to match any color combination of red plus green with yellow indicates absolute color blindness. Protanomaly and deuteranomaly are less severe degrees of protanopia and deuteranopia. The Nagel Anomaloscope[3] is the best known example of such instruments.

The Farnsworth 100 Hue Test[4] consists of eighty-five plastic caps containing a series of graded Munsell papers that the patient arranges in a sequence of look alike or matching colors. Errors in placing the colors in proper order give clues to the anomaly.

The Farnsworth Dichomatous Test[5] is less time-consuming than the 100 Hue Test because it has only fifteen caps that must be arranged in a sequence of similar colors. It gives a clear indication in most cases of the type of defect present.

The American Optical Company Hardy, Rand, and Rittler[6] (A.O.H.R.R.) Pseudoisochromatic test plates are perhaps the best of the book tests for color vision defects. Some indication of the type of defect can be obtained from this test, but this and other book tests, such as the Dvorine and Ishihara Tests, are primarily intended as pass-fail tests.

The lantern test in which the person is asked to name the color displayed, has also been used. It is possible that a color defective person could pass such a test by guessing.

In all tests, one must maintain rigorous adherence to brightness levels and the quality of light used to illuminate the test colors. The recommended lamp source should be used at the prescribed distance. Color vision defects should be noted and the patient warned of the hazards in driving. Color defective persons take longer and make many errors compared to normal sighted persons. If the optometrist is called upon to evaluate a person's ability to drive in the face of a color vision defect, a driving test is perhaps the only way to evaluate the ability of such a person to use the other factors that contribute information and make driving relatively safe in spite of color vision defects. Even so, night driving for color defectives might need to be restricted to well-lighted streets and freeways. A protanopic or protanomalous color defective is very insensitive to red light and will be handicapped when approaching an unfamiliar intersection or an obstacle like a car or truck showing only a red light.

The color defective may be able to analyze a signal light in the day time because the red light is placed above the yellow light. If yellow or green cannot be seen then the signal probably is red, or is not working. At night, when a person can't see the light's position, the primary clue would be the behavior of other traffic.

A person with a color vision defect cannot be licensed to drive a truck in interstate commerce. Japan has long discriminated against the color vision defective citizen in all walks of life starting in grade school (Tagayanagi). Only recently have the multiple, discriminatory restrictions begun to be removed in Japan as a result of Tagayanagi's work. The worldwide use of the Ishihara Color Vision Test indicates Japan's leadership in color vision testing.

Why should we continue to use a system that make second class citizens out of otherwise normal people? It is clear that as soon as possible we need to shape code our red lights used in transportation by adding a white horizontal band across every red signal. This will reduce the driving hazards for all of us.

## C. Stereopsis

Stereopsis is the three-dimensional depth sense mediated through the simultaneous use of two eyes. Stereopsis gives the relative distance of one object compared to another. Perspective and overlay clues are also very important spatial clues which work well for everyone, including people with one eye. Beyond about 3,000 feet, stereopsis is not helpful in judging which object is nearer because of the small separation of the two eyes and the stereo acuity limit of about 12 seconds of arc. In fact, one would expect that objects at infinity would be just noticeably farther away than objects at 3,000 feet.

Chromatic aberration in the eyes coupled with a displaced pupil can create the illusion that lights of different colors are displaced in front of or behind their true position. (For example, a vertical red line between two vertical green lines on a piece of paper, probably will appear to be closer or farther away than the green lines.) That chrome stereopsis is real, is another argument for adding white shape coding to red lights used in our transportation system. White is not subject to a chrome stereopsis error.

Normal stereopsis is highly desirable for maneuvering or driving a bus, truck or automobile when parking, loading or driving in closely spaced traffic. In such situations, the absence of stereopsis means that a driver must obtain spatial information from the perspective clues, from monocular parallax caused by vehicle movements and perhaps by head bobbing. Like color vision, a lack of stereopsis may be evaluated as to its interference with safe driving by a performance test in the vehicle under realistic or actual operating conditions. Stereopsis for high speed highway travel probably is not very important because viewing distances are usually great. Conversely, stereopsis errors in the judgment of the distances of red versus white or green can be very harmful at highway speeds.

Stereopsis testing can be carried out with the classical peg test operated from twenty feet by the subject pulling on a string to bring a movable peg into side-by-side relationship with a fixed peg. The clever ways in which air cadets have defeated this test are legend. It is argued that stereopsis is an all or none phenomenon and that, if you have stereopsis, its excellence depends upon such factors as the accuracy of the binocular vision correction. On this basis, a simple test like the stereo fly or the diastereo test (Hofstetter, 1968) is ample (see Figure 6.6). The latter is a flashlight with a frosted plastic face bearing three spots, one of which is elevated toward the observer. The test criterion may be a simple four correct out of six different presentations at different positions, since, by guessing, one would expect only two out of six correct answers. Hofstetter's studies indicate that those who failed this test, though otherwise normal in superficial appearance, later turned out to be squinters (crossed, or out turning eyes) who had been overlooked in the routine clinic examination.

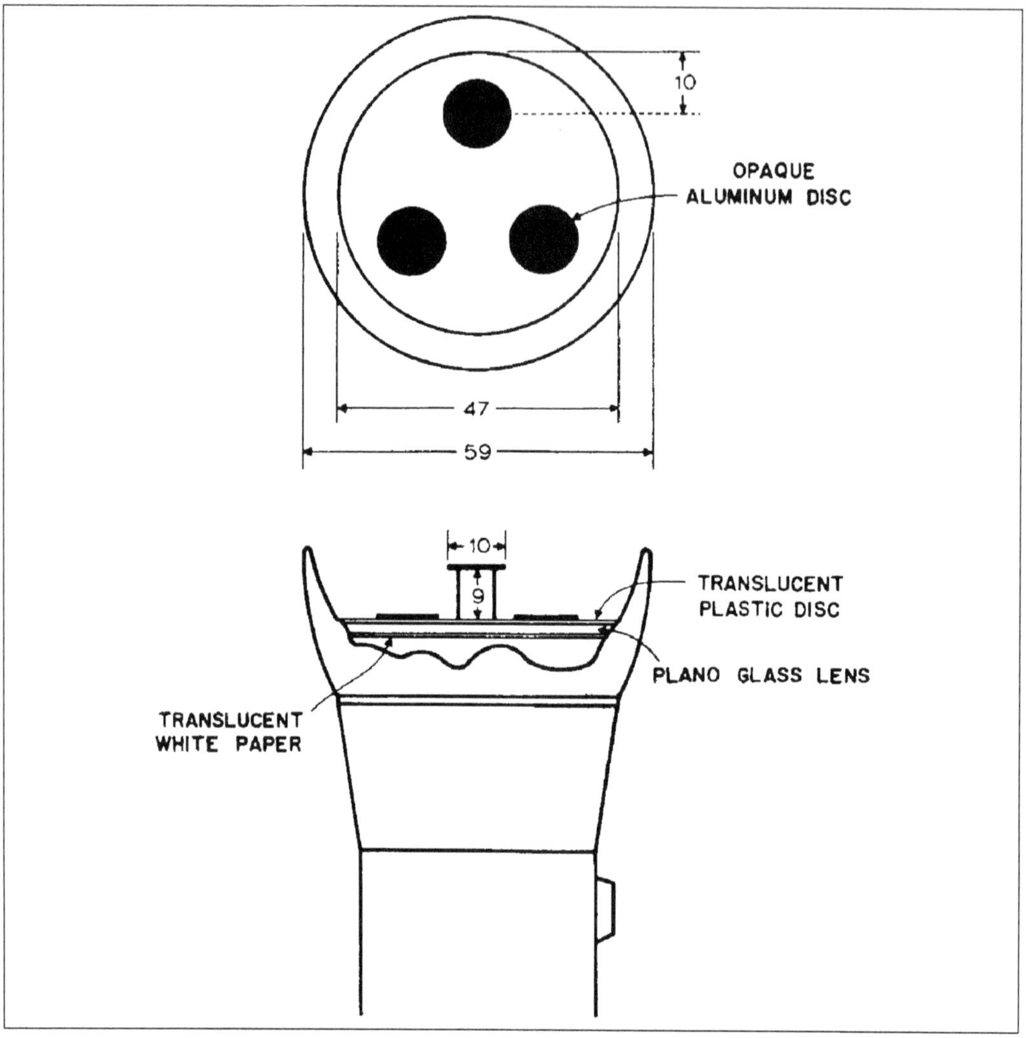


***Figure 6.6*** *Cutaway showing the diastereo test flashlight (the dimensions given are in millimeters). The top view is that seen by the subject, who must select the black spot that appears nearest. A criterion of at least three correct responses out of four presentations at different positions seems adequate to eliminate the chance guess factor, which could give a passing score in the absence of stereopsis.*

## D. Night visual performance

Driving performance at night may be significantly handicapped by the lack of light. This impairment comes about because of the following factors:

a. Reduction in illumination levels at night reduces the visual information available to the driver.
b. Lowered retinal illumination permits pupil dilation, which increases the optical aberrations and reduces the depth of focus.

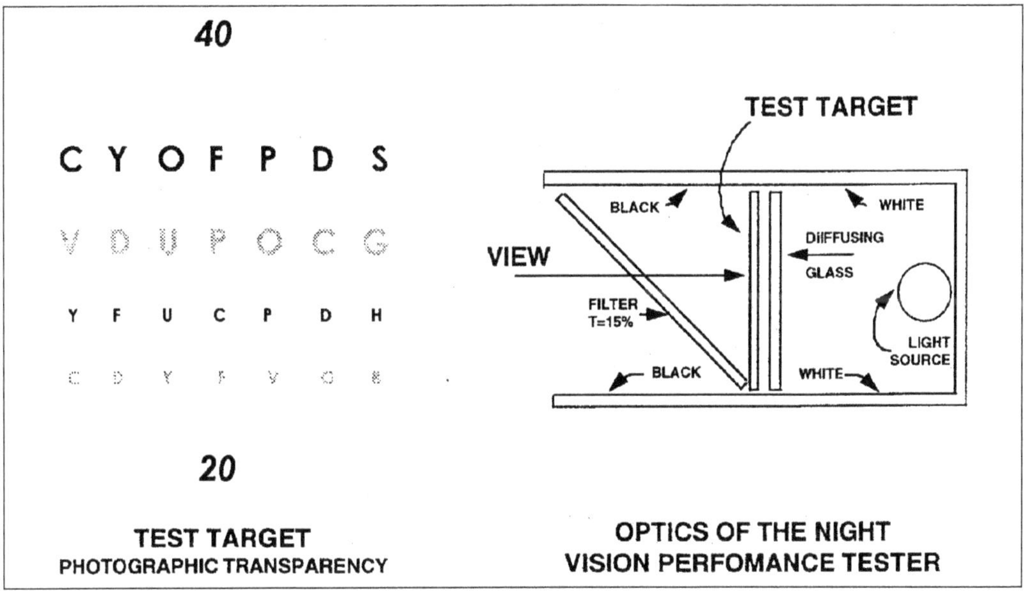


***Figure 6.7*** *The Night Vision Performance Tester provides high and low contrast test letters against a variable luminance background. By covering the chart with a filter, the influence of the room illumination is reduced. By increasing the lamp's light output from zero, the high contrast larger letters will be the first to be readable. More light will be needed to see the smaller letters and those of lower contrast. Similarly when the eye image is reduced in contrast because of cataract, blur, glare light, etc., more light will be required. If the pupil is small, or if excess light absorption occurs in the optical media (cataract), more light will be required. Low contrast test letters and adjustable brightness make this test highly predictable of night driving performance.*

c. Visual acuity falls with lowered light levels so that 20/20 by day will be considerably poorer under night seeing conditions. Acuity deteriorates more with some observers than with others, depending upon the condition of their eyes.
d. Brightness contrast sensitivity is reduced at low levels of illumination; hence easily seen objects of 5 percent contrast at room lighting levels become invisible at roadway illumination levels.
e. Photochemical dark adaptation makes seeing possible at the low levels of night driving. This process is adversely affected by pre-exposure to bright light even up to twelve or more hours beforehand. Hence, it is desirable to protect the driver's eyes from excessive daylight if good performance is desired at night.
f. High altitudes provide lowered oxygen partial pressures in the atmosphere, lowered oxygen tension at the individual body cell, and impaired dark adaptation.

Dark adaptation test performance is adversely affected by vitamin A deficiency, a small pupil, absorption and scatter in the crystalline lens, and the refractive error. The test performance usually can be improved by eating blueberries, taking taurine, taking a zinc supplement as well as vitamin A and other vitamins.

Since night driving requires many facets of vision besides the absolute light sensitivity threshold, called scotopic vision, and since nighttime driving is done at mesopic and low photopic levels rather than at the scotopic levels, a performance test at the levels of night driving, or a predictor of performance at such levels, is needed.

The Night Vision Performance Tester is one such test for predicting night vision performance. Figure 6.7 shows the details of this apparatus, which in essence is a low contrast 20/40 test letter viewed against a background of variable luminance and protected from room illumination by a layer of filters. The normally encountered room reflections from the filter surfaces are eliminated by angling the filters so that they reflect only from a black surface. Two instruments using this principle have been designed. One has a large luminance range and is suitable for office use in measuring age deterioration effects upon vision and in measuring subtle improvements in vision performance due to refractive refinements, diet, or medical treatments. The second instrument is a pass-fail instrument with brightness adjust ability sufficient only to compensate for light source aging. Both instruments contain photosensitive equipment for ensuring specified brightness levels.

Figures 6.8 and 6.9 show the deterioration of visual performance when tested with the Night Vision Performance Tester using lenses to simulate ametropia. Figure 6.10 shows the effect of refractive error upon nighttime visual performance in detecting a black or white obstacle the size of an automobile. Figure 6.11 shows the effect on the test scores of wearing filters.

The Night Vision Performance Tester yields a score in terms of the illumination needed to see a given target; hence, it provides a real indication of the light levels that will be needed for nighttime driving. The tester measures overall visual performance, whatever the factors: these factors are pupil size, ocular transmission, ocular scatter, retinal pathologies, physiological abnormalities, and refractive errors.

The American Automobile Association Glareometer contains a pair of lights simulating headlights and a series of target patterns to be identified. The lower the illumination level on the targets needed to recognize them, the better the performance on the test.

None of the above three tests has been evaluated against the actual driving performance of drivers at night, and, hence, it is not known whether one is superior to another. It is conceivable that they are measuring different things and that one may correlate better with driving performance than another. From the optometric standpoint, the Night Vision Performance Tester or equivalent would seem to be the choice for office use.

## E. Visual fields

All patients, young or old, should have a visual fields check at each eye examination. There is a good correlation between visual field defects and poor health. The mapping of a visual field is analogous to the neurologist mapping the pain and temperature sensitive areas on the skin and studying sensory motor reflexes. Such information permits the expert to pinpoint the location and the probable kind of lesion affecting the nerve pathways. With visual field mapping and checking for other neurological symptoms, brain tumors, abscesses, aneurysms, infarcts, and hemorrhages can be located or ocular pathology revealed. Because visual fields testing is so easy, few realize its tremendous practical value. For example, if "Glaucoma Day" screening efforts were centered around a tangent screen instead of a tonometer, the yield would include nearly three times more actual glaucoma victims than are now detected; and, in addition, brain tumors, retinopathies, cataracts, and such blinding systemic diseases as diabetes would be detected. Another bonus would be a drop in the overreferral rate for glaucoma from such screening.

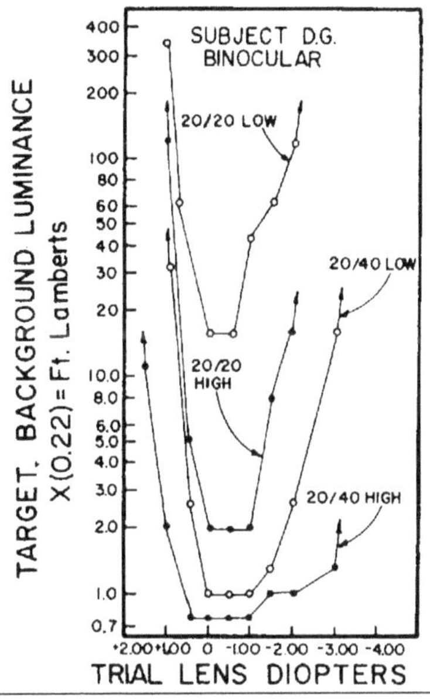


***Figure 6.8*** *The effect of simulated myopia (+ lenses) and simulated hyperopia (– lenses) upon the night vision performance tester back ground luminance for a twenty-year-old binocular subject reading 20/20 high and 20/40 low contrast letters.*

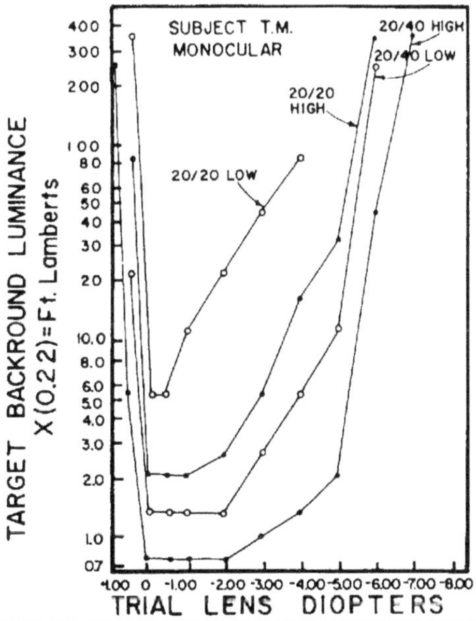


***Figure 6.9*** *The effect of simulated myopia (+ lenses) and simulated hyperopia (– lenses) upon the night vision performance tester background luminance for a forty-year-old subject tested monocularly. Figures 6.8 and 6.9 show the dependence of acuity upon contrast and luminance levels as classically shown in Figure 11.2. In addition, the devastating effect upon visual performance of blur due to refractive errors is shown as a need for more light.*

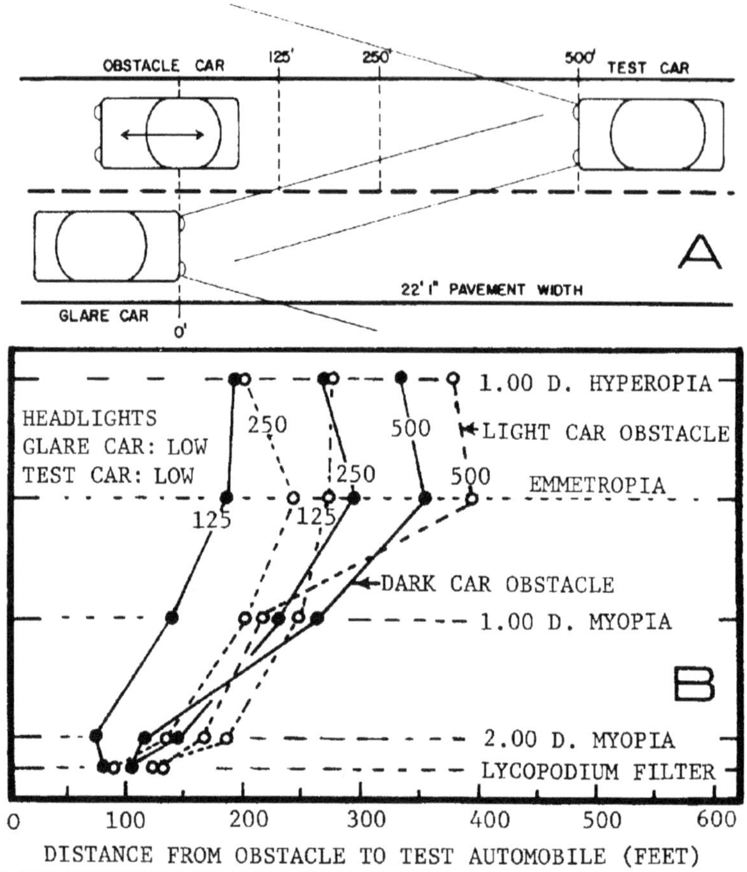


***Figure 6.10*** *Part A shows the experimental arrangement of vehicles used to gather the data in part B. The rear of the obstacle car faced the observer in the test car. A white compact car covered with a white cloth was the light car obstacle. A black compact car covered with a black cloth was the dark car obstacle. The test car was placed at 125, 250, and 500 feet from the glare car. The obstacle car was moved toward the test car until detected. Part B shows that myopia and simulated glaucoma and cataract (lycopodium filter) caused startling losses in the detection distance of an obstacle as large as an automobile. Even the presence of hyperopia reduced performance somewhat in this twenty-six-year-old subject.*

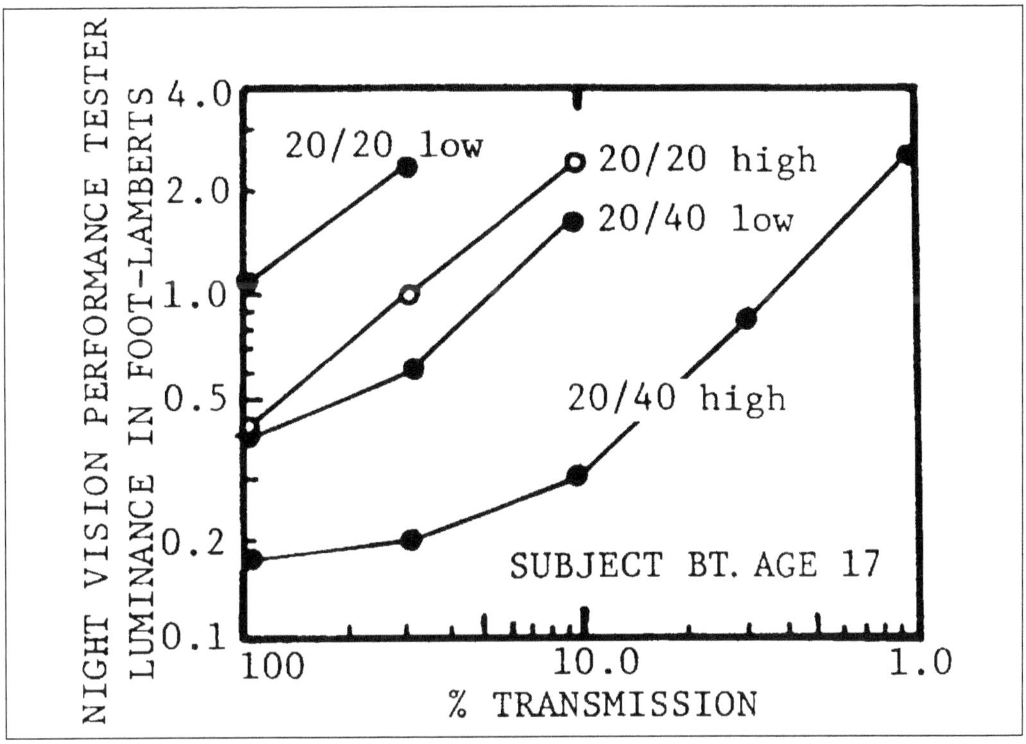


***Figure 6.11*** *The effect of a reduced ocular transmission with age is simulated with neutral density filters before the eyes of a seventeen-year-old subject. One possible reason that a straight line relationship was not obtained is that the pupil tends to compensate for the lowered retinal luminance occurring with the filters. Increased ocular absorption should thus be detected with this instrument. Since about twice as much light is needed to perform the same visual task for each thirteen-year increase in age, a lifetime can cause a need for over 50 times more light compared to a thirteen-year-old. Yet Figure 7.5 shows that the actual transmission change of the eye between a two-year-old and a seventy-five-year-old is not likely to exceed 2.5 times. Probably a degradation in optical image quality and retinal function and a change in pupil size accounts for needing twice the amount of light for every thirteen years of age.*

Projection, self recording, tangent screens; projection photographic recording screens; and pantographic self recording screens are now available to simplify and speed the tangent screen test.

The driver licensing requirement is usually 140 degrees of visual field. Optometric examination can establish the amount of the field defect, its significance for treatment and the possible need to stop driving.

## F. Reaction time

A reaction time test gives information on the total performance potential of an individual. If a sharp, bright retinal image is received and if the neurological components between the eye and the responding skeletal muscles are operating at optimum efficiency, the patient will have a fast reaction time. On the other hand, a blurred, low contrast, low intensity retinal image reduces the strength of the input signal and the reaction time will be longer. Similarly alcohol, drugs, fatigue, and cortical ischemia due to arteriosclerosis or atherosclerosis, will cause a longer reaction time. If, in addition, there is neurological damage or loss of tissue, the reaction time will be further lengthened. Normal young active people have simple visual reaction times, after some practice, of between 0.18 and 0.20 second. If a sound signal is present, the reaction time may become primarily auditory and speed up to 0.15 second. In experimental situations on the highway, visual reaction times from signal change to brake application exceeds 0.5 second. In normal highway traffic, the average reaction time to a clearly visible hazard is 1.64 seconds. 90 percent of all drivers will respond in 2.5 seconds.

Since the reaction time cuts across so many functional systems and gives a measure of performance which can reflect on driving ability, it seems reasonable that licensing agencies should begin testing visual reaction times. Police doing accident investigation could measure driver reaction times as well as blood alcohol levels. It is a simple test, and it will undoubtedly rise to a position of importance in license bureau testing and in optometric offices.

*All detrimental factors in driving, e.g., rain, darkness, excess traffic, poor acuity, defective color vision, etc., can be thought of in terms of an increased reaction time!*

## G. Glaucoma

Optometric testing for glaucoma should include the case history, the optometric examination, the use of some test for visual fields, and the use of a tonometer. Reputable authorities classify chronic simple glaucoma as a symptom and not a disease in its own right. Authorities also agree that it is not clear whether increased intraocular pressure causes the visual field defects, or whether the process causing the field defects is also causing the elevated pressures, which are often, but not always, observed.

Since so little agreement exists on the association of a markedly elevated pressure in the eye with peripheral vision loss, it is essential that a glaucoma detection procedure, or a blindness prevention program, rely upon the case history, fundus examination, central vision, and visual field studies as important prognosticators of health. The tonometer must also be used, for it may indicate an abnormality not noted by any of the other procedures.

The presence of glaucoma presupposes visual field defects, either partial or total. Field defects can make driving hazardous. The larger the defect, and the more it involves both eyes, the more handicapping it is. Glaucoma, using the word to mean elevated pressure, is associated with increased light glare, mostly from the cornea. Stressing the cornea causes a distortion of stromal fibers, reduces corneal transparency and increases the amount of scattered light. The increase in scatter is proportional to the increase in pressure within the eye; hence, a slit lamp or ophthalmoscopic view showing increased corneal scatter, should suggest increased intraocular pressure. Except in an active inflammatory process (or residual clouding from an old one) almost no other cause for increased corneal clouding is commonly encountered. When the pressure reverts to normal ranges, the clouding usually clears up.

Glaucoma affects driving ability by causing visual field defects, by increased ocular scatter, and by reduced night vision capability. The patient treated for glaucoma with pilocarpine has a small pupil which reduces retinal illumination to about 11 percent, assuming a pilocarpine pupil of 2 millimeters compared to the 6 millimeter pupil which is normal under night driving conditions. There is also some evidence that pilocarpine has an adverse effect upon the retina itself. This will further interfere with night vision. One-eyed treatment with pilocarpine will cause severe spatial distortions both by day and night due to the difference in brightness of the right eye, left eye images (the Pulfrich effect).

The treatment of glaucoma by a sympathomimetic drug such as neosyneph-rine causes a large pupil, so there is no handicap for night driving. Combination drugs are available which keep a fairly normal pupil size. Diamox given by mouth will hold pressures in line for long periods, while glycerin given by mouth or intravenously is useful in lowering intraocular pressure in a crisis. *All such treatments are treatments of the symptoms of glaucoma.* For a cure, it appears that other health factors must be evaluated and improved as needed. Improved nutrition and exercise have been shown to favorably affect intraocular pressure.

## Endnotes

1. Made by dusting lycopodium powder over a clean plate of glass bearing a thin film of petroleum jelly and then covering it with a clean cover glass. Lycopodium powder should be available from a pharmacist.

2. The leaf room is a test room whose square corners and flat surfaces have been covered over with leaves hanging by their stems so that the normal appearance of the room is obliterated. Under such conditions, space distortions often become apparent, because the subject does not know what the room is supposed to look like.

3. Distributed in U.S. by Alfred P. Poll, 410 West 55th Street, New York, N.Y., 10019. A similar instrument has been manufactured by Bausch and Lomb Optical Company, Ophthalmic Division, 635 St. Paul Street, Rochester, N.Y., 14602.

4. Munsell Color Corporation Inc., 2441 North Calvert Street, Baltimore, Md., 21218.

5. The Psychological Corporation, 304 East 45th Street, New York, N.Y., 10017.

6. The American Optical Company, Instrument Division, Buffalo, N.Y., 14215.

# Chapter 7

# Eye Disease and Highway Safety

Leslie Weintraub, O.D.

*Synopsis*



## 7.1 Introduction

Most eye diseases cause a reduction in contrast sensitivity, and an increased sensitivity to glare. Since visibility and conspicuity must always be evaluated when reconstructing motor vehicle accidents, contrast sensitivity and glare are major factors. Did the driver see the other motorist, pedestrian, road sign, etc., or not? Visual acuity measurements alone will not determine this. Contrast, glare and other factors need to be evaluated. If a person has decreased contrast sensitivity, decreased color vision and/or increased glare, it may be clearly determined that they could not see the obstruction in the road. This is especially significant in the presence of adverse weather conditions, such as rain, snow, or fog. Water on the pavement alone reduces its contrast by a factor of 5 to 10 times. A person with already reduced visual function may be "blinded" by this. Therefore, in order to evaluate one's ability to drive, ocular disease is a major concern.

## 7.2 Corneal Dystrophies/Degeneration/Scars

The cornea is the first surface through which light enters the eye. It is normally transparent, and regular, or undistorted in shape. The transparency and smooth curvature of the cornea allows the light rays to enter the eye, and bend clearly toward the retina. Any central corneal dystrophies, degenerations or scarring will blur vision by causing aberrations through the irregular or hazy surface. This will decrease visual acuity and increase glare.

## 7.3 Cataracts

Cataracts are any opacity in the lens of the eye. Most commonly, they are age related, but they can also result from trauma, long term oral steroid use, diabetes and other causes. Cataracts diffuse, scatter and back-reflect the light that enters the eye. This means that many aberrant light rays reach the retina, thereby increasing glare and causing a general decrease in visual acuity, contrast sensitivity, and possibly color vision.

A very common complaint of cataract patients is glare from light distortion and "halos" while driving at night. These people commonly suffer from posterior subcapsular type of cataracts, or opacities in the posterior subcapsular region of the lens, which is toward the back of the lens. These people will tend to see better under moderate to subdued lighting conditions, since reflex dilation of their pupils will allow more light to enter the eyes.

Visual acuity in persons with cataracts decreases significantly more than in those without cataracts, when exposed to glaring circumstances. For example, sun reflection, headlights from an oncoming car, and fog will decrease visual acuity and contrast sensitivity at all spatial frequencies even more in persons with cataracts than in persons without. In fact, of all ocular pathologies, cataracts and glaucoma produce the most marked reductions in contrast sensitivity (National Research Council cited in Janke). A person with 20/20 visual acuity, and no cataracts, may "glare" to 20/40, while the person with 20/20 visual acuity and cataracts, may glare to 20/80. Since our contrast sensitivity normally drops off at low spatial frequencies, a low spatial frequency object, such as a truck, will be even more difficult to see through cataracts. This is why, in low contrast circumstances such as fog, an older person may not see a truck. Figure 7.1, adapted from "Dynamic Visual Contrast Sensitivity" (Liebowitz et al.), shows dramatic differences in contrast sensitivity between older and younger drivers, especially in glare conditions.

Cataracts significantly reduce night vision. Night driving and the ability to make out traffic signs becomes much more difficult. For example, an improperly placed traffic sign, or one with poor contrast, will be difficult to see. Low contrast objects will be difficult to view, and in combination with headlight glare, may become completely washed out.

Another possible symptom of cataracts is loss of color vision. "Yellowing" of objects is particularly common in those with nuclear sclerotic cataracts. Nuclear sclerosis, or a yellow to brunescent type discoloration the lens, causes the shorter blue and violet wavelengths to be absorbed, while the longer red and yellow wavelengths are transmitted. A brown or black lens can cause extensive color vision loss.

Patients with nuclear sclerosis also tend to become more nearsighted, and need frequent changes in their eyeglass prescriptions. Cortical opacities, on the other hand, may increase farsightedness. Also, different refractive indexes of the lens may even induce monocular diplopia, or two different images in one eye. This is due to a beam-splitting effect.

Cataracts can cause mild to severe impairments in visual-related driving skills. However, after successful cataract extraction with intraocular implants, these impairments are usually completely resolved.

## 7.4 Glaucoma

Glaucoma is a disease marked by increased intraocular pressure, optic nerve atrophy and visual field loss. This last characteristic, visual field loss, is the most detrimental to driving ability. Since objects of surprise, like a child running after his ball, usually appear from the sides, our peripheral vision is extremely important (see Figure 7.2).

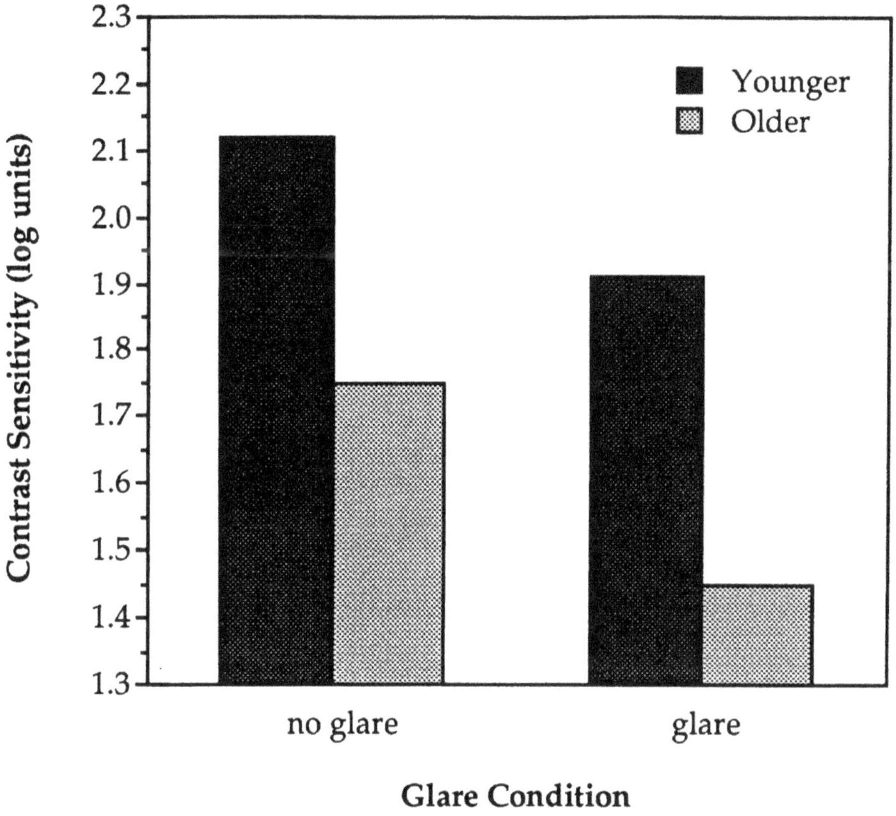


*Figure 7.1 Mean contrast sensitivity for younger men (mean age of 25.7 years) and older (mean age of 68.3 years) observers for the glare and non-glare conditions.*

The amount of peripheral vision loss in a glaucoma patient varies from none to an absolute loss. Generally, we see reductions of sensitivity in various areas of the visual field. This can translate into prolonged reaction times. Johnson and Keltner screened 10,000 volunteers with an automated visual field machine. They found that approximately 13 percent of drivers above 65 years of age showed field loss, and 3.5 percent of them were severe. The most common cause of these visual field losses were glaucoma, retinal disorders and cataracts. They also found that drivers with binocular field loss have traffic accident and conviction rates twice as high as those with normal visual fields, over their three year test (Johnson and Keltner, 1983).

Persons with glaucomatous changes in their peripheral vision will have most difficulties driving at night. The rods, which are used for night vision, are the photoreceptors located in the peripheral retina that are most damaged by glaucoma. Also, contrast sensitivity is markedly reduced in persons with glaucoma (National Research Council, 1987).

## 7.5 Peripheral Visual Field Loss

Visual field tests are not routinely required in order to obtain a driver's license. States usually require a 100–140 degree field of vision with both eyes for a class III drivers license, but rarely test. Also, states do not specify how sensitive that visual field needs to be.

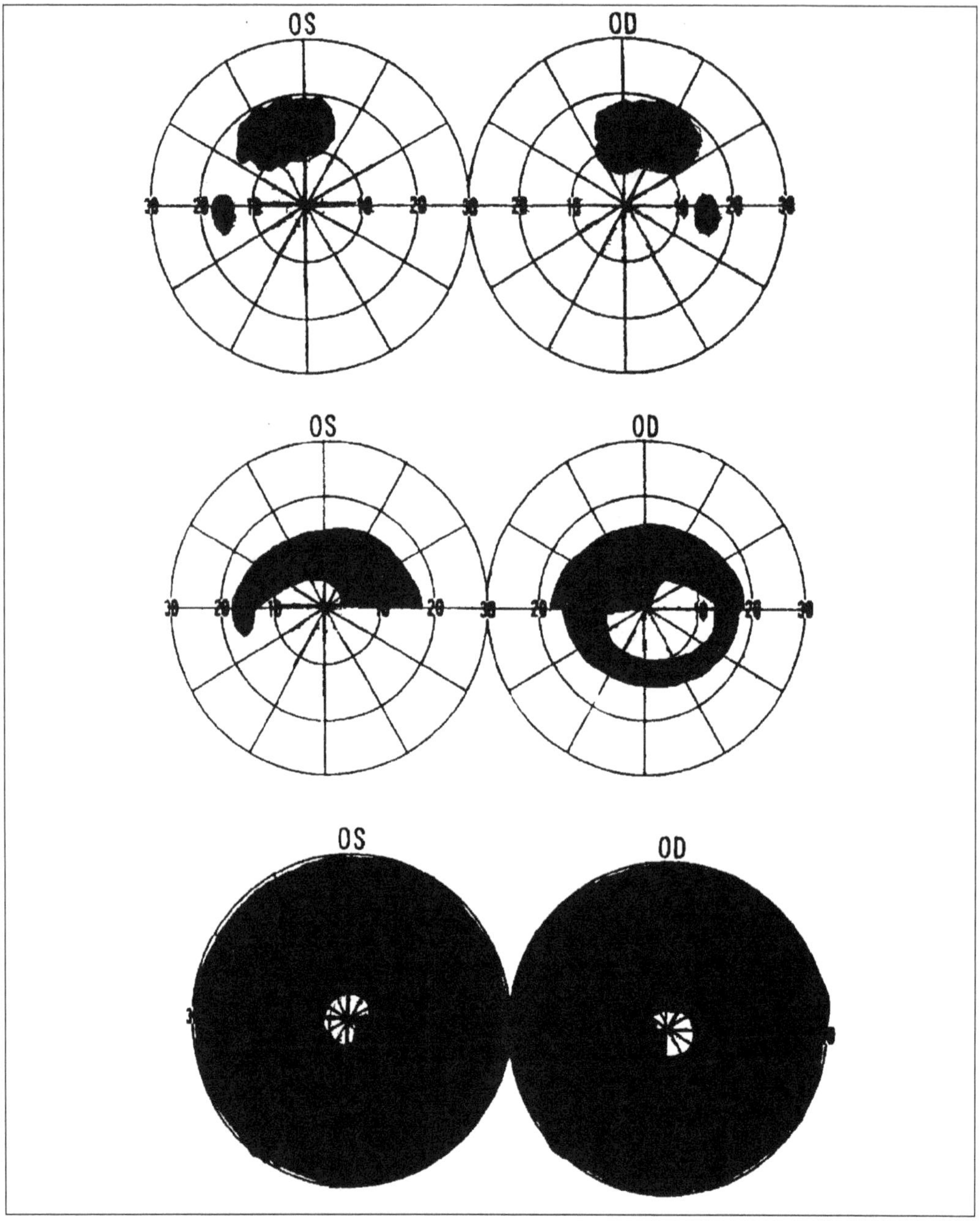


***Figure 7.2*** *Examples of glaucomatous visual fields: Paracentral scotmas (top), Bjerrum or arcuate type scotomas (middle), and advanced glaucomatous fields (bottom). All have 20/20 central vision. Notice how they do not respect the mid-line.*

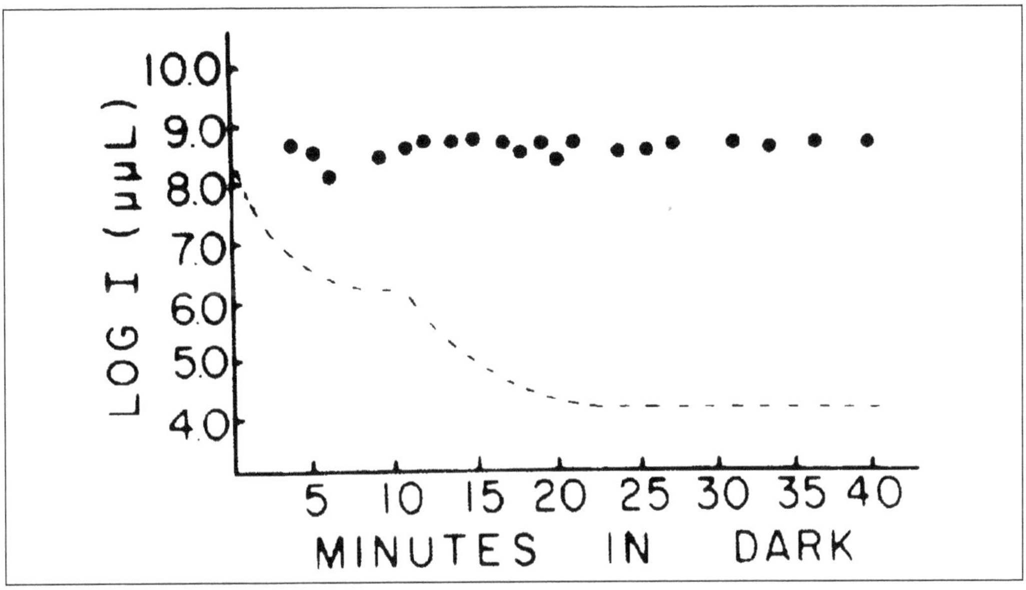


***Figure 7.3** Peripheral dark adaptometry. Dashes show a normal curve following a bleaching light. Dots represent a patient with retinitis pigmentosa, showing abnormalities of both cone and rod function (Duane & Jaeger, Clinical Ophthalmology, Vol. 3, Chap. 24, pg. 5, ©1988 Harper & Row).*

A 1991 study of peripheral vision loss and driving performance shows that real-world accidents, as well as accidents on a driving simulator, increased for those with peripheral vision disabilities (Slyk, Severing, Fishman). They concluded that automobile accidents increased in frequency as the severity of the peripheral vision disabilities increased. Also, they showed that reaction time to peripheral stimuli was prolonged in those persons with peripheral vision loss as compared to people with normal peripheral fields of vision. (See Chapter 8 for more information.)

## 7.6 Macular Degeneration/Maculopathies

Age-related macular degeneration is the leading cause of blindness in the elderly population. However, maculopathies may occur at any age. They primarily involve the central retina. The cones, which are the photoreceptors located in the central retinal region, degenerate. This means they stop sending messages to the brain. This weakens visual acuity and color perception. Peripheral vision normally remains very good. Since static central visual acuity is most affected, persons with significant macular degeneration will probably not be able to pass a driving test.

## 7.7 Retinitis Pigmentosa

Retinitis pigmentosa, RP, are progressive, hereditary retinal diseases characterized by progressive photoreceptor and retinal pigment epithelium degeneration. Usually, rod degeneration is severe, causing drastic reductions in peripheral vision and night vision. The most common symptom is difficulty with dark adaptation, or night blindness. Dark adaptometry shows that in lower levels of illumination, people with RP can only see objects with extremely high luminosity (brightness). The rod and cone threshold are both highly abnormal. See Figure 7.3, adapted from *Clinical Ophthalmology*.

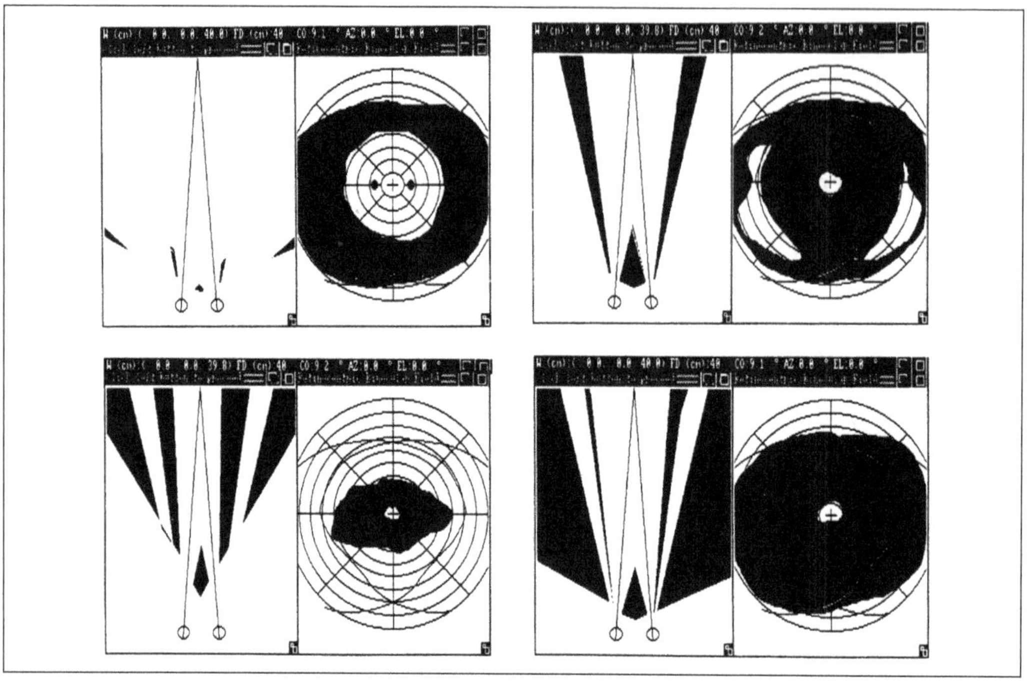

***Figure 7.4*** *Binocular visual fields to the Goldman V/4e target representative of each group profile of RP are shown in the right windows of each figure A–D. A/upper left, Group 1: Concentric partial restriction. B/upper right, Group 2: Concentric loss with residual temporal island. C/lower left, Group 3: Ring scotoma. D/lower right, Group 4: Marked concentric restriction. The left windows in each figure illustrate the three-dimensional perspective of a subject's visual field as the subject fixates straight ahead. Note the volumes of field loss shown in black in the peripheral field which are characteristic of RP.*

Less characteristic RP diseases involve the cone receptors more than the rods. Persons afflicted with this type of disease will have reduced central visual acuity, reduced color vision, or color blindness, and difficulty in bright lights.

RP has been associated with an increased motor vehicle accident rate. Subjects with RP reported significantly more accident involvement than visually normal control subjects, in a five year Illinois study. Total accidents, as well as accidents involving failure to detect peripheral information, was higher in the RP group than in the statistically equivalent in age, gender and years of driving experience group (Szlyk et al., 1991). Examples of binocular visual fields from that study are shown in Figure 7.4.

## 7.8 Diabetic Retinopathy

Diabetic retinopathy is one of the leading causes of blindness in the country, affecting approximately 50,000. It has many stages. Only persons with the initial stage, background diabetic retinopathy (BDR), may have visual driving abilities. Visual changes associated with pre-proliferative and proliferative diabetic retinopathy almost always preclude driving. However, Reuben et al. found 8 percent of diabetic drivers had proliferative diabetic retinopathy, 5 percent were blind in one eye, and 2.4 percent had severe decreases in visual acuity (Reuben et al., 1988).

BDR is usually associated with small intra-retinal hemorrhages. These hemorrhages block the transmission of light to the retina, and may cause small blind spots. The size of these resulting blind spots are proportional to the size of the retinal hemorrhages. Since the retina is unable to be stimulated through them, it follows that less information may reach the brain. Under circumstances with limited visual information, decreased retinal stimulation may result in slower reaction times.

Another characteristic associated with BDR is macular edema. Persons with BDR may develop macular edema, or swelling of the central retina. This causes decreased visual acuity, decreased color vision, and slower dark adaptation. In fact, a common complaint among persons with macular edema is difficulty driving at night. In addition, accommodative ability is reduced in about 20 percent of diabetics.

Also common in diabetic persons is blurred vision caused by fluctuating blood-sugar levels. Patients with hyperglycemia have a tendency toward myopia, while those with hypoglycemia have a tendency toward hyperopia. Blurred vision in the absence of any retinal disease, is associated with changes in the hydration of the lens due to hyperglycemia. As blood-sugar levels fluctuate, visual acuity and refractive error can change, sometimes dramatically. Optimal eyeglass prescriptions may change frequently. This means that a person who has variable blood-sugar levels, whether or not they have been diagnosed with diabetes or not, may see perfectly well to drive safely one day, while on another day may not.

Surgeries, such as photocoagulation of the retina and vitrectomy, have been extremely successful in minimizing visual damages due to neovascularization and vitreal hemorrhages (proliferative diabetic retinopathy). However, regardless of how much vision is salvaged, it is rare that those surgically treated for proliferative diabetic retinopathy will be able to drive safely.

## 7.9 One-Eyed and Spectacle Corrected Aphakes

Persons with only one visually functional eye will have visual field limitations that may result in an increased risk of intersection crashes. Persons who have had their cataracts removed without intraocular lens implantation, who wear aphakic glasses, have visual field limitations as well. Certain aphakic eyeglasses cause ring scotomas, or a circular shaped blind spot in their mid-peripheral vision. Persons driving with this type of eyeglass correction also pose an increased risk for causing an intersection crash.

## 7.10 Postoperative Cataract and Refractive Surgery

Persons who have had their cataracts removed with intraocular lens implantation, as well as those who have had radial keratotomy (RK) or Lasik, experience increased glare. Discomfort and veiling glare may become significantly hazardous to these drivers. Headlight glare at night, is especially disturbing to many of these postoperative patients.

Complications from refractive surgery include irregular astigmatism and decreased contrast sensitivity. Irregular astigmatism will cause decreased visual acuity and may distort images. Decreased contrast sensitivity is a decrease in the ability to distinguish objects from their background. As discussed previously, contrast is a critical factor in determining whether an object is visible. Contrast sensitivity falls dramatically at night. In persons with lower than normal contrast sensitivity, signs or cars with low contrast may not be discernible.

Radial keratotomy weakens the cornea. A weakened cornea is much more susceptible than a normal non-operated cornea to severe corneal trauma, corneal abruptions, hyphemas and resultant cataracts. Automobile crashes and the force of air bags have been shown to more easily cause these types of traumas in post RK persons.

## 7.11 Ocular Muscle Imbalance

Ocular muscle imbalances, or heterophorias, are tendencies of the eyes to become misaligned. There may be an increased strain on these eyes to keep fused, or to maintain single binocular vision. Therefore, these conditions may indirectly cause fatigue. If sudden diplopia (double vision) occurs while driving, it may cause an automobile crash. Uncontrolled or intermittent diplopia represents a driving limitation.

## 7.12 Color Blindness

Most traffic lights have been standardized so that they can easily be distinguished by persons with red-green color deficiencies. Blue has been added to the green lights, and yellow has been added to the red lights, to increase their contrast. Color deficiencies are not considered hazardous for driving, except in severe cases of protanopia (red color blindness), completely color blind, or achromatic persons. Achromatic individuals have very poor vision, and should never drive.

## 7.13 Depth Perception

Stereopsis is the ability to use binocular cues to perceive depth. In other words, it is how well we use both eyes together to distinguish differences in nearness of objects. Stereopsis is significant only at near range, or within two meters. At far range we use mostly monocular cues to determine depth, not binocular cues. If depth perception is poor, it can affect near range driving tasks such as parking. Measurements of depth perception do not correspond with distance visual requirements, such as highway driving.

## 7.14 Age

Normal elderly people have been shown to have a reduction in contrast sensitivity and an increased sensitivity to glare. Whether this is a result of age, or age-related diseases is not definitively concluded. Either way, we all are at risk from their detrimental effects. Anything we can do to help increase visibility and conspicuity on the road would benefit us all.

# References

*Atlas of Clinical Ophthalmology*, J.B. Lippincott Co., Philadelphia, 1988.

Doege and Engelberg, *Medical Conditions Affecting Drivers*, American Medical Association, Chicago, Ill, 1986.

Evans, D.W., and Ginsberg, A.P., "Contrast Sensitivity Predicts Age-Related Differences in Highway Sign Discriminability," *Human Factors*, 27, 637-642, 1985.

Johnson, C.A., Keltner, J.L., "Incidence of Visual Field Loss in 20,000 Eyes and Its Relationship to Driving Performance," *Archives of Ophthalmology*, 101, 371-375, 1983.

Kline, D., "Aging and the Visibility of Highway Signs: A New Look through Old Eyes," AAA Foundation for Traffic Safety, Washington, D.C., 1991.

Leibowitz, Tyrrell, et al., "Dynamic Visual Contrast Sensitivity," AAA Foundation for Traffic Safety, Washington, D.C., June 1993.

Owsley, C., Sekular, R., Seimsen, D., "Contrast Sensitivity throughout Adulthood," *Vision Research*, 23, 689-699, 1983.

Reuben, D.B., Silliman, R.A., Traines, M., "The Aging Driver: Medicine, Policy, and Ethics," *Journal of the American Geriatrics Society*, 36, 1135-1142, 1988.

Stewart, Moore, et al., "Driving Cessation and Accidents in the Elderly: An Analysis of Symptoms, Diseases, Cognitive Dysfunction and Medications," Dept. of Pharmacology and Dept. of Statistics, University of Florida, Gainsville, Fla., AAA Foundation for Traffic Safety, Washington, D.C., January 1993.

Szlyck, Severing and Fishman, "Peripheral Visual Field Loss and Driving Performance," The University of Illinois at Chicago, AAA Foundation for Traffic Safety, Washington, D.C., August 1991.

# Chapter 8

# Drugs and Alcohol Affecting Highway Safety

Leslie Weintraub, O.D.

***Synopsis***



## 8.1 Introduction

Prescription drugs, drugs of abuse, and alcohol may all affect highway safety. Sleepiness is the most common drug and alcohol reaction that causes dangerous driving. The National Highway Traffic Safety Administration (NHTSA) estimates that sleepy drivers cause 50,000 motor vehicle crashes each year. Also, according to The National Transportation Commission, sleepy drivers cause 57 percent of all fatal accidents. Adverse drug and alcohol reactions, overuse of medication, and polypharmacy (consuming many medications that could interact), must all be considered when evaluating one's ability to drive safely.

Medication use and polypharmacy increase with age. They become very common among senior citizens, 65 years and older. According to the 1988 National Disease and Therapeutic Index (NDTI), the 65 and older age group, which was 12 percent of the total population, received 29 percent of all the prescriptions. Medication use increases even more in those aged 75 and above. Three quarters of the population aged 75 and older use prescription medication. The average number of drugs taken daily by patients enrolled in Medicare is ten (Staplin et al., 1987). Elderly people not only take most of the medication, but they also experience three to seven times more adverse drug reactions than younger people do. This is due to a decrease in renal and hepatic functioning with age.

### A. Narcotic analgesics (pain relievers)

Narcotic analgesics include codeine, hydrocodone/Hycodan, oxycodone/Percodan, propoxyphene/Darvon, meperidine/Demerol, hydromorphine/Dilaudid, morphine, opium, heroin, methadone and fentalyls. Heroin is the most commonly abused drug in this category. Methadone is a medication used to treat heroin addicts.

Narcotic analgesics inhibit pain neurons in the central nervous system (CNS) from releasing their neurotransmitters. This decreases the brain's perception of pain. These drugs induce drowsiness and impair driving ability. They also cause varying degrees of euphoria, inability to concentrate, dizziness, apathy, blurred vision and uncontrolled thought. Siegfried and O'Connolly (1986) have noted that opioid analgesics have adverse effects on driving, particularly in the older population. These drugs decrease blood pressure, decrease heart rate, decrease core body temperature, constrict pupils, and may cause eyelids to droop (ptosis). This category of drugs will not affect smooth pursuit eye movements, or nystagmus.

## B. CNS depressants

Central nervous system depressants include: (1) non-barbiturates such as carisoprodol/Soma, cyclobenzaprine/Flexuril and methaqualone/Quaalude; (2) barbiturates such as phenobarbital, alurate and elixin; (3) antianxiety drugs, or the benzodiazepines, such as alprozolam/Xanax, triazolam/Halcion, diazepam/Valium, lorazepam/Ativan, flurazepam, oxazepam and chlordiazepoxide; (4) antidepressants such as amitriptyline/Elavil, imipramine/Tofranil, doxepin/Sinequan, fluoxetine/Prozac, nortriptyline and desipramine; (5)antipsychotics such as haloperidol/Haldol, chlorpromazine/Thorazine, fluphenazine, pericyazine and lithium; and (6) alcohol (ethyl alcohol).

CNS depressants inhibit neural transmission in the brain and spinal cord to varying degrees. Their effects can be additive. Smooth pursuit eye movements and saccades both have control centers at the cerebrum, cerebellum and brain stem. Therefore, these drugs can decrease smooth pursuit eye function, exaggerate normal endpoint nystagmus, and decrease angle of onset of nystagmus. Police officers may detect use of these drugs via horizontal gaze nystagmus (HGN) testing.

All CNS depressants increase the effects of alcohol, and can cause drowsiness, sleep, motor and sensory changes, and also a decrease in psychomotor skills. Small doses used to calm patients' nerves, usually have no affect on driving. However, if these drugs are abused, driving ability will be impaired. In a 1976 study of barbiturates and driving, these drugs were found to increase reaction times, impair motor control, reduce visual motor coordination and impair oculomotor function (Sharma et al., 1976). Also, ataxia, or poor balance and muscular incoordination, can occur with the benzodiazepines. Difficulties with pupillary function, accommodation, image fusion and dark adaptation, which may occur, will especially reduce night driving ability.

These drugs may be particularly dangerous in elderly drivers. Plasma concentrations of antianxiety drugs required for sedation dramatically falls between the ages of 20 and 80 years. Clinically significant drowsiness increases from 4 percent for those aged 40 or less, to 11 percent for those aged over 70 (Ray, Gurwitz, et al., 1992). Also, the benzodiazepines affect psychomotor function in the elderly more markedly than in younger people (Nolan, O'Malley, 1988). Side effects such as morning confusion, drowsiness, ataxia, and a decrease in psychomotor skills in persons taking benzodiazepines the prior evening, increases with age. As high as 39 percent of persons over 70 years old will have these significant side effects.

Many laboratory studies specifically show impaired driving-related skills as a side effect of antianxiety drugs. For example, Seppala, et al., showed increased critical flicker fusion threshold, increased choice reaction time, increased body sway, decreased hand-eye coordination and decreased divided attention, for both middle aged and younger subjects using these drugs. In a three-month study, 38 patients on chlordiazepoxide had ten times the normal amount of traffic accidents (Murray, 1960). Some estimate that accident risk doubles for people taking diazepam/Valium (Janke, 1994).

**Table 8.1**
**Stages of Acute Alcohol Influence**

| BAC (g/100 ml) | Stage of Alcohol Influence | Impairment |
|---|---|---|
| below .05% | subclinical | possible |
| .05% – .08% | euphoria | judgement<br>reaction time<br>muscular coordination<br>driving hazardous |
| .10% or more | excitement | emotional<br>critical judgement<br>visual acuity<br>peripheral vision<br>glare recovery |

Antidepressants and antipsychotics sedate and impair psychomotor function more so in the elderly than in the young (Siegfried and O'Connolly). Antipsychotics, more so than antidepressants sedate their users. This type of sedation increases crash risk. If alcohol is used as well, motor skills become impaired (Scott and Mitchell, 1988). Also, phenothiazines may cause Parkinson-type reactions, such as muscle stiffness, slow reaction times and abnormal nystagmus.

**Alcohol (ethyl alcohol)**

As soon as you start to drink, your blood alcohol concentration (BAC) starts to rise. Driving impairment increases directly with BAC level. This is shown in Table 8.1, adopted from the *Blood Alcohol Concentration Calculator* and *Medicolegal Aspects of Alcohol* of Lawyers & Judges Publishing Company.

It is illegal to drive in all states with a presumptive BAC of .10 percent or above. In California, Florida, Kansas, Maine, Massachusetts, New Hampshire, New Mexico, North Carolina, Oregon, Utah, Vermont and Virginia, the illegal presumptive BAC is .08 percent and above.

Alcohol has been shown to impair vision. Static visual acuity decreased in 54 percent of subjects with BAC levels of .06–.10g/dL, and in 85 percent of subjects with BAC levels of .101–125g/dL (Newman and Fletcher, cited in Garriott, 1993). Other studies show a more significant reduction in dynamic visual acuity. In their 1975 study, Burns et al. showed that although low and high contrast static visual acuity was unaffected by alcohol, dynamic visual acuity was. In their 1993 study of dynamic visual contrast sensitivity, Leibowitz, et al. found that twice as much contrast was needed for detection after subjects imbibed an 8 ounce mixed drink containing 1.4 ml of 190 proof alcohol. This later study found that static visual acuity was also decreased, but to a much lower extent. Loss in both static and dynamic contrast sensitivity is a clear driving hazard.

Decreases in both light and dark adaptation, as well as resistance to glare and impaired color discrimination, have been observed in subjects with BAC levels of .09–.15g/dL (Wallgren and Barry, cited in Garriott). Adams, et al., in 1976 found a decrease in color discrimination in the blue and yellow zones. Also, alcohol may slow the response time to visual stimulation (Suzuki et al., 1957; Lewis et al., 1969; Idestrom et al., 1968).

Impairment of driving related visual skills may occur in persons with BAC as low .03 percent. Brecher demonstrated that in BAC levels as low as .03 percent, binocular coordination is reduced (cited in Garriott, 1993). Also, Moskowitz found decreased visual tracking performances at low BAC levels (Moskowitz, 1974).

Personality changes are associated with alcohol (Barnes, 1974). Alcohol may exaggerate one's mood, increasing depression or aggression. Aggression toward oneself may cause suicide, and aggression toward others may cause violent behavior. If driving, this may turn into suicide and/or homicide by an automobile accident.

Other detrimental effects of alcohol on driving ability include reduction in central processing of information and reductions in short term memory (Burns et al.). A decrease in risk judgement has also been observed (Dott, 1972). Furthermore, alcoholic hangovers have been shown to decrease reaction time, perception and motor performance.

## C. Dissociative anesthetics (PCP and analogs)

This group of drugs includes phencyclidine/PCP, known as "angel dust," and ketamine/Ketalar, which is a veterinary anesthetic. They block pain information to the brain by dissociating the brain from pain information. These drugs stimulate the CNS, increase blood pressure, increase pulse rate, increase body temperature, cause hallucination and insensitivity to pain. These drugs also depress the CNS. They will decrease smooth pursuit ability, exaggerate endpoint nystagmus, and decrease the angle onset of lateral gaze nystagmus. Sometimes these drugs induce an upbeating vertical gaze nystagmus. There is no question that driving under the influence of these drug could be disastrous.

## D. Cannabis (marijuana and hashish)

The active ingredient in cannabis is THC. Marinol and Nabilone are synthetic THC drugs prescribed for cancer and AIDS patients to increase appetite and reduce vomiting. This group of drugs acts within the CNS, but does not affect smooth pursuits or nystagmus. Visual disturbances associated with cannabis use include conjunctival injection (red eyes), a decrease in dynamic visual acuity (Brown et al.), and a decrease in color perception in the blue and red zones (Adams et al.).

Cannabis intoxication is clearly a driving danger. Cannabis reduces eye-hand and hand-hand coordination, increases reaction times and causes incorrect reactions (Kielholz et al., 1973). Cannabis intoxication can also cause incorrect estimates of time and distance, as well as increased brake time (Rafaelsen, et al, 1973).

The primary effects of marijuana are mood changes and disturbances in time perception (Barnes, 1974). It slows central thought processes and impairs short term memory (Burns et al.). Also, people often become oblivious and indifferent to their surroundings. Therefore, chronic marijuana users may have delayed thought processes and become dangerous drivers.

## E. Hallucinogens (psychedelics)

This group includes mescaline, psilocybin (mushrooms), nutmeg, morning glory seeds, Jimson weed, bufotenene, lysergic acid/LSD, methylenedioxylam-phetamine/ecstasy, and dimethoxylamphetamine/STP. These drugs act on the CNS to produce distorted information to the brain. Persons affected by these drugs become distracted, unable to concentrate, and unable to perform skilled tasks such as driving. These drugs will dilate pupils, but do not affect nystagmus or smooth pursuits.

## F. Inhalants

This group includes acetone, toluene, benzene, gasoline, kerosene, hydrocarbons from aerosol containers, and anesthetic gases such as chloroform, nitrous oxide and amyl nitrate. These inhalants depress the central nervous system. Similar to other CNS depressants, using these drugs will show positive HGN test results: decreasing smooth pursuit eye movements, exaggerating endpoint nystagmus and decreasing the angle of onset of lateral gaze nystagmus. High doses may induce vertical nystagmus. These drugs distort the user's perception of time and space, which would be detrimental to driving ability.

### G. CNS stimulants

This group of drugs includes cocaine, amphetamines, methylphenidate/Ritalin, pemoline/Cylert and phenmetrazine/Preludin. These drugs increase the amount of norepinephrine in the body by either inhibiting its uptake or increasing its release. They increase heart rate, increase blood pressure, increase respiration rate and body temperature. People who abuse these drugs will have dilated pupils that react slowly to light and normal HGN responses. Chronic use of amphetamines has been proven to be associated with crash risk (Waller, 1973).

### H. Ophthalmic agents

*Mydriatics and cycloplegics*, such as phenylephrine, hydroxyamphetamine, tropicamide, cyclopentolate, scopolamine, homatropine, and atropine, are drugs that dilate the pupil. Except for phenylephrine and hydroxyamphetamine, they all cause cycloplegia, or inhibit accommodation, as well. They are used diagnostically for routine eye examinations, as well as therapeutically for treatment of certain ocular inflammations. A dilated pupil, and cycloplegia, will both blur vision and increase light sensitivity. Depending on the extent of the dilation and cycloplegia, caution while driving or no driving is recommended.

*Glaucoma medication*

1. *Adrenergics*, such as epinephrine and dipivefrin, cause mydriasis, or dilate the pupil. This may blur vision and cause increased light sensitivity.
2. *Miotics*, such as pilocarpine, carbachol, and echothiophate, and even more so, physostigmine, demarcarium, echothiophate and isofluro-phate, severely constrict pupil size. This decreases peripheral vision, and in the presence of a cataract will also reduce central vision. Persons on topical cholinergic medication should never drive at night, and may not be able to safely drive during the daytime either.

## 8.2 HGN: Horizontal Gaze Nystagmus

The rate of major violations given for driving under the influence of drugs or alcohol is greatest for those aged under 25, and least for the elderly drivers (California Data). Crash risk is directly proportional to blood alcohol concentration, while the relationship between crash risk and drugs of abuse is unknown. However, the combination of even small amounts of alcohol and drugs increases the risk of automobile accidents for all age groups.

Police officers across the nation and in several foreign countries learn to evaluate whether suspected drivers are intoxicated or under the influence of drugs or alcohol (D.W.I. or D.U.I.). Major parts of these drug recognition evaluations are eye tests, or HGN tests. The HGN sequence tests for smooth pursuits, nystagmus at maximum deviation and angle onset of nystagmus. See Table 8.2.

Smooth pursuits are the slow, even eye movements used to track an object. We use them to keep low speed objects of interest on our central retinas. When the central nervous system is depressed, smooth pursuits become uneven or jerky.

**Table 8.2**
**Example of Score Card for HGN Sequence**

Horizontal Gaze Nystagmus Sequence

| | | | | | | |
|---|---|---|---|---|---|---|
| Equal tracking? | Y | N | | | | |
| Equal pupil size? | Y | N | | | | |
| | | | Left Eye | | Right Eye | |
| 1) Smooth pursuits? | | | Y | N | Y | N |
| 2) Normal endpoint nystagmus? | | | Y | N | Y | N |
| 3) Nystagmus onset greater than 45 degrees? | | | Y | N | Y | N |

4 or more "no" marks fails test

Last medications: ______________________________

Comments: ______________________________

______________________________

Nystagmus is an involuntary movement of the eyes. Pendular nystagmus is an involuntary oscillation of the eyes with equal speed in both directions. Jerk nystagmus has a fast phase in one direction and a slow phase in the opposite direction. There are about 45 classifications of nystagmus, but only three types are considered normal. They are fatigue nystagmus, unsustained endpoint nystagmus and sustained endpoint nystagmus. Fatigue nystagmus occurs when eyes are maximally deviated for more than 30 seconds. Unsustained endpoint nystagmus is a few beats of nystagmus at gaze angles of 30 degrees or more. Sustained endpoint nystagmus is nystagmus at gaze deviations greater than 40 degrees. Normal, or physiological nystagmus in most of the population occurs with a very small amplitude of no more than three degrees. It is usually mild, difficult to see, or not visible at all. Whereas horizontal gaze nystagmus is exaggerated when the central nervous system is depressed, and clearly visible.

Before the HGN testing can commence, police officers need to have probable cause, or a reasonable suspicion that the driver is under the influence of drugs or alcohol. According to the NHTSA, the following constitutes reasonable cause:

| *Visual Cues* | *Probability (%) that driver is drunk* |
|---|---|
| 1. Turning with a wide radius | 65 percent |
| 2. Straddling center of lane marker | 65 |
| 3. Appearing to be drunk | 60 |
| 4. Almost striking object or vehicle | 60 |
| 5. Weaving | 60 |
| 6. Driving on other than designated roadway | 55 |
| 7. Swerving | 55 |
| 8. Speed more than 10 mph below the limit | 50 |
| 9. Stopping without cause in traffic lane | 50 |
| 10. Following too closely | 50 |

| | |
|---|---|
| 11. Drifting | 50 |
| 12. Tires on center or lane marker | 45 |
| 13. Braking erratically | 45 |
| 14. Driving into opposing or crossing traffic | 45 |
| 15. Signaling inconsistently with driving actions | 40 |
| 16. Slow response to traffic signals | 40 |
| 17. Stopping inappropriately (other than in lane) | 35 |
| 18. Turning abruptly or illegally | 35 |
| 19. Accelerating or decelerating rapidly | 30 |
| 20. Headlights off | 30 |

After seeing one or more of the signs above, law enforcement officials may begin the HGN sequence. The police officers ask suspects to remove their eyeglasses and follow a slow-moving target, usually a penlight, horizontally at approximately 15 inches from their face. If the suspect tracks the penlight with both eyes moving equally in the same direction, the HGN results should be accurate. If suspects are unable to track objects with both eyes moving equally due to nerve or muscle disease, extreme refractive error, loss of one eye, stroke, medications, and so forth, then HGN testing will not be accurate.

The first part of the HGN sequence is testing smooth pursuits. This is to determine the ability to track a slow-moving object 120 degrees from left to right in four seconds. Smooth pursuits can be no faster than 30 degrees per second. Persons with good vision and binocularity can probably track an object smoothly. If the ocular system is depressed, tracking will be inaccurate, causing eyes to fall behind or jump ahead of their target. The eyes should be tested binocularly, without occluding one eye. The penlight should be held at 12–15 inches from the face, and slightly superior. The target moves from the midline of the face temporally to the maximum lateral deviation of one eye and then back to the midline again. Then, the target moves from the midline of the face temporally to maximum lateral deviation of the other eye and back to the midline. Each eye is graded separately for smooth pursuits.

The second part of the HGN sequence is testing nystagmus at maximum deviation, or sustained endpoint nystagmus. The penlight moves temporally from the midline of the face to maximum deviation and held there. A few beats of nystagmus are perfectly normal at lateral gaze deviation of 30 degrees or more. However, if nystagmus is markedly jerky for four seconds or more, this is considered outside normal limits. Neither eye should be covered, and each eye is tested and graded separately about whether endpoint nystagmus was exaggerated.

The third part of the HGN sequence is measuring the angle of onset of nystagmus, or unsustained endpoint nystagmus. The penlight is moved at a slower pace from the midline of the face temporally, and the angle of onset of nystagmus (AON) is recorded for each eye separately. According to precise laboratory testing, with the use of calibrated visual field devices and precise measuring:

| **51 degrees – 105 × BAC(%) =** | **Angle Onset Nystagmus (AON)** |
|---|---|
| 0.00 percent | 51.00 degrees |
| 0.05 percent | 45.75 degrees |
| 0.10 percent | 40.50 degrees |
| 0.15 percent | 35.25 degrees |

**Table 8.3**
**Ocular Responses to Drugs**

| DRUG | HGN TEST | PUPILS | CONVERGENCE | PTOSIS (droopy eyelids) |
|---|---|---|---|---|
| Narcotic Analgesics | Pass | Constricted | Normal | Present |
| CNS Depressants | Fail | Slow reactions to light | Decreased | Present |
| Alcohol | Fail | Slow reactions to light | Decreased | Present |
| Dissociative Anesthetics | Fail | Normal | Decreased | No |
| Cannabis | Pass | May be dilated | Decreased | No |
| Hallucinogens | Pass | Slow reactions to light | Normal | No |
| Inhalants | Fail | Slow reactions to light | Decreased | No |
| CNS Stimulants | Pass | Dilated Slow reactions to light | Normal | None |

This shows that normal angle onset nystagmus (AON) occurs at 50 degrees or more. AON of 40–45 degrees indicates a BAC between 0.05–0.10, and AON of 0–30 degrees indicates significant intoxication. Police officers will fail a person with endpoint nystagmus of 45 degrees or less. A summary of occular responses to drugs is shown in Table 8.3.

## A. HGN prosecution

The HGN sequence is the most accurate of all the psychophysical roadside sobriety tests for detecting 0.10 BAC. Government studies from 1977–1983 ("Psycho-physical Tests for D.W.I. Arrest," "Developmental and Field Test of Psychophysical Tests for D.W.I. Arrests" and "Field Evaluation of a Behavioral Test Battery for D.W.I.") show about an 80 percent accuracy level. More recently, the statistics show that nystagmus can be 96 percent accurate in detecting 0.10 BAC as the expertise of the police officer increases ("The Scientific Basis for Alcohol Gaze Nystagmus," 1987).

Most of the state courts recognize HGN as a scientific test. In other words, the majority of states accept that there is a scientific relationship between BAC and HGN. The American Optometric Association has passed a resolution endorsing the HGN test as an effective test for detecting alcohol impairment (see Figure 8.1). The scientific community accepts the test as reliable. Expert witnesses confirm to the jury that:

1. There is a scientific relationship between BAC and HGN.
2. The HGN test is a reliable indicator of alcohol impairment.
3. A police officer can be trained to accurately administer the test and measure the results.
4. It is very unlikely to confuse alcohol gaze nystagmus with other forms of nystagmus.

**HORIZONTAL GAZE NYSTAGMUS AS A FIELD SOBRIETY TEST**

WHEREAS drivers under the influence of alcohol pose a significant threat to the public health, safety, and welfare; and

WHEREAS optometric scientists and the National Highway and Traffic Safety Administration have shown the Horizontal Gaze Nystagmus (HGN) test to be a scientifically valid and reliable tool for trained police officers to use in field sobriety testing; now therefore be it

RESOLVED that the American Optometric Association acknowledges the scientific validity and reliability of the HGN test as a field sobriety test when administered by properly trained and certified police officers; and be it further

RESOLVED that the American Optometric Association urges doctors of optometry to become involved as professional consultants in the use of HGN field sobriety testing.

Adopted June 1993
House of Delegates

***Figure 8.1*** *American Optometric Association HGN resolution.*

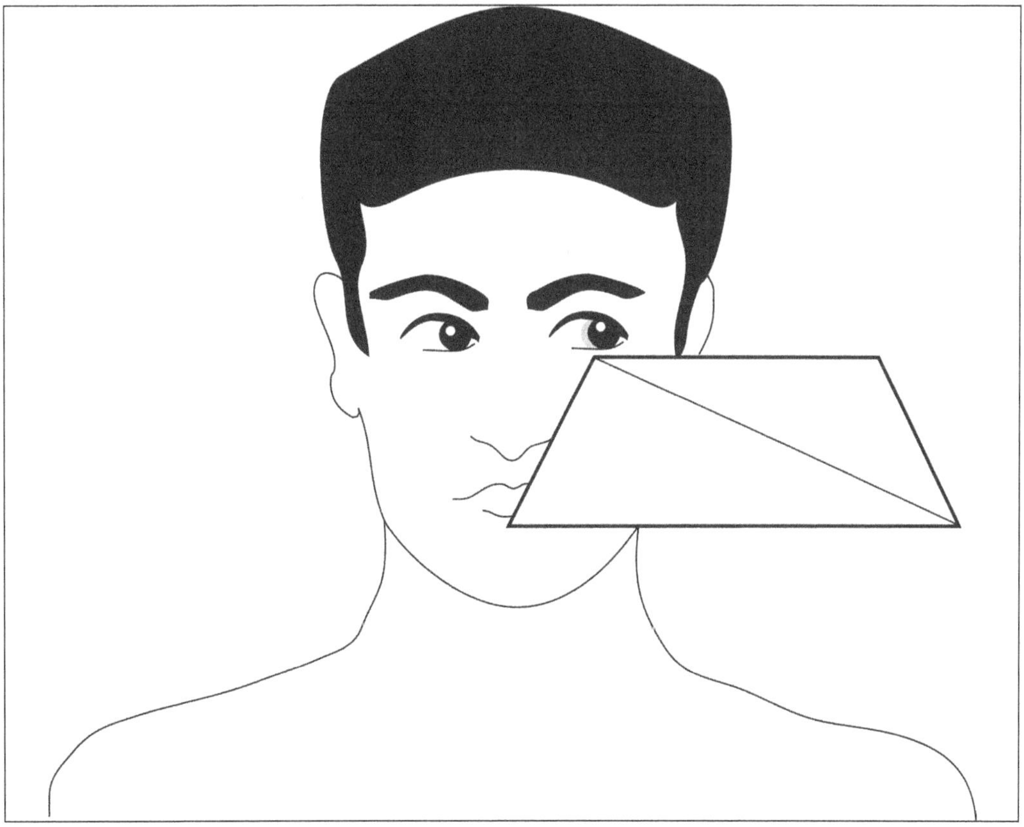

***Figure 8.2*** *45-degree card to score angle onset nystagmus (AON).*

**Table 8.4**
**Average Bifocal Power Needed Focus at 14–18 Inches Based on Age**

| Age | Average Bifocal Power |
|---|---|
| 40 | +1.00 D |
| 45 | +1.50 D |
| 50 | +2.00 D |
| 55 | +2.25 D |
| 60 | +2.50 D |

### B. HGN defense

Defense attorneys usually question the expertise of the police officer. After only one week of training, can they really be so exact in detecting angles of gaze without visual field gauges? Have they used half moon field devices or a 45-degree card to base their measurement on (see Figure 8.2)? How many intoxicated and sober people have they tested? Have they ever been trained at an eye doctor's office? How accurate are the guesstimates the law enforcement officers make as to the angle of onset of nystagmus?

The SFST (standard field sobriety test) manual instructs police officers how to perform the HGN sequence. Any variation from the manual may affect the validity of the test. Also, was the test area illuminated well enough for the officer to see the subject's eyes? How was the area illuminated? Was the subject facing passing cars, blinking lights or any other form of moving objects that can cause optokinetic nystagmus? Certain prescription drugs, such as antihistamines and antiepilepsy drugs, can cause nystagmus. Some people normally exhibit AON of 20–40 degrees.

Defense attorneys should also question the vision of the arresting police officer. HGN test results are based on visual observations of the officer. Not every police officer has 20/20 vision in each eye, normal binocular vision, normal color vision, or a high degree of depth perception. Also, if the police officer is close to forty years old or above, their focusing ability at near is almost always diminished (see Table 8.4). In other words they are not able to see as clearly up close any more due to a decrease in focusing, or accommodative ability. Accommodation decreases rapidly with age. By the mid-forties, most individuals can no longer see clearly at 24 or less inches away without eyeglasses and/or increased illumination. If HGN testing is done by a 45-year-old or older police officer, without his eyeglasses, at night, the results are suspect.

## References

Abrams, Bernard, O.D., "HGN Police Testing and Other Fairy Tales," Feb. 1997, Las Vegas, Nevada.

Adams, Brown, Flom, Jones, and Jampolsky; "Alcohol and marihuana effects on static visual acuity" *American Journal of Optometry and Physiological Optics* 52 729–735, November 1975.

Adams, Brown, Haegerstrom-Portney, Flom, and Jones; "Evidence of the acute effects of alcohol and marihuana on color discrimination," *Perception and Psychophysics*, 20(2): 119–124, 1976.

Austin, Gregory, *Drug Users and Driving Behavior*, National Institute on Drug Abuse, Rockville, Md., 1977.

Barnes, T.H., *Drug Use and Driving*, Addiction Research Foundation, Toronto, 1974.

Bellak, L., and Karasu, T., *Geriatric Psychiatry: A handbook for psychiatrists and primary care*, Grune & Stratton, N.Y.

*Blood Alcohol Concentration Calculator*, Lawyers & Judges Pub. Co., Tucson, Ariz., 1993.

Brown, Adams, Haegerstrom-Portnoy, et al, "Effects of alcohol and marihuana on dynamic visual acuity," *Perception and Psychophysics*, 18(6): 441–446, 1975.

Burns, Marcelline, *Medical Legal Aspects of Drugs, Second Edition*. Lawyers & Judges Pub. Co., Tucson, Ariz., 2006.

Burns, Marcelline, and Sharma, "Marihuana effects of driving: Performance and personality," *Proceedings of the 19th Conference of the American Association for Automotive Medicine*, San Diego, CA, Nov. 20-22, 1975, pp 274–284.

Castledon, C.M., George, C.F., Marcer, D., and Hallett, C., "Increased sensitivity to nitrazepam in old age," *British American Journal*, 274, 10–12.

Clayton, Betts, and Mackay, "A study of the effects of certain tranquilizers and small amounts of alcohol on driving performance," *European Journal of Toxicology*, 5(4): 254–256, 1972.

Council of Scientific Affairs, "Alcohol and the Driver," *Journal of the American Medical Association* (JAMA), January 24/31, 1986, vol 255.

Doege and Engelberg, *Medical Conditions Affecting Drivers*, American Medical Ass., Chicago, 1986.

Dott, A.B., *Effect of Marihuana on Risk Acceptance in a Simulated Passing Task*, Public Health Service Report, DHEW Pub. # HSM-72-10010, Washington, D.C., 197?.

*Drugs of Abuse Calculator*, Lawyers & Judges Publishing Co., Tucson, Ariz., 1993.

Duane and Yaeger, *Clinical Ophthalmology*, Vol 2, J.B. Lippincott Co., Philadelphia, Chapter 11, 1988.

Forkiotis, C.J., "Optometric Expertise: The Scientific Basis for Alcohol Gaze Nystagmus," vol. 59, Curriculum II, No. 7, April 1986.

Garriott, James, *Medical Legal Aspects of Alcohol, Fourth Edition*. Lawyers & Judges Pub. Co., Tucson, Ariz., 2003.

Good, Gregory, and Augsburger, Arol, "Use of Horizontal Gaze Nystagmus as a Part of Roadside Sobriety Testing," *American Journal of Optometry and Physiological Optics*, vol. 63, 467, 1986.

Greenblatt, D.J., Allen, M.D., Shader, R.I., "Toxicity of high dose flurazepam in the elderly," *Clinical Pharmacology and Therapeutics*, 21, 355–361, 1977.

Halpern, Eric and Yolton, Robert, "Is the Driver Drunk? Oculomotor Sobriety Testing," *Journal of the American Optometric Association*, vol. 57, number 9, Sept. 1986.

"HGN test for D.U.I. Under Attack," *American Optometric Association News*, vol. 36, number 11, 12/8/97, pp. 1, 8.

Israelstrom and Lambert, *Alcohol, Drugs, and Traffic Safety*, Addiction Research Foundation, Toronto, 1975.

Kielholz, Hobi, Ladewig, et al, "An experimental investigation about the effect of cannabis on car driving behavior," *Pharmakopsychiatrie Neuro-Psychopharmakologie*, 6(2): 91-103, 1973.

Kosnoski, Yolton, Citek, Hayes, Evans, "The Drug Classification Program: Using ocular and other signs to detect drug intoxication," *Journal of the American Optometric Association*, vol. 69, Number 4, April 1998.

Moskowitz, H., Robinson, C.D., "Effects of low doses of alcohol on driving-related skills: A review of the evidence," U.S. Department of Commerce, National Technical Information Service, Springfield, Va., 1988.

National Highway Traffic Safety Administration, U.S. Dept. of Transportation, "Field Evaluation of a Behavioral Test Battery for D.W.I.," No. DOT-HS-475, Sept. 1983

National Highway Traffic Safety Administration, U.S. Dept. of Transportation, "Development and Field Test of Psychophysical Tests for D.W.I. Arrest," No.DOT-HS-805-864, March 1981.

National Highway Traffic Safety Administration, U.S. Dept. of Transportation, "Psychophysical Tests for D.W.I. Arrest," No. DOT-HS-802-424, June 1977.

National Traffic Law Center, *Horizontal Gaze Nystagmus: The Science and the Law*, July 1999, U.S. Department of Transportation.

Nolan, L., O'Malley, K., "Prescribing for the elderly," Part 1: Sensitivity of the elderly to adverse drug reactions, *Journal of the American Geriatrics Society*, 36, 142–149.

Owens, Alfred, "Differentiation of Visibility and Alcohol as Contributors to Twilight Road Fatalities," *Human Factors*, 38(4), 680-689, 1996.

*Physicians Desk Reference*, Medical Economics Data, 48th Edition, 1994.

*Physicians Desk Reference Side Effects*, Medical Economics Data.

*Physicians Generix,* Data Pharmaceutical, Inc., Smithtown, N.Y., 1992.

Rafaelson, Bech, and Rafaelson, "Simulated car driving influenced by cannabis and alcohol," *Pharmakopsychiatrie Neuro-Psychopharmakologie*, 6(2): 71–83, 1973.

Ray, W.A., Gurwitz, J., Decker, M.D., Kennedy, D.L., "Medication and the safety of the older driver": is there a basis for concern?" *Human Factors*, 34, 33–47, 1992.

Ray, W.A., Thapa, P.B., Shorr, R.I., "Medications and the older driver," *Clinics in Geriatric Medicine*, 9,413–438, 1993.

Scott, R.B., Mitchell, M.C., "Aging, alcohol, and the liver," *Journal of the American Geriatrics Society*, 36, 255–265, 1988.

Siegfried, K., O'Connolly, M., "Cognitive and psychomotor effects of different antidepressants in the treatment of old age depression," *Journal of Clinical Psychopharmacological Research*, 1, 231–243, 1986.

Sharma, and Satanand, "Barbiturates and driving," *Accident Analysis and Prevention*, 8:27–31, 1976.

Vaughn and Asbury, *General Ophthalmology*, Lange Medical Pub., Los Altos, Calif., Chapter 17, 1983.

Willette, Robert, *Drugs and Driving*, Dept. of Health Education and Welfare, Public Health Service, Rockville, 1973.

# Chapter 9

# Visual Aging

J. Vernon Odom, Ph.D. and Marc Green, Ph.D.

*"Grant me the senility to forget the people I never liked anyway, the good fortune to run into the ones I do, and the eyesight to tell the difference."*

—Anonymous

***Synopsis***

## 9.1 Introduction

The frequency of accidents involving the elderly is on the rise. First, it is no secret that society is aging. The elderly represent an increasing proportion of the population, so they will be involved in an accordingly larger percentage of accidents. Some demographic data put the issue into clear relief:

- 13 percent of the population is over 65;
- 25 percent of the population is over 50, the age when decline begins;
- in 30 years, the 65+ population will double (70 million people); and
- over-85 is the fastest growing segment of the population.

Second, aging produces losses in visual, cognitive and motor capabilities. Older viewers do not see as well, think as quickly or respond as fast. In theory, these losses should increase accident involvement.

This chapter provides an overview of changes in visual physiology and function which occur in elderly viewers, focusing on those who have no clinically significant eye disease. In other words, an ophthalmologist or optometrist would say that they were "normal" or "healthy." We do not address the effects of the numerous eye diseases which affect many older viewers. Virtually all older viewers develop some cataracts (although they may not be clinically significant), and many develop age-related macular degeneration, glaucoma, or diabetic retinopathy. Instead, we describe the numerous changes which occur in viewers even if they remain "healthy." Lastly, we do not address the large population of younger viewers with "low vision," impairment due to eye disease or other causes.

## A. Refresher on Visual System and its Function

The visual system consists of two major classes of components: neural components and optical components. Additionally, there are glandular components and muscular components. Viewers "see" with the neural components of the visual system. Light stimulates the rods and cones of the retina. These sensory cells activate a chain of neural cells first in the retina and then, by way of the retinal ganglion cells whose axons combine to form the optic nerve, the brain. Even beginning at the earliest stages of visual processing, different classes of cells in the retina respond to different classes of visual input. Rods respond at very low levels of light at which cones are not active (scotopic levels). As light levels increase, both rods and cones are active (mesopic levels). At very bright levels of light, above about 40 cd/m$^2$, rods are saturated and suppressed; only cones respond differentially to changes in light at higher light levels (photopic levels). Some cells increase their firing rate to increases in light ("on"-cells) while others increase their firing rate to decreases of light level ("off"-cells). These different classes of cells appear to form parallel pathways within the brain. Perhaps, it is not surprising then that by one estimate, the majority of our brains are dedicated to visual processing.

In order for our nervous system to see, a clear image must be focused on the back of the eye. Thus, the eye must have some of the optical characteristics of a camera. The cornea and lens focus light onto the retina by creating what amounts to an adaptive compound lens system. This focused light must pass through largely clear media: cornea, aqueous humor, lens, vitreous humor, and macula lutae (yellow pigment over the macula). The pupil acts as the focal stop or aperture of the eye. It can regulate the light levels reaching the eye to some extent, but its major purpose is probably to adjust image clarity by keeping the pupil as small as is practical at any given light level.

This small pupil increases the range of depths over which an object will be clear (depth of focus) and reduces the influences of corneal and lenticular irregularities (glare) or the clarity of the retinal image.

### B. The Definition of Normal

With age, an increasing percentage of the population has subclinical or clinically significant eye disease. When one discusses normal aging and the vision of normal aging, are such persons to be included in the sample? When one describes changes in vision with age, is one describing the mean of all persons or the mean of only the healthy persons? Another way of thinking of the same issue is to ask, "Which definition of normal does one choose to use?"

One possibility is to think of normal in a purely statistical sense. What are the characteristics of the population of persons of a particular age? Normative studies using this definition describe the characteristics of older persons. Such studies almost always show rapid declines in visual function with age.

A second possibility is to think of normal as meaning healthy or without disease. Studies using these definitions typically are interested in studying the process or mechanisms of aging. Such studies attempt to use some criterion or set of criteria to eliminate portions of the population with disease or in some cases to select special populations who have a specific disease. These special populations will then typically be compared to age-matched controls.

Attempting to eliminate diseased groups from a study population is particularly difficult in an aging population. The most common criterion to classify persons as visually normal is "normal" visual acuity. Clinically, normal is typically defined as an acuity of 20/40 or better with best optical correction. However, statistically normal best corrected visual acuity in younger populations is better than 20/20. Many age-related diseases such as age-related macular degeneration, glaucoma or diabetic retinopathy have effects on visual function years before visual acuity is impaired and have no impact on acuity in their early stages. A second criterion is that the person has no history of ocular disease or systemic disease which affects vision. Diabetes is one systemic disease which affects vision. However, only about 50 percent of persons with diabetes have actually been diagnosed with the disease. Glaucoma is an ocular disease which is difficult to diagnose in its early stages, but which significantly impairs visual function as the visual system is stressed (Yates, Leys, Green, Huang, Charlton, Reed, Di and Odom, 1999). Similarly, we may note that in one study of normal visual function in elderly viewers, more than 50 percent of the initial sample was found to have some sign of age-related maculopathy, a precursor to age-related macular degeneration (Jackson, Owsley and McGwin, 1999). Therefore, using clinically "normal" visual acuity as a criterion or a normal history does not truly eliminate all older persons with ocular disease from a study.

While we raise these issues of definition, we must accept the current literature and use the information which is available as we present information about aging of the visual system. As best we can, we will describe the statistically normal, non-disease related changes in visual function. Lastly, we should also point out that the average or normal person is a statistical construct and the abilities of individuals vary greatly, being much better or much worse than the normal value of a particular age.

## 9.2 Anatomical / Physiological Changes with Age

There are definite changes in visual function with age. A continually disputed question is whether those changes in visual function are a result of optical changes, neural changes or a combination of the two. Prior to examining those changes in visual function we will briefly describe the optical and neural changes associated with age. See Weale (1992) and Sekuler, Kline and Key (1982) for more detailed reviews.

## A. Optical Components

There are well-documented changes in the optical properties of the eye with age. Generally, these changes result in 1) increased light scatter, so that glare is more disruptive, 2) yellowing of ocular tissues so that relatively less blue light reaches the back of the retina, and 3) less light reaching the back of the eye to stimulate the rods and cones.

The role of light scatter is important. Light scatter may be broadly thought of as being of three types: back scatter, transverse scatter and forward scatter. Back scatter is reflected back generally along the path from which the light came; transverse scatter is generally along axes orthogonal to the original direction of the light; and forward scatter is along the original direction of the beam of light.

Even in younger eyes light is scattered by the optics of the eye. Forward scatter is one reason that a point source of light generates a blur circle on the retina. Of major importance in considering scatter is that as transparent or translucent particles in the eye get larger the magnitude of forward scatter increases, i.e., the blur circle will increase. While we will detail the changes at some length, the major result of aging effects on many optical elements of the eye is that the size of translucent or transparent particles increases, increasing the effects of forward light scatter. See recent overviews of the optics of the aging eye (Werner and Schefrin, 2000; Applegate, Donnelly, Marsack, Koenig, and Pesudovs, 2007).

### 1. Cornea

As we age, there is less tear production from the lacrimal glands (Craig and Tomlinson, 1998). While the tear film has a protective function, it also serves an important optical function in providing a smooth interface between the air and the eye, correcting many optical aberrations of the eye. Additionally there is a loss of some cells in the endothelium of the cornea (Yee, Matsuda, Schultz, and Edelhauser, 1985). Because the corneal surface is dryer and less smooth there is an increase in forward light scatter in the eye.

### 2. Lens

Unlike most bodily structures, the lens continues to grow for as long as we live. Somewhat like a tree, it keeps adding layers. The result is that as we age the older layers in the center of the lens receive less and less oxygen because there are no blood vessels in the lens. These central layers become rigid adding to a loss of our ability to accommodate and focus on near objects. Also, the lens tends to become more yellow with age and to develop small, less transparent areas. If these opacities become large enough and intrude on the visual axis we develop a clinically significant cataract. Even if these small opacities do not develop into clinically significant cataracts, lenticular changes result in increased light scatter (Weale, 1992).

Aging also causes "presbyopia," which usually appears between ages 40–50. The lens becomes less elastic, reducing its ability to thicken and increase refractive power. Viewers then require spectacles in order to accommodate to near objects. Some spectacles are bifocal, containing a small area of high refractive power embedded on the lower portion of the spectacle lens. If the viewer is looking down, as during normal reading, then he views the print clearly through the area of extra refractive power. If he is looking straight ahead, as when walking, then the lower part of the visual field will be blurred, since the extra refractive power mis-focuses the distant ground. The bifocals then increase the likelihood of trips and falls because ground obstacles are not as visible. "Progressive spectacles," where refractive power increases gradually toward the bottom of the lens, produce similar effects plus distort the scene as the eyes move.

### 3. Vitreous

Behind the lens is a dense gelatinous, clear body called the vitreous. As we age, the vitreous becomes more liquid. At the same time some small parts become more dense and appear darker. As a result, we develop "floaters," punctuate, nonstationary, moving opacities which may create tiny blind spots ("scotomata") and impair object recognition. Age-related vitreal changes increase forward light scatter (Weale, 1992).

### 4. Macular pigment

A yellow pigment, the macula lutae, covers the central part of the retina where we have our best vision. As viewers age, the pigment becomes more yellow. The yellowness roughly varies with skin pigmentation when viewers are younger. The rate of yellowing is faster for fair skinned individuals so that by the age of eighty there is no difference in yellowness for those of European or African descent. The yellow pigment is thought to protect the central retina from the harmful effects of ultraviolet light. So it is possible that this increased yellowing has some protective value. However, the yellow pigment passes less blue light so that older observers demonstrate greater color confusion on testing than do younger observers (see Pitts, 1982).

### 5. Pupil

Pupillary changes lead to reduced retinal illuminance with age (see Figure 9.1). As viewers age the pupil becomes smaller (miotic). The exact degree of the difference between older and younger people depends on the light level. The difference between younger and older viewers is greater at low light levels. By the age of sixty the change is roughly equivalent to a 0.3–0.5 log unit decrease in retinal illuminance, i.e., the light entering the eye is only about 1/2–1/3 of what it was when the same person was twenty years old (Weale, 1992).

There is one possible positive effect of the reduced pupil size as viewers age. Reduced pupil size makes the eye more like a pinhole camera. This means that although images are less bright, they are less affected by refractive errors, errors of focus (increased depth of focus) or by light scatter (Sloane, Owsley and Alvarez, 1988). One indication of this benefit is that visual functions decline when pupils are dilated (Mangano, Schwartz, Charlton and Odom, 1994; Applegate, Donnelly, Marsack, Koenig, and Pesudovs, 2007).

### 6. Simulating Optical Changes

The eye's optical changes for older observers may be simulated by the combination of three optical elements placed before a young eye: 1) slight abrading of a lens (to simulate increased light scatter), 2) addition of a neutral density filter (to simulate the reduction of light) and 3) addition of a yellow filter (to simulate the yellowing of macular pigment and lens) (Schneck, Adams, Huie and Lee, 1993). For purposes of demonstration, one may place such a lens in front of the projector to demonstrate the relative effects of optical changes of the vision of older adults. The yellow filter and neutral density filter used may be approximated from the published literature. We use a 0.3 or 0.4 ND Wratten filter combined with a light yellow filter (e.g., Wratten 2b or 2e) to provide younger viewers with the impression of age on a visual scene. This technique may provide a rapid intuitive insight as to approximate the visibility to an older observer of an object such as an oncoming vehicle or an object in his or her path.

## B. Neural Components

The magnitude of neural changes with normal aging is disputed. There are reports of reductions in numbers of neural cells at every level of the nervous system. However, "...available anatomical studies in humans and monkeys suggest that aging has only relatively minor effects on the retino-geniculo-striate pathway. Retinal photoreceptor losses are relatively restricted to rods, and there is compensation among the remaining rods for those that are lost. Although some retinal ganglion cells appear to be lost, the loss is small relative to individual-to-individual variability. In addition, there appear to be no massive cell losses in the LGN or striate cortex. Physiological results in the monkey LGN suggest that the functional properties of LGN neurons, and therefore their retinal inputs, are not significantly affected by aging." (Spear, 1993; p. 2589).

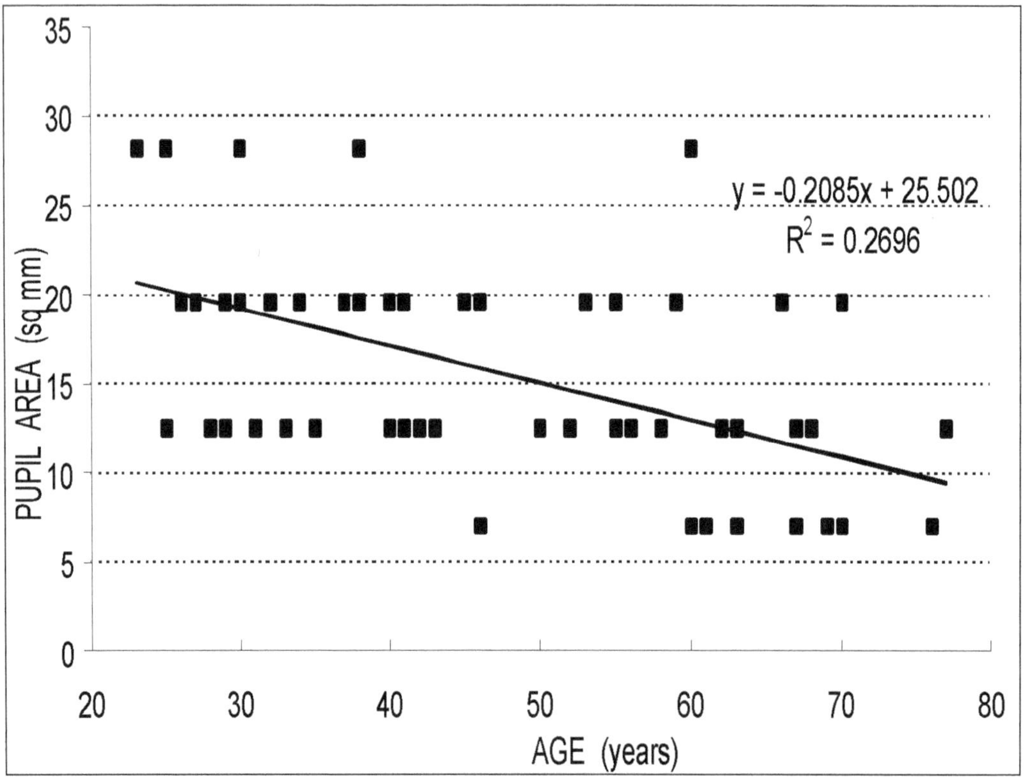


***Figure 9.1*** *Pupil Size and Age (data from Hanna, Chao, Linberg and Odom, 1991.). At any one luminance level the average pupil diameter and area will decrease with age. These data were collected as part of an effort to control retinal illuminance in older viewers. The ambient light level was approximately 68 lux. The relative magnitude of the reduction in pupillary area depends on the ambient light level. Note, however, that even in older viewers there is considerable individual variation in pupillary area and that the pupillary areas of younger and older viewers overlap.*

On the other hand, age-related diseases are associated with the loss of neural cells. The number of ganglion cells lost in Alzheimer's disease is substantial (Sadun and Bassi, 1990; Uylings and de Brabander, 2002). Consequently, one can see increased optic nerve damage in Alzheimer's patients in standard retinal photographs (Nelson, Cruz, Adler, McNinch, Leys, and Odom, 1991). Alzheimer's patients also have impaired visual functions (Cronin-Golomb, Corkin, Rizzo and Cohen, 1991). Age-related ocular diseases cause definite losses of retinal cells. Age-related maculopathy causes increased losses of rods and associated losses of visual functions (Curcio, Owsley and Jackson, 2000) while glaucoma causes losses of photoreceptors (Nork, 2000), ganglion cells and cortical losses (Yücel, Zhang, Weinreb, Kaufman, and Gupta, 2003) with associated losses of visual functions (Odom, Leys, Charlton, Manahilov, and Green, 2006; Yates, Leys, Green, Huang, Charlton, Reed, Di and Odom, 1999).

### C. Extraocular Muscles and Eye Movements

In general, muscle fibers become less elastic with age. The consequence is that the range of eye movements becomes somewhat constricted (Shechtman, Shallo-Hoffmann, Rumsey, Riordan-Eva and Hardigan, 2005). As a result, older viewers must often make head movements in addition to eye movements in order to bring objects from the far periphery into central view (Leigh, 1982).

## 9.3 Visual Function Changes with Age

### A. Functions which Decline with Age

Even when one excludes elderly viewers with observable disease, some visual functions decline with age. Most researchers find that when visual deficits are present, they can largely be explained on the basis of the optical changes which occur in aging, namely the reduced light entering the eye, the increased yellowing of pigments in the eye and increased light scatter within the eye. Usually a residual effect can be attributed to neural changes, but the size of this effect is usually small in a selected disease-free, normal population such that it could also be a result of imprecise estimates of the optical effects.

#### 1. Adaptation / Glare Sensitivity

Adaptation is the process by which the person becomes accustomed to a particular light level and performance at that light level becomes optimal. Generally adaptation comes in two flavors: slow and fast/transient. When lights are turned off, it usually takes as long as 30–45 minutes for the person to adjust to the dark and for light detection thresholds to stabilize. When lights are turned on it takes as long as 10 minutes for the person to adjust to the light and for performance at higher light levels to become optimal. In addition to these slow adaptation processes, there are more rapid changes which occur, for example, the adjustment to rapid changes in light levels.

Slow adaptive processes are usually measured using a "dark adaptometer." Following exposure to a bright light for several minutes, the lights are turned off and the person is asked to indicate when a light is detected in the dark. When the thresholds are plotted, they typically show a rapid decline in threshold which stabilizes and a second rapid decline in threshold which begins after about 5–7 minutes in the dark which stabilizes after about thirty minutes. In general, as people age the thresholds of both the cone (first phase) and rod (second phase) portions of the dark adaptation function are elevated and delayed (Jackson, Owsley and McGwin, 1999).

Glare is an imprecise concept with several meanings. (See Chapter 13.) The first is glare that results from a light being shined onto a surface so that the characteristics of the surface become unclear. Sometimes this is used to great artistic effect as when one sees photographs of the Washington Monument reflected in the Vietnam Memorial; however, it can also be exemplified by street lights reflecting off of wet pavement obscuring line markings indicating lanes or the edge of the road. The second major type of glare is that caused by diffusion of light either by reflection or diffraction of light from small particles, such as headlights from fog or sunlight refracted through smog. Both of these obscure the path ahead. Lastly there is the reduced ability to see as a result of a brighter light source surrounding or to the side of one's line of sight. The most frequently mentioned example of this type of glare is the difficulty some older drivers have driving when the headlights of cars coming from the opposite direction shine in the drivers' eyes. This last type of glare is directly related to the interocular forward light scatter which increases with age in older drivers (van den Berg, 1991; 1995). A number of studies have demonstrated that people's acuity or contrast thresholds are reduced when a glare source is present and that the reduction in acuity or contrast increases as people age (Elliott and Bullimore, 1993). See Chapter 13 for methods of computing the effect of glare on contrast sensitivity.

### 2. Color Vision

Older viewers make increased numbers of errors on tests of color matching (Shinomori, Schefrin, and Werner, 2001). The color matching errors that the very elderly make are much like those made by younger persons who view the same stimuli through yellow filters. Such yellow filters have two effects, one is a change in luminance, and the other is reducing the amount of blue light which reaches the eye. Another way of describing the same effect is to say that older observers' color matching errors resemble those of persons without blue cones or of younger observers tested under lower light levels (Knoblauch, Saunders, Kusuda, Hynes, Podgor, Higgins and de Monasterio, 1987).

### 3. Visual Acuity

Visual acuity is a measure of the ability to resolve small details. Visual acuity declines with age on average. Clinicians and researchers typically say that visual acuity of 20/20 is normal and any acuity that is 20/40 or better is within the normal range. However, when one tests young adults, their average best corrected visual acuity is better than 20/20 (Pitts, 1982; Frisén and Frisén, 1982; Ohlsson and Villarreal, 2005; Malmer and Martin, 2005). This remains true up until about fifty years of age. At about fifty-five or sixty the average visual acuity is about 20/20. Later, average visual acuity of viewers without clinically significant cataracts declines sharply, reaching about 20/80 by ninety years of age (Pitts, 1982; See Figure 9.2 adapted from Pitts, 1982). Groups of carefully selected healthy older viewers (i.e., over sixty years) will have acuity in the range of 20/25–20/20; the average acuity including all viewers is usually better than 20/40 (Frisén and Frisén, 1982; Malmer and Martin, 2005).

### 4. Contrast Sensitivity

A very important aspect of the visual system is our ability to detect small changes in the contrasts of objects. Under optimal conditions viewers can detect a contrast of 0.02 percent. In older adults this ability declines, even in viewers without ophthalmic disease so that by the age of seventy, the typical best threshold is 0.1 percent (Higgins, Jaffe, Caruso, and de Monasterio, 1988). The contrast sensitivity changes are spatial frequency dependent (see Figure 9.3 adapted from Huang, Odom, Green and Colvin, 1997). The greatest losses occur at high spatial frequencies. The second greatest losses occur at low spatial frequencies with little or no loss in the middle spatial frequencies. The low spatial frequency losses are enhanced at low luminance levels. Because low spatial frequency changes are difficult to explain on the basis of optical changes, they have been interpreted as evidence of neural changes in normal aging (Sloane, Owsley and Alvarez. 1988; Schefrin, Tregear, Harvey and Werner, 1999).

### 5. Visual Field, Visual Search and "Useful Field Of View"

Medical exams have long included perimetry, a visual field measurement that tests detection of small lights flashed at various locations in the visual field. As viewers age, their perimetry tests show a visual field loss of 10–15 degrees on either side. Most, if not all, of this decrease can be attributed to the reduced light entering the eye. Even younger viewers have narrower visual fields in dimmer light (Seiple, Szlyk, Yang, and Holopigian, 1996).

Surprisingly, standard perimetry has found only a weak connection between visual field losses in aging (e.g., Johnson, Adams, and Lewis, 1989) and accident rates (Johnson and Keltner, 1986) unless the loss is huge. Still, the International Council of Ophthalmology recommends minimum visual field width of 120° for unrestricted licensing. Required binocular field widths vary greatly across states, from 70° to 140°, while some states have no specific limit.

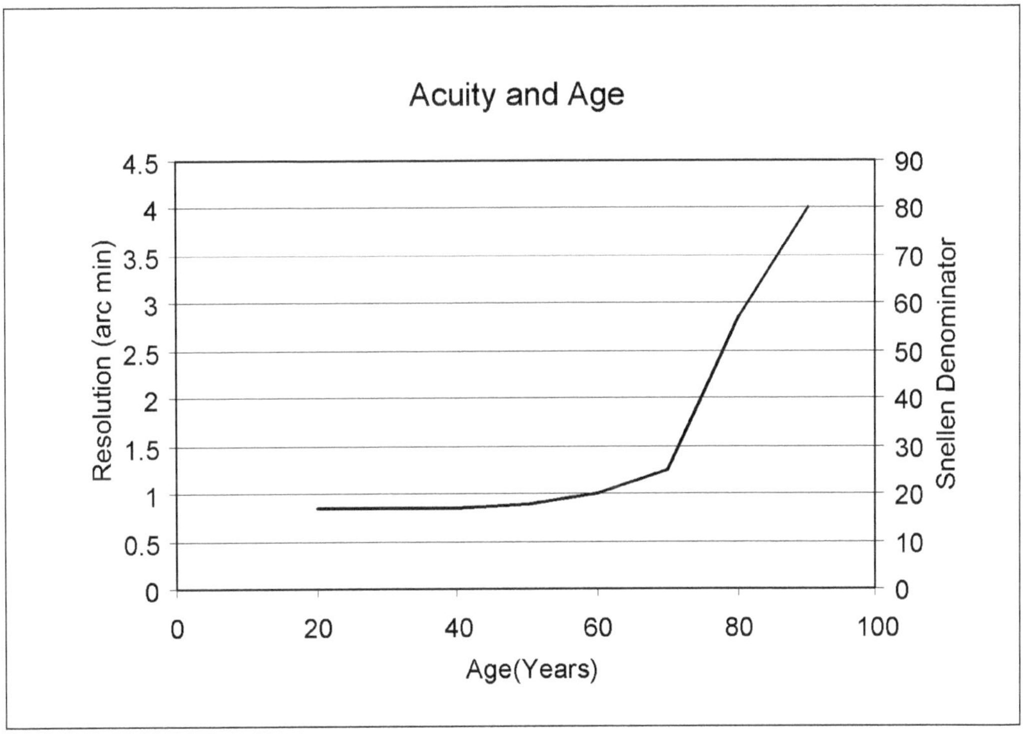


*Figure 9.2 Visual Acuity and Age (graphed data from Pitts, 1982). Visual acuity remains stable during most of adulthood. However, it declines rather rapidly after age fifty-five to sixty even in the absence of clinically significant cataracts. The studies on which Pitts based his data may have included viewers with subclinical pathology as more recent studies indicate that even at age eighty carefully selected viewers with no evidence of ophthalmic disease have visual acuities better than 20/40 (see Frisén and Frisén, 1982; Malmer and Martin, 2005)*

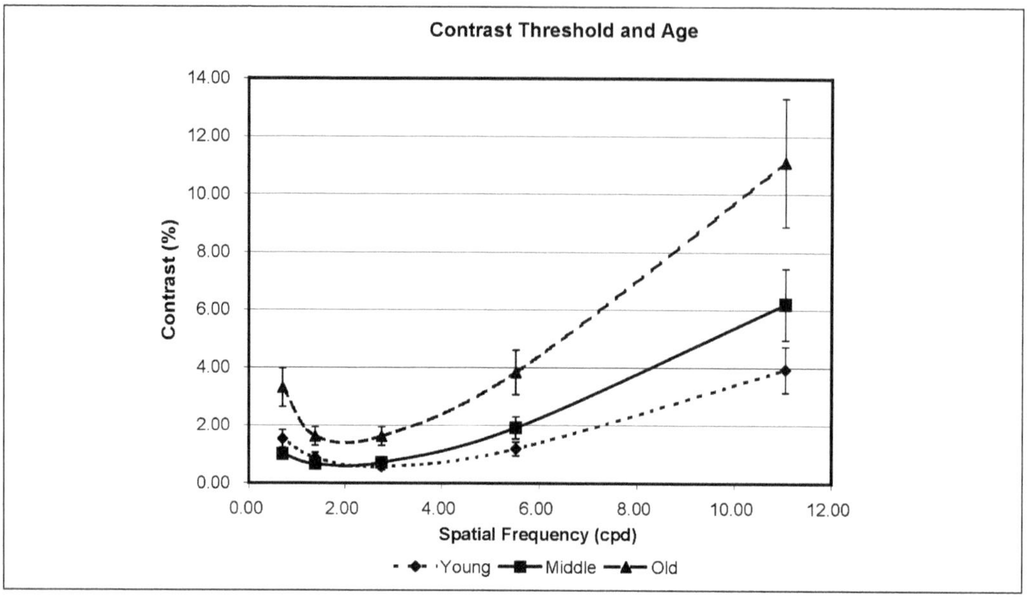


***Figure 9.3*** *Contrast Sensitivity and Age (data from Huang, Odom, Green and Colvin, 1997). Young observers were aged eighteen to twenty-five years, middle-aged observers were aged thirty to fifty years, and older observers were aged more than sixty-five years. Older observers were selected based on visual acuity better than 20/30 and normal performance on a test of cognitive functioning. Contrast thresholds were measured using a four alternative spatial forced choice paradigm. The screen size was 11.59 arc degrees at the viewing distance of 1 m. The mean screen illuminance was 68 lux.*

Burg and Hills (1977) concluded accident rates would be better predicted by perceptual rather than sensory tests, such as standard perimetry. (Once again, the sensation-perception distinction is important.) In fact, more recent evidence suggests that perceptual factors make real visual field losses greater than those suggested by standard perimetry. Sanders (1970) defined the concept of "functional field of view" as the area of space from which a viewer can acquire information at a glance and without head or eye movement. This visual field, now more commonly called the "useful field of view" (UFOV), differs from the traditional sensory-defined field by involving cognitive abilities. The UFOV requires not only detection but also recognition, localization and possibly reaction time to suprathreshold targets. A person with a reduced UFOV may detect targets but will have less ability to switch attention and react. Since objects on a collision course generally appear first in the peripheral field, reduced UFOV is likely a significant factor in crashes. Owsley, Ball, Sloane, Roenker, and Bruni (1991) concluded that reduced UFOV was responsible for 13 percent of the variance in crash data for older drivers and 29 percent specifically for intersection crashes.

While older viewers have a reduced UFOV, the cause is not entirely clear. Several studies (Seiple, Szlyk, Yang, and Holopigian, 1996; Gillard, 2002 ) have found that older viewers have impaired perception relative to younger viewers but that the relative loss does not change with visual field location. In other words, the apparently reduced UFOV follows directly from a generalized loss of attention, slowing, etc. rather than a loss that is specific to the peripheral field. However, these studies used alerted drivers who already had high arousal and knew that targets would appear. Real-world tests may have produced different results.

### 6. Motion Sensitivity and Speed Estimation

Older viewers have a reduced ability to detect rapidly moving objects. Many studies have found that older viewers have deficits in motion perception, a judgment critical in many collision avoidance scenarios. Older viewers have higher motion detection thresholds (Buckingham, Whitaker and Banford, 1987; Whitaker, Elliott and MacVeigh, 1992), higher motion discrimination thresholds (Raghuram, Lakshminarayanan, and Khanna, 1999; Odom and Leys, 2007) and longer reaction times to motion onset (Porciatti, Fiorentini, Morrone, and Burr, 1999).

### 7. Bisection Acuity

Hyperacuity is a class of visual tasks which younger viewers can perform much better than standard visual acuity tasks. Under the best conditions, the ability to tell whether one line is exactly in the middle between two other lines (bisection acuity) is about 2 arcsec or thirty times better that standard visual acuity. As viewers age bisection acuity becomes much worse (Whitaker, Elliott and MacVeigh, 1992; see Enoch, Werner, Haegerstrom-Portnoy, Lakshminarayanan, and Rynders, 1999).

One model of bisection acuity would suggest that it is equivalent to being able to tell the relative phase or position of two objects. We tested this hypothesis by determining the relative phase discrimination of viewers with normal visual acuity. Indeed their phase discrimination was impaired as they became older (Odom, Green, Cutlip, Chao, Yao, and Charlton, 1989).

### 8. Texture Discrimination

The ability to discriminate changes in texture is one of the major cues for discriminating objects and their location in depth. At least three texture discrimination tasks are impaired with age: the ability to distinguish differences in the number of dots (Huang, Leys, Green, Yates and Odom, 1997), the ability to detect line segments of an orientation different from the line segments surrounding them (Huang, Leys, Green, Yates and Odom, 1997), and relative phase of a higher frequency grating superimposed on a lower frequency grating (Odom, Green, Cutlip, Chao, Yao, and Charlton, 1989). Let us consider briefly just one of these, the ability to tell which area has more dots. When viewers look into the distance, more distant objects have a finer grain, in other words there are more dots than closer objects. Therefore, these monocular cues of depth such as texture density are impaired as people age.

### 9. Depth Perception and Stereopsis

There are many cues for depth including monocular cues such as texture and shadow. However, binocular depth perception or stereopsis has long been of special interest because it requires normal cortical neural function. Stereopsis (see Chapter 3) is usually divided into local stereopsis which appears to depend at least in part on matching object edges and global stereopsis which is usually thought to be independent of object detection per se (Julesz, 1971).

A number of studies have found that local stereopsis for near objects is reduced with age (see Pitt, 1982). In large part one may explain these results on the basis of reduced accommodative power with age. A few studies have employed dynamic random dot stereograms presented on a television screen to examine the effects of age on global stereopsis. Few of these studies have actually corrected for the 1–2 diopter of refractive error introduced for older observers by placing the stimulus at a 1/2–1 meter distance from the observer. The assumption has been that a 1–2 diopter error will have no effect on stereo thresholds, because of data presented by Julesz (1971) that low pass filtering did not remove the stereo percept. However, stereo thresholds are impaired by reduced retinal illuminance (see Figure 9.4; Hanna, Chao, Linberg and Odom, 1991) and by refractive error (see Figure 9.5; Odom, Chao, and Leys, 1992). Typically these studies have found a more modest age-related decline in the sensitivity to global stereoscopic stimuli (see Figure 9.6; Chao, Hanna, Linberg and Odom, 1990) which largely disappears when optical factors are corrected (Hanna, Chao, Linberg and Odom, 1991).

## 10. Optic Flow and Heading

Optic flow is the relative change in the positions of objects at different places in the visual field as one moves. Since the pioneering work of Gibson (Gibson, 1950; 1986; also see Calvert, 1950; Lee, 1980), optic flow has been identified as a major determinant of people's ability to successfully navigate in their environment. A number of components of the optic flow field have been identified, including radial inward or outward flow, laminar left or right flow, rotational clockwise or counterclockwise flow and deformation (Koenderink, 1986). In an optic flow field there is a stationary point from which all of the changes flow. The stationary focus of expansion (FOE) is the point toward which the person is heading. Thus, the insight of Gibson was that detecting the FOE was sufficient to determine a person's heading. The simplicity of defining the FOE has lead to considerable research to determine the conditions under which normal observers can accurately detect the FOE and use it to determine their heading.

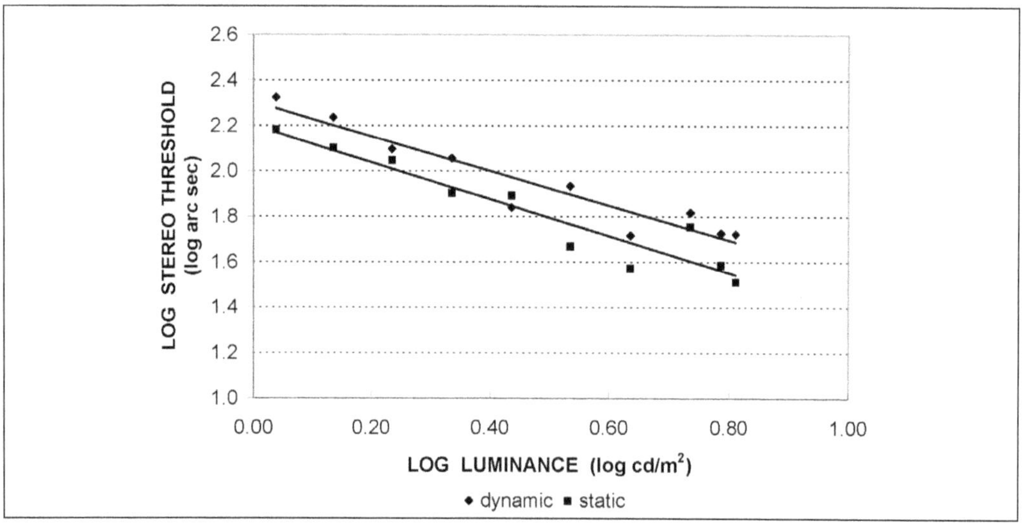


***Figure 9.4*** *Effects of Luminance on Stereo Acuity (data from Hanna, Chao, Linberg and Odom, 1991). Viewers looked at an anaglyphic dynamic random element stereogram (ADRES) through colored filters (red = Wratten 29 and green = Wratten 65) at a distance of two meters. The ADRES had the appearance of eight horizontal bars in depth which had a hypercyclopean spatial frequency of 0.63 cpd. The horizontal bars were either stationary or seemed to reverse positions in depth 3.7 times per second. The screen subtended a visual angle of 7.6 x 5.6 deg and had a luminance of 6.5 cd/m² when viewed through the chromatic filters.*

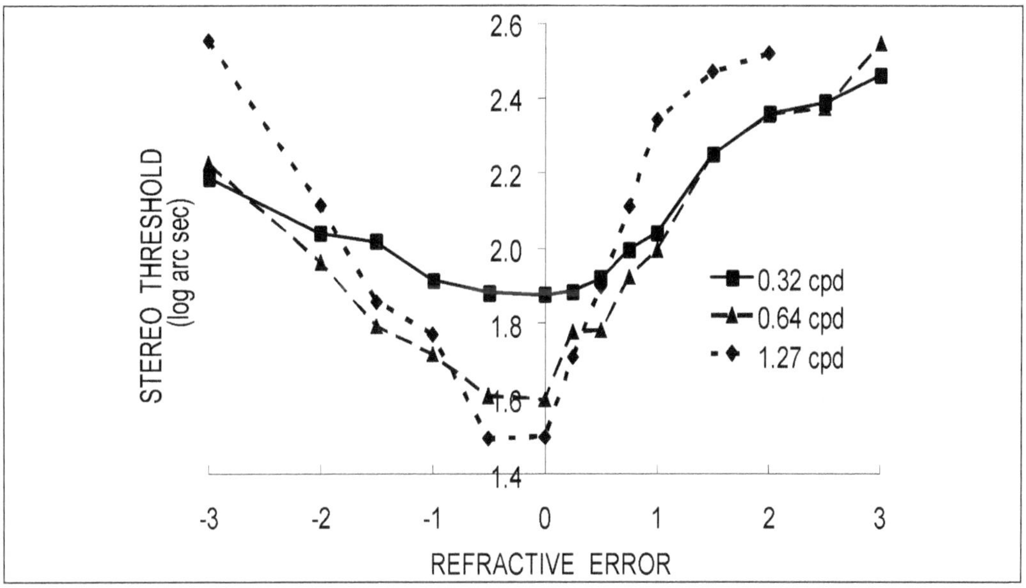


***Figure 9.5*** *Effect of Refractive Error on Stereo Thresholds (data from Odom, Chao, and Leys, 1992). Viewers looked at an anaglyphic dynamic random element stereogram (ADRES) through colored filters (red = Wratten 29 and green = Wratten 65) at a distance of two meters. The ADRES had the appearance of stationary horizontal bars in depth which had a hypercyclopean spatial frequency of 0.32, 0.64, or 1.27 cpd. The screen subtended a visual angle of 7.6 x 5.6 deg and had a luminance of 6.5 cd/m² when viewed through the chromatic filters.*

Theoretical analyses have indicated that optic flow information is sufficient to inform people, animals and machines of the spatial layout of their environment and the direction and heading of themselves and moving or stationary objects (see Koenderink, 1986; Koenderink and van Doorn, 1987; Longuet-Higgins and Pradzny, 1980). Physiological studies have indicated areas of the brain that appear to be specialized for retrieving optic flow information (Greenlee, 2000; Morrone, Tosetti, Montanaro, Fiorentini, Cioni, and Burr, 2000; Vaina and Rushton, 2000).

There are numerous potential visual sources of information about heading in natural environments, including egocentric direction (Rushton, Harris, Lloyd, and Wann, 1998; Warren, Kay, Zosh, Duchon, Sahuc, 2001; Harris and Carre, 2001; Harris and Bonas, 2002), environmental features which serve as landmarks (Warren, Kay, Zosh, Duchon, Sahuc, 2001; Harris and Carre, 2001; Duchon and Warren, 2002; Cutting, 1986), and textural characteristics (Duchon and Warren, 2002). Additionally, detection of the FOE can be easily obscured by eye movements or motion along a curvilinear path (Royden, Banks and Crowell, 1992; 1994; Royden, 1994) and is also subject to illusory effects (Duffy and Wurtz, 1993; Meese, Smith, Harris, 1995; Lappe, Bremmer, and van den Berg, 1999). Consequently, people use multiple cues in determining heading and controlling their direction of motion (Cutting, 1986; Duchon and Warren, 2002). Although optic flow is not the only cue to heading and direction in wayfinding, there is substantial evidence that viewers can use the FOE present in optic flow to determine their heading and direction of self-motion (Warren and Hannon, 1988; 1990; Royden, Banks and Crowell, 1992; 1994). Heading detection as indicated by the threshold for detecting the FOE is impaired with age. Comparing young normals to viewers with normal visual acuity and no evidence of glaucoma or age-related macular degeneration, there is an almost twofold increase in the threshold for heading detection (see Figure 9.7; Humble, Ghude, Leys, and Odom, 2006).

### 11. Visual Masking and Clutter

Environmental conditions can magnify the age-related acuity and contrast sensitivity losses found in typical laboratory studies. As noted in Chapter 14, laboratory tests use uniform backgrounds, but real viewers may see targets against contoured, structured backdrops. Older viewers show particularly large contrast sensitivity deficits in this clutter (e.g., Green, Huang and Odom, 2004).

Other studies have found that clutter impairs the ability of older viewers during search for suprathreshold targets. Rabbitt (1965), for example, found that elderly viewers required longer to perform a card sorting task but that the biggest effects occurred when the cards contained distractors, elements not relevant to performing the task. Rabbitt concluded that the elderly have trouble in search tasks where there are irrelevant distractors and that the effect was due to an inability to focus selective (spatial) attention. Other research (e.g., Plude and Hoyer, 1986) suggests that the elderly exhibit more susceptibility to clutter when target location is not known in advance.

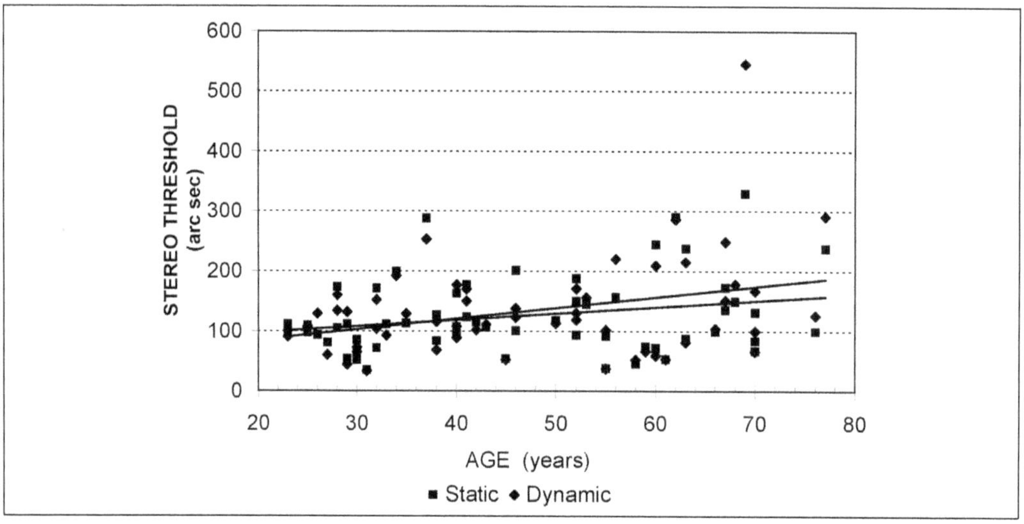


***Figure 9.6*** *Stereoacuity and age (data from Hanna, Chao, Linberg and Odom, 1991). Squares represent stereothresholds for dynamic random dot stereograms with stationary cyclopean bars. The diamonds represent stereo thresholds of stereograms which reversed in depth. Viewers aged twenty-three to seventy-seven years participated in the study. Over the age range tested their stereothresholds increased from about 100 arcsec to almost 200 arcsec for bars reversing in depth to about 150 arcsec for static stereo bar patterns. Stimulus conditions were the same as those indicated in Figure 9.4.*

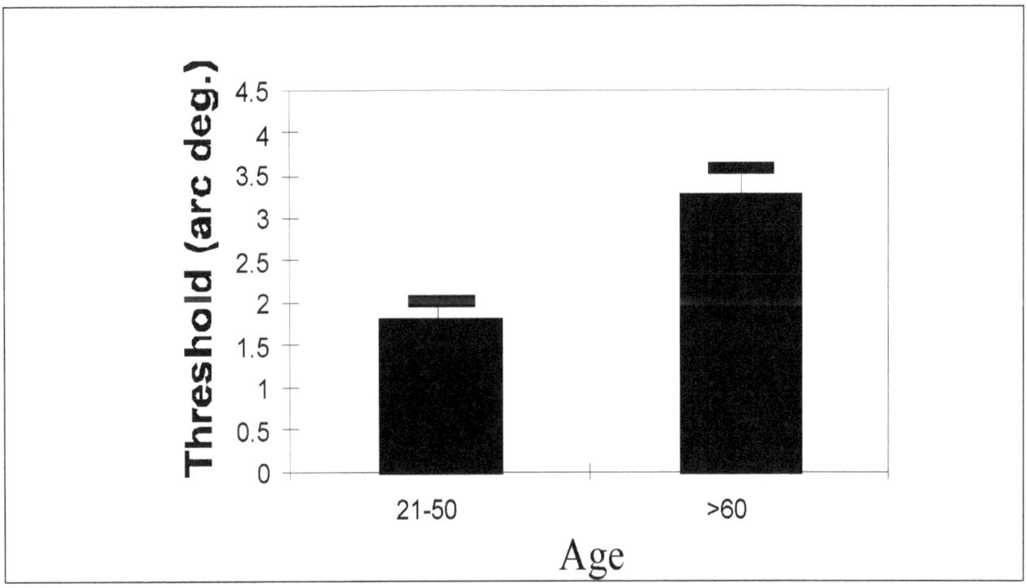


*Figure 9.7* Effect of Age on Heading Thresholds (data from Humble, Ghude, Leys, and Odom, 2006). The stimulus subtended 44.6 arc deg in the horizontal dimension at a viewing distance of 50 cm. 100 light dots appeared on a dark background. The dots appeared at random locations and moved away from a focus of expansion (FOE). Dots had a lifetime of 467 msec or were replaced as they moved off of the screen. Thresholds were determined using a dual two alternative forced choice staircase procedure.

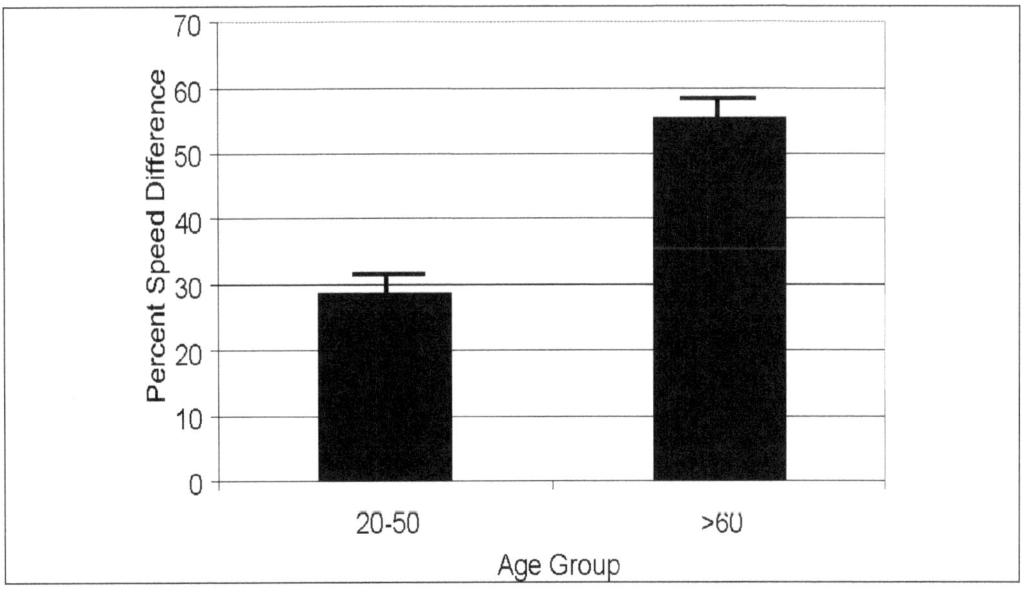


*Figure 9.8* Speed Discrimination (unpublished data, Odom and Leys, 2007). The display consisted of four regions of randomly placed dots. In two regions dots moved to the left and in two they moved to the right. The observer's task was to indicate the direction in which dots were moving faster. Against a baseline speed of 15.69 deg/sec, younger observers required a 28 percent change in speed while older viewers required a change of 55 percent before correctly identifying the direction of faster motion 70 percent of the time.

### 12. Visual Reaction Time

Scientists have used two approaches to conceptualizing aging effects. One assumes that aging affects each ability differently. Aging losses in detection, perception, attention, memory, etc. are separate dysfunctions with different underlying causes. The alternate approach explains aging effects by a single overarching factor that cuts across all sensory and motor performance. One such longstanding explanation (Welford, 1958) is that age-related deficits are due to increased internal noise which lowers the signal/noise ratio. (See the Chapter 2 discussion of Signal Detection Theory.) Response slows because the older person must gather more information to increase signal strength against the background noise. This creates a "generalized slowing," (Salthouse, 1985; Cerella, 1990) of all sensory and cognitive functioning. Reaction time also slows because the older person needs to collect more information to increase signal strength to the required signal-noise ratio (Salthouse, and Lichty, 1985). Loss of muscle strength and flexibility may further slow reaction times.

However, Chapter 17 noted that reaction time studies have had difficulty in demonstrating slower response for older drivers. The apparent paradox occurs because older responders only slow under some circumstances. To explain why, we digress to a brief discussion of reaction time theory.

Uncertainty is a key variable in reaction time. The main enemy of quick response for all responders, regardless of age, is the increased amount of cognitive processing that uncertainty creates. Donders (1868) proposed a reaction time task classification based on degree of inherent uncertainty.

*Simple (Type A):* Simple reaction time occurs when there is a single signal and a single response. The observer waits for a known signal and makes a predetermined response as fast as possible. In the classic laboratory procedure, the observer sits with his finger on a telegraph key and waits for a light to flash. When it does, he releases a telegraph key as fast as possible. Reaction time is the time between light onset (signal) and release of the key (response).

*Choice (Type B):* Choice reaction time occurs when there are multiple possible signals, each requiring a different response. The responder must decide which signal was present, and then choose the appropriate response. This requires two processes not present in simple reaction time: 1) signal discrimination—decide which signal occurred and 2) response selection—choose the response based on which signal occurred. The amount of uncertainty increases with the number of possible signals and responses. Choice reaction time more resembles actual driver decision. There is uncertainty as to what might appear and where. In low visibility, there can be a large uncertainty gap between detection on the one hand and recognition and situation awareness on the other. There can also be a response uncertainty—brake/swerve, swerve left/right, etc.

*Disjunctive (Type C):* There are multiple possible signals but only one response. In this case, the responder makes the response when one stimulus occurs but withholds response when the others appear. Uncertainty increases with the number of possible signals. Type C has more uncertainty than Type A but less uncertainty than Type B.

When laboratory research (e.g., Gottsdanker, 1982) has used a simple Type A task, then older viewers exhibit little slowing. However, Type A tasks have little uncertainty and cognitive processing complexity, so all viewers tend to approach the "irreducible minimum," the fastest possible response times. In such cases, there is little discrimination among responders of different capacity. It's like giving a very easy final exam that allows all students to score 100 percent, revealing nothing about the relative abilities of different students. Tests need to have some degree of difficulty before they can separate responders of differing ability. Type B and C reaction times contain uncertainty that slows reaction time from the irreducible minimum. When tested in a more complex diagnostic task, such as Type B, then older viewers show significant slowing (e.g., Simon and Pouraghabagher 1978).

Other research also demonstrated the effect of uncertainty on reaction time by manipulating probability and expectation. Many studies (e.g., Stelmach, Goggin and Amrein, 1988) have found older viewers showed little deficit if they had foreknowledge of the correct target location, time of arrival, and appropriate response. Uncertainty in any of these factors created larger deficits.

In sum, younger and older viewers have similar reaction times when conditions are simple, visibility good and uncertainty minimal. As uncertainty and complexity increase, both younger and older responders slow, but older viewers slow more. These observations allow some possible predictions about driver behavior. For example, an older driver following near a lead vehicle that flashes its brake lights should show relatively little deficit since it is a highly overlearned Type A-like situation—if the red light illuminates, then brake. An older driver who looks down a dark road at night and sees the dim shape of a trailer blocking the road, would be in a Type B or possibly C task and show a very large deficit due to the recognition uncertainty, violated expectation and response uncertainty among swerving left or right or braking.

## B. Visual functions which remain relatively unchanged with age

When one excludes elderly viewers with observable ocular disease, some visual functions do not appear to decline with age. The functions which are relatively unimpaired in older persons are functions involved in localizing objects.

### 1. Vernier Acuity

Vernier acuity is the ability to tell whether two objects are lined up as on a Vernier dial. (See Chapter 14.) Odom, Vasquez, Schwartz, and Linberg (1989) first demonstrated that vernier acuity did not decline with age in viewers with normal visual acuity and normal ophthalmic examinations. This observation has subsequently been confirmed by other investigators (Whitaker, Elliott and MacVeigh, 1992; see Enoch, Werner, Haegerstrom-Portnoy, Lakshminarayanan, and Rynders, 1999; but see Garcia-Suarez, Barrett, and Pacey, 2004). The fact that vernier does not change greatly with age and is also minimally affected by optical characteristics has led to its being proposed as a useful test of visual function in older viewers (Enoch, Werner, Haegerstrom-Portnoy, Lakshminarayanan, and Rynders, 1999).

### 2. Orientation Discrimination

One way of conceptualizing vernier acuity is to suggest that vernier acuity is a special case of orientation discrimination. If this were true, one would expect that viewers with normal visual acuity would have little or no reduction in their ability to discriminate orientation of parallel lines or gratings. We have demonstrated that orientation discrimination for gratings is not altered in older viewers (Odom, Green, Cutlip, Chao, Yao, and Charlton, 1989).

## C. Relation of Sensory to Perceptual and Cognitive Deficits

The relationship of sensory to cognitive deficits has long been a controversial topic. However, it is not surprising perhaps that those older viewers who have difficulty following conversations in groups may also have more difficulty recognizing faces or changes in facial expressions. Viewers who are confused as they wander in the hospital or lose their way in traffic may be the same viewers who have reduced contrast sensitivity or visual acuity. Several lines of evidence do in fact point to strong correlations between sensory abilities and cognitive abilities in aging. The Alabama group has found that performance on search tasks and "useful field of view" are very good predictors of driving performance and accident rates (see discussion above). The Berlin group reports that as much as 93 percent of the variance in declines in cognitive performance in aging can be accounted for by individual differences in sensory abilities (Baltes and Lindenberger, 1997). Lastly, sensory deficits have been observed in older viewers with Alzheimer's disease (see discussion above on neural deficits). The interpretation of these studies remains controversial but clearly they do point out a relationship between the neural substrates of cognition and sensory ability.

## 9.4 Implications of Visual Aging Changes for "Normal" Behavior and Environmental Design

### A. Summary and General Solutions

Older persons may have relatively severe visual losses even in the absence of eye diseases such as age-related macular degeneration, glaucoma, or diabetic retinopathy. These visual problems are largely related to optical changes in the aging eye which cause things to be appear darker, more yellow, and more subject to glare.

The general solutions to these optical problems is to counteract them by using brighter lighting, higher contrast objects, more saturated colors (generally avoid pastels), and to demarcate borders and edges clearly. Here is a general summary: (See Green, 2002 for more information.)

- The absolute amount of required illumination cannot be specified without task analysis because needed light level is a function of the size and physical contrast of the critical visual details. Any requirements for speed and/or accuracy also increase needed illumination;
- The illumination should increase without creating glare, which occurs when viewing a bright light or a bright reflection off a glossy surface. Instead of using a few intense light sources, the best strategy is use many smaller ones. Moreover, ambient lighting should be indirect, hiding intense light sources from direct view. Diffusing surfaces over the lights also will help reduce glare. Similarly, reduce glare from sunlight with shades and awnings. Put carpets over polished hardwood or tile floors, and minimize glass display cases and other reflective surfaces.
- Put the light where it does the most good. Higher illumination means higher energy costs, but it is not necessary to dramatically increase illumination everywhere. The ambient illumination can remain moderate, as long as the lighting at task areas is sufficiently high.
- Provide adjustable light sources. Where there is a combination of younger and older workers, this may be impractical for ambient sources, but it should be feasible for task lighting. However, there is research to suggest workers do not always choose optimal levels.
- Older viewers light and dark adapt more slowly, so keep the light from one area to another at a similar level. If the older person works at a computer, make sure the area surrounding the computer screen has similar brightness. The Illuminating Engineering Society recommends a brightness difference of no greater than 3:1.

### B. Mobility

1. Stairs, escalators and ladders are a special problem. The changes in optics result in poor ability of normal older viewers to discriminate beginning and end of stairs, resulting in increased falls. One solution is to clearly demarcate the edges of steps.

2. Maintaining objects in the field of view can be difficult. Because of the reduced field of view older viewers are more prone to "bump" into things especially in new environments. One solution in many situations is to clearly place high-contrast borders around objects on walkways, etc. Another is to have a clear brightness and color demarcation between floor and walls.

## C. Driving: Are Older Drivers Really Worse Drivers?

The many visual losses documented above suggest that older drivers should be unsafe drivers. According to most sources, accident statistics (e.g., Cerelli, 1989; OCED, 2001) seemingly confirm the prediction because older drivers have more accidents per mile/km. Closer examination, however, tells a very different story, one which highlights the need to interpret epidemiological data and accident statistics with great caution (e.g., Green, 2001).

Most studies comparing accident rates for younger and older drivers contain hidden biases. The "frailty bias" occurs because older drivers are frailer and more prone to injury when a collision occurs. Since injury accidents are more likely to be included in databases, collisions involving older drivers have a higher likelihood of being reported. Li, Braver and Chen (2003) found that when corrected for the frailty factor, the apparent overrepresentation of older drivers in accident statistics dropped significantly.

The "low mileage bias" (Janke, 1991) is the fact people who drive more miles have fewer accidents on a per mile basis. This is likely due to several factors. Long trips (on freeways and between cities, etc.) which build up total mileage are less hazardous. Accidents on interstates are spectacular but relatively low per mile because traffic is lighter, attentional demands lower and quick reaction is less often required. There are few complex intersections and traffic is almost invariably going in the same direction. In contrast, short trips on congested city streets with vehicles approaching from many different angles put a higher premium on rapid perception, peripheral vision, attention and decision-making. Lastly, people who drive more are likely more practiced and more prepared to handle emergencies.

The low mileage bias inflates the percentage of accidents involving older drivers since they travel fewer miles (e.g., Planek, 1972). Recent studies (e.g., Hakamies-Blomqvist, Raitanen, and O'Neill, 2002; Langford, Methorst, and Hakamies-Blomqvist, 2006) that have corrected accident data for the low mileage bias found no evidence of higher crash involvement by older drivers.

There are several explanations for the apparent paradox between these results and the unquestioned visual and cognitive impairment of aging. Older drivers risk compensate in many ways (Preusser, Williams, Ferguson, Ullmer, and Weinstein, 1998). They travel more slowly and drive less often at night and in other hazardous conditions. They are less likely to drive under the influence of drugs and alcohol. Moreover, their experience gives them better ability to anticipate hazardous conditions. In sum, they tend to compensate for impairment by avoiding situations where their diminished capacity is taxed.

These newer studies, however, should not be taken to mean that older drivers are as good as younger drivers. There are specific situations where the impairments of normal aging as well as the diseases of aging are likely to be a causative factor. As already noted, loss of acuity and contrast sensitivity *per se* are not highly related to accident occurrence. Of course, the meaning of this epidemiological finding is also unclear. Driving license exams test for acuity and likely weed out potential drivers with losses big enough to be a significant factor. People with poor acuity probably risk compensate.

There are some instances where aging deficits are likely be a factor. One obvious case is at night when the increased glare susceptibility and the slower dark adaptation can create large detection impairments. The UFOV discussion suggested that older drivers will also exhibit especially large deficits with objects located in the peripheral field, which is the case for most pedestrian and right-angle collisions. Older viewers are also more impaired by background clutter and masking. In many accidents, the cause is due more to cognitive than sensory factors, since older people exhibit general cognitive slowing, poorer memory and less ability to divide attention. Older drivers will exhibit especially large deficits in situations that are complex or ambiguous because they take longer to gain situational awareness. For example, an older driver on a dark road sensing an ambiguous shape may take longer to realize that it is a trailer blocking the roadway. When making turns at intersections, the older driver may have difficulty keeping track of vehicles approaching from different directions.

These predictions are consistent with the results of the National Institute on Aging symposium where 400 older drivers discussed their biggest difficulties in driving. They had greater difficulty with speed judgments and found that vehicles moved too quickly (as might be expected from generalized slowing), and they had especially large difficulties merging with traffic. They also had problems seeing the peripheral field, and they had difficulty noticing unexpected appearances of vehicles away from the direct line of sight. Moreover, research studies have confirmed these introspections and have further identified several driving tasks that cause older drivers significant difficulty:

- Judging whether a rear-end collision will occur;
- Judging correct speed;
- Braking rapidly;
- Steering smoothly;
- Judging when to merge into traffic; and
- Judging when to turn corners.

## 9.5 Conclusions

Research on visual aging has grown dramatically in recent years as the demographic shift toward an older population accelerates. This chapter has provided only a brief overview on the vast amount of available research. To very quickly summarize the reams of research, both optical and neural visual components degrade, and both psychophysical and cognitive abilities fade. Older viewers exhibit reduced acuity and contrast sensitivity, smaller visual fields, increased glare susceptibility, slowed light adaptation, generalized slowing of cognition, and impairment in ability to focus and divide attention. They also exhibit other losses in a wide range of motor abilities. The functional losses first become apparent in the early forties (e.g., Green, Huang and Odom, 2004), although the impairment does not usually become significant until the sixties. Moreover, much of the older population also suffers further losses from eye diseases, such as glaucoma, age-related macular degeneration, diabetic retinopathy and retinitis pigmentosa. This chapter, however, has addressed only "normal," healthy vision.

Older drivers are well aware of their limitations and perform some degree of risk compensation. When corrected for frailty and low mileage biases, accident rates for the elderly are no worse than for younger drivers. Moreover, situational variables modulate the magnitude of many perceptual and cognitive losses. In relatively simple situations, older viewers may perform almost as well as younger ones. However, complex and ambiguous situations decrease performance for all viewers, but the elderly exhibit relatively greater loss. Interestingly, the same pattern occurs in other impaired populations, such as intoxicated, drug-using and distracted drivers. Are older drivers equivalent to drunk drivers?

Lastly, "normal" visual aging raises issues in the assignment of blame. If an older person has an accident because of a "normal" visual loss, is he at fault? Should the same standards of normality be applied to a twenty-five year old and a seventy year old driver? Should the elderly person be held responsible for failing to compensate for his losses through less risky behavior (not driving at night, etc.)? Should the licensing authority be held accountable for granting him a license? Should designers of products/environments, like roadways, used by the elderly be responsible for designing to their lower perceptual and cognitive abilities?

These are legal rather than scientific or human factors questions, so we have no answers. However, we can say that design is (or should be) based on the visual capabilities of the user population. If those visual capabilities change due to a demographic shift, good design says that the designs should change too. Organizations, such as the Illuminating Engineering Society of North America, have begun recognizing the need to design for the older person by including specific guidelines in their recommendations.

## References

Administration on Aging. 2006. *A Profile of Older Americans: 2006*. Accessed at http://www.aoa.gov/prof/Statistics/statistics.asp. January 4, 2008.

Applegate, R. A., W. J. Donnelly, III, J. D. Marsack, D. E. Koenig, and K. Pesudovs. 2007. Three-dimensional relationship between high-order root-mean-square wavefront error, pupil diameter, and aging. *Journal of the Optical Society of America A*. 24, 578-587.

Ball, K., and R. Sekuler. 1986. Improving visual perception in older observers. *Journal of Gerontology* 41, 176-182.

Ball, K., B. Beard, D. Roenker, R. Miller, and D. Griggs. 1988. Age and visual search: Expanding the useful field of view. *Journal of the Optical Society of America A*. 5, 2210-2219.

Ball, K., C. Owsley, and B. Beard. 1990. Clinical visual perimetry understates peripheral field problems in older adults. *Clinical Vision Science* 5, 113-125.

Ball, K., D. Roenker, J. Bruni, L. Jackson, R. Dahl, and M. Rowan. 1990. Age and visual search: bases for shrinkage of the useful field of view. *Investigative Ophthalmology and Visual Science*. 31 (ARVO Suppl.), 356.

Baltes, P. B. and U. Lindenberger. 1997. Emergence of a powerful connection between sensory and cognitive functions across the adult life span: a new window to the study of cognitive aging? *Psychology and Aging*. 12, 12-21.

Buckingham, T., D. Whitaker, and D. Banford. 1987. Movement in decline? Oscillatory movement displacement thresholds increase with age. *Ophthalmic and Physiological Optics*, 7, 411-413.

Calvert, E. S. 1950. Visual aids for landing in bad visibility with special reference to the transition from instrument to visual flight. *Transactions of the Illuminating Engineering Society. London*. 15, 183-219.

Cerella, J. 1990. Aging and information-processing rate. In (J. E. Birren and K. W. Schaie Eds.), *Handbook of the psychology of aging* (3rd Ed.), 201-211. San Diego: Academic Press.

Cerrelli, E. 1989. Older drivers, the age factor in traffic safety. *NHTSA, DOT HS 807 402.*

Chao, G. M., F. Hanna, J. V. Linberg, and J. V. Odom. 1990. Static and global stereo acuity: effects of age. *Technical Digest Series (Optical Society of America)* 21, 42.

Craig, J. P. and A. Tomlinson. 1998. Age and gender effects on the normal tear film. Advances in Experimental Medicine and Biology. 438, 411-5.

Cronin-Golomb, A., S. Corkin, J. Rizzo, and J. Cohen. 1991. Visual dysfunction in Alzheimer's disease: Relation to normal aging. *Annals of Neurology* 29, 41-52.

Curcio, C. A., C. Owsley, and G. R. Jackson. 2000. Spare the rods, save the cones in aging and age-related maculopathy. *Investigative Ophthalmology and Visual Science*. 41, 2015–18.

Cutting, J. E. 1986. *Perception with an Eye for Motion*. Cambridge, Mass: *The MIT Press.*

Donders, F. C. 1868. On the speed of mental processes. Translated by W. G. Koster, 1969. *Acta Psychologica* 30: 412-431.

Duchon, A. P. and W. H. Warren, Jr. 2002. A visual equalization strategy for locomotor control: of honeybees, robots, and humans. *Psychological Science*. 13, 272-278.

Duffy, C. J, and R. H. Wurtz. 1993. An illusory transformation of optic flow fields. *Vision Research*. 33, 1481-1490.

Early, F., and A. Smith. 1990. Spatial frequency discrimination in normal ageing and in one case of Alzheimer's disease. *Clinical Vision Science* 56, 59-64.

Elliott, D. B. and M. A. Bullimore. 1993. Assessing the reliability, discriminative ability, and validity of disability glare tests. *Investigative Ophthalmology and Visual Science*. 34, 108-19.

Enoch, J. M, J. S. Werner, G. Haegerstrom-Portnoy, V. Lakshminarayanan, and M. Rynders. 1999. Forever young: visual functions not affected or minimally affected by aging: a review. *Journal of Gerontolology A Biological Science and Medical Science*. 54, B336-51.

Frisén, L., and M. Frisén. 1981. How good is normal visual acuity?. A study of letter acuity thresholds as a function of age. *Albrecht Von Graefes Archiv fuer Klinische und Experimental Ophthalmologie*. 215, 149-57.

Garcia-Suarez, L., B. T. Barrett, and I. Pacey. 2004. A comparison of the effects of ageing upon vernier and bisection acuity. Vision Research. *44*, 1039-1045.

Gibson, J. J. 1950. *The Perception of the Visual World.* Boston: *Houghton Mifflin.*

Gibson. J. J. 1986. *The Ecological Approach to Visual Perception.* Hillsdale, NJ: *Lawrence Erlbaum Associates.*

Gillard, J. 2002. Evaluation of Driver Useful Field Of View (UFOV): Effects Of Age And Eccentricity. Unpublished Master's Thesis, University of South Dakota.

Gottsdanker, R. 1982. Age and Simple Reaction Time. *Journal of Gerontology* 37, 342-348.

Green, M., W. Huang, and J. V. Odom. 2004. Aging vision in visual clutter. *The Human Factors and Ergonomic Society Meeting*, New Orleans, LA.

Green, M. 2001. Lies, Damned Lies and...Controls, *Risk Management* Nov 8–9.

Green, M. 2002. Safe Environments for the Older Worker," *Occupational Health & Safety*, January.

Greenlee, M. W. 2000. Human cortical areas underlying the perception of optic flow: brain imaging studies. *Internationl Review of Neurobiology*. 44, 269-292.

Hakamies-Blomqvist, L., T. Raitanen, and D. O'Neill. 2002. Driver ageing does not cause higher accident rates per km., *Transportation Research Part F: Traffic Psychology and Behaviour*, 5, pp. 271-274.

Hanna, F., G. M. Chao, J. V. Linberg, and J. V. Odom. 1991. Static and dynamic global stereo acuity: effects of age. *Investigative Ophthalmology and Visual Science*. 32 (ARVO Suppl.), 709.

Harris, J. M. and W. Bonas. 2002. Optic flow and scene structure do not always contribute to the control of human walking. *Vision Research*. 42, 1619-1626.

Harris, M. G. and G. Carre. 2001. Is optic flow used to guide walking while wearing a displacing prism? *Perception*. 30, 811-818.

Higgins, K., M. Jaffe, R. Caruso, and F. DeMonasterio. 1988. Spatial contrast sensitivity: Effects of age, test-retest, and psychophysical method. *Journal of the Optical Society of America A* 5, 2173-2180.

House, P., M. Schulzer, and G. Douglas. 1991. Characteristics of the normal central visual field measured with resolution perimetry. *Graefe's Archive for Clinical and Experimental Ophthalmology*. 229, 8-12.

Huang, W., M. J. Leys, M. Green, J. T. Yates, and J. V. Odom. 1997. Influences of noise on adult age differences in dot numerosity and orientation discrimination thresholds. *Investigative Ophthalmology and Visual Science*. 38 (ARVO Suppl.), S67.

Huang, W., J. V. Odom, M. Green, and A. Colvin. 1997. Effects of noise on age differences in contrast thresholds. Proceedings of the Annual APA Meeting. Chicago, IL. American Psychological Association.

Humble, H. L., P. Ghude, M. J. Leys, and J.V. Odom. 2006. Effects of visual noise on heading perception in optic flow patterns. *Investigative Ophthalmology and Visual Science*. 47, E-Abstract 2305.

Jackson, G. R., C. Owsley, and G. McGwin, Jr. 1999. Aging and dark adaptation. *Vision Research* 39, 3975-3982.

Jaffe, G., J. Alverado, and R. Juster. 1986. Age-related changes of the normal visual field. *Archives of Ophthalmology* 104, 1021-1025.

Janke, M. K. 1991. Accidents, mileage, and the exaggeration of risk. *Accident Analysis and Prevention*. 23, 183-188.

Johnson C., A. Adams, and R. Lewis. 1989. Evidence for a neural basis of age-related visual field loss in normal observers. *Investigative Ophthalmology and Visual Science* 30, 2056-2064.

Johnson, C., A. Adams, and R. Lewis. 1989. Evidence for a neural basis of age-related visual field loss in normal observers. *Investigative Ophthalmology and Visual Science* 30, 2056-2064.

Johnson, C., and J. Keltner. 1986. Incidence of visual field loss in 20,000 eyes and its relationship to driving performance. *Archives of Ophthalmology* 101, 371-375.

Julesz, B. 1971. *Foundations of Cyclopean Perception*. Chicago: The University of Chicago Press.

Knoblauch, K., F. Saunders, M. Kusuda, R. Hynes, M. Podgor, K. E. Higgins, and F. M. de Monasterio. 1987. Age and illuminance effects in the Farnsworth-Munsell 100-hue test. *Applied Optics* 26, 1441–1451.

Koenderink, J. J., and A. J. van Doorn. 1987. Facts on optic flow. *Biological Cybernetics,* 56, 247-254.

Koenderink, J. J. 1986. Optic flow. *Vision Research*. 26, 161-179.

Langford, J., R. Methorst, and L. Hakamies-Blomqvist. 2006. Older drivers do not have a high crash risk: A replication of low mileage bias. *Accident Analysis and Prevention* 38, 574-578.

Lappe, M., F. Bremmer, and A. V. van den Berg. 1999. Perception of self-motion from visual flow. *Trends in Cognitive Science*. 3, 329-336.

Lappe, M. 2000. Computational mechanisms for optic flow analysis in primate cortex. *International Review of Neurobiology*. 44, 235-268.

Lee, D. N. 1980. The optic flow field, the foundation of vision. *Philosophical Transactions of the Royal Society of London B Biological Sciences*. 290, 169-179.

Leigh, R. J. 1982. The impoverishment of ocular motility in the elderly. In *Aging and Human Visual Function* edited by R. Sekuler, D. Kline, and K. Dismukes, 173-180. New York, NY: Alan R Liss, Inc.

Li, G., E. Braver, and L. Chen. 2003. Fragility versus excessive crash involvement as determinants of high death rates per vehicle-mile of travel among older drivers. *Accident Analysis and Prevention* 35, 227–35.

Lindenberger, U. and P. B. Baltes. 1997. Intellectual functioning in old and very old age: cross-sectional results from the Berlin Aging Study. *Psychology and Aging* 12, 410-432.

Lindenberger, U. and P. B. Baltes. 1994. Sensory functioning and intelligence in old age: a strong connection. *Psychology and Aging* 9, 39-355.

Loewenfeld, I. E. 1979. Pupillary changes related to age. In: H. S. Thompson, R. Daroff, L. Frisen, J. S. Glaser and M. D. Sanders (eds.), *Topics in neuro-ophthalmology*, Williams and Wilkens, Baltimore, MD.

Longuet-Higgins, H. C., and K. Prazdny. 1980. The interpretation of moving retinal images. *Philosophical Transactions of the Royal Society of London B Biological Sciences*. 208, 385-397.

Malmer, L., and L. Martin. 2005. Micro dot test of foveal function. A comparison with visual acuity at high and low contrast. *Ophthalmic and Physiological Optics* 25 (2), 81–86.

Mangano, L., T. L. Schwartz, J. F. Charlton, and J. V. Odom. 1994. The effect of cycloplegia on visual acuity and contrast sensitivity. *Investigative Ophthalmology and Visual Science*, 35 (ARVO Suppl.), 2202.

Meese, T. S., V. Smith, and M. G. Harris. 1995. Induced motion may account for the illusory transformation of optic flow fields found by Duffy and Wurtz. *Vision Research*. 35, 981-985.

Morrone, M. C., M. Tosetti, D. Montanaro, A. Fiorentini, G. Cioni, and D. C. Burr. 2000. A cortical area that responds specifically to optic flow, revealed by fMRI. *Nature Neuroscience*. 3, 1322-1328.

Nelson, T. R., R. A. Cruz, S. A. Adler, D. McNinch, M. J. Leys, and J. V. Odom. 1991. Some Alzheimer's viewers show atrophied optic nerves clinically. *Society for Neuroscience Abstracts* 17(Part 1), 695.

Nork, T. M. 2000. Acquired color vision loss and a possible mechanism of ganglion cell death in glaucoma. *Transactions of the American Ophthalmological Society*. 98, 331–363.

OCED. 2001. Organization For Economic Co-operation And Development. *Ageing And Transport: Mobility Needs And Safety Issues*. Paris, France.

Odom, J. V., and M. J. Leys. 2007. Effects of age and age-related degeneration on speed discrimination. Unpublished data.

Odom, J. V., G. M. Chao, and M. Leys. 1992. Symmetrical refractive error elevates stereo thresholds. *Investigative Ophthalmology and Visual Science*. 33 (ARVO Suppl.), 1375.

Odom, J. V., M. Green, C. Cutlip, G. M. Chao, K. Yao, and J. F. Charlton. 1993. Aging impairs spatial discrimination of phase but not orientation. *Society for Neuroscience Abstracts* 19 part 1, 385.

Odom, J. V., M. J. Leys, J. Charlton, V. Manahilov, and M. Green. 2006. Detecting glaucomatous damage: evaluation with contrast independent tasks. *Journal of Modern Optics*, 53, 1373-1385.

Odom, J. V., R. Vasquez, T. Schwartz, and J. V. Linberg. 1989. Adult vernier thresholds do not increase with age, vernier bias does. *Investigative Ophthalmology and Visual Science* 30, 1004-1008.

Ohlsson, J., and G. Villarreal. 2005. Normal visual acuity in 17-18 year olds. *Acta Ophthalmologica Scandinavica.* 83, 487-491.

Owsley, C., K. Ball, M. Sloane, D. Roenker, and J. Bruni. 1991. Visual/cognitive correlates of vehicle accidents in older drivers. *Psychology and Aging.* 6, 403-415.

Pitts, D. G. 1982. The effects of aging on selected visual functions: Dark Adaptation, Visual acuity, stereopsis, and brightness contrast. In *Aging and Human Visual Function* edited by R. Sekuler, D. Kline, and K. Dismukes, 131-159. New York: Alan R. Liss, Inc.

Planek, T. 1972. The aging driver in today's traffic: a critical review. In (T. Planek, W. Mann and E. Wiener, eds.) *Aging And Highway Safety: The elderly In A Mobile Society.* Nighway Safety Research Center: Chapel Hill, N.C.

Plude, D., and W. Hoyer. 1986. Age and the selectivity of visual information processing. *Psychology and Aging.* 1, 4–10.

Porciatti, V., A. Fiorentini, M. C. Morrone, and D. C. Burr. 1999. The effects of ageing on reaction times to motion onset. *Vision Research* 39, 2157-2164.

Preusser, D., A. Williams, S. Ferguson, R. Ullmer, and H. Weinstein. 1998. Fatal crash risk for older drivers at intersections. *Accident Analysis and Prevention* 30, 151-159.

Rabbitt, P. M. A. 1965. An age decrement in the ability to ignore irrelevant information. *Journal of Gerontology*, 20, 233-237.

Raghuram, A., V. Lakshminarayanan, and Ritu Khanna. 1999. Psychophysical estimation of speed discrimination. II. Aging effects. *Journal of the Optical Society of America A.* 22, 2269-2280.

Royden, C. S. 1994. Analysis of misperceived observer motion during simulated eye rotations. *Vision Research* 34, 3215-3222.

Royden, C. S., M. S. Banks, and J. A. Crowell. 1992. The perception of heading during eye movements. *Nature* 380, 583-585.

Royden, C. S., M. S. Banks, and J. A. Crowell. 1994. Estimating heading during eye movements. *Vision Research* 34, 3197-3114.

Rushton, S. K., J. M. Harris, M. R. Lloyd, and J. P. Wann. 1998. Guidance of locomotion on foot uses perceived target location rather than optic flow. *Current Biology.* 8, 1191-1194.

Sadun, A. A., and C. J. Bassi. 1990. Optic nerve damage in Alzheimer's disease. *Ophthalmology* 97, 9-17.

Salthouse T., and W. Lichty 1985. Tests of the neural noise hypothesis of age-related cognitive change. *Journals of Gerontology*, 40, 443-50.

Salthouse, T. 1985. *A Theory of Cognitive Aging*. Elsevier: Amsterdam.

Sanders, A. 1970. Some aspects of the selective process in the functional field of view, *Ergonomics* 13, 101-117.

Schefrin, B. E., S. J. Tregear, L. O. Harvey, and J. S. Werner. 1999. Senescent changes in scotopic contrast sensitivity. *Vision Research* 39, 3728–3736.

Schneck, M. E., A. J. Adams, K. Huie, and E. Lee. 1993. A filter for simulating color and spatial vision of the elderly. In *Color Deficiencies XI* edited by Bruce Drum, 357-367. Dordrecht, Netherlands: Kluwer Academic Publishers.

Seiple, W., J. Szlyk, S. Yang, and K. Holopigian. 1996. Age related functional field losses are not eccentricity dependent. *Vision Research* 36, 1859-1866.

Sekuler, R., R. Kline, and D. Key. 1982. *Aging and Human Visual Function*. New York: Alan R. Liss, Inc.

Shechtman, D., J. Shallo-Hoffmann, J. Rumsey, P. Riordan-Eva, and P. Hardigan. 2005. Maximum angle of ocular duction during visual fixation as a function of age. *Strabismus* 13, 21-26.

Shinomori, K., B. E. Schefrin, and J. S. Werner. 2001. Age-related changes in wavelength discrimination. *Journal of the Optical Society of America A*. 18, 310-318.

Simon, J., and A. Pouraghabagher. 1978. The Effect of Aging on the Stages of Processing in a Choice Reaction Time Task. *Journal of Gerontology 33*. 553-561.

Sloane, M., C. Owsley, and S. Alvarez. 1988. Aging, senile miosis and spatial contrast sensitivity at low luminance. *Vision Research* 28, 1235–1246.

Spear, P. D. 1993. Neural bases of visual deficits during aging. *Vision Research*. 33, 2589-609.

Stelmach, G. E., N. L. Goggin, and P. C. Amrhein. 1988. "Aging and Reprogramming: the Restructuring of Planned Movements." *Psychology and Aging* 3, 151-157.

Uylings, H. B. M., and J. M. de Brabander. 2002. Neuronal Changes in Normal Human Aging and Alzheimer's Disease. *Brain and Cognition* 49, 268-276.

Vaina, L. M., and S. K. Rushton. 2000. What neurological viewers tell us about the use of optic flow. *Internationl Review of Neurobiology* 44, 293-313.

van den Berg, T. J. 1995. Analysis of intraocular straylight, especially in relation to age. *Optometry and Vision Science*, 72, 52–59.

Warren, Jr., W. H., and D. J. Hannon. 1988. Direction of self-motion is perceived from optical flow. *Nature* 336, 162-163.

Warren, Jr., W.H., and D. J. Hannon. 1990. Eye movements and optical flow. *Journal of the Optical Society of America A*. 7, 160-169.

Warren, W. H., B. A. Kay, W. D. Zosh, A. P. Duchon, and S. Sahuc. 2001. Optic flow is used to control human walking. *Nature Neuroscience* 4, 213-216.

Weale, R. A. 1992. *The Senescence of Human Vision.* Oxford: Oxford University Press.

Welford, A. T. 1958. *Ageing and human skill.* London: Oxford University Press.

Werner, J. S., and B. E. Schefrin. 2000. Optics and vision of the aging eye. In J. M. Enoch, *OSA handbook of optics*, vol. III. New York: McGraw Hill.

Whitaker, D., D. Elliott, and D. MacVeigh. 1992. Variations in hyperacuity performance with age. *Ophthalmic and Physiological Optics* 12, 29-32.

Yates, J. T., M. J. Leys, M. Green, W. Huang, J. Charlton, J. Reed, B-Z Di, and J. V. Odom. 1999. Parallel Pathways, Noise Masking and Glaucoma Detection. *Documenta Ophthalmologica* 95, 283-289.

Yee, R. W., M. Matsuda, R. O. Schultz, and H. F. Edelhauser. 1985. Changes in the normal corneal endothelial cellular pattern as a function of age, *Current Eye Research* 4, 671–678.

Yücel, Y. H., Q. Zhang, R. N. Weinreb, P. L. Kaufman, and N. Gupta. 2003. Effects of retinal ganglion cell loss on magno-, parvo-, koniocellular pathways in the lateral geniculate nucleus and visual cortex in glaucoma. *Progress in Retinal and Eye Research* 22, 465-481.

Yücel, Y. H., Q. Zhang, R. N. Weinreb, P. L. Kaufman, and N. Gupta. 2003. Effects of retinal ganglion cell loss on magno-, parvo-, koniocellular pathways in the lateral geniculate nucleus and visual cortex in glaucoma. *Progress in Retinal and Eye Research* 22, 465-81.

# Chapter 10

# Visual Problems in the Automobile

Merrill J. Allen, O.D., Ph.D.

***Synopsis***



## 10.1 Eye Position on the Highway

The trend of automobile design is toward a lower silhouette. Few cars can provide an eye height of 48 inches even for above average height drivers. The low frontal area of an automobile is desirable for high speeds to reduce wind resistance, and the associated lowering of the center of gravity provides a greater resistance to rollover. On the present highways and at the present highway speeds, however, it does not seem to be necessary to lower the vehicle profile for safety from rollover, and therefore current trends appear to be almost entirely based upon styling, to build a sports car image, and to reduce wind resistance to save fuel.

Practical considerations of passenger comfort and safety require that the size of the passenger automobile be about that of the New York Safety Sedan (Hildebrand and Wakeland, 1966), whose dimensions are as follows: wheel base, 123 inches; tread, 62 inches; overall length, 220 inches; overall width, 80 inches; overall height loaded, 58 inches; weight loaded, 5100 pounds; engine, 260 horsepower.

These dimensions provide room for an average family plus room for thick, energy absorbing doors, for interior padding, for energy-absorbing sheet metal in front and behind the passenger compartment, and for excellent roll over protection. The eye height would be about 48 inches, depending on the driver and the seat adjustment. No American or foreign automobiles are as large as the New York Safety Sedan.

Complications of rakish styling and lowered height are the loss of driver's eye height and problems of head lighting the roadway. The horizon of a six foot man is almost three miles away. When he sits in any of the low American and European cars, he loses about a mile in seeing distance. For safety, a greater seeing range is needed with increasing speed; hence the eye height in automobiles should go up!

Distance judgments depend upon perspective clues, which are improved with increasing height. The time available for a motorist to recognize a hazard and react to it is less as speed increases. Similarly, the ability to determine whether a situation is hazardous is reduced as the eye height is lowered. No one likes to be of short stature at a sports event or on a crowded sidewalk.

Headlight performance is dependent upon height. The higher the headlight, the greater its range. On the other hand, the nearer the headlight is to the driver's eye level, the greater the atmospheric back scatter from dust, smoke, rain, snow, fog, and haze. Hence, the light must be both as far below the line of sight as possible and yet be as high above the roadway as possible.

The headlight system requires careful aiming to avoid glare in the eyes of the oncoming driver and yet provide illumination far ahead along the roadway. When the driver's eyes, the headlights and the roadway are all very nearly in the same plane, rain, snow and fog glare cannot be avoided.

On level ground, the effect of eye height upon the distance to the horizon, is as shown in Table 10.1.

If the drivers' eyes are 42 inches, and headlights are 24 inches above the pavement, and aimed down 1.5 degrees and to the right 1.5 degrees, a change in vehicle load enough to tilt the front up by more than 1.5 degrees will place the headlight beam in the oncoming driver's eyes. High speed and low eye height are not a safe combination for the American highway.

It is essential that the aim of the headlights be independent of vehicle load. This can be done by stabilizing the headlights themselves or by stabilizing the level of the vehicle. The driver's seat needs to be raised in future production, and/or a mirror system installed which effectively raises the eyes two or three feet.

**Table 10.1**

| Eye Height | Horizon | |
|---|---|---|
| Feet | Feet | Miles |
| 1 | 6,499 | 1.23 |
| 2 | 9,191 | 1.74 |
| 3 | 11,257 | 2.13 |
| 4 | 12,998 | 2.45 |
| 5 | 14,533 | 2.75 |
| 6 | 15,920 | 3.02 |
| 7 | 17,195 | 3.26 |
| 8 | 18,383 | 3.48 |
| 9 | 19,498 | 3.69 |
| 10 | 20,552 | 3.89 |

## 10.2 Glare

*The Dictionary of Visual Science* (Schapero et al., 1968) lists ten kinds of glare which may be condensed to three principal types: sensory overload, optical image degradation, and psychological annoyance.

*Sensory overload* begins to occur when the average luminance level exceeds 1,000 foot lamberts. By 7,000 to 10,000 foot lamberts, tearing and eye spasms occur, and visual performance falls. Optically, the image quality is the same or somewhat better at the higher luminances because of the smaller pupil.

*Optical image degradation*, veiling glare, can occur via a uniform "film" of light scattered across the retina from a single bright glare source, or from every point of the white portion of this printed page. Multiple glare sources, such as chromium, mirrors, window glass, etc., cause a "veiling glare" which reduces the contrast in the retinal image and reduces visual performance, perhaps even to zero. The image degradation is known to be worsened by pathology, refractive errors, and age; what may be a compensatable glare to some may be incapacitating to others.

*Psychological annoyance* glare is also called discomfort glare. This is typified by the western sky in the late afternoon, which brightens as the sun comes down toward the horizon. A driver traveling west will ultimately find that the increasing sky brightness becomes uncomfortable. It is generally felt that discomfort glare has little relationship to veiling glare, although veiling glare also occurs in all such situations. Discomfort glare tolerance can be very low in certain refractive and pathological conditions.

Each of the foregoing three types of glare results in reduced visual performance. Only for sensory overload can ordinary nonpolarizing sunglasses be helpful. For best vision the optimum scene luminance should average about 400 foot lamberts. An improvement in performance occurs if luminances of several thousand foot lamberts are reduced to about 400.

Veiling glare reduces performance proportionally according to the equation:

$$B_v = \frac{KB_0}{\phi^n}$$

where $B_0$ is the illuminance falling on the pupil from the glare source, $\phi$ is the distance of the glare source away from the line of sight in degrees, and constants $K$ and $n$ are approximately equal to 10 and 2 respectively. Differences in the formulas reported in the literature, are largely due to age differences, and to other ocular conditions of the subjects, as well as to the different methods of specifying the amount of glare light entering the eye.

Discomfort glare reduces performance three ways, see Figure 10.1. Often there is an element of sensory overload when discomfort is experienced. The glare source scatters a veil of light throughout the eye. Deterioration in performance can be expected by sensory overload and image contrast reduction. The discomfort itself reduces performance by providing a perceptual interference that may even reach the emotional level of anger or crying.

The driver's glare resistance is enhanced by a clean windshield, clean glasses, clean and properly aimed headlights, an optimum correction for refractive errors, no vertical and lateral imbalances, and by the driver's optimum state of health and minimal perceptual load. Experiments indicate that the effects of glare on performance will be about five times worse on the highway than in an experimental situation. Either the perceptual load is increased, or attention to driving is reduced, or both.

Glare light entering the driver's eyes comes from several sources, of which the windshield is the most important (Allen, Aug. 1969). Figure 10.1 shows that the primary source of glare light is the windshield.

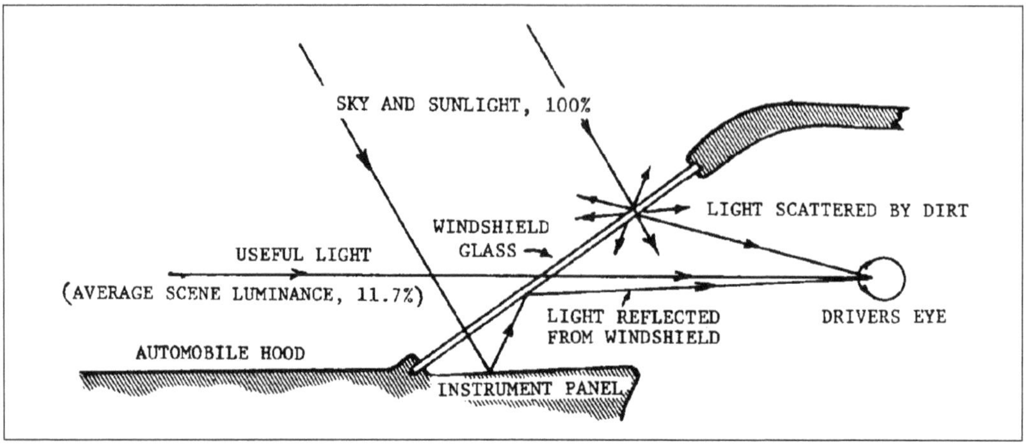


***Figure 10.1*** *Sources of glare from the windshield and related structures. Note that average useful light from the scene is 11.7 percent. Dirt in full sunshine and/or the instrument panel top and windshield may easily direct enough light toward the eyes to be greater than the useful light.*

**Table 10.2**
**Average Scene Reflectivity**

| Sky Ft. Lamberts | Scene Ft. Lamberts | % Scene Reflective | Terraine Measured |
|---|---|---|---|
| 6900 | 1080 | 15.65 | Concrete Road |
| 7000 | 880 | 12.57 | Dirt |
| 7100 | 500 | 7.04 | Green Field |
| 7200 | 900 | 12.50 | Blacktop |
| 7200 | 1380 | 19.17 | Gravel parking |
| 7300 | 1040 | 14.25 | Concrete |
| 7400 | 950 | 12.84 | Dirt |
| 7700 | 380 | 4.93 | Green Field |
| 7800 | 1280 | 16.41 | Gravel Road |
| 8000 | 570 | 7.41 | Blacktop |
| 8150 | 830 | 10.18 | City Street |
| 7850 | 680 | 8.66 | City Street |
| **Avg. 7466** | **Avg. 872** | **Avg. 11.7** | **Avg. scene** |

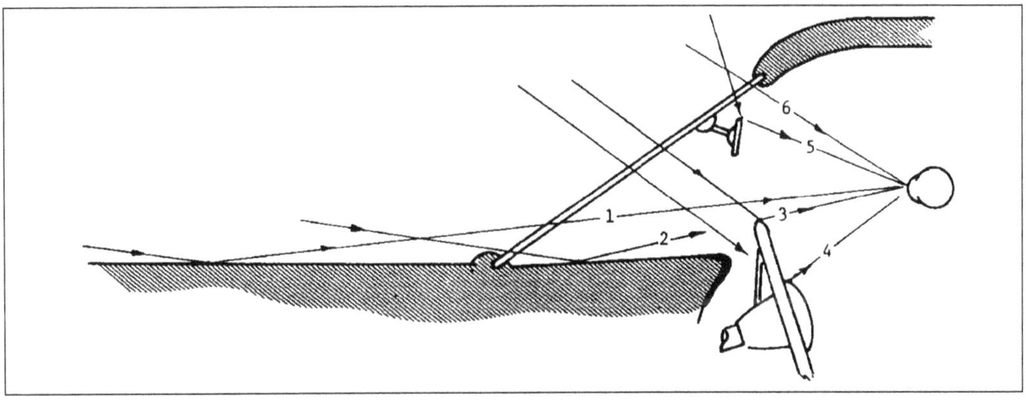


*Figure 10.2* Nonwindshield sources of glare. The numbered rays are from glare sources as follows: (1) from the glossy hood paint, hood chromium, and fender chromium; (2) from the windshield trim, wiper hardware, speaker grille, and glossy dash panel top (especially pre-1967 automobiles); (3) glossy reflections from the rim of some steering wheels; (4) reflections from bright steering wheel hardware; (5) reflection from mirror hardware and pillar post (windshield corner post); and (6) glare light directly from the sun and/or sky.

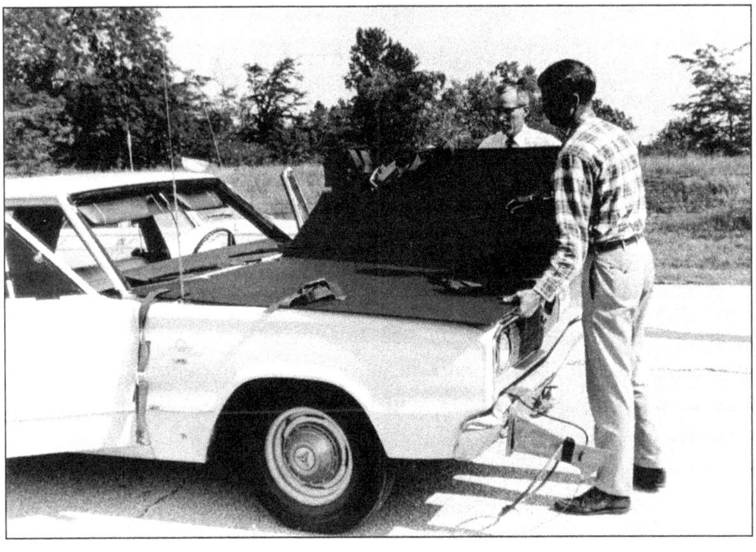

*Figure 10.3* Test automobile for the study of vehicle glare. The windshield has been removed and the sun visors enlarged. The hood is being covered with a flat black material. Roadside targets were triggered by the vehicle 325 feet in advance and the reaction times needed for their detection by each of three observers in the front seat were recorded. The device on the bumper tripped a string across the road to raise the target.

In Table 10.2, the average scene reflectivity of 11.7 percent was determined by using a light meter pointed upward to measure the illumination falling on a horizontal plane on the earth, and by directing the meter horizontally to measure the light from the trees, houses, fields, etc. When measuring the light from the environment, a flat black shield was placed on top of the light meter to block out the light from the sky. Because the shield obstructed half of the receptive field of the photocell, its readings were doubled to get the values tabulated.

Figure 10.2 shows the other factors involved in automobile glare in addition to those of the windshield. Ray 1 is reflected from the hood paint and hood or fender ornaments. Ray 2 is reflected from the dash panel, windshield trim, and wiper hardware. Ray 3 is reflected from the steering wheel structure. Ray 4 is reflected from the trim of the horn rim and steering wheel hub. Ray 5 is reflected from the mirror hardware, and Ray 6 is directly from the sun or from the open sky.

Figure 10.3 shows an instrumented vehicle with a detachable windshield used to evaluate the effect of glare encountered in typical daytime driving. A study of forty-five drivers of all ages (Allen, Spring 1968) revealed that the most comfortable and efficient daytime driving occurred when all possible sources of glare had been removed. The windshield generally afforded the most predictable and important glare of all sources tested. At times, sky glare, hood glare, and chromium glare were serious. When all sources gave maximum glare at the same time, the driver's performance was the most adversely affected.

Tables 10.3 and 10.4 give the variations in sky luminance with the earth's latitude, the time of year, and the time of day, for a clear, and for an overcast sky. In Table 10.3 the values are taken so that the area around the sun and the sun itself are not measured. Note that on June 21 at 8 a.m., looking east, and at 4 p.m., looking west, the sky is very bright. In March and September at 10 a.m., and at noon looking south, the sky is also very bright.

In Table 10.4 when the sky is overcast, the luminances of the sky are more uniform so that directional effects are not significant. Because sky luminances are low, the illumination at ground level is likely to be much lower than when the sun is visible. Furthermore, the loss of shadows when the sky is overcast causes a loss of contrast which increases the visual handicap imposed by sky glare. Thus, overcast days are more annoying to a motorist than a day of full sunshine. Motorists will turn on their headlights earlier at the end of an overcast day compared to a clear day. The new automatic daytime running lights will ensure adequate daytime vehicle conspicuity.

To summarize, daytime glare is of multiple types and causation. Excessive overall illumination can be reduced with sunglasses, and visual performance will be increased. Specific glare objects that are excessively bright, such as chromium, hood paint, sky, and sun adjacent to the normal visual task, cannot be toned down very much with sunglasses without a loss in visual performance. Sunglasses may actually reduce visual performance, because they may reduce the useful light below optimum values, still leaving the proportion of glare to useful light unchanged. They also add a veiling glare of their own from dirt and surface reflections. Discomfort glare is a function of total luminance, differential luminance, area, and distance from the visual task. Glare from the windshield and dash panel is apt to approach the discomfort level even on overcast days in the daytime. For this type of discomfort, sunglasses may be helpful, but visual performance may not improve.

Sky glare, road glare, water droplets, and dirt on the windshield all contribute significant amounts of glare, the total of which may be over powering. Sun visors are a simple and effective means to control the sky glare. Some glare control comes from the color band at the top of the windshield. The windshield washer is an excellent means for reducing glare in bright sunshine by removing dust and dirt.

**Table 10.3 Equivalent Sky Luminance in Foot Lamberts—Clear Days***

| | December 21 | | | | | March and September 21 | | | | | June 21 | | | | |
|---|---|---|---|---|---|---|---|---|---|---|---|---|---|---|---|
| Latitude | 8 a.m. | 10 a.m. | Noon | 2 p.m. | 4 p.m. | 8 a.m. | 10 a.m. | Noon | 2 p.m. | 4 p.m. | 8 a.m. | 10 a.m. | Noon | 2 p.m. | 4 p.m. |
| **North** | | | | | | | | | | | | | | | |
| 30° N | 450 | 600 | 600 | 600 | 450 | 700 | 1000 | 1050 | 1000 | 700 | 1550 | 1400 | 1000 | 1400 | 1550 |
| 34° N | 350 | 550 | 550 | 550 | 350 | 800 | 800 | 900 | 800 | 800 | 1350 | 1400 | 950 | 1400 | 1350 |
| 38° N | 300 | 550 | 550 | 550 | 300 | 750 | 800 | 900 | 800 | 750 | 1350 | 1300 | 950 | 1300 | 1350 |
| 42° N | 250 | 500 | 500 | 500 | 250 | 700 | 750 | 800 | 750 | 700 | 1300 | 1300 | 950 | 1300 | 1350 |
| 46° N | 150 | 450 | 500 | 450 | 150 | 700 | 750 | 750 | 750 | 700 | 1300 | 1250 | 950 | 1250 | 1300 |
| **South** | | | | | | | | | | | | | | | |
| 30° N | 1100 | 1950 | 2250 | 1950 | 1100 | 1700 | 2300 | 2800 | 2300 | 1700 | 1200 | 1600 | 2400 | 1600 | 1200 |
| 34° N | 1100 | 1900 | 2200 | 1900 | 1100 | 1700 | 2650 | 2900 | 2650 | 1700 | 1350 | 1650 | 2300 | 1650 | 1350 |
| 38° N | 900 | 2300 | 2200 | 2300 | 900 | 1700 | 2700 | 2950 | 2700 | 1700 | 1350 | 1650 | 2300 | 1659 | 1350 |
| 42° N | 600 | 2100 | 2150 | 2100 | 600 | 1700 | 2700 | 2450 | 2700 | 1700 | 1350 | 2000 | 2500 | 2000 | 1350 |
| 46° N | 400 | 1900 | 2100 | 1900 | 400 | 1700 | 2700 | 2900 | 2710 | 1700 | 1350 | 2100 | 2700 | 2100 | 1350 |
| **East** | | | | | | | | | | | | | | | |
| 30° N | 1550 | 1500 | 1000 | 700 | 400 | 2000 | 2500 | 1500 | 900 | 700 | 2800 | 2650 | 1400 | 1000 | 700 |
| 34° N | 1350 | 1400 | 950 | 700 | 400 | 2400 | 2600 | 1600 | 950 | 650 | 2800 | 2700 | 1450 | 1000 | 700 |
| 38° N | 1200 | 1300 | 900 | 650 | 350 | 2500 | 2600 | 1500 | 900 | 600 | 2800 | 2700 | 1400 | 1050 | 700 |
| 42° N | 750 | 1200 | 850 | 600 | 250 | 2400 | 2400 | 1450 | 800 | 600 | 2900 | 2600 | 1400 | 1000 | 700 |
| 46° N | 500 | 1100 | 800 | 500 | 150 | 2300 | 2100 | 1400 | 700 | 600 | 2850 | 2600 | 1400 | 1000 | 700 |
| **West** | | | | | | | | | | | | | | | |
| 30° N | 400 | 700 | 1000 | 1500 | 1550 | 700 | 900 | 1500 | 2500 | 2000 | 700 | 1000 | 1440 | 2650 | 2800 |
| 34° N | 400 | 700 | 950 | 1400 | 1350 | 650 | 900 | 1600 | 2500 | 2400 | 700 | 1000 | 1400 | 2700 | 2800 |
| 38° N | 350 | 650 | 900 | 1300 | 1200 | 600 | 900 | 1500 | 2600 | 2500 | 700 | 1050 | 1400 | 2700 | 2800 |
| 42° N | 250 | 600 | 850 | 1200 | 750 | 600 | 800 | 1450 | 2400 | 2400 | 700 | 1000 | 1000 | 2600 | 2800 |
| 46° N | 150 | 500 | 800 | 1100 | 500 | 600 | 700 | 1400 | 2100 | 2300 | 700 | 1000 | 1400 | 2600 | 2850 |

* Average values, direct sunlight excluded.

**Table 10.4**
**Equivalent Sky Luminance in Foot Lamberts—Average Overcast Day**

| Latitude | 8 a.m. | 9 a.m. | 10 a.m. | 11 a.m. | |
|---|---|---|---|---|---|
| | 4 p.m. | 3 p.m. | 2 p.m. | 1 p.m. | Noon |
| December 21 | | | | | |
| 30° N | 420 | 740 | 1020 | 1210 | 1270 |
| 32 | 350 | 700 | 960 | 1150 | 1200 |
| 34 | 320 | 650 | 910 | 1100 | 1140 |
| 36 | 260 | 600 | 840 | 1020 | 1070 |
| 38 | 230 | 550 | 790 | 940 | 1000 |
| 40 | 190 | 500 | 740 | 900 | 930 |
| 42 | 150 | 450 | 660 | 820 | 860 |
| 44 | 100 | 380 | 600 | 760 | 790 |
| 46 | 60 | 340 | 550 | 680 | 730 |
| 48 | 40 | 290 | 470 | 630 | 650 |
| 50 | 0 | 240 | 420 | 560 | 580 |
| March 21 or September 21 | | | | | |
| 30° N | 910 | 1320 | 1710 | 2010 | 2140 |
| 32 | 880 | 1290 | 1650 | 1940 | 2070 |
| 34 | 860 | 1250 | 1600 | 1870 | 1980 |
| 36 | 840 | 1220 | 1560 | 1800 | 1900 |
| 38 | 800 | 1200 | 1500 | 1740 | 1840 |
| 40 | 790 | 1140 | 1460 | 1670 | 1760 |
| 42 | 760 | 1120 | 1410 | 1600 | 1690 |
| 44 | 740 | 1080 | 1340 | 1540 | 1620 |
| 46 | 710 | 1030 | 1290 | 1470 | 1550 |
| 48 | 690 | 990 | 1240 | 1410 | 1480 |
| 50 | 650 | 940 | 1180 | 1330 | 1400 |
| June 21 | | | | | |
| 30° N | 1270 | 1730 | 2250 | | |
| 32 | 1280 | 1730 | 2240 | | |
| 34 | 1290 | 1730 | 2220 | | |
| 36 | 1290 | 1730 | 2200 | 2960 | |
| 38 | 1290 | 1720 | 2160 | 2840 | |
| 40 | 1290 | 1700 | 2120 | 2650 | 3060 |
| 42 | 1300 | 1690 | 2080 | 2540 | 2860 |
| 44 | 1290 | 1670 | 2050 | 2430 | 2660 |
| 46 | 1290 | 1640 | 2010 | 2330 | 2520 |
| 48 | 1290 | 1620 | 1960 | 2250 | 2400 |
| 50 | 1260 | 1590 | 1900 | 2160 | 2280 |

Polarizing sunglasses will protect the motorist against the sun glare reflected from the roadway and the top of the hood. They will also reduce the windshield glare from the top of the dash panel. The better solution for the dash panel is a piece of black velvet cloth laid on top of it. (Be sure to cut openings for the hot air ducts that defrost the windshield.)

*Automobile stylists are beginning to learn that the top of the dash panel is optically a part of the windshield* and should be strictly off limits to decorators, painters, and artists. In this case, as in many others, doing it right will lend beauty as well as safety.

The author had a research car with a modified dash panel covered with black nylon flock. The nylon fibers were electrostatically propelled onto the wet epoxy adhesive. Each nylon fiber was at right angles to the surface and produced a durable equivalent of velveteen cloth. This surface treatment was truly dead black, looked nice, and did not show dirt. This finish was also applied to the hood. After twenty-four months the dash panel was still perfect, but the sun had bleached the nylon flock on the top of the hood.

The process seems ideal for dash panels and, if the material can be made sun resistant, its application to hoods is nothing short of a stylist's dream. *No other feature on Indiana University's research automobiles ever attracted so much attention as the black nylon flock on the hood of that white Coronet!*

On visiting new and used car lots in 1999, no dash panels were flock coated or painted black. However, to my surprise, I discovered that *flock finishes*, similar to the one above, but not in black, have been put *under the rear window of all passenger cars, new and used! All manufacturers know how but none are installing it on the dash panel.* The omission of this important safety feature indicates extreme bureaucratic indifference to safety. As a result of news items, and, television shows (KGO-TV News, San Francisco, Nov. 1995 and 20/20 News, Feb. 1999) which discussed and demonstrated the seriousness of the problem, it seems reasonable that antiglare dash panel finishes will soon become standard and motor vehicle safety will be significantly improved.

## 10.3 Dirt and Scratches on the Windshield

One solution to some of the more serious windshield problems is to tilt the windshield top forward, or opposite to its present tilt (Figure 10.4). The glass would then reflect the shaded portions of the inside of the roof structure instead of the sun-illuminated dash-panel top. Such a tilt would also eliminate much of the problem of the dirty windshield by shading the dirt. Dirt absorbs useful light, and reflects glare light toward the driver. The present windshield tilt exposes the dirt to full sunshine for over two-thirds of the day.

The reverse tilt of the windshield would make it easier to get to the inside surface to keep it clean, an often neglected consideration. Outside cleaning would be somewhat more difficult, but the windshield would be inherently cleaner than it is now since it would not frost or collect dew at night as readily, or trap air borne dust and dirt.

The only contraindication to such a design is aerodynamic. However, since vehicle stability at high speed is a serious problem, an air foil like upper contour of the automobile produces lift and can be dangerous. A number of land and water race drivers have died in vehicles that became airborne without ailerons, rudder, or horizontal stabilizer. An unknown number of passenger vehicle occupants have been injured or killed when they became airborne when caught in a strong wind at high speed in a lightweight vehicle. Since conventional automobile configurations do not assure ground hugging at high speeds, a windshield redesign could be the lift spoiler needed to help maintain vehicle stability. Lift spoilers are already in use on production automobiles as well as on racing cars.

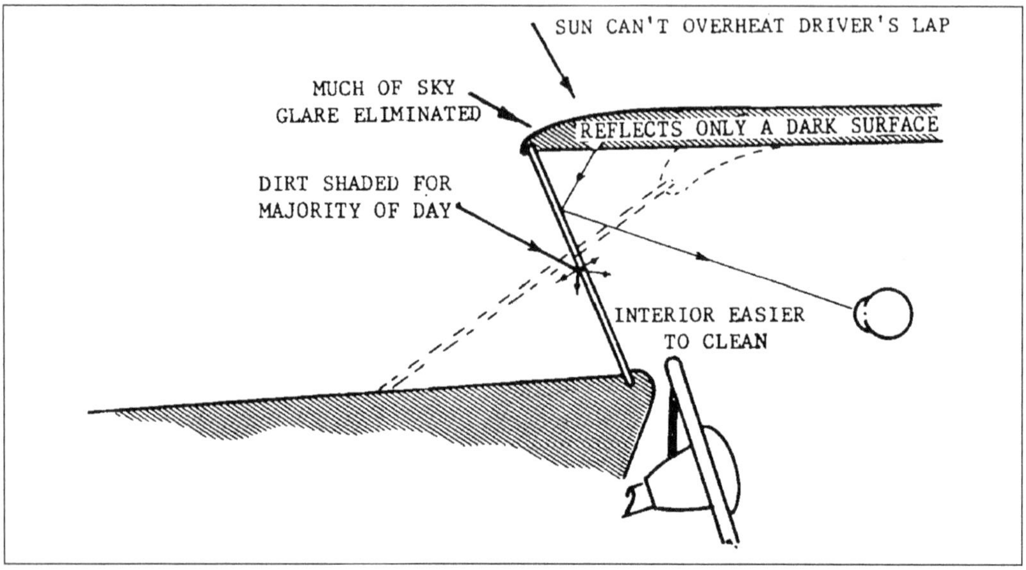


***Figure 10.4*** *Characteristics of a windshield with a reverse tilt. Air cushion crash protection will keep passengers away from the windshield during a crash; hence the only design considerations are optical and aerodynamic. This design is optically superior.*

Glare at night is mostly a problem of windshield dirt and scratches (see Figure 10.4). Allen (August 1969) has shown that the number of miles driven correlates with the number and severity of windshield scratches resulting from windshield wiper operation. At roughly 50,000 miles the windshield should be replaced or repolished to restore optimum vision at night against headlight glare.

Some cleaning procedures and some environmental factors, such as sandstorms, abrasive air pollutants, sand used in winter on ice and snow, etc., can quickly cause severe windshield damage. A test for scratch deterioration can be made by observing the reflection of the sun in the windshield (see Figure 10.19). New glass will show a bright sun image on a clear sky background. An older glass will show bright scratch rings around the sun's image. These will extend out several inches from the edge of the solar image. Driving an old car and a new car against headlights at night will illustrate the greater spread of headlight glare and the greater difficulty of seeing when looking through the older glass. Resurfacing is able to restore new windshield performance.

## 10.4 Windshield Tint

The popular misconception that a tinted windshield reduces glare at night may stem from comparing the old, scratched, nontinted windshield with the new unscratched tinted windshield at the time of buying a new car. When new untinted glass is compared with new tinted glass, however, the untinted glass gives a superior performance at night (Blackwell, 1954; Haber, 1955; McFarland and Domey, October 1958).

It is often argued that daytime comfort offered by the tinted windshield off-sets the extra nighttime hazard. Such arguments do not hold up. (1) There is evidence that comfort leads to inattention and, in the proper circumstances, to sleep. (2) The question of comfort is relative because tinted automobile glass removes less than 50 percent of the direct solar heat energy. (3) The nighttime hazard due to losing about 40 percent of the visible light is greater than usually claimed. The experimental method used to show that tinted windshields do not reduce seeing at night was improper. On my testimony, the research report was withdrawn.

Many studies on tinted windshields have been conducted on the detectability of objects on the roadway as illuminated by low-beam headlights. Low-beam headlights are aimed down 1.5 degrees and give a sharp cutoff in light pattern on the roadway ahead. An object is not likely to be seen until it is close enough to enter the bright portion of the headlight pattern. At the forward edge of the headlight pattern the inverse square law does not hold, and a few feet of change in distance of the automobile from the object can dramatically change the illumination on that object at pavement level. Hence the reduction in seeing of a tinted windshield, which reduces light at the eye about 40 percent, compared to a clear windshield would be compensated for by allowing the object to move a few feet nearer into the headlight pattern. Thus, promoters of tinted windshields are able to say that only a 1 to 3 percent loss in seeing distance occurs due to a tinted windshield.

If an object on the highway is not seen considerably prior to entering the low-beam headlight pattern, it will probably be struck when traveling at 60 miles per hour. We are overdriving our low-beam headlights from 40 miles per hour up! Windshield tint interferes most with the detection of unlighted vehicles or pedestrians on or near city streets, on country roads, and on highways. Obstacles in front and to the left will not come into the bright portion of the low-beam headlight pattern as soon and will be rendered even less visible by a tinted windshield.

As retinal luminance levels are reduced toward the absolute threshold, for example, by old age and by windshield tint, the ability of the eye to discriminate subtle brightness differences falls off precipitously. At high levels a 1 percent brightness difference can be detected, whereas at the absolute threshold an object exhibiting a brightness difference from its background of 100 percent might not be detected.

A plate of glass loses light by surface reflection. Figure 10.5, Curve B, shows how the loss is dependent upon the angle of incidence of the light for a single surface. For two surfaces the loss is nearly doubled. Modern windshields are tilted to about 60 degrees from vertical. Figure 10.5 shows that a loss of about 20 percent due to reflection alone will occur with an untinted glass. Further inspection of Figure 10.5 reveals that the present windshield angle of American cars polarizes almost 100 percent of the light which it reflects. The amount reflected by a plate of clear glass at 60 degree incidence angle is about 20 percent; hence 80 percent is transmitted. This 80 percent is composed of 60 percent of the original amount of light which is unpolarized and 20 percent which is polarized. Hence, 25 percent of the light is polarized. Light reflected into the driver's eyes from the street, hood, etc., is partially polarized in the same plane as the light reflected from the windshield. In the daytime the angled windshield filters out some of the polarized component of specular glare from the pavement. However, by night, street lighting engineers rely on specular glare from the pavement to give efficient silhouette seeing with minimum wattage sources. The 60-degree angled windshield unfortunately removes a portion of the polarized component of that light also.

The transmission curve of a tinted windshield shows the relative efficiency of the windshield in removing heat radiation compared to visible light (see Figure 10.6). Solar energy is distributed about equally between visible and invisible radiation (see Figure 10.7); hence a windshield that absorbs all of the infrared and ultraviolet energy still transmits 50 percent of the solar energy. From Figure 10.7 it is apparent that the infrared and ultraviolet energy absorption is not perfect, nor is visible light transmission perfect. Figure 10.8 gives the ideal windshield tint, which would transmit all of the visible light available and remove all of the solar energy that does not contribute to vision. Only uncolored glass can come near the 100 percent transmission ideal in the visible portion.

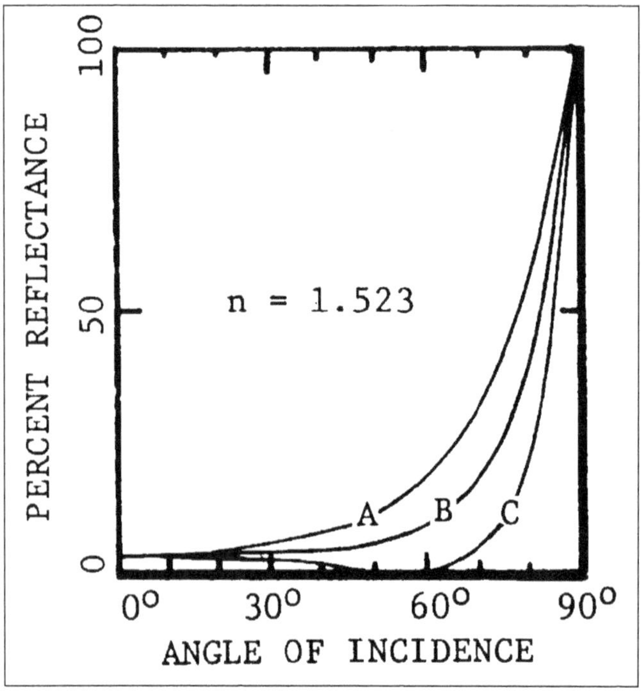


***Figure 10.5*** *Effect of angle of incidence of light striking a single glass surface upon percent of light reflected. Curve B is the average reflectance of the ordinary and extraordinary rays striking the surface. On Curve C the reflectance drops to zero near 55 degrees; thus only the A curve component of the light is reflected. In other words, the reflected light is completely polarized.*

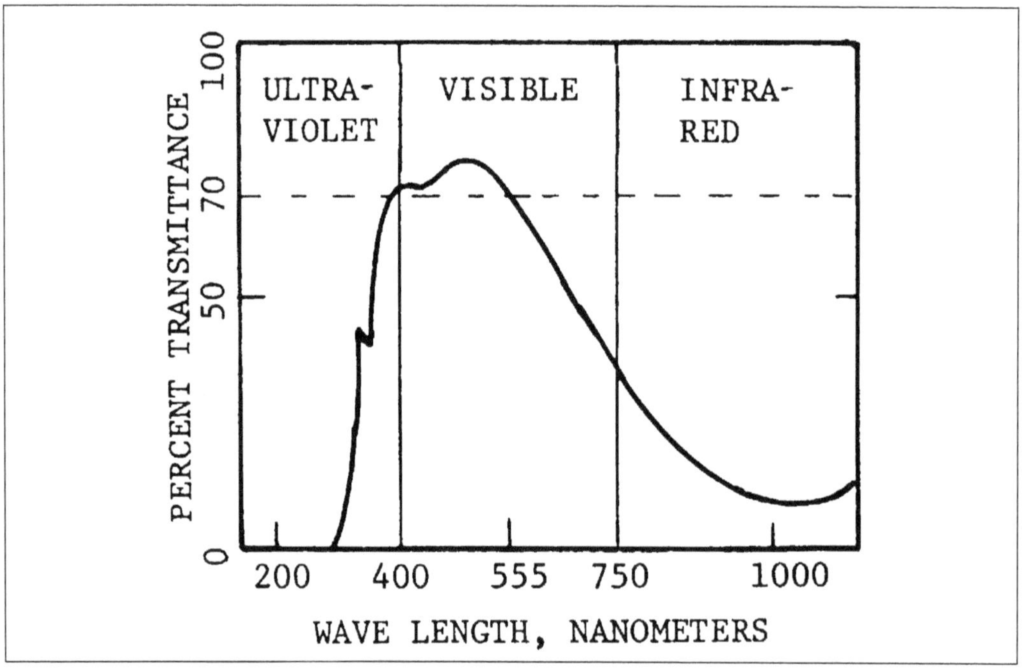


***Figure 10.6*** *The transmission curve of a modern heat absorbing automotive windshield (Whittemore, 1965). The bluish green color of this glass results from the lowered red light. Visible light lies between 400 and 750 nanometers (millimicrons).*

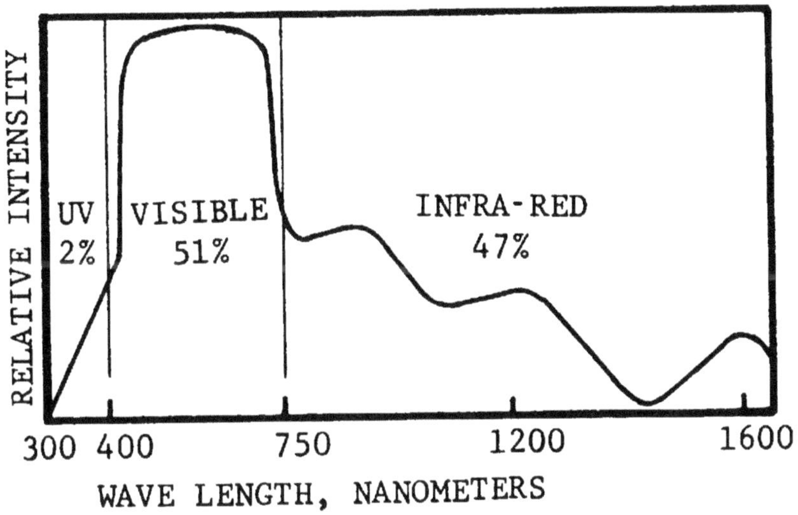


***Figure 10.7*** *The relative intensity of solar radiation at each wavelength (Whittemore, 1965). The heat content of the visible portion of solar radiation is 51 percent, while for infrared (the "heat" radiation) only 47 percent is present.*

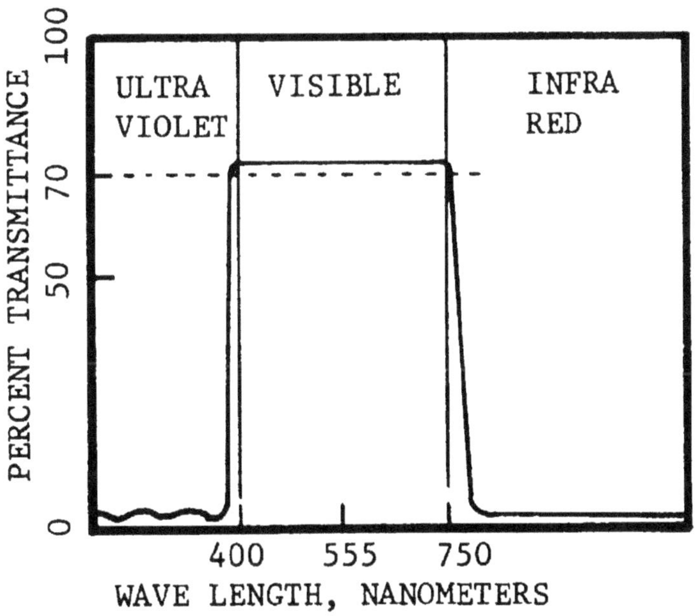


***Figure 10.8*** *An "ideal" automotive glass (Whittemore, 1965) would absorb all of the infrared and ultraviolet and only 70 percent across the spectrum of visible radiation's. Such a glass would absorb about 64.3 percent of the solar energy. In practice only about 50 percent is absorbed. The arbitrary choice of 70 percent transmission across the visible spectrum is challenged in this book as hazardous at night and inadequate during the day.*

When windshield tint is present, angling the glass will increase the distance that the light has to travel in the glass; hence the absorptive effect of the tint on the light will be increased. Figure 10.9 gives the results of measurements with a Pritchard Spectra Photometer on samples of clear and tinted windshield glass supplied by the Ford Motor Company.

At 60 degrees tilt angle, the clear windshield sample transmitted 79 percent while the tinted windshield sample transmitted 65 percent of the white light from a tungsten source. At 60 degrees, when the red filter in the photometer was used, the clear windshield transmitted 75 percent, whereas the tinted windshield transmits only 49 percent of the red light from a tungsten source. The red filter in the Pritchard Spectra Photometer is tristimulus red, and will not necessarily match the red filter in a given taillight or stop signal. A deeper red (longer wavelength), will be attenuated below the 49-percent measurement obtained, see the windshield transmission curve, Figure 10.6.

From these data it is clear that the Society of Automotive Engineers' specification that a tinted windshield shall transmit not less than 70 percent visible light is misleading. The SAE specification holds for vertical windshields and not for windshields in automobiles, and ignores the selective absorption of tinted windshields for red light. If we are to hold to a 70 percent minimum allowable transmission, which most authorities have agreed to, it is apparent from Figure 10.9 that, even vertically, a tinted windshield cannot pass when tested for red light transmission! Furthermore, when installed in an automobile, the sample tested indicates that only 65 percent overall transmission for visible light is possible.

*It is not possible to meet the minimum SAE specification of 70 percent transmission with the present tinted glass. Hence all American automobiles with tinted windshields violate the intent of this specification!*

A protanopic or protanomalous color-defective person is insensitive to red light (see Figure 10.10). A normal person looking through a tinted windshield has a reduction in red sensitivity similar to being a protanope. A protanope who is already insensitive to red, will suffer even greater handicap viewing red lights through a tinted windshield (see Figure 10.10).

The curves in Figure 10.10 are for a vertical windshield. To determine the effects of tilting the windshield, the data in Figure 10.9 should prove useful. The selectively greater loss of red light by a tilted and tinted windshield is evidence that it is hazardous in the daytime, since red signal and brake lights may not be bright enough at best to be seen quickly in full daylight. The effect of the tint is to make the daylight relatively still brighter than the red signal light.

Another undesirable aspect of tinted window glass is that it reduces the chances of seeing the occupants of another automobile, thus further reducing the chances for social interactions. Social interactions are known to discourage antisocial behavior. I feel that a person's bad driving manners would improve if other drivers could talk about him or to him, as with a bull horn or a radio communications system. Driving mistakes could be discussed, and a sort of an on-the-job training would result. Since we do not have this, the eye-to-eye contact of drivers on occasion can be very useful.

Another adverse feature of tinted automobile glass is the inability to see through two or more cars if their windows are tinted. In regard to tilt angle, heat absorbing efficiency goes down the more nearly the glass faces the sun. At the same time the amount of glare light reflected from the sky toward other drivers increases. This increased sky or sun reflection from the windshield tends to obscure the view of the people in the car, accentuating the obscuration due to tint.

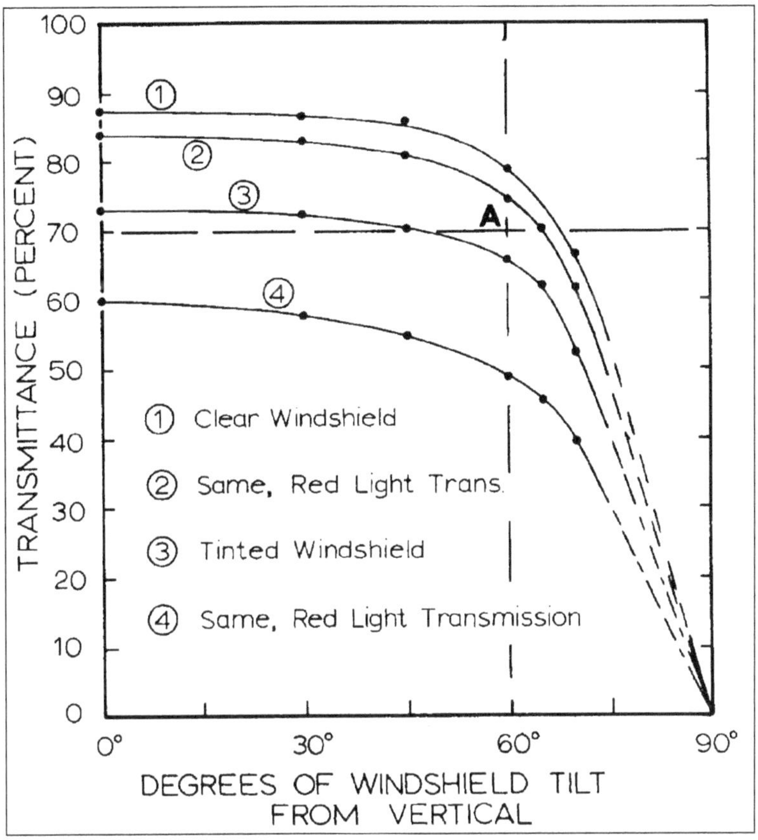


***Figure 10.9** Plot of transmission of a clear and tinted (heat absorbing) windshield for various tilt angles, and for red and white light transmission. Note that point A, the intersection between the tilt angle of 60 degrees and the Society of Automotive Engineers' lower limit of transmission, is above both the white light and the red transmission curves for a tinted windshield. These measurements were made on new one-foot-square samples.*

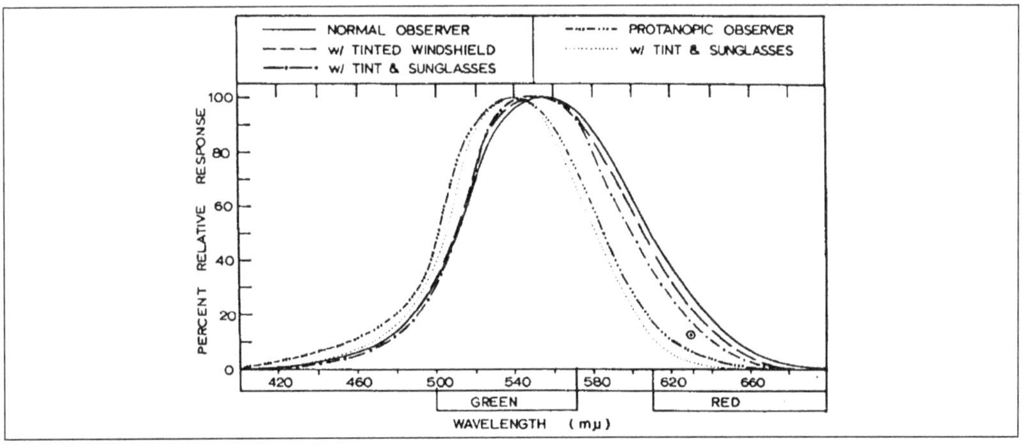


***Figure 10.10** The effect of windshield tint and green sunglasses upon normal and protanopic (red insensitive) luminosity curves when the windshield is vertical. Tilt of the windshield to 60 degrees from the vertical will reduce the red end of the tinted windshield curves by about 26 percent (see Figure 10.9). The encircled dot at 639 millimicrons indicates the effect of tilting a tinted windshield to 60 degrees when green sunglasses are worn by a normal observer. This figure shows that if a protanopic driver wears green sunglasses and peers through a tinted windshield it will be virtually impossible for him to see any red light!*

## 10.5 Distortions

Distortions may exist in front, rear, and side windows. Orange peel like irregularities, show up as blurred vision, while major surface defects produce gross displacements and distortions of objects from their true location and shape. Microscopic defects, such as inadequate surface polish or metallic deposits can cause light scatter and blurred vision.

The major surface defects are most serious when trying to see through the vehicle ahead. The combination of rear window and front window distortions may be considerably greater than the simple sum of the two distortions; hence rear window distortions as well as windshield distortions need to be minimized.

Quality control of gross distortions is improving. Most cars have reasonably good see through ability. Windshield distortions of vision can occur and are found to some degree among each manufacturer's products. Variations in sheet glass production, in heat forming, in lamination procedures, and in materials, combine to produce one windshield of reject quality while the next one will be acceptable. Whether the rejects are rejected is a matter of company quality control standards.

Distortions near the right side of the windshield, in effect, enlarge the corner post obstruction. When entering a roadway, vehicles approaching from the right and viewed through even slight distortion can be misjudged both as to speed and distance, and the distortion may cause driver behavior similar to that of not having seen the approaching vehicle at all. Major distortions near the straight ahead position can cause double images, eye fatigue, headache, and nausea. These symptoms may or may not interfere with driving efficiency, depending upon the person and the severity of the distortion. Distortions near the left corner post are especially hazardous when turning left and in detecting pedestrian and vehicle traffic approaching from the left. In effect the left corner post is enlarged by glass distortions.

Side window distortions do not seem to be as hazardous to the driving operation. However, these distortions do impair see through ability by other drivers in numerous instances, and generally a car is labeled as low quality if obvious distortions are present. It is probable that children and other passengers are more likely to have car sickness when side and rear windows are distorted.

Often we hear that the curved windshield is the cause of all manner of distortions and that a flat windshield would be better. Actually a curved windshield with the eye at the center of curvature is the more ideal arrangement (see Figure 10.11). Viewing through a flat plate of glass at an oblique angle, reduces transmission and exaggerates any irregularities in the surface and optical media, as well as creating an astigmatic like blur of the object viewed. The gentle curvature of the modern windshield is a reasonable compromise. However, the slope angle of 60 degrees backward tilt away from the vertical is a major source of light loss, dirt deposits, internal reflections, glare, heat build up, optical distortions and reflections from the dash panel. Our present windshields are not ideal.

## 10.6 Obstructions and the Rear-View Mirror

The largest single obstruction in the driver's forward field of view is usually the inside rear-view mirror. The placement of this mirror seems not to be determined by the eye height of the 95th-percentile driver but by the position of the rear window. As a result, most hard tops and almost all sedans have a serious obstruction to forward view due to the low position of the rear-view mirror. A survey of 1960 to 1962 automobiles (Allen, December 1962) showed that the rear view mirror occupied 14 to 18 degrees of the field of view and was between 32 to 53 degrees to the right side of straight ahead. In comparison the left windshield corner post varied between 5 and 17 degrees in lateral dimension and was located between 10 and 26 degrees to the left of straight ahead of the driver's eyes. The right windshield corner post was about 5 degrees in thickness and was about 75 degrees away from straight ahead.

The styling trends in 1996 have made these visual obstructions worse. In addition, designers have cramped the driver and passengers.

The outside rear-view mirror is improperly located on some vehicles. Federal standards first required in 1967 that outside rear-view mirrors be installed on all automobiles.

Outside rear-view mirrors in many 1996 automobiles, occupy most of the area that used to be the vent window in the front door glass (see Figures 2.3, 2.4). For short drivers, these obstructions are very serious. The seating height must be raised and the corner-post obstruction reduced.

A properly designed periscopic rear view mirror could eliminate the need for the outside mirror and reduce obstructions to the drivers side vision. Periscopic and other exotic rear view mirror designs have been around for 50 years or more. They range from the simple convex single mirror through complex lens-reflector designs using astigmatic elements. Experimental systems include television displays, radar detectors, and laser ranging devices.

Flat mirror systems are more desirable than other systems because they are inexpensive; they are not subject to distortion; they give no inherent enlargement or reduction in the image viewed, and space perception is normal. They permit a wide range of head and eye movements. If properly arranged, they permit rearward view by looking upward slightly, thus not interfering seriously with forward vision.

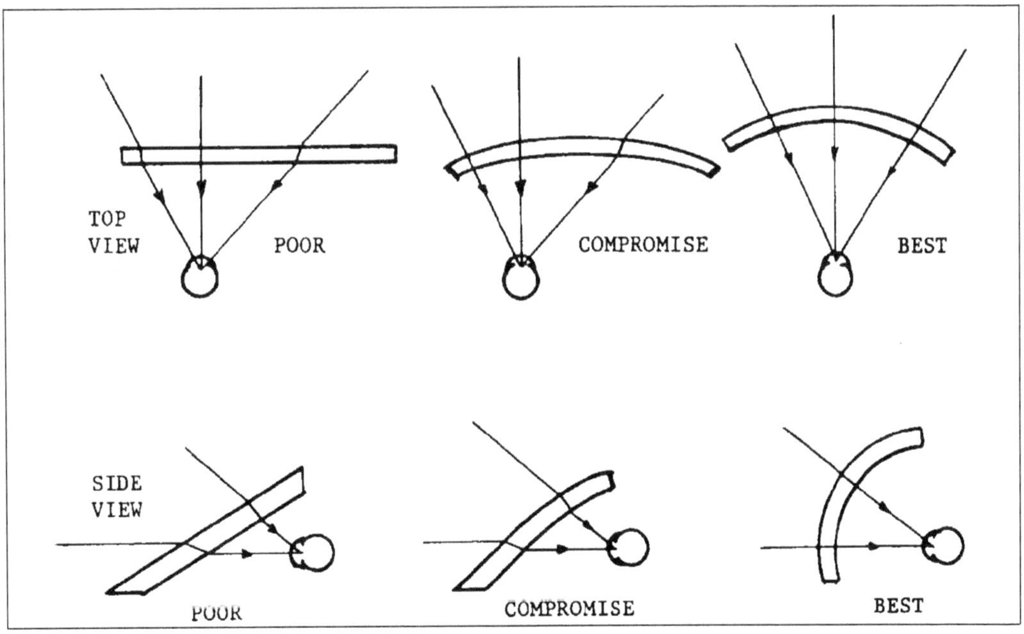


***Figure 10.11*** *Schematic diagram of some possible windshield designs. In general a concentric design would give zero distortion and negligible refractive power if the thickness were small.*

All other systems suffer from disadvantages. For example, the television display of rearward scenery must of necessity be confined to a small area on the dash or elsewhere. This means that size and distance information are grossly distorted and resolution is reduced by the amount of the size reduction needed to get a large field of view. Being a near task, the driver must focus the eyes when looking at the miniature display. Those drivers over 45 years of age may not be able to focus on the display. This is not to say it cannot be done, but at present a television rear view display loses more than it gains. Training would be needed to get the most out of the information provided.

It is not possible to interpret accurately what is "out there" by what you see in that little TV window. Almost the same problems exist with the convex rear view mirror which is commonly placed adjacent to a flat mirror to help compensate for its limitations.

Principles to be observed in the construction of periscopic systems with flat mirrors are as follows: (1) an even number of reflections is needed for forward vision, (2) an odd number of reflections is needed for rearward vision, (3) the system should be as short as possible from the eye to the exit aperture to ensure the largest field of view, (4) filters should be avoided and as few optical elements used as possible because of light losses, (5) direct sun on components, and sky glare in the field of view should be avoided, and (6) the mirror should be placed directly ahead and above the line of sight of the driver to avoid obstructions in the field of view.

A windshield tilted forward at the top would provide space for the rearward and forward periscopic components. Figures 10.12 and 10.13 give the essentials of two designs of periscopes for automobile use. These combine forward and rearward visibility, with selection of view being based upon a simple movement of the eyes, or a forward movement of the head to look forward.

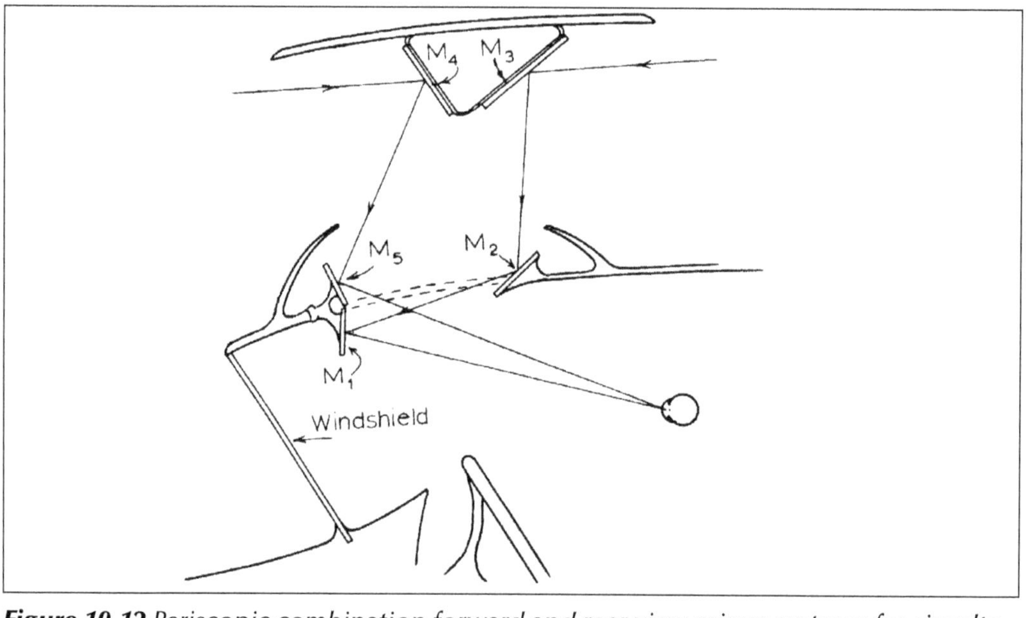


***Figure 10.12*** *Periscopic combination forward and rear view mirror systems for simultaneous viewing from one eye position.*
*$M_1$ Mirror is adjustable about horizontal axis for rear view.*
*$M_2$ Mirror is fixed for rear view.*
*$M_3$ Mirror is fixed for rear view.*
*$M_4$ Mirror is fixed for forward view.*
*$M_5$ Mirror is adjustable for forward view.*

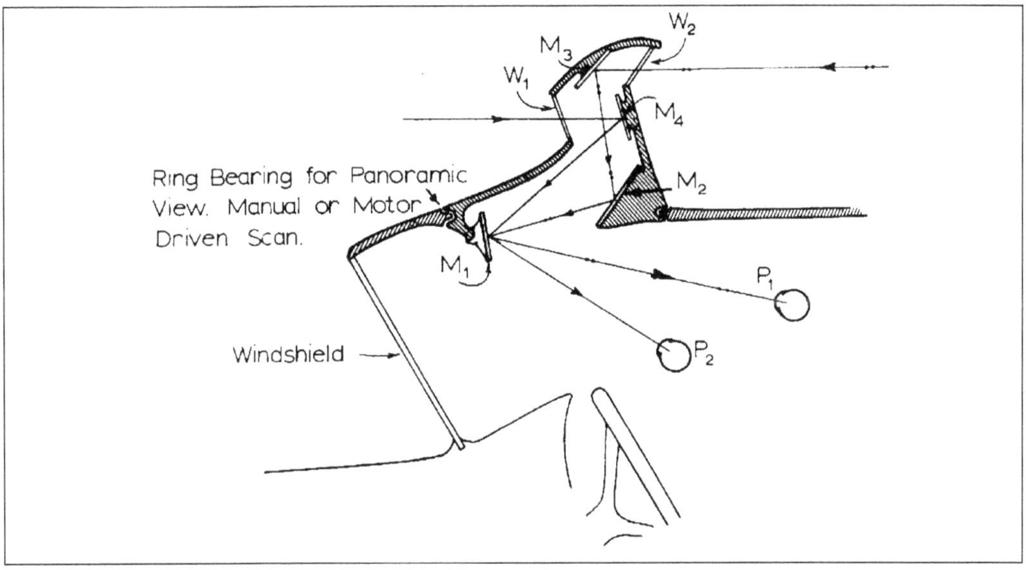


***Figure 10.13*** *Periscopic combination forward and rear view mirror systems requiring two position viewing. The normal eye position, $P_1$, would permit a periscopic rearward view, whereas movement of the head forward to $P_2$ would provide a periscopic forward view. Mirror $M_1$ is adjustable to allow for driver height. Fixed mirrors $M_2$ and $M_3$ provide a rearward view through window $W_2$, while fixed Mirror $M_4$ provides a forward view through Window $W_1$.*

## 10.7 Instrument Panel Visibility

The major factors contributing to the speed and accuracy of instrument panel readability in the daytime are: the illumination on the display compared to the illumination on the road, the size of the numerals or letters, the contrast of the numerals or letters with their background, the accommodative ability of the eyes of the driver, and the placement of the seat and the steering wheel.

The speed of recognition of the critical dial or gauge is increased with larger sizes, greater illumination, greater contrast, and a younger driver who can focus his eyes more quickly.

A study on 1960, 1961 and 1962 automobiles (Allen, February 1963) showed that the average eye-to-dash-panel distance was 72 centimeters in fifty-six automobiles with the seat in the position in which it was found. The height of each of the numbers on the speedometer averaged 1 degree 16 minutes, and each odometer numeral averaged 20 minutes in height. (A 20/20 letter is 5 minutes high.) At that time the illumination on the dash panel ranged from 46 to 1,640 foot candles. In average daytime conditions.

A study (Allen, October 1964) of 50 new 1963 automobiles in dealer stocks measured the time required to look from the sun lighted exterior scene to the dash panel and recognize a speedometer numeral. The two observers were seventeen years of age and pretrained for five days to build up their reaction time skills, The average time of these *practiced* subjects to clear the dash panel without sunglasses was 0.717 seconds, while the same task required 0.781 seconds with fit over sun glasses. In addition to this first recognition time a driver would still have to search until he found the speedometer needle or other gauge of importance. Following this he must return his eyes to the outside scene. It may be conservatively estimated that a normal driver of 35 to 40 years of age will require more than two seconds to inspect the average dash panel and return attention to the highway. Some panels and some conditions would greatly lengthen this time.

Improvements have been made in dash panel design in general, but daytime illumination is a problem in some automobiles and displays are not standardized. A pair of glasses tinted in the upper portions and clear in the lower portions, combined with a properly powered bifocal for older drivers, makes a significant improvement in the speed of inspecting the dash panel and returning vision to the highway.

Dash panel visibility at night depends upon the same factors as for daytime visibility, except that panel lighting is supplied artificially. The best color depends upon the nature of the driver's refractive error. Because of chromatic aberration in the eyes, a hyperope and an emmetrope would see the instrument panel best with green or blue light, whereas a myope or a bifocal wearer, might see it better with red light, assuming normal color vision. At night the loss of surround lighting can contribute to disorientation, double vision, and drowsiness. This effect can be reduced by increasing the instrument panel illumination, and by turning on the inside overhead light.

Vision and Human Factors experts should optimize and standardize the information, location, size, brightness and color to be displayed on all motor vehicle dash panels. They should also standardize the location of control levers, buttons, etc. that control the seats, windows, door locks, door handles, turn indicator, gear shift lever, steering wheel controls, emergency signals, etc.

## 10.8 Headlights

### A. Aim

Improper headlight aim, because of lamp replacement, bent fenders, broken or sagging springs, or unusual vehicle load, is a major cause of glare at night, but for a reason different from what most people think. Improper headlight aim reduces the illumination pattern in front of the automobile to less than optimum. This means that for a low beam aimed too low, the seeing distance is reduced, and the brightness of the illuminated road surface is higher than normal. If the low beam is aimed too high, a greater seeing range is provided, but the illumination on the pavement needed for vehicle guidance will be lowered. Within limits, in either case, there is not much difference in glare to oncoming motorists on a straight highway, because of the shape of the low-beam pattern of American headlights. However the loss in head lighting range with a beam that is too low, and the loss in pavement illumination when the beam is too high, renders the driver with poorly aimed headlights more susceptible to ordinary glare light from other cars (see Table 9.12).

Glare at night is more a matter of the difference in luminance levels between the glare source and the visual task than of the intensity of the glare source alone. Anything which destroys the headlight aim or distribution built into the lamp will seem to increase oncoming headlight glare at night. Dirt and scratches on the headlight lens also produce important degradations in headlight efficiency. The light that is diverted from the roadway is scattered in part toward the oncoming driver's eyes, at the same time the losses of light on the roadway make oncoming headlights appear brighter or more glaring.

Gadgets sold to be attached to headlights are almost always harmful. For example, yellow filters absorb blue light as well as lose about 8 percent of the white light by reflection. "Sleepy-eye" chromium covers used over the top half of the head lamp lens are especially detrimental since they destroy the headlight pattern, thereby increasing the glare into oncoming drivers' eyes and reducing the useful illumination. Dark filters to fit over the headlights are for sale in auto supply stores! All of these should be banned along with add-on window tint. They can kill!

Improving the light pattern and increasing the headlight light output will definitely be of benefit for night time driving. The importance of headlight aim should be emphasized in new car literature and in automotive magazines. Warnings should be clearly stated about the hazards of covering the head lamp with anything, including dirt.

Many automobiles are so sensitive to load that two male adults in the rear seat are enough to require reaiming of the headlights. In 1969, manufacturers made it possible to reach headlight adjustment screws without removing chromium trim. This was an important improvement because it speeded up headlight adjustments and permitted the motorist to adjust head lamps to correct for an overload of his vehicle.

The new headlight designs make adjusting the headlight aim more difficult. The next step needed is to provide headlight adjustment from the driver's seat to match the load, or to provide a load stabilized vehicle that maintains the same headlight level whether loaded or empty. Improved head lighting means less highway glare and fewer accidents.

## B. Filament shields

High beam head lamps used in four headlight arrays do not have filament shields to prevent upward scatter into rain, snow, and fog, whereas low beams do. These shields are the result of an invention by Orville Stamm who, personally, for seventeen years extolled their virtues and attempted to interest the automobile industry and the several large manufacturers of lamps. In 1955, the year that his patent expired, the lamp manufacturers began to advertise an improved fog penetrating head lamp incorporating his shield. All low-beam headlights use similar shields. Certainly, the United States Patent Office protects the inventor, but it has, on occasions such as this, deprived the public of safety advancements for seventeen years while the inventor wastes his time, effort, and money trying to find a manufacturer willing to pay a royalty on a patent.

## C. Sleepy eye shields

Headlight sleepy eye shields (see Figure 10.14), seen occasionally in 1996, were not adopted or endorsed by automobile manufacturers, nor did the manufacturers strongly oppose them, or dozens of other "sucker trade" accessory items offered for sale on the "after market." The sleepy eye shield increased glare and reduced roadway illumination because it destroyed the SAE standard headlight beam pattern (Allen, January 1967). They are especially dangerous in snow, rain and fog. The results of the study of these shields were sent to the Federal Trade Commission. The FTC completely ignored this study. Sleepy eye shields are no longer readily available in stores. Apparently, this headlight problem is about to disappear.

## D. Disappearing headlights

Headlights that are covered when not in operation are a true salesman's gimmick which has hazardous complications. Being mechanical, they are subject to failure and wearing out. Thus interferences with aim as well as the chances for mechanical failure exist. Such headlights are absolutely contraindicated when air flow streamlining, and fuel economy are important.

Complications occur even when they are operating properly. The lamps are exposed only when hot and road splatter dries on them. When the lights are turned off they are automatically stored, hot and dirty. When they would be washed in the rain or in the service station, they are covered. The dirt builds up and destroys the headlight distribution pattern and reduces the light output, thereby increasing the glare to oncoming motorists. (I asked a salesman of a used car dealer to open the headlights of a beautiful, clean used car. The headlights had a one-eighth-inch deposit of road dirt on them!) Less light where it belongs on the pavement, makes approaching headlights seem more glaring.

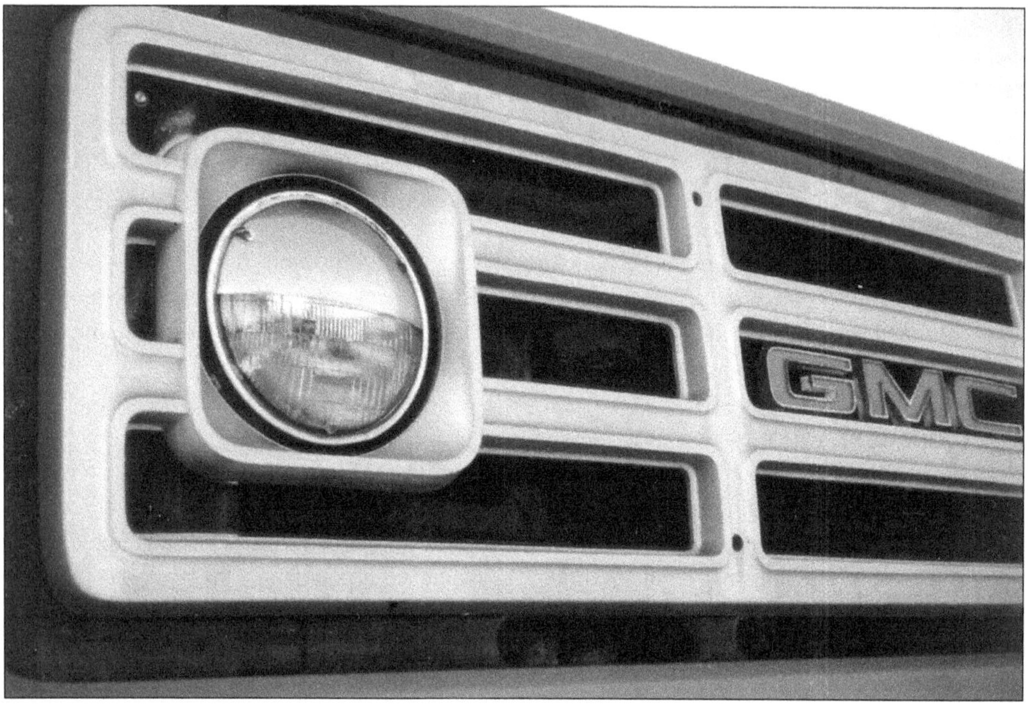


*Figure 10.14* *Sleepy eye shields have long been improperly promoted as reducing glare and improving visibility. They have virtually disappeared because of new headlamp designs. Unbelievably, dark filters covering the headlights are now being sold. All such gimmicks should be illegal because they violate the headlight aim and brightness standards.*

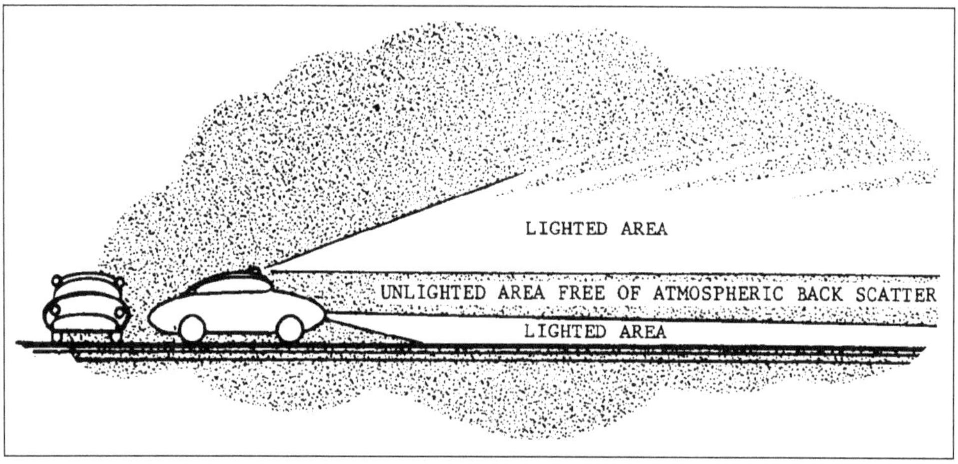


*Figure 10.15* *Recommended vehicle lighting for forward vision. Regular headlights would be designed to have a limited upward component to prevent lighting particulate matter in the atmosphere before the driver's eyes. To permit reading freeway signs and stop signs, which are usually above eye level, the smaller top-mounted lights would be used.*

Disappearing headlights cannot be used in the daytime to signal an approaching driver. The lights are allowed up to three seconds to open (U.S. Department of Transportation, 1968). Let us assume two seconds. Two automobiles approaching each other at 60 miles per hour, will travel 352 feet closer in two seconds! Hence disappearing headlights are as useless for signaling in the daytime as the horn is for warning oncoming drivers on the highway.

There appears to be no justification for covering the headlights. We have few gravel roads and we are not a nation of race drivers. The only advantage seems to be styling. Styling also can be hazardous because the front and rear of the automobile now look almost identical when the headlights are covered. The disappearing headlight was put on the market at a time when great resistance was shown by the manufacturers to such things as energy-absorbing steering columns and dual brakes. The development cost for disappearing headlight designs probably equaled or exceeded the cost of each of the safety features that the industry was required to install and to which they objected so loudly, at least in the beginning.

Starting in 1995, all automobiles in the USA came equipped with daytime running lights. Low-beam headlights, or half voltage high beam headlights are reasonably well suited for use as daytime running lights (Allen, September 1965). Disappearing headlights seemingly will have no place in future car production, thus disappearing headlights will disappear.

### E. All weather head lighting system

An ideal all weather system installed in self leveling automobiles would be one that puts no light at all into a zone between three and five feet above the road (see Figure 10.15). There would be very little back scatter from fog, rain, or snow and the seeing range would be increased. Since such a headlight cannot light signs overhead. Headlights mounted above eye level are needed. These would be aimed so that no light drops below five feet. Because they would be nearer to the driver's eyes than conventional headlights, they could be less powerful and still provide adequate illumination for seeing overhead retroreflectorized signs.

In addition, such roof-mounted headlights, one at each side, would shape code the front of the automobile with a rectangular pattern of white lights which would not be confused with present taillight patterns or with the compatible proposed future taillighting system described in the next section.

## 10.9 Signal Visibility

### A. Front signals

American automobiles suffer from a poorly designed signal system. For instance, front turn signals are not visible to adjacent cars in multilane traffic because they are placed too low and are aimed only in the forward direction. Except for being in a desirably shaded location, all other evidence indicates that turn signals should be raised to the top of the fender. This would permit visibility of the signal from all angles, front and side.

A desirable feature is that the parking lights in front are illuminated when the headlights are on. When one headlight is burned out, the parking light identifies the vehicle as an automobile and not a motor cycle. Recent surveys indicate the number of defective headlights to be about one out of seventy-five motor vehicles. Counts in Bloomington, Indiana, a college town, show about one out of 25 passenger cars has only one headlight!

Unfortunately, having the parking lights on reduces the signal value of the turn signal, which usually has its filament within the same bulb. Amber has been used both on the front and rear for turn signals. Among color defectives as well as normal people, amber is often confused with red (Heath and Schmidt, 1959).

Of the signal colors red, green and yellow (amber), the yellow is the weakest and produces the most mistakes in color recognition. It is sometimes called white, red, or green. In the daytime, body styling confuses the front and rear appearance of automobiles. The use of amber on the front may add to this confusion. At night when only the parking lights are on, the use of amber on the front also confuses the front and rear of an automobile.

The use of new lighting technology can provide signal lights operating at five to ten flashes per second. Such flash rates are very powerful in getting a driver's attention in a very short time. Normal flash rates are clearly inadequate.

## B. Rear signals

### 1. Color

Rear lighting suffers significant deficiencies. Two percent of male drivers have a reduced sensitivity to red light of 20 percent or less (depending upon the wavelength composition of the red light), compared to a color-normal individual. Furthermore, tinted windshields, which are estimated to be in more than half of American automobiles, further reduce the transmission of red light compared to white or green light. To correct for these losses, taillights would need to be five times brighter or of a color other than red. The sensitivity to green is not adversely affected by windshield tint, by any of the common color vision defects, or by space perception aberrations (Allen, December 1964); hence its use for a rear running light is highly recommended.

The front turn signals should be amber but with a high flash rate. The brake light needs to be red, but shape coded with a white bar so that we do not discriminate against color blind drivers.

### 2. Position

For an open highway with low traffic density, taillights and brake lights need to be low for maximum appearance of nearness. When traffic becomes heavy, a high position for taillights and brake lights at the roof line of a passenger car is needed to permit them to be seen through other cars and to reduce the chances of a multiple rear-end collision. Thus these lights need to be at both low and high positions on each motor vehicle.

When automobiles are traveling close behind one another on a straight, level stretch of roadway, a slight change in velocity of the lead car can cause a touch of the brake for the second and third cars, a panic braking for the fourth and fifth, and a rear-end collision for most of the rest. Thus is born the spectacular freeway pile-up.

If the second driver could signal the fifth driver behind him that he had touched his brake, that driver would know of the hazard just as soon as the drivers who are nearer. By thus increasing the range of brake lights by five cars, the first rear-end accident would not occur until the twenty-fifth car back instead of the fifth, a saving of twenty cars! Furthermore, the severity of the collisions that did occur would not peak as quickly, and more vehicles would escape with light damage.

In a study (Allen et. al., February 1967) using auxiliary taillights mounted near the top of the rear window of a station wagon, the signal was found to penetrate to at least the third driver behind the lead car without time attenuation, whereas ordinary taillights required that each driver see the brake light ahead of him and put on his brakes to signal the man behind him to put on his brakes.

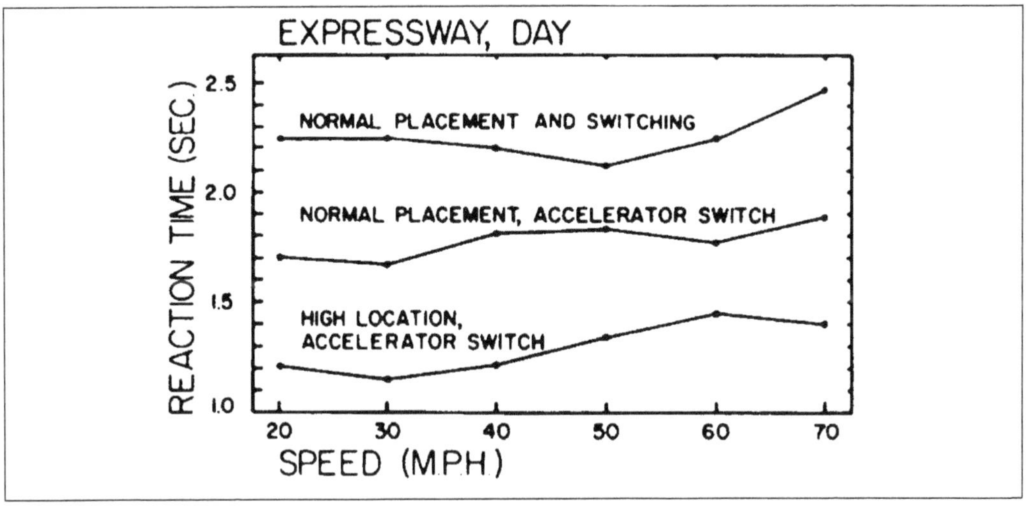


***Figure 10.16*** *Drivers' reaction times at various speeds on the daytime expressway following test vehicles with two rear lighting arrangements and with brake and accelerator switching.*

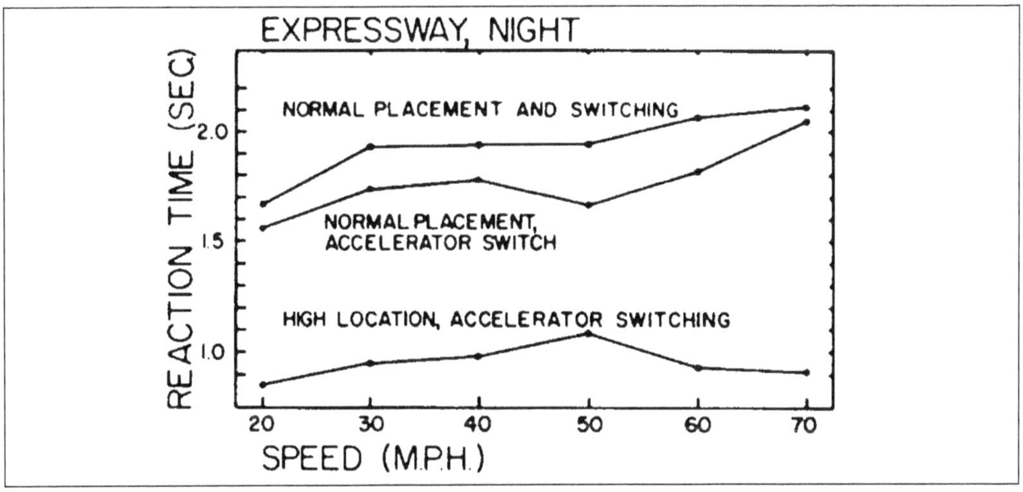


***Figure 10.17*** *Same as Figure 10.16 except that data were taken at night.*

Figures 10.16 and 10.17 show the improvements in performance obtained in following behavior when the taillights were raised, and when a switch was put on the accelerator which lighted the taillights before the foot could get to the brake pedal. It is apparent that performance is best when the driver can see through the car ahead. It is also improved by accelerator switching of the brake light. In this experiment three drivers and a timer operator had to react when the lead vehicle applied its brakes. By subtracting a simple reaction time of 0.2 second for the timer operator, the average driver reaction time using the stock brakes was 0.58 second. With the high positioned accelerator switched brake light system, the individual driver reaction time averaged 0.25 second. In other words, high placement of brake lights can transmit information to closely following drivers much quicker than the stock brake lights can.

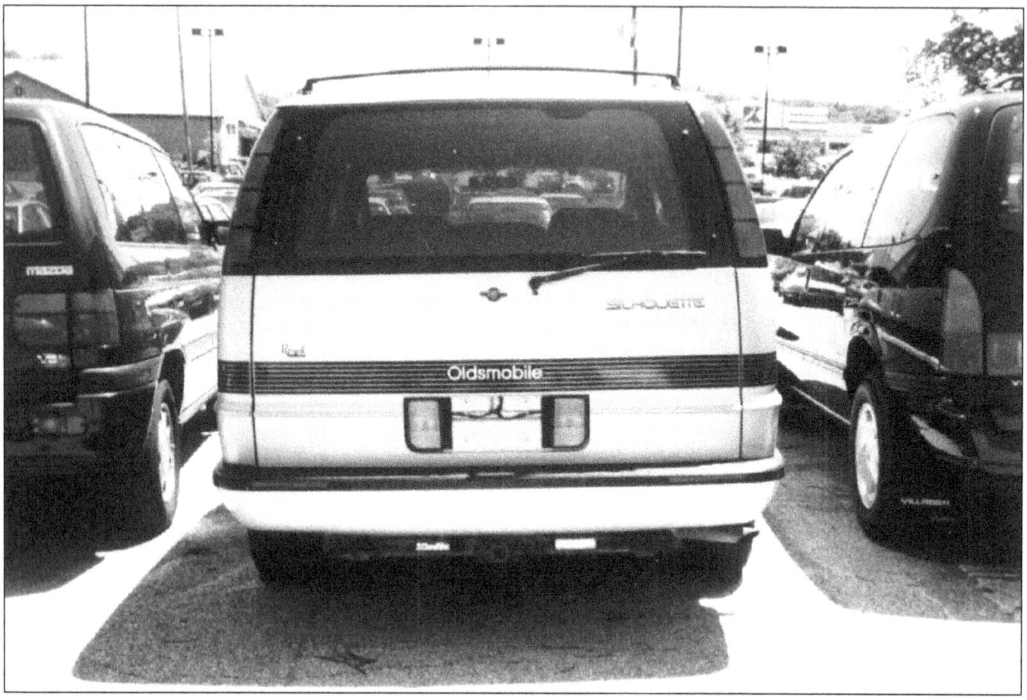


*__Figure 10.18a__ GM's Silhouette has tail, turn and brake lights placed on either side of the rear window. The only lights near the pavement are the back up lights near the license plate. This photo is of a white van which compensates partially for the poor taillighting design. With dark bumpers and dark body colors, this taillight design is hazardous.*

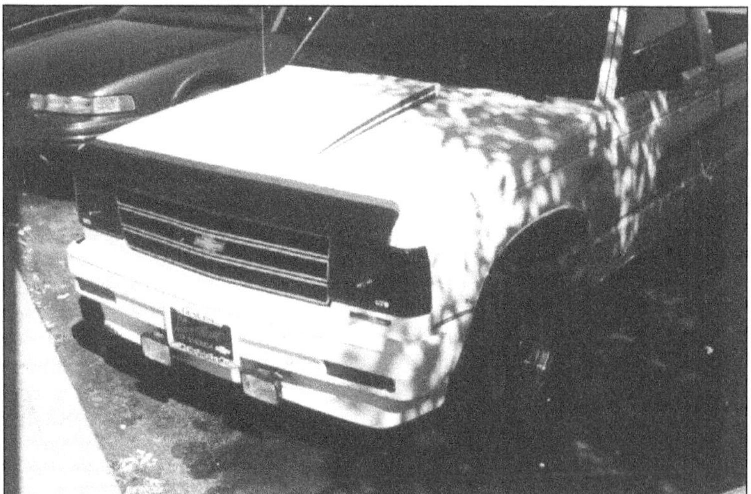

*__Figure 10.18b__ Black add-on filters over the headlights combined with the dark colored shield across the front of the hood, reduce the visibility of this vehicle and reduces headlight brightness about 50 percent. Every 13 years, we need twice as much light to do the same task as we did before. A 50 percent filter makes us 13 years older!*

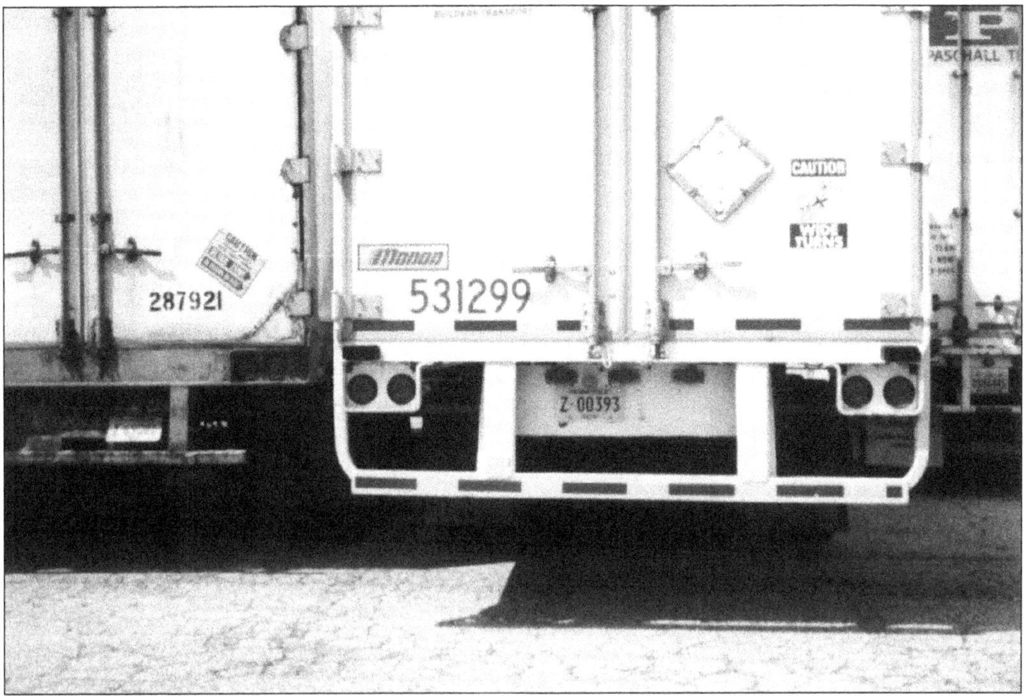


***Figure 10.18c*** *Two truck trailers. The one on the right is relatively clean and has the new multiple strips of reflective tape to improve its visibility. It shows the newer, lower and stronger rear bumper with reflectors on it close to the pavement. In contrast, the trailer at the left is dirty and has none of the new safety features. Even though the trailer on the right has a new lower bumper, it needs to be still lower because it is higher than passenger vehicle bumpers.*

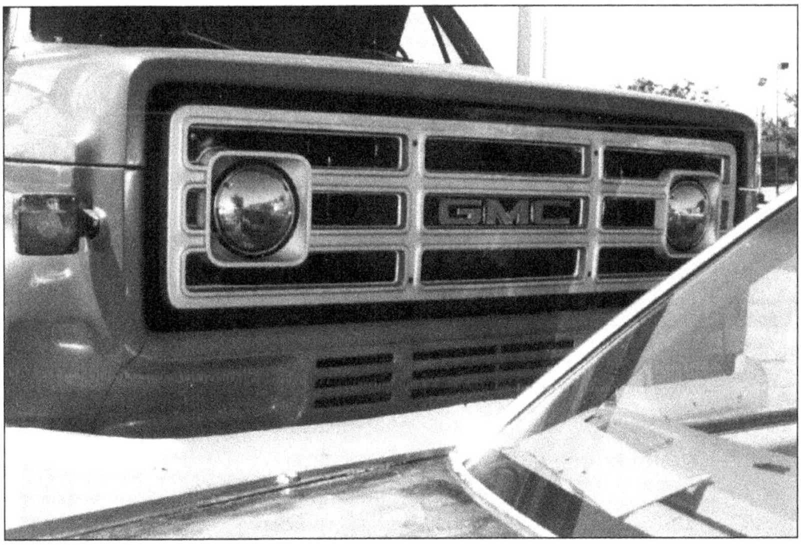


***Figure 10.18d*** *A pickup truck's bumper is at the height of the bottom of the side window of a full size passenger vehicle. This pickup's headlights are at or above the eye level of most motor ists. This causes excess glare at night. In addition, this pickup has glare producing sleepy eye shields on the headlights.*

While there is a clear superiority of placing the brake light at eye level when cars are traveling close together, as on freeways, it is not proper to assume that the present taillights should be replaced with roof mounted lights. The taillight function is best located below eye level, to localize the position of the vehicle with respect to the pavement and the horizon. The high position brake light should be in addition to the stock brake lights and not a substitute for them. Since roof heights vary among vehicles, the high signal light placement should be at a standardized height above the pavement; for example, 60 inches.

In keeping with space perception cues it is desirable to make the car ahead of you appear as close as possible. This is done by lowering the regular tail (presence) lights and by increasing their luminance, their size, and their lateral separation. When brakes are applied it is desirable to increase still more the apparent nearness of the stopping vehicle. This is done by increasing the spacing and the intensity and by reducing the height of the brake lights compared to the taillights. Thus, brake lights should be outside of the taillights and should be larger, brighter, and lower. Appendix A (on supplementary CD-ROM to this book), Figure A.2, shows the brake lights at the same level as the presence lights, because the presence lights have been placed as low as practicable to enhance their location fixing value.

#### 3. Shape coding

As indicated in the preceding section, higher placed lights also must be added to help prevent freeway collisions. These are in effect high placed repeater lights, but they could serve another most valuable function. They would increase the apparent size of the rear end of a vehicle and would provide the means for effective shape coding (see Appendix A—on supplementary CD-ROM to this book—Figure A.2). For example, a midline green light at the top of a passenger automobile would form the apex of a green triangle for taillights. A red brake light at each outer edge of the top, combined with the regular brake lights, would form a distinctive square (see Appendix A—on supplementary CD-ROM to this book—Figure A.2). The separate turn signal lamp in the conventional lower location should be supplemented by a lamp adjacent to the high-mounted red brake light.

By shape coding the red lights with a horizontal white bar, the brake lights would be easily seen and recognized by all drivers including those with a color vision defect.

#### 4. Dual intensity

Other deficiencies in present day taillighting are the use of the same intensity for daytime brake and turn signaling as is used at night, and the use of bright trim surrounding and covering over the taillights. Even the use of bright red paint for automobile colors makes an already inadequate daytime brake light virtually useless. In the daytime, a red brake light surrounded by red paint of an equal or greater intensity, becomes a flashing black signal and doesn't have any attraction or warning value unless one is looking directly at it. Tail and brake lights that brighten as the daylight increases are the answer and are easy to manufacture.

### C. Flash rate

Special attention must be directed toward signal lights that now flash at pleasant frequencies rather than efficient frequencies. Flash rates of 120 per minute or less are recommended by the Society of Automotive Engineers. Old flashers and bulbs often combine to give flash rates of ten to fifteen per minute. Such a slow rate gives the light an on and an off phase of about 2.5 seconds each. Since a visual fixation takes only 0.20 to 0.25 second, a person could look at a light four or five times, always catch it in the dark or light phase, and thus not be sure it was flashing. Preliminary study indicates that a light that flashes five to ten times per second, gives a signal that is far more effective than the current system. Solid state lights perform very well at high flash rates.

## D. Dirt

A major defect in modern automobile lighting is dirt. Styling dictates changes in lamp housing details, but changes to reduce dirt pickup and moisture penetration are not notable. The collection of dust and road mud is a function of position and air flow past the light (see Figure 10.19). Attention to air flow patterns should be a part of lighting design as well as a factor in wind resistance and effective lateral body area distribution. Until such is the case, the motorist and the trucker must make a lamp cleaning tour around the car or truck at each stop.

Head and taillights have been observed to have water in them! Even slight water and dust penetration spoils the efficiency of the retroreflector prism faces on the inside of the plastic lens. Paint and plastic materials deposited on the inside of the plastic lens from the heat of the lamp further destroy the retroreflector efficiency. Moisture damage to painted or aluminized reflective surfaces and moisture caused corrosion on electrical contacts are of importance because they reduce lamp light output. Old style sealed beam headlights did not have these problems.

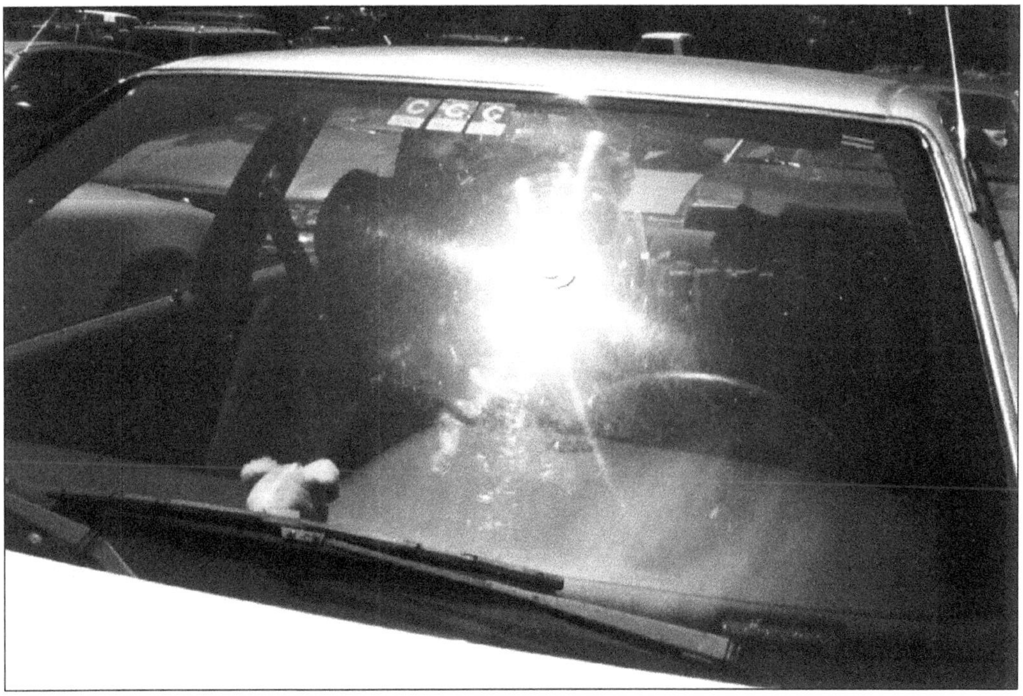

***Figure 10.19*** *A simple test for windshield condition. Look at the reflected image of the sun as you view the windshields in a parking lot on a clear, bright day. There will be a few new, unscratched windshields and there will be some seriously scratched windshields as shown above. Light from damaged windshields added to light scattered from dirt and light reflected by the windshield from the top of the dash panel can cause an accident by preventing seeing a pedestrian, cyclist, automobile, bus, truck or train in time. (The circular object on the glass was intended but failed to block out the main image of the sun for the camera.)*

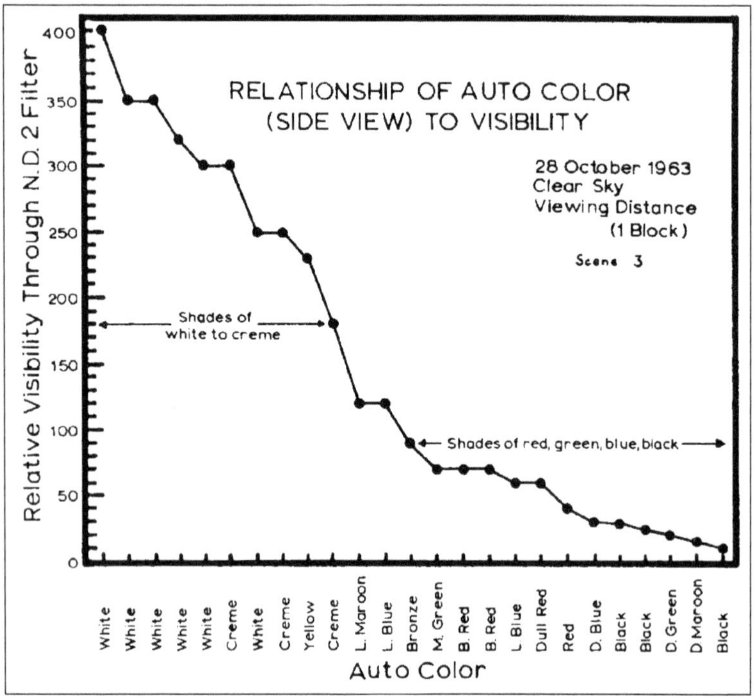


***Figure 10.20*** *Actual field measurements with a Luckiesh-Moss visibility meter of automobile color visibility. Automobiles were observed from a position in front about 45 degrees off the line of travel, much as would be the case in a developing intersection collision. Without question the shades of red, green, blue, and black were more camouflaged than the shades of yellow, cream, and white.*

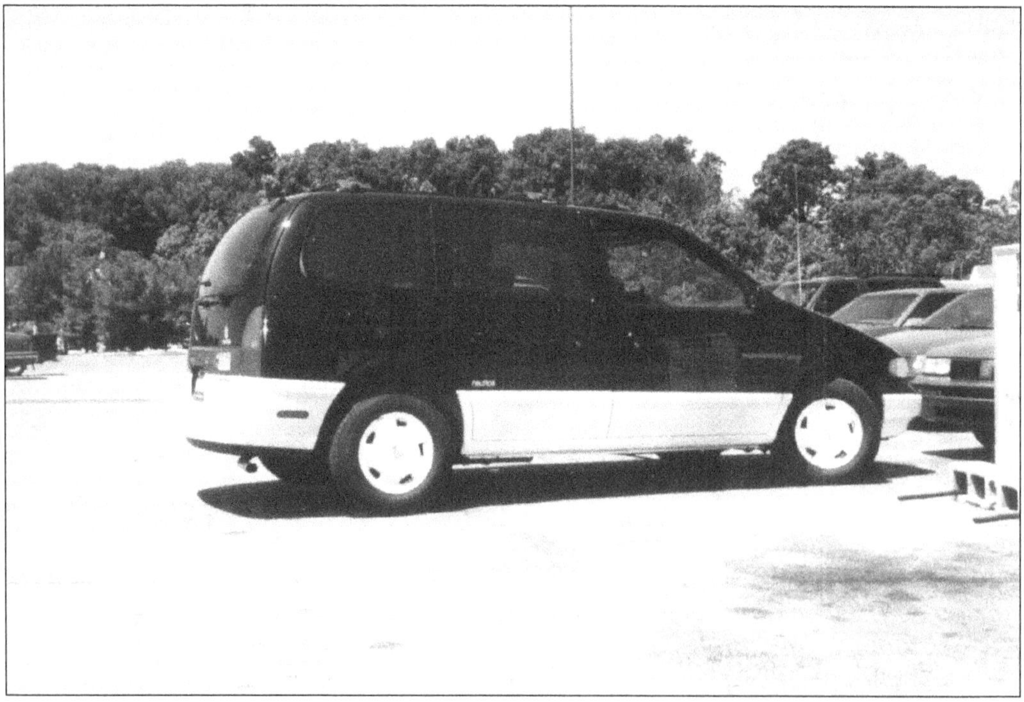

***Figure 10.21*** *If it had white side wall tires, this van would be the perfect example of the Ban Black safety concept for all motor vehicles. Even so, this photo shows elements of camouflage. The main body, which is black with tinted windows, matches the trees while the top of the white lower portion lines up with the bottom of the trees and looks like the pavement! All white and no window tint would be best.*

## 10.10 Vehicle Visibility

After over fifty years of manufacturing automobiles in all conceivable colors, the automobile manufacturers still produce car colors in terms of what will sell, not what is safe. Studies have shown that up to ten times as many accidents happen to black cars as to white. Other data indicate white cars are up to forty times more visible than black (see Figure 10.20). Still other data indicate that greater visibility means fewer and less severe accidents. Red and black have the lowest visibility of all colors. Cream, yellow, and white are the most visible.

Along with statistics on color, it is known that the small, powerful sports car has the highest accident rate and greatest death rate compared to full sized automobiles. The higher death rate is no surprise because of the small amount of protective metal surrounding the passengers. The higher accident rate could be due to speed alone, but indications are that speed is only an indirect factor.

The most probable causes of more sports car accidents are the use of dark colors, including red, and their small size (see Figure 10.21). We recognize an object's nearness in part by its size, and we recognize its approach speed almost entirely by the rate of increase in size. Therefore, a small vehicle is judged to be farther away and its approach speed is judged to be slower than it really is. The driver of a sports car cannot rely upon the help of those other drivers who reduce the overall number of accidents by compensating for the mistakes of others. The sports car driver, with his low vantage position, excessive speed potential, low visibility, and reduction of the amount of Good Samaritan Protection from other drivers, must rely almost entirely upon his own skills to avoid accidents. Obviously, from the accident statistics and insurance rates, his own skills alone are not always enough.

It is hoped that the automobile manufacturers will find it expedient to protect the motoring public from the misfit sports cars by at least improving their conspicuity.

It is hoped that manufacturers will adopt white bumpers, white tires, white mud guards, white lower side panels, etc., as standard equipment for all production vehicles, including passenger cars, sports cars, trucks, buses and construction equipment. This would eliminate about 70 percent of the accidents.

# Chapter 11

# Visual Hazards on Streets and Highways

Merrill J. Allen, O.D., Ph.D.

***Synopsis***



## 11.1 Nighttime Hazards

### A. Inadequate illumination and blacktop pavements

The human eye is capable of an extreme range of adaptation to changes in the ambient light level. However, such flexibility does not tell the whole story. A major part of this adaptability comes from the ability to change the "grain" of the retina; that is, to group photoreceptors and bipolar, ganglion, and other cells into larger functional units as the light level falls, and into smaller units as the light level rises. The result is a dependency of visual acuity upon light level. See Figure 11.1.

Other important visual functions such as color vision, speed of perception reaction time, binocular fusion, and stereopsis are adversely affected by the increasing retinal grain at lower luminance levels. The contrast sensitivity also is degraded and is of importance in detecting objects as distinct from their background. The greater the contrast sensitivity, the easier it is to detect an object. Figure 11.2 shows the minimum contrast of an object which will make it perceptible at each luminance level. Contrast is defined by the equation:

$$C = (B_1 - B_2) \div B_1$$

where $C$ is the contrast, $B_1$ is the background luminance, and $B_2$ is the test object luminance. Contrast sensitivity is the reciprocal of contrast. Increasing illumination increases the sensitivity to contrast and makes object detection easier. Conversely, Figure 11.2 shows that at nighttime roadway luminance levels of one foot lambert or less, an object must be considerably brighter or darker than its background to be seen. Thus reading road signs, and the detection of an object such as a pedestrian becomes more difficult. Also the times for detection, recognition, and response increase.

Since the amount of light present is the distinguishing difference between night and day, the problems of night driving would be reduced if more light were available. It has been shown that visibility even in the daytime is improved by adding lights to vehicles (Allen, May 1964, March 1965; Port of New York Authority, 1968). That more light at night is beneficial, using the same system of automobile and highway head lighting as we now have, is predicted from the behavior of the human eye with changing light levels (see Figures 11.1 and 11.2). This has been verified by a number of studies (Roper and Meese, 1964; Christie, 1968) involving accident experience vs. highway lighting and field testing of vehicles with increased headlight output.

Because of the need for more light at night, the blacktop (asphalt) highway, due to its low reflectance, is an uninspired design. The amount of light returned from headlight beams depends upon the composition and aging of the blacktop surface and may vary from virtually zero when the pavement is new or wet to nearly the same as Portland concrete when the blacktop mixture includes a large proportion of light colored stone and the asphaltic cement has been worn away. Much of seeing at night is by silhouette or back lighting; that is, a dark object is seen against a light background. Portland cement gives good visibility because it provides a light background for objects. Pedestrians usually wear dark clothing and are best seen in silhouette; hence blacktopped roadways impair the seeing of pedestrians. Any light colored object will stand out better on black, but unfortunately not many roadway hazards are light in color, and few are as important as the pedestrian.

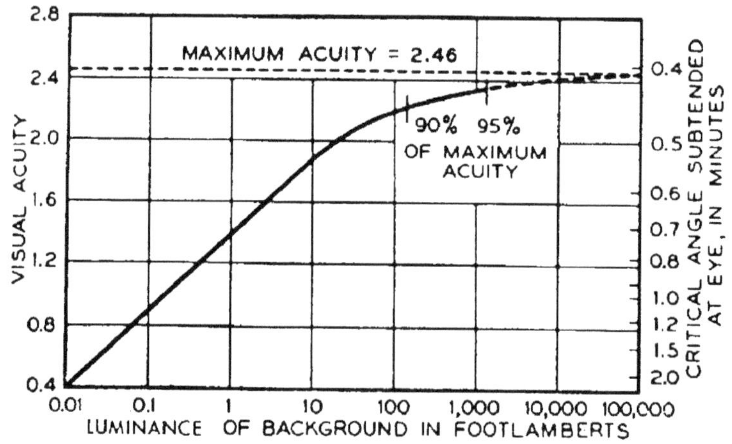


***Figure 11.1*** *The effect of illumination on visual acuity. A high contrast black Landolt ring was displayed on a variable luminance background and was observed with normal pupils and binocular vision. (From IES Lighting Handbook, 4th ed., Figure 2.14, pp. 2–8.) (Note: The dotted extension of the curve is somewhat misleading as the acuity does not rise past about 900 foot lamberts, and 20,000 foot lamberts is reported to be intolerable to the eye.)*

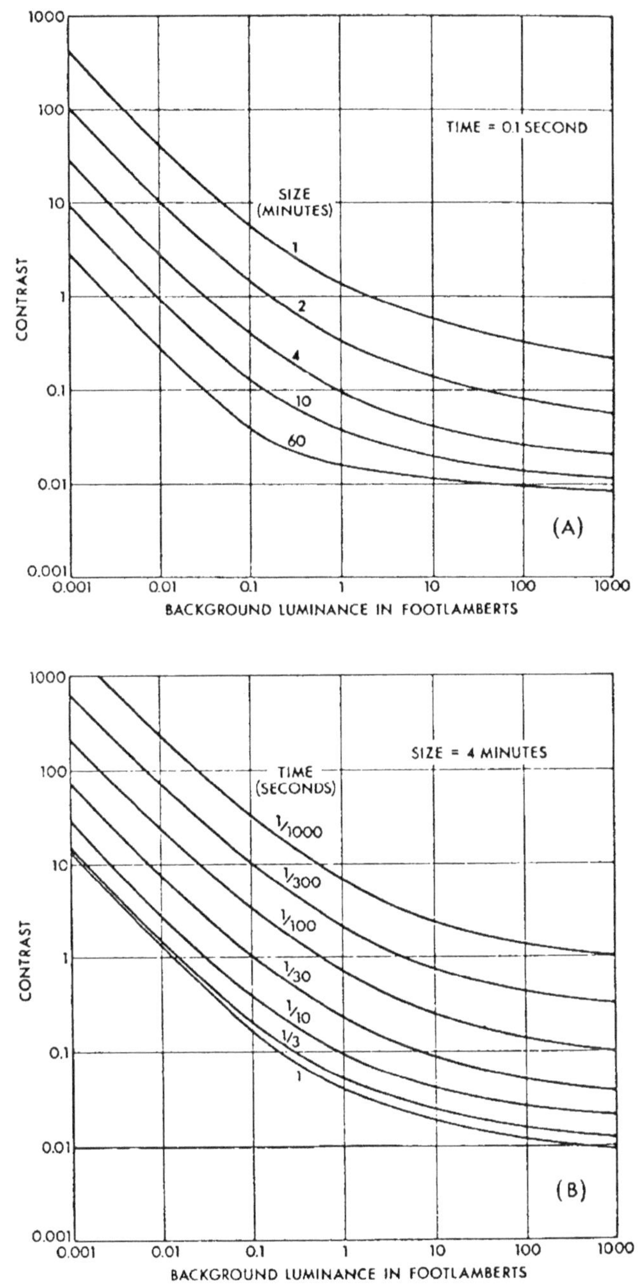


***Figure 11.2*** *The relationship between size, contrast, background luminance, and exposure duration for threshold seeing. Contrast is $\Delta L/L$, where L is the luminance of the background and $\Delta L$ is the difference between the luminance of the target and the background. Contrasts above 100 are possible when the test object is brighter than the background (from IES Lighting Handbook, 4th ed., Figure 2.16, pp. 2–8).*

A person's alertness depends upon the amount of stimulation he receives. When alone on a highway at night, the lowered light level, especially from a new blacktop road, reduces alertness and increases the risk of falling asleep.

On the positive side, for dry blacktop pavements, reflectorized center and edge lines stand out more clearly. These reflectorized lines greatly assist night driving because they make the task of staying on the road in the proper lane easier. In addition, continuous edge marking could help reveal a pedestrian near the edge of the pavement at a greater than normal distance.

With the onset of rain the advantage of blacktop disappears in supplying contrast to edge and center reflectorized paint lines. Wet blacktop pavement becomes even blacker, and the currently used reflectorized paint loses most of its unique properties. The film of water prevents rays, which approach at grazing incidence, from penetrating to the pavement. The water defocuses the glass beads used in the reflectorized paint destroying their reflective ability. Hence at the time when headlight output is less due to dirt and rain drops, and cause more glare to oncoming motorists, the blacktop itself and its markings are significantly less visible.

On the other hand, the glossy surface reflectance when pavements are wet effectively extends the headlight range! Objects placed in the roadway may be illuminated at greater than dry weather conditions due to the pavement reflecting light like a mirror. Water reflectance is demonstrated by the red light reflected from the pavement as you approach a reflectorized stop sign at night!

Your headlights are reflected up to the sign, and the sign sends the light back in the direction from which it came. Thus the pavement glows red.

The motorist's ability to localize his own vehicle properly in his own lane is seriously impaired because of the loss of wet pavement edge detail, and because of the rain droplets in the atmosphere. The amount of obscuration is not dependent on the size of the droplets, but on the number falling on a unit of area in one second (Middleton, 1958). Thus obscuration depends upon the number of drops per unit volume of air at any given instant.

The combination effect on vision of drop obscuration in the atmosphere, water splatter on the windshield, and back scatter of light from the headlights by water drops in the air, results in a seeing condition that is unusually poor and hazardous in the rain at night.

## B. Improper use of reflectors

The retroreflector, composed of internally reflecting cube corner prisms is an efficient practical means for alerting a motorist to its presence. Placed on automobiles, bicycles, trucks, trains, and pedestrians, these reflectors can be seen three to ten times farther away than unreflectorized objects. However, a retroreflector is just a spot of light in a field of blackness until the motorist is near enough to have his headlights reveal the nature of the object supporting the reflector. To aid in quick identification, reflectors placed on the rear of vehicles are red (except for reflectorized license plates) and those near the front are amber. To identify the type of vehicle or even where it is, requires the motorist to approach close enough for head lighting to reveal the details. The goal of marking a vehicle by reflectors is to provide a passive system at night that always reveals its presence and location.

Unfortunately, things do not work so well in practice because of a general lack of understanding of and how to use them. For example, nonhazardous driveways along a roadway are often marked with red reflectors, while bridge abutments within inches of high-speed traffic, even on new interstate highways, may not be reflectorized. A person may wish to identify his own driveway, and he should be permitted to do so, but not with red, which is supposed to mean danger.

Another example are the highway delineators, retroreflectors on top of four foot posts parallel to the edge of the roadway. The retroreflector color is normally white, with amber being used to mark exit ramps on divided highways, thus duplicating the reflector color on the front of an automobile or truck. Since the eye level of the driver of a modern automobile rarely exceeds forty-eight inches, most motorists must look up to see these reflectors.

If the road curves, the motorist can see the curve only by the apparent changes in reflector spacing and by the fact that the reflectors that are the farthest away are the dimmest. The normally powerful perspective cues to space are completely missing, or are reversed, if the reflectors are at or above the driver's eye level. At 48 inches in height the reflectors are in a less intense portion of the headlight beam pattern and hence cannot reflect much light.

The ideal location for such reflectors is attached to the pavement surface at the edge of the highway. If they must be moved back into the grass they should be placed within twelve inches of the ground. Perhaps the four-foot post is needed to prevent a mower from striking it, but the reflectors should be near the bottom. The presence of these delineator posts is an unnecessary obstruction. They are often struck, generally provide no useful information, and the reflectors divert the eyes from the road and are often deceptive. To ensure their low visibility, the posts themselves are usually painted a camouflaging green!

Reflectors placed on trucks and on slow moving vehicles are too high for accurate localization on the highway by perspective clues. In fact, on trucks the high placement and the narrow spacing of lights and reflectors, plus the dirt may deceive even the sophisticated motorist into believing that a slow moving truck is far away when in reality a collision may be imminent. Many rear-end accident drivers show little or no effort to brake prior to collision, and in many instances the motorist has actually left the highway, following the lights of a parked vehicle to collide with it.

One early morning on a four-lane divided highway, I saw two cars side by side about 600 feet ahead of me. I wondered which one I should get behind as I was gaining on them. Several seconds later I asked myself again which one I should follow. I was now about 300 feet behind them. As I studied these cars, I began to see something in the upper part of my windshield. It was the back of an unreflectorized truck about 90 feet away (instead of 300 feet away) and moving slowly. I only had time to swerve! I shook for 15 minutes! There were two taillights on the left of the truck and two on the right. Each pair appeared to me to be a car far down the highway! White mud guards and strip reflectors outlining the back of the truck would have solved this perceptual problem.

There are two classes of retroreflectors used on automotive equipment. Class A retroreflectors are defined by their light output distribution and intensity, which are given in Table 11.1

The entrance angle is the angle formed by the incident light beam with the normal to the surface of the reflective device, e.g., a sign or license plate; or from the optic axis, e.g., a taillight lens with integral retroreflector.

**Table 11.1**
**Minimum Candlepower per Incident Foot Candle for Class A Red Reflex Reflector**

| | Entrance Angles, Degrees | | | | |
|---|---|---|---|---|---|
| **Observation Angle, Degrees** | **0** | **10 up** | **10 down** | **20 left** | **20 right** |
| 0.2 | 4.5 | 3.0 | 3.0 | 1.5 | 1.5 |
| 1.5 | 0.07 | 0.05 | 0.05 | 0.03 | 0.06 |

**Table 11.2**
**Minimum Candlepower per Incident Foot Candle for Class B Red Reflex Reflector**

| | Entrance Angles, Degrees | | | | |
|---|---|---|---|---|---|
| **Observation Angle, Degrees** | **0** | **10 up** | **10 down** | **20 left** | **20 right** |
| 0.2 | 0.50 | 0.40 | 0.40 | 0.20 | 0.20 |
| 1.5 | 0.01 | 0.01 | 0.01 | 0.01 | 0.01 |

The observation (divergence) angle is the angle formed by the observer's line of sight and the illuminating beam where these two lines intersect at the reflector.

A Class B retroreflector must meet the requirements shown in Table 11.2.

The usual size for the Class A and B reflectors is four inches in diameter. Thus, the candlepower per square foot of reflector surface is quite high (12.6 times greater than the values given for the four-inch size). Even though the Class A reflector has a very high light returning ability, it does this only along the axis or normal to the surface. At 20 degrees off axis the light returned is down to one-third. Hence for wide angle usage as on the sides of automobiles the Class A reflector must be redesigned. Reflective sheeting, on the other hand, is composed of imbedded glass spheres instead of internally reflecting prisms and has as its great virtue a high efficiency at a large entrance angle.

Table 11.3 permits comparisons of reflective sheeting of various colors and efficiencies with cube corner Class A reflectors. In Table 11.3, candle power per foot candle per square foot is a measure of the efficiency of the reflector under certain standard conditions such as a divergence angle of 0.5 degree with an incidence angle of -4 degrees or +30 degrees, as used in retroreflective license plate testing.

The following formula gives the essential relationships:

$$CP_R = \frac{I_R d^2}{I_E A}$$

$CP_R$ is the candle power of the reflector, $I_R$ is the illumination falling on the plane of the reflector in foot candles, $d$ is the distance between the source of illumination and the reflector, $I_E$ is the illumination falling on the eye or the photo detector in foot candles returned from the reflector, and $A$ is the area of the reflector in square feet.

The Federal Motor Vehicle Safety Standards (U.S. Department of Transportation, 1968) called for Class A retroreflectors for rear application and Class A retroreflectors or reflective sheeting for side markers. More recent standards require that truck trailers be outline reflectorized both on the sides and the rear. This is important safety improvement is beginning to be seen on trucks.

Highway reflectorized paint is a different problem, as will be seen in Figure 11.3. This figure details the role played by the left and right headlights in the typical automobile at the upper limit of the low beam head lamps. Since the 300 feet is not to scale with the height and spacing of the lamps, the angles are not true; however, they do indicate the grazing nature of the illuminating and viewing rays. Such tiny angles make the measurement especially difficult.

Figure 11.4 shows the optics of a portable pavement-marking photometer built by the 3M Company. Note the folded light path needed to make the optical path long enough to permit reasonable aperture spacing to provide the 0.35 degree and 0.78 degree angles between the incident and view rays.

**Table 11.3**

TABLE 9-3
COMPARATIVE BRIGHTNESS OF 3M SCOTCHLITE BRAND
SHEETING AND CUBE-CORNER REFLECTORS
*(candle power per foot-candle per square foot)*

| *Incidence Angle Degree* | *Divergence Angle Degree* | *3070 (3M) White* | *3170 (3M) White* | *3270 (3M) Silver* | *3870 (3M) Silver* | *3M Signal Del. Silver* | *SAE Class A Cube Corner (White)* | *3171 (3M) Yellow* | *3271 (3M) Yellow* | *3274 (3M) Orange* | *3870 Type Amber (3M)* | *3M Signal Del.-Amber* | *SAE Class B Cube Corner (Amber)* | *3272 (3M) Red* | *3870 Type Red (3M)* | *3M Signal Red* | *SAE Class A Cube Corner (Red)* |
|---|---|---|---|---|---|---|---|---|---|---|---|---|---|---|---|---|---|
| −4 | 0.2 | 30 | 45 | 60 | 155 | 187 | 224 | 25 | 30 | 16 | 60 | 112 | 140 | 12.5 | 30 | 56 | 56 |
| +10 | 0.2 | | | 55 | | 180 | 144 | | 25 | 15 | | 108 | 90 | 11.5 | | 54 | 36 |
| +15 | 0.2 | | | 50 | 100 | | | | 25 | 13.5 | 42 | | | 10.5 | 21 | | |
| +20 | 0.2 | | | 40 | | 173 | 72 | | 20 | 11 | | 104 | 45 | 8.5 | | 52 | 18 |
| +30 | 0.2 | | | 25 | 50 | 144 | | | 15 | 7 | 17 | 86 | | 5.5 | 8.5 | 43 | |
| +40 | 0.2 | 7.0 | 7.5 | 12.5 | 25 | 72 | | 5.5 | 6.0 | 2.8 | | 43 | | 1.9 | | 21 | |
| +45 | 0.2 | | | 5.0 | 10 | | | | 4.0 | 2.5 | 6 | | | 1.5 | 3.0 | | |
| +50 | 0.2 | | | 3.5 | | | | | 2.5 | 1.2 | | | | 0.9 | | | |
| −4 | 0.5 | 18 | 23 | 25 | 65 | 72 | | 12.5 | 15 | 8 | 20 | 43 | | 6.5 | 10 | 21 | |
| +10 | 0.5 | | | 25 | | 72 | | | 14 | 7.5 | | 43 | | 6.0 | | 21 | |
| +15 | 0.5 | | | 25 | 50 | | | | 12 | 6.5 | 17 | | | 5.5 | 8.5 | | |
| +20 | 0.5 | | | 20 | | 65 | | | 10 | 5.5 | | 39 | | 4.5 | | 19 | |
| +30 | 0.5 | | | 15 | 25 | 50 | | | 8 | 3.5 | 10 | 30 | | 3.0 | 5.0 | 15 | |
| +40 | 0.5 | 4.5 | 5.0 | 7.5 | 15 | 29 | | 3.0 | 4 | 2.0 | | 17 | | 1.2 | | 8.5 | |
| +45 | 0.5 | | | 3.5 | 5.0 | | | | 2.8 | 1.2 | 2.5 | | | 1.0 | 1.2 | | |
| +50 | 0.5 | | | 3.0 | | | | | 1.5 | 0.5 | | | | 0.4 | | | |
| −4 | 1.5 | 2.5 | 3.0 | 4.0 | 8 | | 3.4 | 2.0 | 2.5 | 1.2 | | | 2.1 | 1.0 | | | .84 |
| +10 | 1.5 | | | 3.5 | | | 2.4 | | 2.5 | 1.1 | | | 1.5 | 0.9 | | | .60 |
| +15 | 1.5 | | | 3.0 | | | | | 2.5 | 1.0 | | | | 0.8 | | | |
| +20 | 1.5 | | | 2.5 | | | 1.4 | | 2.3 | 0.8 | | | 0.9 | 0.7 | | | .36 |
| +30 | 1.5 | | | 2.0 | | | | | 1.8 | 0.5 | | | | 0.5 | | | |
| +40 | 1.5 | 1.5 | 1.5 | 1.6 | 2.0 | | | 0.8 | 0.9 | 0.4 | | | | 0.4 | | | |
| +45 | 1.5 | | | 1.1 | | | | | 0.8 | 0.2 | | | | 0.1 | | | |
| +50 | 1.5 | | | 1.1 | | | | | 0.5 | 0.1 | | | | 0.1 | | | |

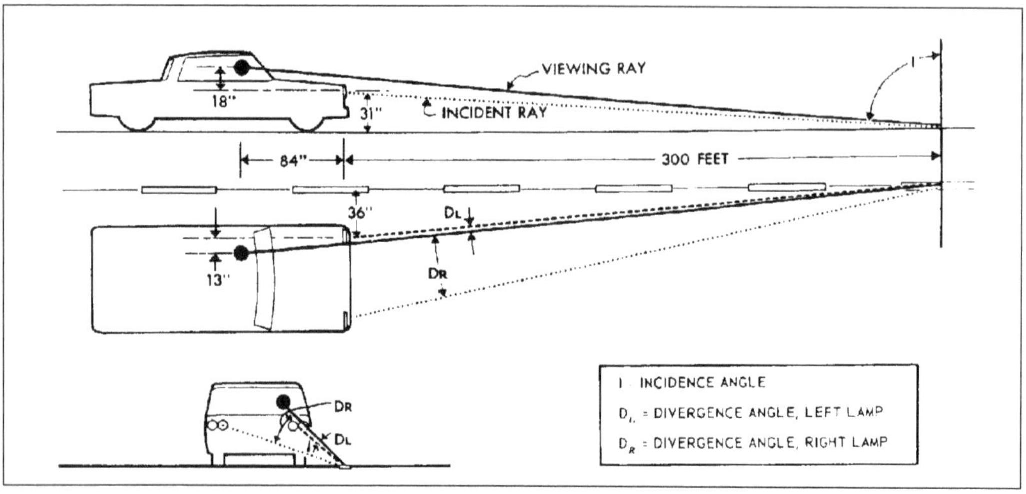


***Figure 11.3*** *Relationship between driver, head lamps, and pavement marking. Geometry involved in reflectivity from center line point at 300 feet distance, using representative dimensions for a dual head lamp vehicle. (From Harrington et al., 1962.)*

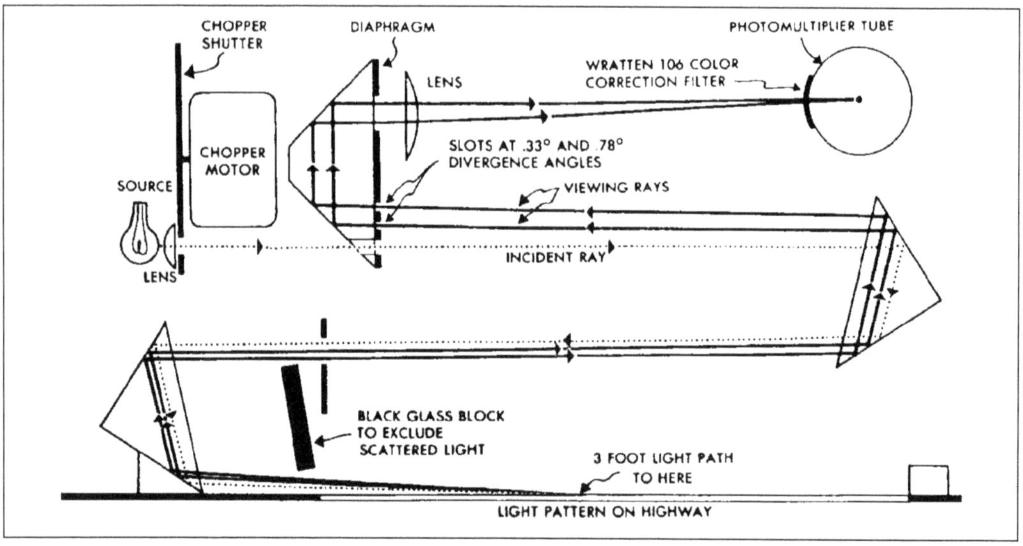


***Figure 11.4*** *Principal components of pavement marking photometer optical system. (From Harrington et al., 1962.)*

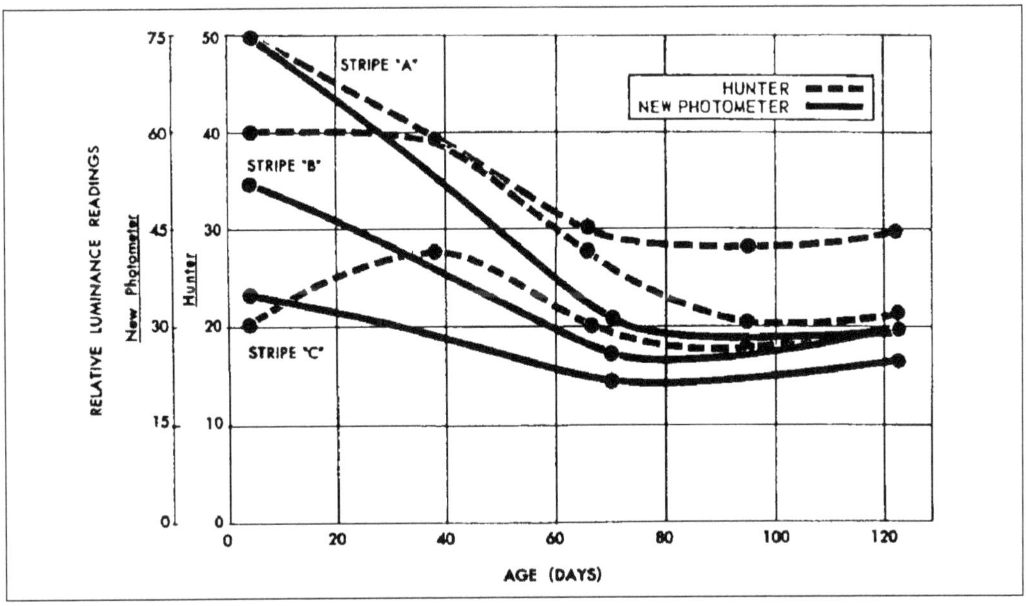


***Figure 11.5*** *Relative luminance readings vs. age of reflectorized highway paint. Comparison of reflectorized transverse test stripes for three representative 1.5 index beaded markings as measured by the Hunter and the new photometer. (Wisconsin Highway Department annual performance test stripes.) (From Harrington et al., 1962.)*

Figure 11.5 gives the aging characteristics of three different beaded paint stripes exposed to highway traffic as measured by the 3M instrument and the Hunter Night Visibility Meter, a fairly widely used instrument. Paint reflectance varies as beads wear away and new beads are exposed, which is not necessarily a linear effect.

A different device has been employed by the author to make paint stripe measurements. It uses the highly versatile Pritchard Spectrophotometer (Photo Research Corporation) as a photo detector and an automobile bulb as a light source. The optics are similar to those in a retinoscope. They are cheap, rugged, and self-aligning.

## C. Pedestrians: A double hazard and a double right

A pedestrian has the right to be protected from careless motorists. Similarly, a motorist has a right to be protected from careless pedestrians. That headlights at night do provide the pedestrian with warning of an approaching automobile as well as helping the motorist is indicated by the report of a 14.1 percent drop in pedestrian vehicle accidents after the change over was made to low-beam headlights instead of parking lights within the New York City limits on February 4, 1952.

Unfortunately, the motorist usually has no warning of the presence of a pedestrian because of the normal low reflectivity of clothing. An illustration of the difficulty is the following incident which occurred early in our testing of pedestrian visibility. The experimenters found that cardboard boxes, spray painted black, were visible at considerable distances because of surface reflections.

To evaluate quickly the visibility of cloth, one of the graduate students volunteered to stand in the roadway, while a second student approached in an automobile at 20 miles per hour. The plan was to stop as soon as the driver saw the pedestrian's dark clothing. The pedestrian stood in line with the driver's side of the approaching car and waited, anticipating the driver's stop. It finally became necessary to leap out of the way as the car continued down the road at 20 miles per hour. When the driver returned to the pedestrian's location, he asked, "Where were you?" A simple question indeed, but one of great significance. Keep in mind the slow speed, the motorist's sure knowledge that a pedestrian was out there, the absence of glare, and the driver's ready to stop attitude.

In the nighttime pedestrian accident reports on record in the Indiana Department of Motor Vehicles for 1966, 87 percent of the drivers whose automobile struck a pedestrian at night claimed difficulty in seeing the pedestrian, while only 11.8 percent made the same claim during the daytime. Furthermore, 23.4 percent of the drivers at night claimed they heard the impact before they saw the pedestrian!

Since the percentage of blood alcohol is higher among dead pedestrians than among the population at risk at the same location as the accident (Haddon et al., 1961; Indiana University, 1964), pedestrians obviously are not always able to avoid an automobile even though headlights do offer a warning. The motorist also deserves some warning sign to help protect the pedestrian and to protect himself. There are signs that announce a curve ahead, road repairs in progress, a dead end, or a stop sign, but the sign that flashes only when a pedestrian is present has not yet been invented.

Table 11.4 gives the reaction distance plus the stopping distance, called critical visibility distance, for an automobile with safe tires and brakes, traveling on dry pavement and driven by an individual with an assumed reaction time of 0.75 seconds.

**Table 11.4**

| Miles Per Hour | Critical Visibility Distance (ft.) |
|---|---|
| 20 | 45 |
| 30 | 72 |
| 40 | 123 |
| 50 | 185 |
| 60 | 261 |
| 70 | 349 |
| 80 | 450 |

Table 11.5 indicates the percentage of pedestrians that were detected by four sober researchers at distances equal to or greater than the critical visibility distance based on a 0.75 second response time instead of the 1.64 to 2.5 seconds needed for 50 to 90 percent of the people actually driving on our streets and highways (AASHTO). The pedestrian was a tall cardboard box, 1 foot by 1 foot by 4 feet, covered with cloth. The cloth reflectances were: black 9 percent; gray 16 percent; white 75 percent; and reflectorized tape, 1 inch by 12 inches, reflecting 50 candles per square foot per foot candle of illumination. The black cloth pedestrian was the least visible while the reflectorized pedestrian was the most visible.

Table 11.6 shows the adverse effect of alcohol (.06 percent to 0.10 percent) on the driver's ability to detect these targets. Except for the black cloth pedestrian at 20 miles per hour, the detection of all pedestrian targets was reduced by alcohol. If AASHTO's 1.64 or 2.5 seconds response times had been used instead of 0.75, the ability to detect all targets would have dropped dramatically, sober or intoxicated. Had there been oncoming headlight glare, the detection rate would have been still further reduced. Keep in mind that a 97 percent probability of seeing 100 pedestrians still leaves 3 that were not.

**Table 11.5**
**Percent Targets Detected Sober**

| | Miles per hour | | | | | | |
|---|---|---|---|---|---|---|---|
| | **20** | **30** | **40** | **50** | **60** | **70** | **80** |
| Black P | 86.4% | 68.2% | 45.4% | 15.9% | 0% | 0% | 0% |
| Gray P | 100 | 100 | 47.2 | 13.9 | 5.5 | 5.5 | 0 |
| White P | 100 | 100 | 100 | 100 | 97.2 | 91.7 | 52.7 |
| Reflectorized P | 100 | 100 | 100 | 100 | 100 | 100 | 100 |

**Table 11.6**
**Percent Targets Detected Alcohol**

| | Miles per hour | | | | | | |
|---|---|---|---|---|---|---|---|
| | **20** | **30** | **40** | **50** | **60** | **70** | **80** |
| Black P | 90.8% | 63.6% | 15.2% | 0% | 0% | 0% | 0% |
| Gray P | 97.2 | 73.2 | 14.2 | 2.7 | 0 | 0 | 0 |
| White P | 100 | 100 | 94.4 | 88.9 | 80.5 | 61.1 | 25 |
| Reflectorized P | 100 | 100 | 100 | 100 | 100 | 100 | 94.5 |

The message is clear. The pedestrian must never depend on the oncoming driver to see him/her. White clothes, reflective material and a flash light should be standard for night time wear on streets and roadways. The pedestrian should always walk facing oncoming traffic to improve self protection.

Since men traditionally wear dark clothing, and since twice as many men are killed as women, who tend to dress more colorful, clothing appears to be a factor in accident statistics. However, more men are at risk than women, and such a conclusion is somewhat speculative. Certainly the pedestrian should be on guard at all times, and avoid trusting the oncoming driver to stop or turn.

Tables 11.5 and 11.6 show the remarkable benefit from a 1 by 12-inch piece of cloth, factory treated with reflective beads. The cloth appears silver gray to a driver until lighted by his headlights, then it appears to glow brightly. Pedestrian protection also could be provided by using reflectorized buttons, shoes and dangle tags.

Though not available, the motorist who has just been demoted to pedestrian status by a flat tire, could obtain increased visibility at night by using a side lamp directed to light the ground around the vehicle. About 1928, L. D. Bridge was issued a patent on a Safety Side Light to assist people entering and leaving an automobile. It provided considerable light for tire repairs, for illuminating the pedestrian, for localization of the vehicle, for entering driveways, and even was of some benefit in fogs. These lights were not adopted for passenger automobiles, though some manufacturers have a turn light that resembles the original Bridge light.

In 1928, Charles A. Sims invented the Sims Side Lamp (see Figure 11.6). His announcement began, "The Sims Side Lamp. At Last! After thousands have sacrificed their lives, after science has dug deep, and industry spent fortunes, a simple idea solves the glaring headlight trouble." His idea was never taken up by the auto industry, either. Decisions about head lighting were made, but they were for the high low-beam headlight system we have today.

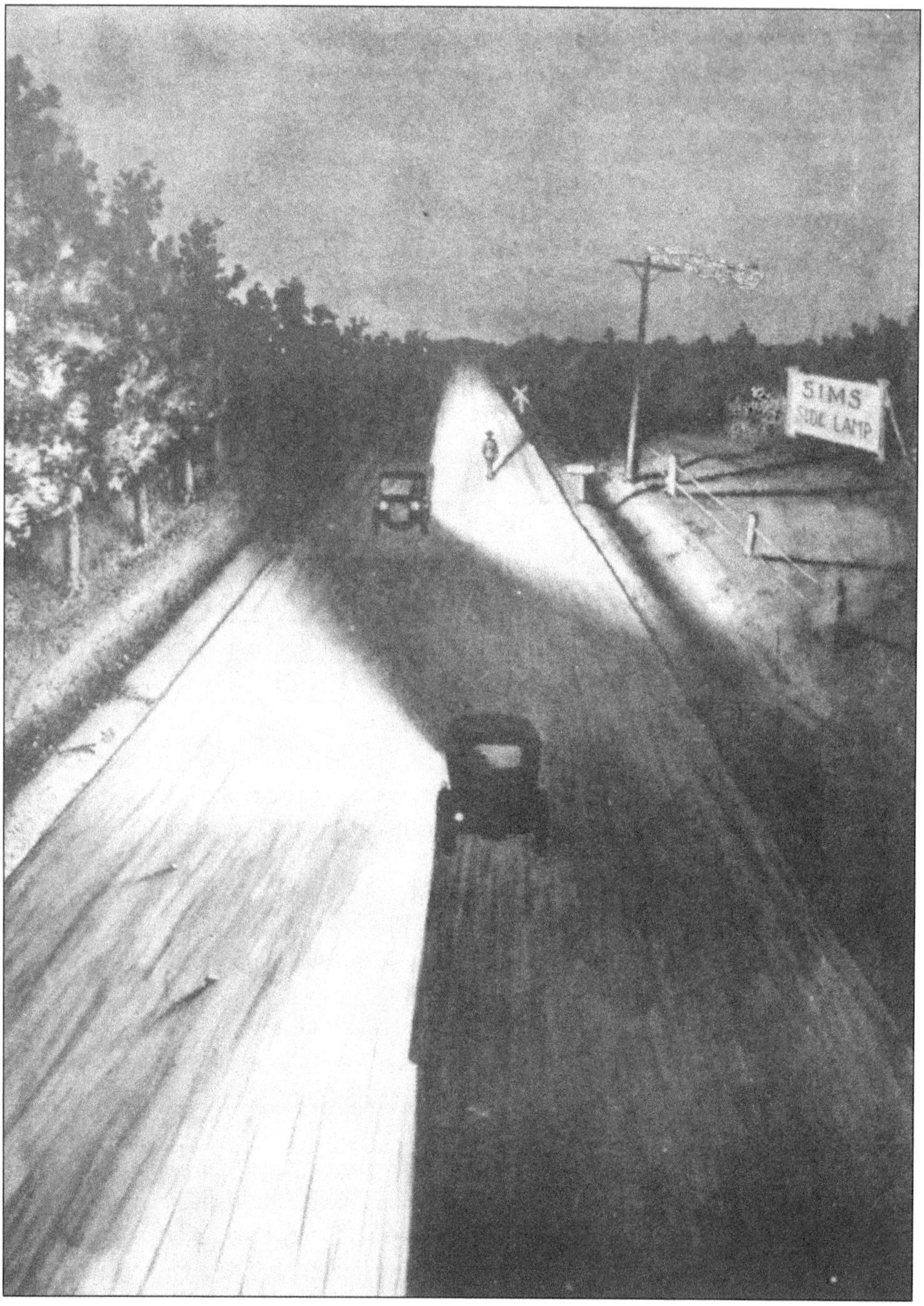


**Figure 11.6** *Side lamps for aiding oncoming motorist, patented by Charles Sims, January 10, 1928. Mr. Sims described the intended method of operation as follows: "As shown above when two cars approach each other the operators switch off their front lights entirely, and automatically switch on the side lights which illuminates the roadway for each other. Instead of shooting the light at each other, you reverse it and shoot it from each other. It's done instantly without vibration or flickering, no refocusing of the eyes to penetrate a different degree of light or darkness. You are still looking after the light and not into it." (Taken from materials describing the Sims patent, with permission.)*

Without knowledge of the work of these early inventors, the author proposed a side light system (Allen, October 1962) to light the way for the oncoming driver. This involved lights in a number of positions, including the top of the car. The most efficient was at bumper height, aimed backward to light the pavement adjacent to the test vehicle. Figure 11.7 shows lights mounted on the front bumper on each side. The rear fender behind the rear wheel is probably the optimum place to set the light into the body work. The light on the right side is of some benefit, but practical considerations might limit the system only to the lights at the left rear. Figures 11.8 and 11.9 show the benefits of the system in overcoming the glare of oncoming automobiles.

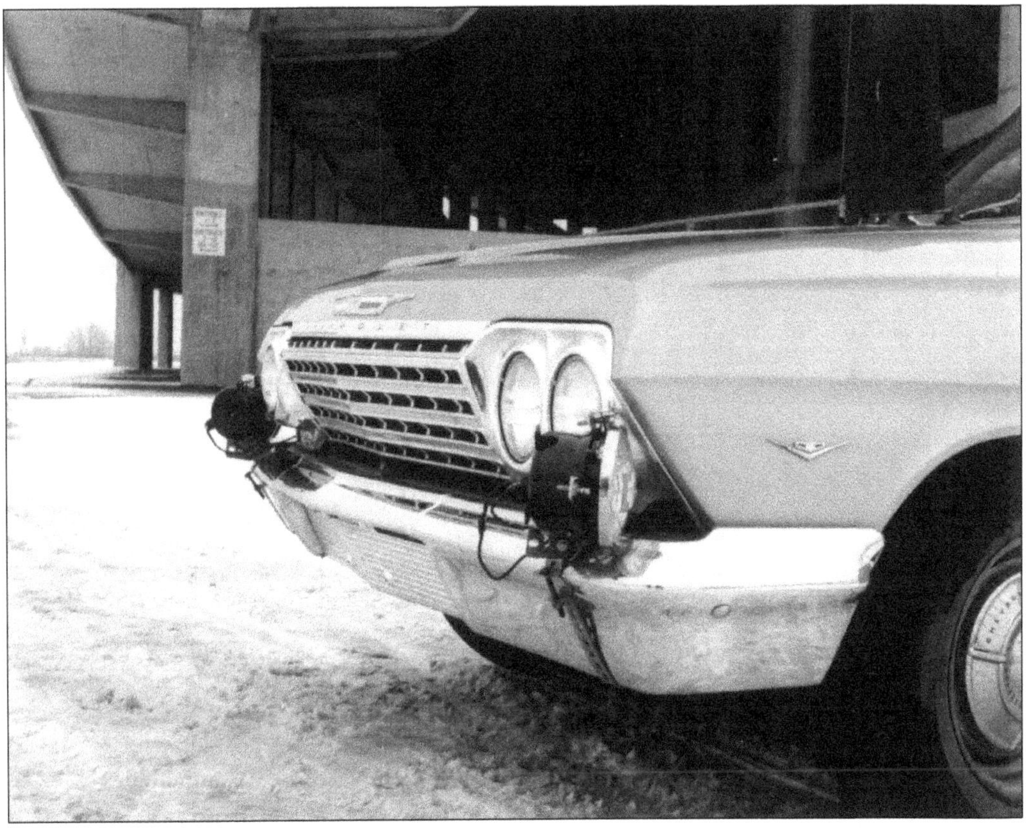

***Figure 11.7*** *Backward aimed headlights to aid the oncoming driver. A 5.5-inch sealed-beam headlight was mounted on the front bumper at each side. These lights were aimed backward as shown. The lower and more nearly straight back they were placed, the better they lighted the pavement for the oncoming driver.*

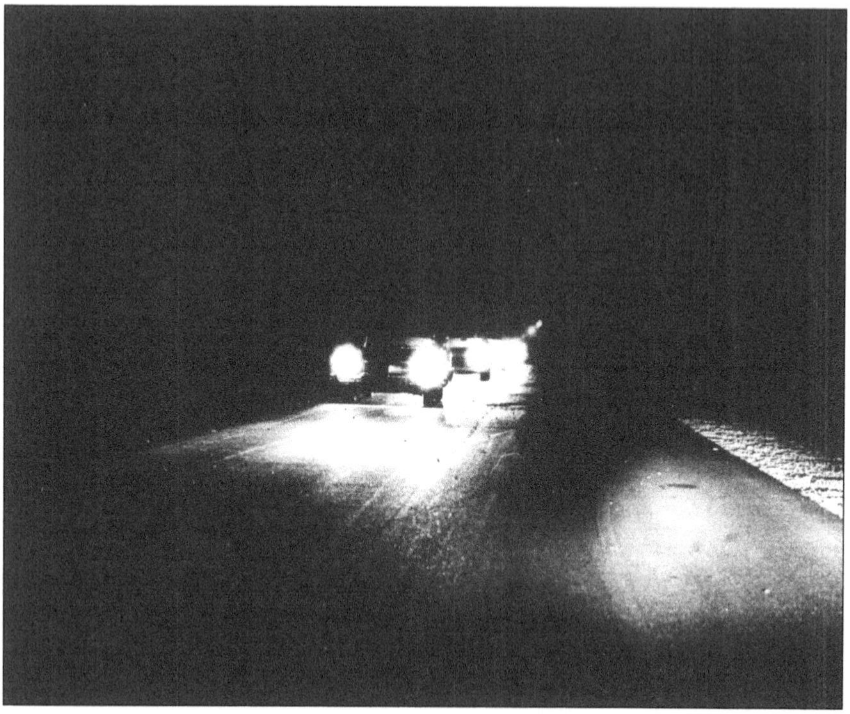

***Figure 11.8*** *Unseen pedestrians stand on the pavement beside four approaching cars on low beams. The camera car's low beams do not reveal the presence of the hazard.*

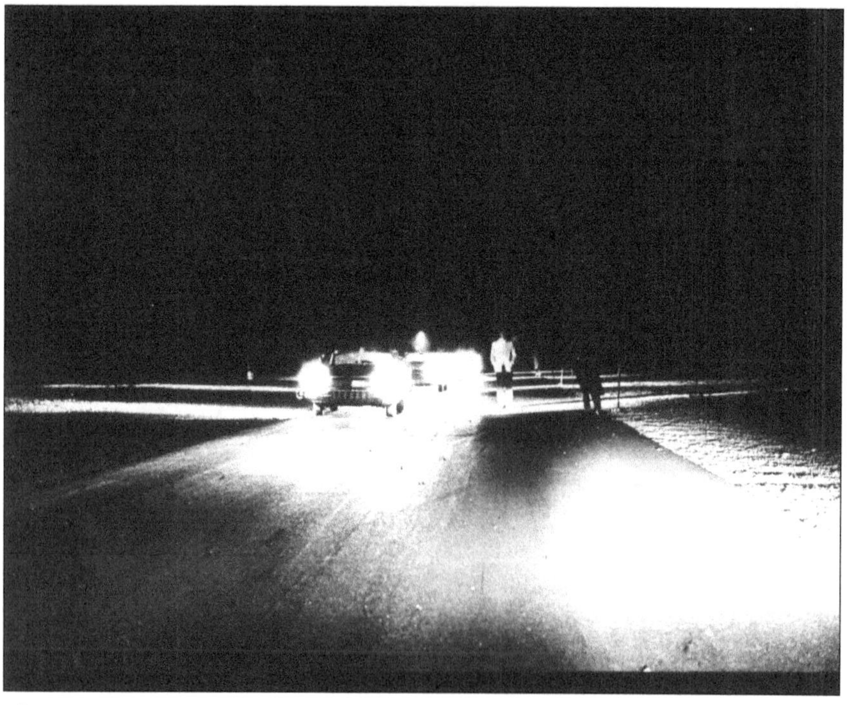

***Figure 11.9*** *Silhouette and direct lighting provided by side lights. The three pedestrians now become visible. Note the increased size of the field of view compared to Figure 11.8. The driver of a side-lighted automobile finds the increase in peripheral field of view a help in maintaining orientation and alertness.*

The idea for such a system came from using the light spilled laterally across the road by automobile headlights. Earlier headlight design and wrap around fenders eliminated this weak but valuable clue. In fact, the shielding of head and taillights from side view prompted the General Services Administration and later the Department of Transportation to require both side marker lights and reflectors on all new passenger cars, trucks, and buses by 1970.

Considerable experience was gained using the side light system shown in Figure 11.7. Twenty automobiles were equipped and sent out on a quiet highway in a caravan. Motion pictures were taken of the effects of meeting, passing, and following such vehicles. The results were considered to be highly favorable. The system was recommended as a means of providing glare free illumination on the streets and highways which increases as traffic increases and does not require the cost and upkeep of extensive stationary highway lighting.

This is not a proposal to do away with conventional highway lighting or the very high mounted lighting advocated by the Texas Transportation Institute, but such lighting can never be everywhere or enough. The side lighting would provide ambient light when needed to reveal pedestrians and other road hazards. It would be turned off automatically when no cars were present. The lone motorist operating on high beams would be reasonably able to see hazards if speeds were not excessive. As soon as the driver dropped to low beams because of other automobiles, the side lights would come on to help oncoming motorists; at the same time the approaching motorists' side lights would come on when they dimmed their lights.

## D. Rain and fog hazards

Water particles between 2 and 100 microns are found in fog. Figure 11.10 shows that for practical purposes fog is not found with particle sizes less than about 10 microns, and this only in clouds. Particles below 2 microns produce haze. Water particles do not exist below about 0.2 microns, as seen in Figure 11.11.

Fog and cloud particles scatter visible light uniformly without regard to wavelength. Even haze does not scatter blue and green much more than red. Rayleigh's theory of light scatter leads to the following equation, where *S* is the total scattered light from a unit of illu
mination of wavelength λ, n is the refractive index, and *V* is the volume of the particle.

$$S = 24\pi^2\left[\left(\frac{n^2-1}{n^2+2}\right)\frac{V^2}{\lambda^4}\right]$$

Table 11.7, derived from Rayleigh's theory, gives the relative amounts of scattering by clean dry air at 1013.2 millibar pressure and 0 degrees Centigrade temperature for each wavelength in nanometers.

Rayleigh scatter holds for spherical particles up to 0.1 wavelength. As the particle sizes increase, the scattering function becomes more complex; and for certain particle sizes it is possible to have even more red scatter than blue. However, in general, clean atmospheric transmission favors the longer wavelengths. The table above shows that for automobile travel this is probably of no significance because the range usually involved is less than a half mile (800 meters).

The smallest cloud particles are encountered in stratus clouds which average 4 microns, with cumulus clouds averaging 5 microns and nimbostratus 10 microns, (Middleton, 1958). These sizes are significantly larger than the 0.55 micron wavelength of visible light; hence selective absorption of various wavelengths is practically non existent. Certainly, the average ground fog with particle sizes from 15 to 100 microns will act impartially upon all visible wavelengths.

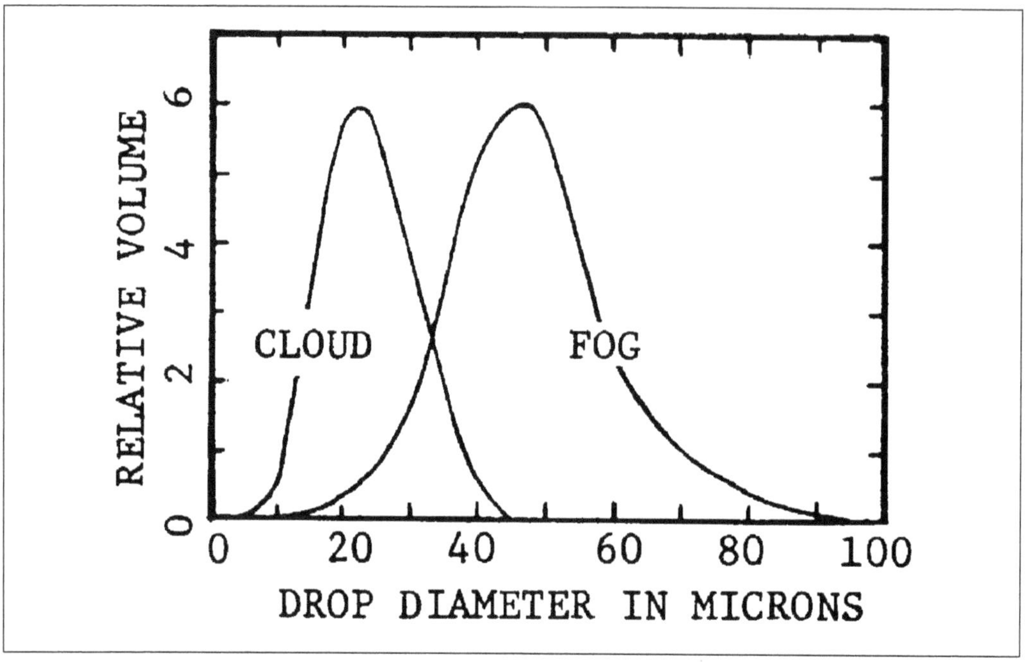


***Figure 11.10*** *Typical drop size distributions for a coastal fog and for a cloud (mountain fog). The curves are plotted to show how the liquid water is distributed (by volume) among the various drop sizes. (After Houghton [1939], from Middleton [1958], Figure 3.18.)*

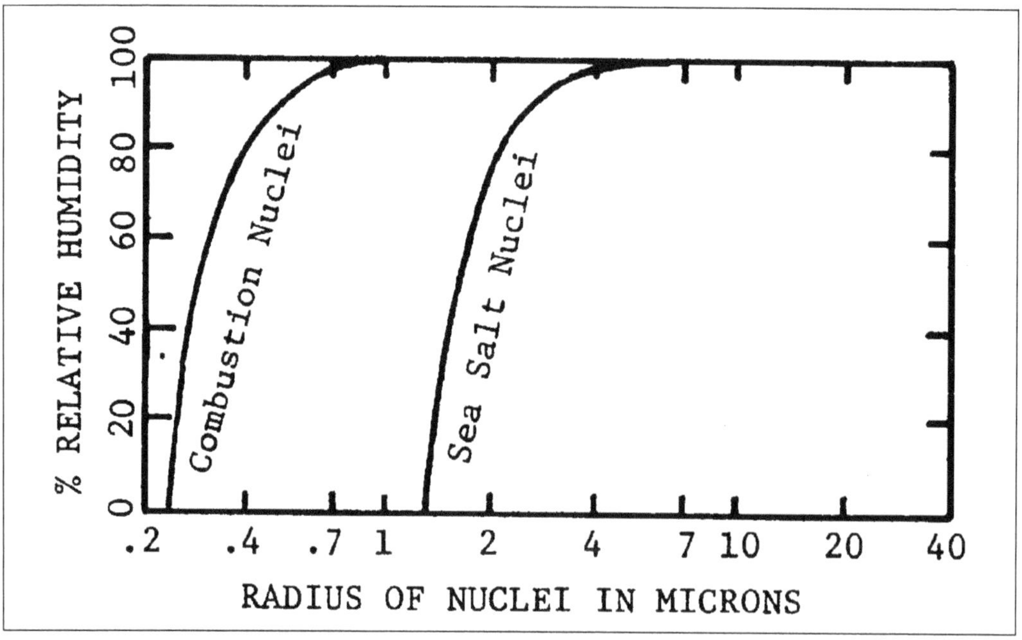


***Figure 11.11*** *Variations in the radius of combustion nuclei and sea salt nuclei with relative humidity. (After Wright [1939], from Middleton, [1958], Figure 3.1)*

**Table 11.7**

| λ wavelength | 400 | 500 | 600 | 700 |
|---|---|---|---|---|
| **Relative scatter** | 4.358 | 1.750 | 0.833 | 0.466 |
| **Loss at 800 meters** | 3.2% | 1.4% | 0.67% | 0.361% |

Thus, automobile fog light color has no scientific basis, and the superior performance claimed for fog lights must result from secondary factors such as the narrow beam spread and remote location of the beam away from the line of sight. Similarly, arguments as to the benefits or disadvantages of one color over another in penetrating fog or rain have no substance for automobile signal systems. A proper signal system can be chosen only after evaluating the physiological, psychological, and systems aspects of the driving problem.

Daytime fog is dangerous for driving because it scatters, or attenuates the useful light coming from the object, and substitutes random light from elsewhere. This reduces the contrast of the object without changing the sharpness of its borders. Increasing distance increases the attenuation of the useful light and increases the veiling light added. The attenuation function is that of any filter; that is, a percentage is lost per unit of distance the light travels. The veiling effect, however, makes the daytime seeing evaluation somewhat more complex, while the nighttime situation involving headlights is even more complex.

Without nearby headlights, an automobile's headlights or taillights can be seen at a considerable distance in fog, because, no matter how dense the fog, theoretically some light will get through to the observer.

If the intervening fog is illuminated by one's own headlights, the amount of light coming through the fog from the oncoming automobile must exceed the just noticeable brightness difference at the level of illumination caused by one's own lights. Of course, as fog density goes up, the greater is the nearby fog illumination from one's own lights and the smaller is the amount of light penetrating through the fog from the oncoming car.

The classification of fog is difficult, but Table 11.8 provides an operational definition of the several subjective terms that are often used. The daylight visual range is for the detection of dark objects about the size of an automobile as seen against a light background. The atmospheric transmission is given for each type of fog for various distances and would be useful in calculating the range at which a light could be seen through fog, assuming that the minimum contrast for detection between the light and its background needs to be 4 percent or more.

The visibility of roadway details falls off more quickly than is the case for light sources. The following analogy will illustrate the principles involved. If one looks through a handkerchief held very near to the eyes he/she will be able to see large objects, but will have lost the ability to see detail. The white cloth transmits some light from the objects, but it also is itself an object, brightly illuminated by the ambient light. Now consider that the room is dark and that the objects you are trying to see are illuminated only by the light that has penetrated the handkerchief from a flashlight you hold in your hand. The handkerchief is equivalent to an impenetrable "fog" and you must change it to something like a nylon stocking of loose mesh, to pass enough light to be able to see through to the objects. If you hold the flashlight beyond the handkerchief or stocking so it illuminates the objects directly, without illuminating the cloth, visibility will be improved.

**Table 11.8**
**Atmospheric Transmission**

| | | | Maximum % Transmission at Ranges Indicated. | | | | | |
|---|---|---|---|---|---|---|---|---|
| Code No. | Weather | Maximum Daylight Visual Range (ft.) | 3280 ft. | 1640 ft. | 820 ft. | 410 ft. | 205 ft. | 102 ft. |
| 0 | Dense fog | 164 | | | | $1\times10^{-6}$ | 0.1 | 3 |
| 1 | Thick fog | 658 | $32\times10^{-8}$ | .005 | .71 | 8.41 | 29 | 54 |
| 2 | Moderate fog | 1640 | .004 | 0.63 | 7.9 | 28 | 53 | 72 |
| 3 | Light fog | 3280 | 2 | 14 | 37.5 | 61 | 78 | 88 |
| 4 | Thin fog | 6560 | 14 | 37.5 | 61 | 78 | 88 | 94 |
| 5 | Haze | 26,240 | 37 | 61 | 78 | 88 | 94 | 96 |
| 6 | Light haze | 32,800 | 68 | 82 | 91 | 95 | 98 | |
| 7 | Clear | 65,600 | 82 | 91 | 95 | 98 | | |
| 8 | Very clear | 164,000 | 93 | 96 | 98 | | | |
| 9 | Extra clear | 164,000+ | 93+ | | | | | |

Data adapted from Illuminating Engineering Society Hanbook, 1952, pp. 9–44.

Thus, a fog light should illuminate no fog between the driver's eye and the object viewed. However, in practice, secondary scattering from fog particle to fog particle, and limitations as to where lights can be placed on the car, limit the performance of fog lights. To achieve the best possible vision in fog, the fog lamp should be low and to the extreme right corner of the vehicle away from the driver. The lamp should produce a concentrated beam with no upward scatter above the horizontal. In effect, it should be in a tube about two feet long to eliminate all spill light that could illuminate the fog particles in front of the driver's eyes.

## E. Railroad crossings

Railroad crossings are a significant hazard. The Department of Transportation (DOT, 1968) reports as follows:

- Of the 3,932 crossing accidents of all kinds in 1967, 3,733 involved collisions between railroad movements and motor vehicles and resulted in 1520 deaths and 3,726 injuries. In 2,456 collisions, 65.79 percent, trains struck motor vehicles, resulting in 1,158, or 76.18 percent, of the deaths and in 2, 218, or 59.53 percent, of the injuries. In the other 1,277 collisions, 34.21 percent, motor vehicles struck the sides of train movements, resulting in 362, or 23.82 percent, of the deaths and in 1,508, or 40.47 percent, of the injuries.
- Of the 3,733 collisions, 1,617, or 43.32 percent, occurred at crossings which were especially protected by one of the following: lowered gates, train man, watchman, audible and visual signals, audible signals, or visible signals. The other 2,116, or 56.68 percent, occurred at crossings protected by signals or signs that did not indicate the approach of trains.

- The latest available statistics show a total of 214,417 rail highway crossings at grade. Of these crossings, 44,432 or 20.72 percent, were specially protected; 169,985, or 79.28 percent, were not specially protected.
- Of the 3,733 crossing collisions, 2,273, or 60.89 percent, occurred in daylight, and 1,460, or 39.11 percent, took place at night. There were 2,564 collisions, or 68.68 percent, in clear weather, and 1,169, or 31.32 percent, under cloudy or inclement weather conditions.
- Of the 3,733 collisions between trains and motor vehicles, automobiles were involved in 2,906, or 77.85 percent; busses in 11, or 0.29 percent; motor trucks in 780, or 20.89 percent, and motorcycles in 36, or 0.96 percent.

Very little modern technology has crept into railroading if the signals at 79.28 percent of the intersections are any criterion. At most crossings the only signal present is the typical railroad cross buck. Often only one is present and in design, color, and size of lettering is just as it was years ago. Nevertheless about $190 million per year was spent on railway crossings from 1963 to 1967 (Insurance Institute for Highway Safety, 1970).

In the past the railroads have lost few lawsuits and have been slow to make improvements. This is partly because accidents at a particular crossing are infrequent, and partly because it is difficult to convince a jury that a train can be unnecessarily difficult to see and hear. Of course, failure to provide locomotives and rolling stock with maximum visibility paints, reflectors, and lights, as well as failure to keep signs and signals in top condition, can be considered to be contributory negligence in many accidents. Because families and friends of motorists who have died in train accidents have not been able to organize effectively to loudly express their righteous indignation, we continue to live with the hazard.

A law suit in Kalamazoo, Michigan in which the railroad lost, and in which I testified, resulted in an increase in brightness of all railroad red signal lights across America.

Some railroads are incorporating lights mounted low on the front of the locomotive to help the engineer see land slides across the tracks. These improve locomotive visibility to motorists. The 275,000 candle power high mounted headlight on locomotives is used as a defense in court by the railroads. It is little realized that such brightness is only in the central ±5 degrees of the beam which is high above the driver and aimed to light the tracks.

The problem is manifold. (1) On the average the accident probability at a crossing is one every ten years (Schoppert et al., 1968), or so infrequently that it does not seem to be a problem to the local citizens. (2) A fast train on a collision course with an automobile must be looked for at angles ranging from 45 to 90 degrees from straight ahead or, for the most part, must be looked for through the side windows. (3) Trains provide their bulk above the line of sight, so that for a slow or stopped train it is often possible to view a seemingly unobstructed roadway beneath a railroad car, especially at night. (4) Trains are usually not painted in bright colors, are not reflectorized, are not lighted, and are not clean. (5) The active as well as the passive railroad crossing signals are archaic and hence not ideally designed to use all the clues of spatial localization, attention getting, maximum visibility, and signal information free of ambiguity.

Every railroad crossing could be signalized by using a strobe light on the locomotive and freight cars. They would greatly increase the conspicuity of the train and would light the trees and houses to alert the motorist. Strobes were being used for several years but were abandoned by the railroads in spite of strong supportive data. Apparently the Union Workers objected.

The evidence is that modern technology is ignored by the railroads. The railroad bureaucrats seem to believe that all accidents are due to the "nut behind the wheel." Abandoning the strobe flasher widely used elsewhere, is but one example. A second is that laser technology seems to have escaped them. A laser beam in each locomotive aimed at reflectors placed at each crossing would signalize all intersections across America with high intensity, high conspicuity flashing light, that would come on only when a train was coming. This laser system would cost only a tiny fraction of the archaic signal system now in use by the railroads.

We need the railroads! Let's help them figure out how to stop killing people. When an accident occurs, talk to the news media about it. This will help attract the attention of local citizens and of the railroad.

## F. Trucks

Trucks on the streets and highways represent a special hazard to passenger automobile drivers because of their poor visibility. This is another instance of virtual protection or immunity being extended to trucks because of their economic importance and legislative lobbying ability. No lobby of the relatives of the dead is present in the legislative halls to counter truck lobbies. Part of their immunity comes from law. It is a fact that the vehicle striking the rear of another vehicle is held to be at fault automatically unless partially relieved of that fault by contributory negligence on the part of the struck vehicle. So long as the inadequate Interstate Commerce Commission requirements for lights and reflectors on trucks are adhered to, the stopped or slow moving truck is not held to be contributory, and hence there is little incentive to improve the visibility of trucks. Such protection also leads to inadequate under run protection, which leads to a high fatality rate for car truck collisions. Since there are fewer survivors of collisions with the rear or side of a truck compared to other types of collisions, because the passenger vehicle runs under the frame of the truck and shears off the top, the insurance or court proceedings are simpler and the amount of damages claimed are usually less.

Truckers operate their vehicles under the rules of the Interstate Commerce Commission, which seems to work closely with industry to set so called "realistic" standards, including those for vehicle lighting. That these standards might pose a hazard to passenger vehicles is difficult to prove in a court of law trying to assess who is to blame in a particular accident. Judges and juries are not naturally aware of highway and vehicle design deficiencies and are likely to assume that meeting federal regulations provides the best that there is. Though federal regulations are intended to represent the minimum, they often end up being the maximum in practice.

Federal lighting requirements for 1998 for trucks and trailers of 80 inches or wider are shown in Tables 11.9 through 11.12 (U.S. Department of Transportation, 1998). These standards offer some improvements. For example, two taillights and turn signals are now required on truck tractors instead of the previous one and none respectively. However, significant inconsistencies persist, such as, the amber brake, turn, and hazard warning signals permitted on the rear along with amber park, turn, and hazard warning signals on the front. Retention of other hazardous specifications indicate that more revisions are needed.

Such hazardous specifications include permitting headlights to be as high as 54 inches, when the average eye height of an automobile driver is below 48 inches; permission to place taillights and stop lights as high as 72 inches above the road; permission to place reflex reflectors as high as 60 inches when automobile head lamps are about 28 inches high and aimed downward; permission to place side marker lamps and turn signal lamps anywhere above 15 inches; and the continued use of identification and clearance lights whose respective purposes have little if anything to contribute to safe operation of the trucking equipment in traffic.

## Table 11.9
## Originals from National Highway Traffic Safety Administration, DOT 49 CFR Ch. V (10–1–98 Edition)

TABLE I—REQUIRED MOTOR VEHICLE LIGHTING EQUIPMENT OTHER THAN HEADLAMPS

Multipurpose Passenger Vehicles, Trucks, Trailers, and Buses, of 80 or More Inches Overall Width

| Item | Multipurpose passenger vehicles, trucks, and buses | Trailers | Applicable SAE standard or recommended practice (See S5 for subreferenced SAE materials) |
|---|---|---|---|
| Taillamps | 2 red | 2 red | J585e, September 1977. |
| Stoplamps | 2 red | 2 red | SAE J1398, May 1985. |
| License plate lamp | 1 white | 1 white | J587 October 1981. |
| Reflex reflectors | 4 red; 2 amber | 4 red; 2 amber | J594f, January 1977. |
| Side marker lamps | 2 red; 2 amber | 2 red; 2 amber | J592e, July 1972. |
| Backup lamp | 1 white | None | J593c, February 1968. |
| Turn signal lamps | 2 red or amber; 2 amber | 2 red or amber | SAE J1395, April 1985. |
| Turn signal operating unit | 1 | None | J589, April 1964. |
| Turn signal flasher | 1 | None | J590b, October 1965. |
| Vehicular hazard warning signal operating unit. | 1 | None | J910, January 1966. |
| Vehicular hazard warning signal flasher.. | 1 | None | J945, February 1966. |
| Identification lamps | 3 amber; 3 red | 3 red | J592e, July 1972. |
| Clearance lamps | 2 amber; 2 red | 2 amber, 2 red | J592e, July 1972. |
| Intermediate side marker lamps. | 2 amber | 2 amber | J592e, July 1972. |
| Intermediate side reflex reflectors. | 2 amber | 2 amber | J594f, January 1977. |
| Conspicuity | See S5.7 | See S5.7 | See S5.7 |

The nature of the remaining hazards becomes clear if one encounters a truck trailer crossing an intersection. The lights at the top are of no value in locating the truck; they might seem to be, for example, on a television antenna tower miles away. The reflectors on the sides are usually dirty and are above the beams of the standard automobile headlight and most truck headlights as well. The side marker lamps have no specified height above 15 inches and most usually are mounted high; hence they are of little utility in localizing the vehicle. Most truck trailers have a high bed permitting unobstructed vision beneath it, especially for those seated in an automobile. Upon seeing the roadway unobstructed, and with the weak ambiguous side lights mounted high overhead, the motorist may be lured into a side collision which will have a high probability of being fatal.

From the rear view the hazard is similar. Closely spaced taillights, as sometimes used, covered with dirt and mounted high, appear to be significantly farther away than they actually are and tend to lure the unwary motorist in too close. If the speed difference is great enough, a collision will result. With his lights on and reflectors in place, the trucker is not legally negligent, but the motorist who died is, even though he couldn't see the truck or misjudged its location and speed. Keeping one's vehicle under control as required by law is one thing, and having a fighting chance to know of the hazard one faces from the low visibility and deceptiveness of modern trucks is another. Mo torists should not have to continue to pay with their lives to keep the trucks rolling in their present design condition and thus to save the owners and manufacturers a few dollars. There should be under run guards at passenger vehicle bumper height, and side and rear lights and reflectors at no higher than 15 inches above the pavement, where they can be seen and localized on the roadway. Truck and trailer wheels should be better shielded to reduce road spray and dirt collection. Mud guards as now used are only partially effective.

## Table 11.10
## Originals from National Highway Traffic Safety Administration, DOT 49 CFR Ch. V (10–1–98 Edition)

### Table II—Location of Required Equipment

Multipurpose Passenger Vehicles, Trucks, Trailers, and Buses, of 80 or More Inches Overall Width

| Item | Location on— | | Height above road surface measured from center of item on vehicle at curb weight |
|---|---|---|---|
| | Multipurpose passenger vehicles, trucks, and buses | Trailers | |
| Headlamps | On the front, each headlamp providing the upper beam, at the same height, 1 on each side of the vertical centerline, each headlamp providing the lower beam, at the same height, 1 on each side of the vertical centerline, as far apart as practicable. See also S7. | Not required | Not less than 22 inches (55.9 cm) nor more than 54 inches (137.2 cm). |
| Taillamps | On the rear, 1 on each side of the vertical centerline, at the same height, and as far apart as practicable. | On the rear, 1 on each side of the vertical centerline, at the same height, and as far apart as practicable. | Not less than 15 inches, nor more than 72 inches. |
| Stop lamps | ......do | ......do | Do. |
| License plate lamp | At rear license plate, to illuminate the plate from the top or sides. | At rear license plate, to illuminate the plate from the top or sides. | No requirement. |
| Backup lamp | On the rear | Not required | Do. |
| Turn signal lamps | At or near the front—1 amber on each side of the vertical centerline, at the same height, and as far apart as practicable.<br>On the rear—1 red or amber on each side of the vertical centerline, at the same height, and as far apart as practicable. | On the rear—1 red or amber on each side of the vertical centerline, at the same height, and as far apart as practicable. | Not less than 15 inches, nor more than 83 inches. |
| Identification lamps | On the front and rear—3 lamps, amber in front, red in rear, as close as practicable to the top of the vehicle, at the same height, as close as practicable to the vertical centerline, with lamp centers spaced not less than 6 inches or more than 12 inches apart. Alternatively, the front lamps may be located as close as practicable to the top of the cab. | On the rear—3 lamps as close as practicable to the top of the vehicle at the same height, as close as practicable to the vertical centerline, with lamp centers spaced not less than 6 inches or more than 12 inches apart. | No requirement. |
| Clearance lamps | On the front and rear—2 amber lamps on front, 2 red lamps on rear, to indicate the overall width of the vehicle, one on each side of the vertical centerline, at the same height, and as near the top as practicable. | On the front and rear—2 amber lamps on front, 2 red lamps on rear, to indicate the overall width of the vehicle, one on each side of the vertical centerline, at the same height, and as near the top thereof as practicable[2,3,4]. | Do. |
| Intermediate side marker lamps. | On each side—1 amber lamp located at or near the midpoint between the front and rear side marker lamps. | On each side—1 amber lamp located at or near the midpoint between the front and rear side marker lamps. | Not less than 15 inches. |
| Intermediate side reflex reflectors. | On each side—1 amber located at or near the midpoint between the front and rear side reflex reflectors. | On each side—1 amber located at or near the midpoint between the front and rear side reflex reflectors. | Not less than 15 inches nor more than 60 inches. |
| Conspicuity | See S5.7 | See S5.7 | See S5.7 |
| Reflex reflectors | On the rear—1 red on each side of the vertical centerline, as far apart as practicable, and at the same height.<br>On each side—1 red as far to the rear as practicable, and 1 amber as far to the front as practicable. | On the rear—1 red on each side of the vertical centerline, as far apart as practicable, and at the same height.<br>On each side—1 red as far to the rear as practicable, and 1 amber as far to the front as practicable. | Do. |
| Side marker lamps | ......do | ......do | Not less than 15 inches, and on the rear of trailers not more than 60 inches. |

**Table 11.11**
**Originals from National Highway Traffic Safety Administration, DOT 49 CFR Ch. V (10–1–98 Edition)**

TABLE III—REQUIRED MOTOR VEHICLE LIGHTING EQUIPMENT

All Passenger Cars and Motorcycles, and Multipurpose Passenger Vehicles, Trucks, and Buses, of Less Than 80 Inches Overall Width

| Item | Passenger cars, multipurpose passenger vehicles, trucks, and buses | Trailers | Motorcycles | Applicable SAE standard or recommended practice (See S5 for subreferenced SAE materials) |
|---|---|---|---|---|
| Headlamps | See S7 | | 1 white | For motorcycles only, J584, April 1964, J566, January 1960. |
| Taillamps | 2 red | 2 red | 1 red | J585e, September 1977. |
| Stoplamps | 2 red | 2 red | 1 red | SAE J586, February 1984. |
| High-mounted stoplamp. | 1 red | Not required | Not required | J186a, September 1977. |
| License plate lamp. | 1 white | 1 white | 1 white | J587, October 1981. |
| Parking lamps | 2 amber or white | None | None | J222, December 1970. |
| Reflex reflectors | 4 red; 2 amber | 4 red; 2 amber | 3 red; 2 amber | J594f, January 1977. |
| Intermediate side reflex reflectors. | 2 amber | 2 amber | None | J594f, January 1977. |
| Intermediate side marker lamps. | 2 amber | 2 amber | None | J592e, July 1972. |
| Side marker lamps | 2 red; 2 amber | 2 red; 2 amber | None | J592e, July 1972. |
| Backup lamp | 1 white | None | None | J593c, February 1968. |
| Turn signal lamps | 2 red or amber; 2 amber | 2 red or amber | 2 amber; 2 red or amber. | SAE J588, November 1984. |
| Turn signal operating unit.[3,4] | 1 | None | 1 | J589, April 1964. |
| Turn signal flasher | 1 | None | 1 | J590b, October 1965. |
| Vehicular hazard warning signal operating unit. | 1 | None | None | J910, January 1966. |
| Vehicular hazard warning signal flasher. | 1 | None | None | J945, February 1966. |

New regulations require retroreflective materials to outline the side and rear of trucks. This is a step forward. The next step is to move the reflective material down 15 inches above the pavement!

Black should be banned. White tires, white mud guards and a white painted under run protection panel all around the truck should be standard.

## G. Black versus white tires

One possible improvement in visibility at very little if any cost would be the use of tires made of white rubber throughout. If this were done, the tire tread against the pavement would provide a gleaming white surface for easy seeing by the motorist as he approaches from the rear. Although the side walls would get dirty, they would be better reflectors than the current black tires now in use.

## Table 11.12
## Originals from National Highway Traffic Safety Administration, DOT 49 CFR Ch. V (10–1–98 Edition)

TABLE IV—LOCATION OF REQUIRED EQUIPMENT

All Passenger Cars and Motorcycles, and Multipurpose Passenger Vehicles, Trucks, Trailers, and Buses of Less Than 80 Inches Overall Width

| Item | Location on— | | Height above road surface measured from center of item on vehicle at curb weight |
|---|---|---|---|
| | Passenger cars, multipurpose passenger vehicles, trucks, trailers, and buses | Motorcycles | |
| Headlamps | On the front, each headlamp providing the upper beam, at the same height, 1 on each side of the vertical centerline, each headlamp providing the lower beam, at the same height, 1 on each side of the vertical centerline, as far apart as practicable. See also S7.. | On the front, on the vertical centerline, except that if two are used they shall be symmetrically disposed about the vertical centerline. | Not less than 22 inches (55.9 cm) nor more than 54 inches (137.2 cm). |
| Taillamps | On the rear—1 on each side of the vertical centerline, at the same height, and as far apart as practicable. | On the rear—on the vertical centerline except that if two are used, they shall be symmetrically disposed about the vertical centerline. | Not less than 15 inches, nor more than 72 inches. |
| Stoplamps | On the rear—1 on each side of the vertical centerline, at the same height, and as far apart as practicable. | On the rear—on the vertical centerline except that if two are used, they shall be symmetrically disposed about the vertical centerline. | Not less than 15 inches, nor more than 72 inches. |
| High-mounted stoplamp. | On the rear, on the vertical centerline [See S5.1.1.27, S5.3.1.8, and Table III], effective September 1, 1985, for passenger cars only. | Not required | See S5.3.1.8 for passenger cars. Not less than 34 inches for multipurpose passenger vehicles, trucks, and buses. |
| License plate lamp | At rear license plate, to illuminate the plate from the top or sides. | At rear license plate | No requirement. |
| Parking lamps | On the front—1 on each side of the vertical centerline, at the same height, and as far apart as practicable. | Not required | Not less than 15 inches, nor more than 72 inches. |
| Reflex reflectors | On the rear—1 red on each side of the vertical centerline, at the same height, and as far apart as practicable.<br>On each side—1 red as far to the rear as practicable, and 1 amber as far to the front as practicable. | On the rear—1 red on the vertical centerline except that, if two are used on the rear, they shall be symmetrically disposed about the vertical centerline.<br>On each side—1 red as far to the rear as practicable, and 1 amber as far to the front as practicable. | Not less than 15 inches, nor more than 60 inches. |
| Backup lamp | On the rear | Not required | No requirement. |
| Turn signal lamps | At or near the front—1 amber on each side of the vertical centerline, at the same height, and as far apart as practicable.<br>On the rear—1 red or amber on each side of the vertical centerline, at the same height, and as far apart as practicable. | At or near the front—1 amber on each side of the vertical centerline at the same height, and having a minimum horizontal separation distance (centerline of lamps) of 16 inches. Minimum edge to edge separation distance between lamp and headlamp is 4 inches.<br>At or near the rear—1 red or amber on each side of the vertical centerline, at the same height and having a minimum horizontal separation distance (centerline to centerline of lamps) of 9 inches. Minimum edge to edge separation distance between lamp and tail or stop lamp is 4-inches, when a single stop and taillamp is installed on the vertical centerline and the turn signal lamps are red.. | No requirement.<br>Not less than 15 inches, nor more than 83 inches. |
| Side marker lamps | On each side—1 red as far to the rear as practicable, and 1 amber as far to the front as practicable. | Not required | Not less than 15 inches. |
| Intermediate side marker lamps. | On each side—1 amber located at or near the midpoint between the front and rear side marker lamps. | Not required | Not less than 15 inches. |
| Intermediate side marker reflectors. | On each side—1 amber located at or near the midpoint between the front and rear side marker reflectors. | Not required | Not less than 15 inches, nor more than 60 inches. |

The benefits in increased visibility for all vehicles would be worthwhile, and especially for trucks. White tire treads would provide localization clues superior to anything we have available today, and their visibility would improve with adverse weather because of their self cleaning properties. So far the tire industry has ignored this safety feature.

## H. One to four a.m.

The incidence of fatal one car accidents is extremely high in the early morning hours. The confirmed explanation of this phenomenon is not at hand; however, a look at some of the factors is in order. First is the matter of fatigue and the need for sleep.

One should never drive after his normal bedtime, because about 2 hours after normal bedtime it becomes difficult if not impossible to stay awake. By about two o'clock in the morning one enters a sleep producing driving environment. The traffic on the highway is sparse; therefore the bright points of light from tail and headlights are missing most of the time. All that remains is the dark of the night, with a gradual brightening in the lower field of view as the pavement comes nearer to the headlights. Neither vegetation nor the surface of the pavement can be clearly focused upon because of the low illumination and their steady "movement" as the automobile proceeds. Darkness allows pupil dilation, which tends to cause blurring due to aberrations. Darkness may also allow accommodation to increase, sometimes as much as 1.5 diopters, further blurring the limited detail available. The rapidly reducing strength of the visual stimulation because of increased blurring and lowered illumination is similar to that encountered with the eyes closed, when sleep readily occurs.

A hypnotic effect at night is undoubtedly involved; however, the distinction between a hypnotic trance and real sleep is difficult to make when a subject is unduly fatigued past his bedtime. Alcohol, carbon monoxide (cigarettes and automobile exhaust), and a full stomach are all predisposing factors. Each or all may team up with fatigue, the absence of detail in the roadway scene, and the hypnotic nature of the driving task, and can overcome even the best driver.

The loss of visual control is real. It appears that a nystagmus develops which lowers acuity. This is accompanied by a loss of fusion and an extreme urge to close the eyes. Such danger signs cannot be ignored! On the highway, one should open the window, turn up the radio, turn on the dome light, turn up the dash light, and indulge in singing and isometrics, and stop at the nearest stopping point.

The use of the interior lighting of the vehicle, including brightening the dash panel, is most comforting when driving for long periods at night. Fusion recovers, acuity improves, and the darkness seems literally to be pushed away when it had been in danger of engulfing the tired driver. The fear of destroying dark adaptation by having extra light in the car should be overbalanced by the fear of the complete loss of orientation which occurs with fatigue under low levels of illumination. Actually, dark adaptation to levels lower than the roadway will not occur, and normal interior lighting can have very little effect on the level of adaptation needed for the external scene. The only precaution is to be sure that the dash panel does not reflect into the windshield and that the windshield is clean. Observations indicate a very slight loss of visual range with interior lighting. At the same time vision seems clearer, probably due to a smaller pupil.

A number of ideas to add detail in the outside scene at night have been proposed. Small points of light on posts at the front edges of the hood would provide an ocular focus and would help maintain vehicle and driver orientation. A bright reticule or cross hair, as used in military gun sights, could be optically projected into the roadway, perhaps off the windshield's back surface. Such a target would be excellent for keeping convergence and accommodation under control. However, it would have to have a large aperture of perhaps twelve inches to permit freedom of head movement, and it would be both difficult to install and expensive to build. Nevertheless, plastic Fresnel lens components might provide the breakthrough needed.

The ultimate goal for night driving is more light. Both the Sims side light and the proposed side lighting (see Figure 11.7) supply surround light with a noticeable increase in comfort. Increasing headlight brightness will improve night driving safety.

Of course, the ideal admonition is to avoid driving during the early morning hours if one normally sleeps then. Avoid large meals, alcohol, and smoking (Adams and Belvin, 1966; MacFarland and Moseley, September 1954). Keep lights on bright as much as traffic will allow. If drowsiness seems to be occurring, change body position, change temperature in the car, turn on the radio and the dome light, and slow down five or ten miles per hour; at least do not go faster "to get there sooner." If out of control of your body physiology, stop well off the pavement, at a service station, roadside park, or other protected location. If you stop along the highway, move at least ten feet off the pavement, turn off your headlights, set your emergency four-way flasher into operation, turn off your engine, and take a nap.

The hazard of roadside stopping without the four way flasher is that your normal red taillights may lure another sleepy driver to follow you right off the pavement and collide with you. Above all, do not take a walk on the pavement, because few drivers will be looking out for a pedestrian. Even if they were, the chances are against the pedestrian being seen in time. If the shoulders are muddy, or if the roadway is not wide enough to pull off at least 10 feet, drive carefully until you find a service station or other safe location.

### I. Headlight laws

A driver will have trouble seeing oncoming cars against the setting or rising sun, while oncoming drivers will be able to see perfectly well with the sun behind them. However, they should have their headlights on to help them to be seen. Many states require headlights to be turned on by 30 minutes after sunset to thirty 30 before sunrise. Such legislation should be changed to ensure that headlights must be turned on at least one hour before sunset and not turned off sooner than one hour after sunrise, if then. This would require headlights to be on any time the sun is lower than 15 degrees from the horizon. It is hoped that legislators would require headlights to be on all day long.

The use of daytime running lights now being installed in new cars will solve this problem. The only negative is that older cars without daytime headlights will be at still greater risk among the lighted cars.

Certainly, the rule of headlights on 30 minutes after the sun sets and off 30 minutes before the sun rises is archaic and unrealistic for today's driving. Figure 11.10 indicates that motorists themselves find driving without lights after sunset unacceptable. The far north, as in Alaska, has a poorly defined sunset and prolonged poor seeing, hence a safer rule for all states is to have headlights on anytime the engine is running. Since accidents are more frequent in the late afternoon hours and since this time is very difficult for drivers, especially on two-lane free access roads and highways, the motorist would be wise to stop and have a light supper and, if necessary, continue the trip after the sun has set.

## 11.2 Daytime Hazards

### A. Sun and sky glare

On a bright sunny day who would think visibility could be a problem? Yet, as discussed in Chapters 2 and 8, numerous factors degrade vision in the daytime. Accident statistics show clear dry days to be especially hazardous. The most disabling circumstance in the daytime occurs when the sun is in the driver's forward field of view. The nearer it is to the line of sight of the driver, the more disabling. The eye becomes adapted to the high luminance levels. It is hampered by the stray light in the eye and the fact that all hazardous objects on the ground are viewed from their dark or shadowed side. Polished concrete or asphalt pavement may gleam like a ribbon of fire from a low-hanging sun. Seeing people, cars, or even trucks becomes impossible under certain situations and difficult under virtually all situations with a low sun. Nonpolarizing sunglasses make the seeing situation against the sun worse because they reduce the visibility of the already inadequately lighted objects in the field of view. Polarizing sunglasses will reduce pavement glare and windshield reflections and should improve vision.

Sky glare and sun glare usually are efficiently controlled with the sun visor provided in most cars. This has proven to be the most useful device in glare experiments for improving visual performance. Among the many sources of glare, sky glare seems to be as serious or more serious than any other. Reflection from the top of the hood can be distressing if the hood is of light color and highly polished. There are paints which remove the gloss without changing the appearance of the paint. They might be helpful, especially among police and fleet owners.

Reflections from the top of the dash panel off the back side of the windshield are still excessive in all new automobiles. As mentioned before, an adequate solution is a piece of black velveteen cloth draped over the top of the dash. Dirt on the windshield or on spectacles provides an amount of glare proportional to the amount of dirt and direction of the sun. The solution is to clean the spectacles and operate the windshield washer. Don't forget to clean the inside of the windshield.

## B. Atmospheric boil

This condition is seen on hot days as a shimmering and unsteadiness of objects at a great distance. The effect is due to shifting of the optical density of the air due to wind and temperature differences. This phenomenon reduces the visual acuity for objects seen outdoors through several hundred feet of atmosphere compared to clinical acuity. The reduction in acuity depends upon the amount of atmosphere between the eyes and the target and the thermal discontinuities in the atmosphere. Under most conditions where highway signs are involved, acuity should not fall very much. However, conditions can vary widely in the atmosphere, and if one needs to know the acuity possible in a given circumstance, his best approach is to measure it. Atmospheric boil is at a minimum right after sunrise and just before sunset. It is maximum when the solar radiation is greatest. It is at a constant second maximum during the night hours. The effect is present winter or summer and is least on overcast days.

Atmospheric attenuation and sky light also tend to reduce the contrast of distant objects; hence for optimum visibility a sign or an object must have a high contrast with its background. With increasing speeds we need some signs to be legible from 2,000 feet or more. Certainly, this kind of visibility, cannot be provided in every kind of weather, no matter how big we make the sign. The freeway sign that slips by in the fog without being seen in time to read it, is a case in point.

Thus, it seems that a series of advance warning information signs, in addition to the main sign, are imperative to ensure that the motorist is informed of decisions to be made or actions to take. Visibility through short sections of the atmosphere will always be superior to that through longer sections, and perhaps the ideal sign system would be that placed nearby on the pavement itself. Color coding of lanes or of lane marking paint stripes has been shown to be of great value, at least in the daytime. Reflectorized paint colors would be necessary at night to permit enough light to be returned to the eyes to make seeing of the colors. Pavement rumble strips are highly desirable especially prior to signalized crossings on a highway.

## C. Mirage effects

Mirages occur regularly on the highways. While typically seen in the daytime as shimmering white light resembling water on the distant pavement surface, mirages also are seen for several hours after sunset. Then they behave like a base up prism, refracting part of the rays from oncoming headlights to make them appear double as if two cars were approaching, one above the other. In the early morning hours, after the pavement has cooled more than the air, the surface air works like a base down prism, bending light downward, thus somewhat increasing visibility over hills.

Probably the most significant hazard from daytime mirages is the delayed appearance of a vehicle approaching on the crest of a hill. The heated air near the pavement surface bends light upward so that the rays of light from an oncoming automobile do not travel in a straight line. Hence the automobile beyond the crest of a hill must come closer, so that the bent light rays from it will arrive at our eyes, instead of going over our heads.

The heated air near the pavement also causes distant vehicles to disappear or to be so poorly defined that they cannot be accurately located or judged for speed. Sometimes a vehicle may be completely covered over by the bright sky light appearing to come from the boundary layer of air over the pavement. Others may lose some of their parts, such as their lower half or a portion in the middle.

Since the mirage of water on the highway is really a refracted image of the sky, a most unbearable glare from the pavement occurs when the part of the sky seen on the roadway contains the sun! Such a situation cannot be remedied effectively by any sunglasses, and the luminance level may become so high that the motorist will be forced, in the interest of safety, to pull into a rest area and wait 15 or 20 minutes until the condition subsides before continuing to drive.

## D. Camouflage effects

The difference in luminance between an object and its background is a clue to an excellent camouflage technique. The smaller the luminance difference between an object and its background, the less likely will be the detection of the object. For example, when viewed from the air at low altitude, the highways are full of cars. As altitude increases, fewer cars are seen, and they are the lighter colored ones only. The lightest colors are the last to disappear at very great altitude. When earth scenery is viewed from a car, its average luminance is about the same as a well-worn highway. Against this average background, measurements with a Luckiesh Moss Visibility Meter show that light colored automobiles are significantly more visible. Thus, gray or dark colored automobiles have an element of camouflage built in. The fact that 21 candle power running lights or 4 candle power parking lights reduce the number and the severity of daytime accidents proves that such camouflage effects really do exist and do contribute to accidents.

A spotted Dalmatian dog sitting in the spotty shade of a tree will be camouflaged. This illustrates a second principle in camouflage: namely, the characteristic shape of an object can be disguised by adding meaningless spots, areas, and lines that could easily be confused with the background. Measurements on aircraft visibility both in the air and on the surface of the earth have shown that when an airplane was a single solid color it was the most detectable. When various patterns were used, the detectability was reduced in proportion to the amount of variegation, even for uniform sky viewing. Thus, two tone paint patterns on automobiles are likely to be less visible than a single color, especially a light one.

Automobile surfaces are already composed of large areas of glass, which average about the same luminance as the background. The popular vinyl top and black bumpers, used with all conceivable paint colors, adds to the two-toning effect provided by the windows and is not a wise color choice because of a severe reduction in the visibility of the car and an increase in the heat uptake inside the car in the summer.

Chromium reflects about 50 percent of the light falling on it. Because it is usually highly polished, it sparkles and brightly images the sun. Under many conditions the reflections from chromium make a car very visible. However, since chromium behaves like a mirror, there may be reflections from dark-colored objects at a given moment, whereupon the chromium looks dark or even black.

Chromium, therefore, cannot be relied upon to provide the visibility that a dark-colored automobile needs. On the other hand, bright metal surfaces on one's own car that reflect the sun tend to interfere with vision and to increase the effectiveness of camouflage on streets and highways.

The most effective camouflage technique is to hide the object rather than to disguise it. The automobile discovered in front of the truck one is passing, was hidden from view. An automobile in a fog is hidden. The pedestrian or vehicle partially or completely covered by the windshield corner posts or the rearview mirror is hidden. Even the dirt spots on the windshield and the dangling toys in some cars will hide or partially obscure an object on a collision course. As shown earlier, an object on a collision course does not change its position in the field of view of the driver. It just gets larger. Since objects attached to the car, such as windshield dirt spots, do not change their position either, they interfere with detecting the outside object.

Hiding tail and headlights from oblique view by forward and rearward jutting fenders led the government to require reflectors and/or side marker lights beginning with the 1968 models. Darkness is itself great camouflage.

Modern styling modifies the estimate of speed and direction of an object. Strong slanting lines will confuse the real size and shape of an object. Styling has thinned the roof line, which reduces the apparent height of a passenger automobile and makes it appear farther away and thus to be going slower. Window, fender, and grill lines are slanted in various directions and give the illusion of motion. The prevalence in accident reports of the statement, "I didn't see!" indicates the effectiveness with which camouflage operates in driving a motor vehicle.

## E. Rain, mist, snow, and fog

Daytime rain, mist, snow, and fog serve to reduce the contrast of objects seen from a motor vehicle, They increase the already existing effects described above. Windshield dirt and water droplets tend to increase the detrimental effects which occur during rain due to the absence of shadows, atmospheric scattering, and dirt on roadway objects.

An especially significant hazard in adverse weather is the pedestrian. When getting wet, a human being becomes preoccupied. They will cover their head and run or walk in front of an automobile. Pedestrians seem to picture the motorist as an inconsiderate person, sitting dry and comfortable in the car, watching the poor pedestrian getting wet. The pedestrian believes the motorist can see him, can stop, and will stop if there is any question about the pedestrian getting hurt.

The motorist, on the other hand, has his/her own problems. The windshield wipers do not sweep all of the windshield area; the vision through what is wiped is not good; side windows, rear windows, and major parts of the windshield often are fogged. The motorist feels closed in. Because traffic moves slowly, he may become annoyed. Because pedestrians are taking unusual risks, the driver may feel that they are being "pushy" and are imposing, since the driver has so many other problems, many of them due to the weather. The confusion and poor visibility may be so adverse that the pedestrian may not be seen at all and an accident occurs.

Under adverse weather conditions, it is imperative that vehicles have their lights on so that pedestrians and motorists can see them. Umbrellas should be transparent so the pedestrian can see approaching automobiles. Each person must be taught that, in the final analysis, he/she is the only person to be depended upon for personal safety. Never walk with your back to oncoming traffic, be convinced of the difficulties of being seen, and act intelligently and safely. Understand that hair, hats, glasses, clothing, and anything else that interferes with side vision, can cost you your life.

The growing use of daytime headlights will reduce the dangers described above.

# Chapter 12

# Measurement and Evaluation of Motor Vehicle Lighting: A Systematic Approach

Developed by Bernard S. Abrams, O.D.
Measurement and Case Example by Sgt. Gregory Vandenberg
Graphics Designed for: The Institute of Vehicular Safety
by Charles H. Matthews, Evidence Research Services

***Synopsis***



## 12.1 Preface

The objective of this block of instruction is to familiarize the reader with a methodology whereby vehicle lighting systems may be tested accurately, and useful application may be made of the data collected. We have designed a testing platform, together with programmed data collection and presentation formats, which provide a consistent approach throughout the process, from the establishment of a testing range, through the final courtroom presentation. It is assumed that the reader is already proficient in certain skills necessary in the technical evaluation and reconstruction of traffic crashes, particularly with regard to the taking of routine field measurements, the subjective evaluation of road surface characteristics, and, most especially, proper mechanical drawing or engineering graphics techniques.

While not discussed in the main text, we would add that conditions of adverse weather (rain, snow, fog) should be avoided in the testing of lighting profiles. Equally, the testing would ideally be conducted during a no-moon period (this does not necessarily mean a new moon; rather, a period during which moonrise allows for sufficient dark periods, or there is sufficient heavy overcast to obscure the moon). We assume that you are all innovators, or you would not be reading this book.

As a final word, we would note that while we have made every effort to simplify this process, the underlying precepts have a certain degree of complexity. These can best be overcome through patience and scrupulous attention to detail, both cornerstones on which good science is founded.

## 12.2 Establishing the Test Range

### A. Desirable qualities of the test range

Before establishing a range for the testing and measurement of vehicle lighting systems, a suitable site must be chosen. If the basic qualities presented below are met at the test site, the chances of consistent, accurate test results are greatly improved.

The surface material on the test range should closely duplicate that found in the vehicle's usual highway environment. In most instances, this means an asphalt concrete material. Probably the best surface selection is what is commonly termed a "travelled" surface (i.e., one on which the sharp edges of the stone have been degraded somewhat, and the surface color appears generally as a dull gray-brown), as this is the most likely surface to be encountered in the field. Newly-applied asphalt has an excessively high surface content of tar, and thus reduced reflectivity, while a badly worn ("traffic polished") surface develops a sheen, thus increasing reflectivity.

The surface contour should be as flat as possible. If it is necessary to conduct testing on a grade, the grade must be maintained throughout the length of the test range. Any drainage crowns or slopes should be minimal or absent.

It is helpful to imagine a plane projected horizontally through the centers of the beams of a vehicle's headlamps. On the ideal test range, this plane would be parallel to the ground with the vertical height between the ground and the imaginary plane being equal at all points of measurement. The ideal facility to meet this requirement may be a drag strip or unused runway.

The ambient lighting (i.e., light from sources other than the source being measured) must be kept at a minimum. Any adjacent light sources must be sufficiently distant, or of sufficiently low intensity, to prevent skewing of the test measurements. The headlamps of passing vehicles may severely skew the test results; thus, the site should be selected with a view to minimize or eliminate the effect of such traffic.

The access to the test range should allow for the greatest flexibility, as testing dates must be adjusted to accommodate the vagaries of weather, priority demands, and so forth. Ideally, we would have exclusive access and control over the test facility, thus enabling us to make adjustments to the surface conditions, range dimensions, and so on, as may be required by individual circumstances.

### B. Construction of the test range

Having located a suitable site for out test range, the next step is to construct the facility. You should refer to *Instruction Packet Drawing 1* (Figure 12.1), which provides the layout and dimensions of the surface markings which constitute the test range. In addition, we have enclosed an actual case example.

This design contemplates the construction of a permanent facility, with a 600 foot length and a 24-foot breadth, providing for a variety of potential testing requirements.

The vehicle staging area is intended to aid in the proper alignment of motor vehicles to the measurement area and should be of sufficient depth to accommodate even large, commercial vehicles. As noted, this area may be marked with any suitable highway-striping paint, as surface reflectivity is not critical here.

The Downrange, or measurement area, must be given different treatment. Obviously, highly reflective paints would not be suitable here. In the case of a permanent test range, we would suggest the use of a flat, "red oxide" type primer for markings in this area. This has reasonable durability and low reflectivity, yet it provides reasonable contrast to the surface to allow the testing personnel to locate the measurement station with the aid of a flashlight.

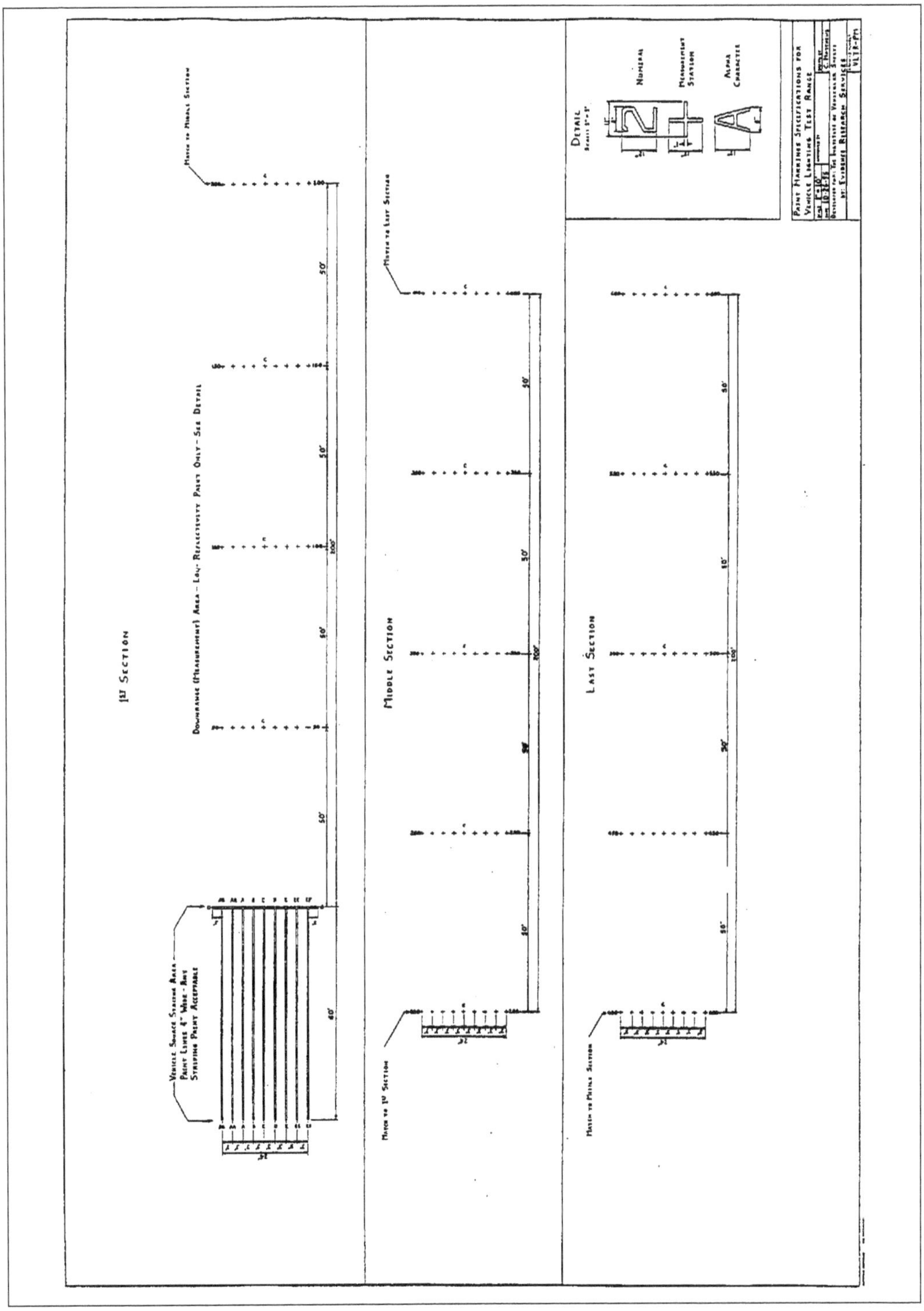


***Figure 12.1*** *Instruction Packet Drawing 1.*

When a field-expedient test range is used, chalk, crayon, or similar temporary markings may be used.

Ultimately, the objective is to position a uniform set of measurement stations at known distances from the light source, thus providing for a consistent method of taking the required measurements on every occasion.

In the case of a permanent test range, we would recommend that the layout be done with the aid of a transit level. This will not only ensure that the various lanes are established parallel to one another, but allow for the discovery of substantial departures from level for the various stations. If such a departure is found, the difference should be noted for later use in the actual conduct of the light measurements.

Fully recognizing that the ideal, permanent facility may not be such an easy matter to establish, we will also offer some guidance for the construction of a field-expedient test range. The layout is best done in daylight.

A field-expedient test range requires the same basic characteristics as the permanent facility in the way of surface material, ambient light, and surface contour, but it may be used anywhere these conditions are found.

In this case, the Vehicle Staging Area is omitted. The downrange area is established to permit the testing required for the particular circumstance.

This range is constructed around the test source; the first step being to position the test source (usually a vehicle) at one end of the contemplated range.

The next step is to define a centerline extending through the centerline of the source. This can easily be done with the aid of an assistant sighting along the centerline of the vehicle, and directing you right or left, as may be necessary, as you move downrange.

Along this centerline, mark small crosses every 50 feet (the front of the vehicle is considered to be "0" feet), and label each with a letter "C." Continue this to the desired length of the range.

Having done this, measure distances in increments of three feet to either side of the crosses mentioned above, taking care that these lie along lines that are perpendicular to the established centerline. At each of these incremental distances, also make a small cross, but do not label these.

Once you have measured to the desired distance on both sides of the centerline, move up the extreme edge of the range on each side, and label the edge crosses with the appropriate depth (50', 100', etc.) and with the lane designator as taken from Instruction Packet Drawing 1.

As an example, let us assume that we are using a conventional automobile as a source and wish to establish a field-expedient test range that is 250 feet long and 12 feet wide; we will be testing the headlamp pattern.

We park the vehicle at one end of the selected surface with the front of the vehicle facing downrange, assuring that we have at least 250 feet of surface ahead of the vehicle and six feet of surface to either side of its centerline.

We position an assistant behind the vehicle; he looks through the car and establishes a line-of-sight using the "third" brake light and the mounting post of the rear-view mirror.

Starting at the front of the vehicle, using either a conventional tape measure or wheel measure, we measure a distance of 250 feet and stop here. Our assistant directs us to the right or left, as necessary, until we are standing on the centerline projected through the vehicle.

At our feet, we make a cross, labelled with a "C"; we then measure back toward the vehicle, stopping every 50 feet, and mark identical crosses, taking direction from the assistant to assure that we remain on the centerline. Note that it is helpful to orient the crosses such that one bar lies directly on the centerline and the other perpendicular to the centerline.

We then measure distance of three feet and six feet, respectively, to either side of the centerline, taking care to move at a perpendicular to the centerline, and mark a cross at each of these locations; this is repeated at each of the centerline crosses.

Standing at the front of the vehicle and facing downrange, we now move to the far left-hand cross at 50 feet downrange. This is labelled "A 50." The far right-hand cross at 50 feet is labelled "E 50." You will note that this corresponds to the lane designators on the referenced drawing.

Moving downrange, the farthest outside crosses are similarly labelled, with the numeric figure corresponding to the downrange distance in feet.

The example cited above is typical of a field-expedient test range established to measure the headlamps of a car in the confines of an ordinary traffic lane.

If the circumstances require a "bias" to one side of a traffic lane (e.g., in a circumstance involving a pedestrian or animal outside of the travel lane), it will be necessary to add measurement lanes to the appropriate side of the test source. This is accomplished by either adding a lane farther away from "C," as specified on the drawing, or by establishing the centerline of the vehicle on an alternate measurement lane to one side or another of "C."

Please note that, whatever type of test range is established, it is necessary to use the lane designators indicated to successfully utilize the measurement system presented here.

## 12.3 Taking Measurements

Having previously established our test range, we will now proceed to take measurements of the light produced by our test source.

We will continue with the example set forth in the previous section, "Establishing the Test Range." For the purposes of this discussion, we will assume that we are using a 1991 Cadillac Brougham, around which we constructed the field-expedient test range previously discussed. During this discussion, you should refer to the completed sample of Form VLP-FM, which is part of the instruction packet (Figure 12.2).

To take and record measurements, we will require a copy of *Form VLP-FM*, a clipboard, a small flashlight, a tape measure or folding rule (the latter gives better service), a pencil, a wheel measure, and, naturally, a reliable light meter. The light meter is to be calibrated in accordance with the instructions you have received previously.

It is very helpful to have an assistant or two to aid in taking the measurements and recording the results. We highly recommend that whoever records the results be chosen with a consideration of good penmanship.

You will note that the form VLP-FM consists primarily of a matrix upon which the test results are recorded; along the margins are areas where additional data is requested. At this point, our primary concern is with the sections marked "*Vertical Stations*" and "*Target Value* =."

The Vertical Stations are designated numerically and, in the case of stations 2 through 5, arbitrarily. Station 1 will always be ground level as it forms the foundation line for other vertical measurements.

Stations 2 through 5 may be any height above ground level which the particular testing program may require. In our example, Station 2 is the vertical height of the center of the headlamp beams (assumed to be symmetrical-if actual measurement of a vehicle reveals minor differences in the dimension, an average of the two will probably suffice), and Station 3 is the height of the driver's eye (measured on-site). In our example, Station 2 is 26 inches above ground level, and Station 3 is 46 inches above ground level. Stations 4 and 5 are not used in this instance, and are lined through.

DATE: [illegible] TIME: 1745 PAGE 01 OF 01 PAGES

VEHICLE LIGHTING FIELD MEASUREMENTS

| Station | | 0′ | 50′ | 100′ | 150′ | 200′ | 250′ | 300′ | TARGET (○) AT: |
|---|---|---|---|---|---|---|---|---|---|
| AB | 5 | | | | | | | | |
| | 4 | | | | | | | | |
| | 3 | | | | | | | | |
| | 2 | | | | | | | | |
| GROUND | 1 | | | | | | | | |
| AA | 5 | | | | | | | | |
| | 4 | | | | | | | | |
| | 3 | | | | | | | | |
| | 2 | | | | | | | | |
| GROUND | 1 | | | | | | | | |
| A | 5 | | | | | | | | |
| | 4 | | | | | | | | |
| | 3 | | .295 | .094 | .050 | .035 | .021 | | 50′ |
| | 2 | | .684 | .143 | .060 | .041 | .025 | | 71′ |
| GROUND | 1 | | 3.78 | .563 | .107 | .057 | .037 | | 116′ |
| B | 5 | | | | | | | | |
| | 4 | | | | | | | | |
| | 3 | | .291 | .190 | .052 | .034 | .029 | | 50′ |
| | 2 | | .912 | .145 | .067 | .042 | .029 | | 75′ |
| | 1 | | 4.55 | .611 | .116 | .058 | .038 | | 114′ |
| C | 5 | | | | | | | | |
| | 4 | | | | | | | | |
| | 3 | | .315 | .112 | .131 | .034 | .023 | | 50′ |
| | 2 | | 1.52 | .192 | .072 | .042 | .024 | | 80′ |
| GROUND | 1 | | 5.34 | .920 | .054 | .055 | .039 | | 125′ |
| D | 5 | | | | | | | | |
| | 4 | | | | | | | | |
| | 3 | | .338 | .126 | .056 | .032 | .021 | | 56′ |
| | 2 | | 3.23 | .278 | .088 | .039 | .028 | | 87′ |
| GROUND | 1 | | 4.61 | 1.60 | .201 | .078 | .036 | | 130′ |
| E | 5 | | | | | | | | |
| | 4 | | | | | | | | |
| | 3 | | .305 | .132 | .071 | .041 | .036 | | 59′ |
| | 2 | | 1.43 | .409 | .103 | .058 | .036 | | 106′ |
| GROUND | 1 | | 4.95 | .219 | .368 | .087 | .028 | | 150′ |
| EE | 5 | | | | | | | | |
| | 4 | | | | | | | | |
| | 3 | | | | | | | | |
| | 2 | | | | | | | | |
| GROUND | 1 | | | | | | | | |
| EF | 5 | | | | | | | | |
| | 4 | | | | | | | | |
| | 3 | | | | | | | | |
| | 2 | | | | | | | | |
| GROUND | 1 | | | | | | | | |

COMPLETED SAMPLE

RANGE TYPE / LOCATION: FIELD EXPEDIENT / ADAMS CO. AIRPORT

PERSONNEL: TPR. B. JONES, SGT. R. ROE

SOURCE: 1991 CADILLAC BROUGHAM 4-DR. (EXEMPLAR) VIN: 1G6DW53A6MB700001

CASE TITLE / NUMBER: STATE vs DOE / 01-2345

VERTICAL STATIONS:

5 = N/A
4 = N/A
3 = DRIVER HEIGHT-OF-EYE – 46″
2 = CTR. OF HEADLAMP BEAM – 26″

TARGET VALUE = .3 Fc ± 5% (.285 – .315 Fc)

NOTES: CTR.-TO-CTR. DISTANCE BETWEEN HEADLAMPS 53″
LOW BEAM LAMPS TESTED

***Figure 12.2*** *Completed sample of form VLP-FM.*

The Target Value is determined to be 0.2 foot candle, plus or minus 5 percent. The range is, therefore, from .285 to .315 foot candle. Note that whatever target value is selected, it is best to hold the error tolerance to as small a value as possible. For reasons which will become apparent in a later section, even the 5 percent tolerance we have used in this example is too great.

Recorded in the "Notes" section is the horizontal, center-to-center distance between the headlamps, in this case 53 inches; it is also noted that this is a test of the low-beam lamps. Other marginal data blocks are relatively self-explanatory.

The main data area consists of a matrix on which the measured values are recorded. There are nine primary horizontal rows, lettered from "AB" through "EF"; you will note that these designators correspond to the lane designators specified in Instruction Packet Drawing 1.

Lanes AB, AA, EE, and EF are not used in this example; therefore, they are lined through.

Each of the primary horizontal rows is subdivided into five individual rows, each labelled "1" through "5." These correspond to the "Vertical Stations"; again 4 and 5 are not used in this example and are lined through.

The matrix uses eight vertical columns. The first seven columns are designated, in increasing order, with the downrange distance of the measurement stations in fifty-foot increments. In this instance, we have not taken measurements at either 0 feet or 300 feet, and these columns are lined through.

The eighth column is for recording target value and will be discussed in a later paragraph.

In our example, we will begin at 50 feet along lane "A" and commence to take and record measurements. A measurement is taken at the ground at this point and recorded in Row A, subdivision 1, in the 50 foot column. Using the tape measure or folding rule, we take a second measurement 26 inches above the ground, and record this in the space immediately above the last value (i.e., row A, subdivision 2, 50 foot column). We next measure to 46 inches above ground and repeat the procedure, with the value being recorded above the last.

When an assistant is recording the measurements for you, we recommend that the assistant read back each value as it is recorded, to assure that it is correct.

If you have followed this example, you should find values at Vertical Stations 1, 2 and 3 of .295, .684, and 3.78 respectively, in Row A of the 50 foot column.

Having recorded these measurements, we move to Lane B on the test range (still at 50 feet downrange), and repeat the process; we continue this until all values are obtained.

Once we have obtained measured values for each of the pre-established measurement stations, we must seek the target values.

It can be easily seen that we found values meeting the target parameters at Vertical Station 3, 50 feet downrange, along Lanes A, B, and C. Equally, we found a target value at ground level (Vertical Station 1) along Lane E at 150 feet downrange.

In our example, we can observe that for Vertical Station 3, along Lanes D and E, we would expect to find a .3 foot candle value between 50 and 100 feet downrange. Moving along the lanes and taking measurements every foot or so, we find that this is indeed true; we find our target value at 56 feet on Lane D, and at 59 feet along Lane E.

Moving to the "*Target Value*" column on the work form, we record the downrange distance at which we found the target values at Vertical Station 3. Again, if you have followed along with the example, you will note that for Vertical Station 3, we recorded target values at 50 feet for each of Rows A, B and C and at 56 feet and 59 feet, respectively, for Rows D and E.

The same procedure is followed for the remaining vertical stations on each lane, and the figures are recorded in the appropriate columns.

It should be noted that assistants must not be between the light source and the measuring instrument. Equally, while it will be necessary to use a light to read the instrument and record data, all lights should be extinguished while the instrument is actually directed at the source.

In the case of field-expedient ranges, a lookout must be kept for passing vehicles, as lights from which may skew the test results.

As a final note, all personnel should clearly hear the measured values and take note of them in relation to previously-obtained values. Any station at which a suspect value is obtained should have sufficient repeated tests to assure that the value obtained is accurate. (For example, if we find a reading of .9 foot candle in a field of .2 or lower values, we would tend to suspect that this was inaccurate and probably the result of an unnoticed, passing vehicle. Certainly, this must be retested.)

## 12.4 Final Presentation of Data-Profile Plots

Now that we have collected the measurements of the light produced by our source, we must present the data in a useful form. Here again, we will continue with the example we have begun in previous sections. In this section we will make use of *Form VLP-1*; a blank version of this form is included as *Instruction Packet Drawing 2* (Figure 12.3), and a sample completed version, in accordance with our example, is included as *Instruction Packet Drawing 3* (Figure 12.4).

This form is a representation of 300 feet of the downrange portion of the test range; the original scale is 1 inch =10 feet, which we find to be a very convenient scale in which to work for crash reconstruction purposes. You will note that we use a graphic scale; we do this against the possibility that we may later wish to enlarge or reduce the drawing, in which case the graphic scale allows for accurate measurements without the need of developing "odd" scale.

The *Plan View* section of the drawing represents the horizontal plane of measurement. All of the measurement lanes are represented here; downrange distances have been left blank, as it may be necessary to use two forms if more than 300 feet of downrange distance is used for testing.

In the *Side Views* section, we have divided the range into nine vertical planes, each corresponding to one of the test lanes. Allowance is made for vertical stations to a maximum of 10 feet above ground; you will note that the ground level foundation line is pre-established.

The *Data and Notes* section contains a reproduction of the data area of *Form VLP-FM* (Figure 12.2), as well as pre-established lines for the recording of Vertical Station and Target Value information. Ample space is provided for additional notes which may be required. The form is to be set up on a drawing board, and brought into square with either a T-square or drafting machine.

To complete the form, we begin by carefully recording the data we obtained in our measurements. These are simply copied into the appropriate locations in the data area.

We will next carefully record the approximate downrange distance figures in their respective locations. In the case of our example, these range from 0 feet through 300 feet.

The next step is to define the boundaries of the test range on the drawing. This is done with the use of long-dashed lines drawn *just outside* the area in which measurements were made. This is done on both the Plan and Side views, with ample space being allowed on the latter for the plotting of Vertical Stations.

The source lamps are then represented to scale on the Plan View; we have used a small letter "x" to represent each of these. As the headlamps in the example are located at Vertical Station 2, 0 feet, their location is assumed in the Side Views.

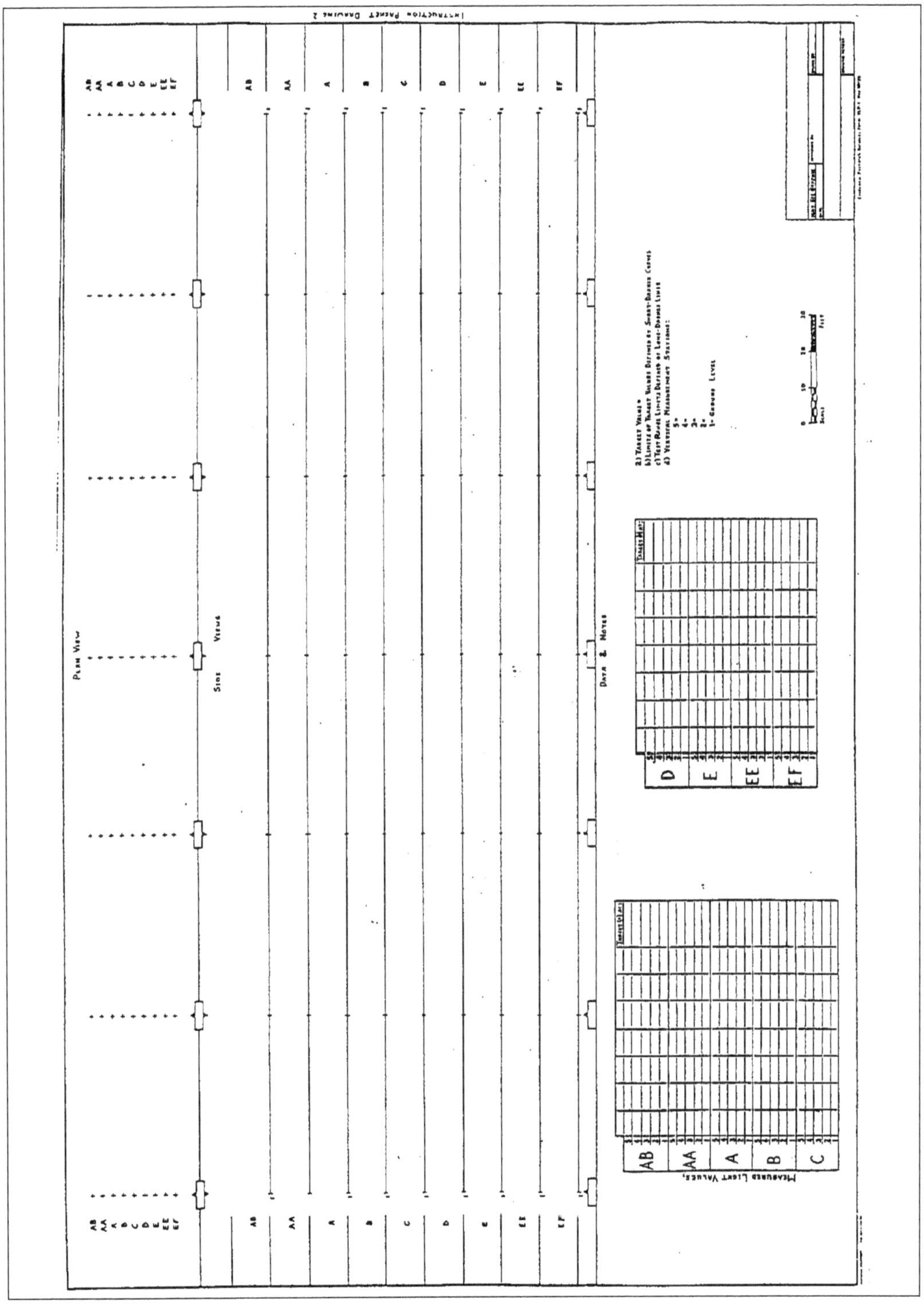

*Figure 12.3* Instruction Packet Drawing 2.

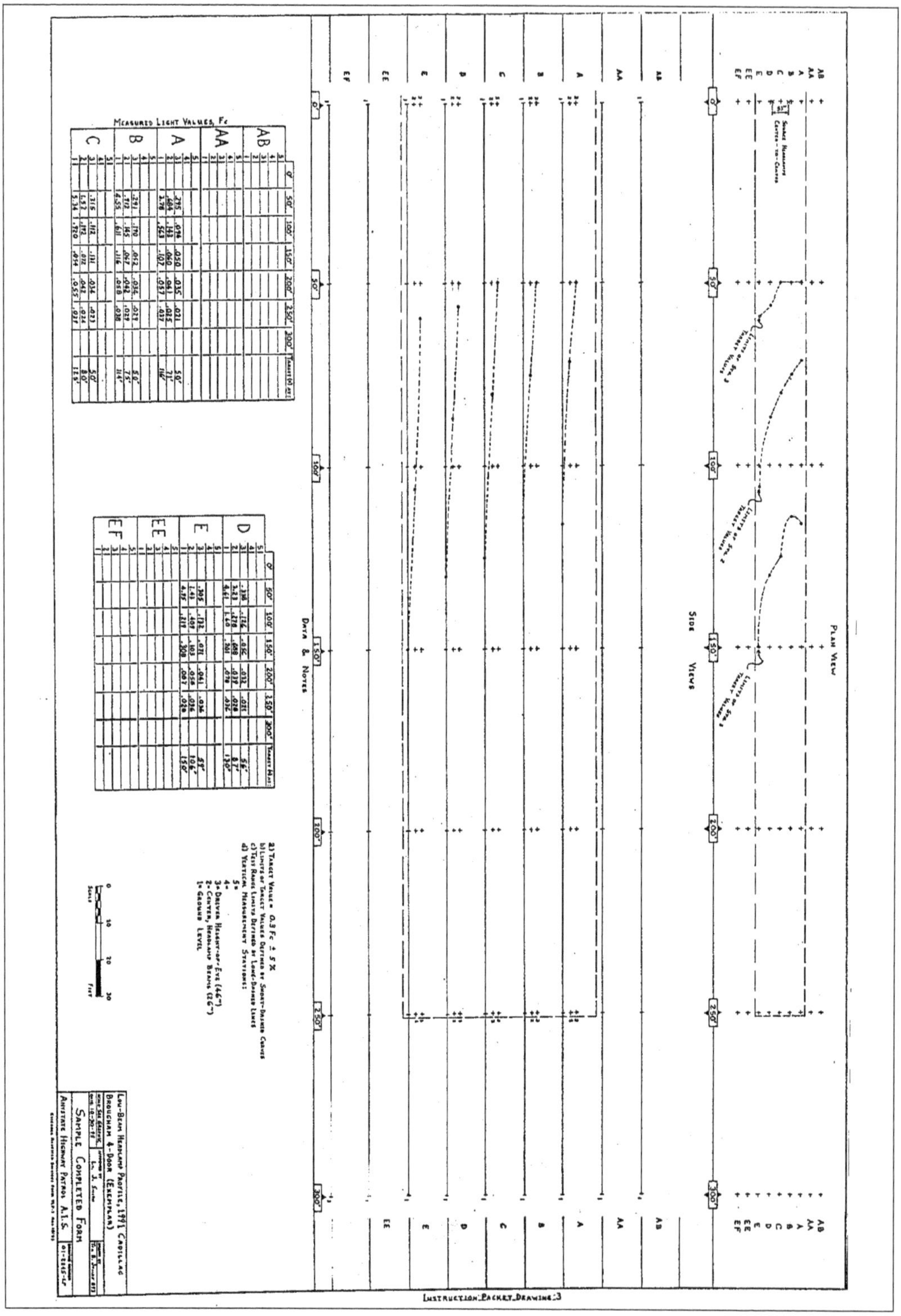


***Figure 12.4*** *Instruction Packet Drawing 3.*

We now plot, again to scale, the vertical stations on each of the Side Views, in this case on Views A through E. Each pre-established vertical station is represented by a small cross, as was the case with the horizontal stations. There will be a vertical station at each 50-foot downrange increment, on each Side View, for every vertical station used. These stations are pre-plotted for Station 1, Ground, but must be individually plotted for Stations 2 and 3.

Next, we establish construction lines between the downrange increments where we will have Target Values on both the Plan and Side Views. (Note that these should be very light, erasable lines.)

We measure along these lines in the Plan View to the appropriate location at which we found target values for each lane and for each Vertical Station. At these locations, a small circle is plotted. It is helpful to place a small number adjacent to these circles to identify the respective vertical station of each. This may be erasable.

The target value locations thus established on the Plan View are simply projected down to their respective locations on the appropriate Side View.

This done, our next task is to illustrate the approximate limits of the target values in each view. This is done by drawing the best smooth curve through the target values within the same measurement plane.

In the case of the Plan View, a curve is drawn through all target value circles designated Station 1, then another through Station 2 circles, and, finally, through Station 3 circles.

It is here that we will further address the subject of the selection of target values. In our example, you will recall, we selected a target value of 0.3 foot candle, with an error tolerance of plus or minus 5 percent, which yielded a range of from .285 to .315 foot candle. You will also recall that we found values within these tolerances at 50 feet downrange, along Lanes A, B, and C, at Vertical Station 3 for each lane.

Look closely at the plot example in the Plan View on Instruction Packet Drawing 3, where the Vertical Station 3 plot is indicated.

The "best smooth curve" through the values specified for Lanes A, B, and C is a straight line! If we had accepted the default value for this station in Lane E (you will see that we found a .305 foot candle value at 50 feet here), all of our plot points but one would have been in a line. The resulting "best smooth curve" would have appeared as essentially a straight line across the 50-foot marker, punctuated by a sort of "spike" extending to 56 feet downrange and lying between Lanes C and E; hardly an accurate representation of the true limits of the target value area!

With this in mind, we will reiterate the importance of selecting the narrowest error tolerance possible for the target value, particularly when dealing with very small values in the first instance. In this example, the difference between the default value of .305 foot candle and the true target of .3 foot candle is only about 1.64 percent, but we found the true value nine feet downrange from the default value location, which made a considerable difference in our resultant plot.

The search for precise values entails considerable effort, patience, and attention to detail, but is necessary.

To return to the completion of the plots, we next direct our attention to the Side Views. Here again, we simply draw the best smooth curve through the target value locations in each measurement plane. These curves are readily observable on the example.

Once this is done, the construction lines are erased, the title block completed, and the drawing is complete. The curves we have plotted can now be used as the basis for evaluation of visibility in crash reconstructions and for the construction of models to illustrate the dynamics of visibility issues in court.

With the availability of low cost Computer Aided Drawing (CAD) software programs, isocandella maps of headlamp patterns can be quickly and easily constructed as an alternative to the hand drafting method described.

By plotting the target values and drawing a curved line through the target value control points, an acceptable scale representation of the pattern can be constructed. This headlamp pattern, attached to a vehicle symbol, can in turn be placed in a CAD site diagram to provide a graphic representation of the vehicle's headlight pattern for evaluation purposes.

Following are two examples of field-expedient headlamp profiles where only the target value foot candle readings (.3 foot candle) are recorded (Figures 12.5 and 12.6) and plotted (Figures 12.7 and 12.8). These examples were created using a CAD program. Although both examples document low-beam headlamps, note the differences in the patterns due to headlight condition, age, and aim.

**0.3 Foot Candle Isocandella Map of 1988 Chevrolet Cavalier Low Beam Headlamps**

| | 10 ft Left | 6 ft Left | 3 ft Left | Center | 3 ft Right | 6 ft Right | 11 ft Right |
|---|---|---|---|---|---|---|---|
| @ Ground | $91^{\underline{10}}$ | $110^{\underline{7}}$ | $127^{\underline{0}}$ | $157^{\underline{3}}$ | $191^{\underline{1}}$ | $213^{\underline{11}}$ | $228^{\underline{10}}$ |
| @ 25 in. | $66^{\underline{0}}$ | $66^{\underline{10}}$ | $73^{\underline{6}}$ | $127^{\underline{5}}$ | $170^{\underline{0}}$ | $191^{\underline{6}}$ | $203^{\underline{11}}$ |
| @ 43 in. | $36^{\underline{10}}$ | $50^{\underline{8}}$ | $59^{\underline{7}}$ | $71^{\underline{10}}$ | $107^{\underline{10}}$ | $138^{\underline{2}}$ | $58^{\underline{9}}$ |

Measurements taken at ground level, center of headlamp (25 inches), and driver's eye level (43 inches).

All measurements listed in feet and inches.

***Figure 12.5***

| Isocandella Map for Pontiac 6000 | | | | | |
|---|---|---|---|---|---|
| Distance from Vehicle | 6ft Left | 3 ft Left | C/L of Vehicle | 3 ft Right | 6 ft Right |
| 50 @ Ground | .635 | 1.53 | 3.70 | 2.18 | 2.75 |
| @ Headlamp | .265 | .300 | .410 | .40 | .308 |
| @ Eye Level | .200 | .215 | .236 | .224 | .206 |
| 100 @ Ground | .115 | .160 | .230 | .271 | .276 |
| @ Headlamp | .083 | .097 | 1.01 | 1.16 | .095 |
| @ Eye Level | .065 | .072 | .078 | .071 | .070 |
| 150 @ Ground | .052 | .061 | .065 | .078 | .094 |
| @ Headlamp | .042 | .048 | .054 | .055 | .056 |
| @ Eye Level | .036 | .040 | .041 | .044 | .041 |
| 200 @ Ground | .030 | .050 | .051 | .057 | .042 |
| @ Headlamp | .026 | .029 | .031 | .031 | .031 |
| @ Eye Level | .025 | .025 | .026 | .027 | .028 |
| 250 @ Ground | .021 | .021 | .024 | .025 | .026 |
| @ Headlamp | .019 | .020 | .021 | .022 | .023 |
| @ Eye Level | .017 | .018 | .019 | .019 | .022 |
| .3 fc @ Ground | 62 ft | 71 ft | 87.5 ft | 92.5 ft | 64 ft |
| .3 fc @ Headlamp | 41 ft | 50 ft | 55.5 ft | 57.5 ft | 51.5 ft |
| .3 fc @ Eye Level | 10 ft | 38 ft | 40 ft | 38 ft | 22.5 ft |

All values are given in foot candles.

***Figure 12.6***

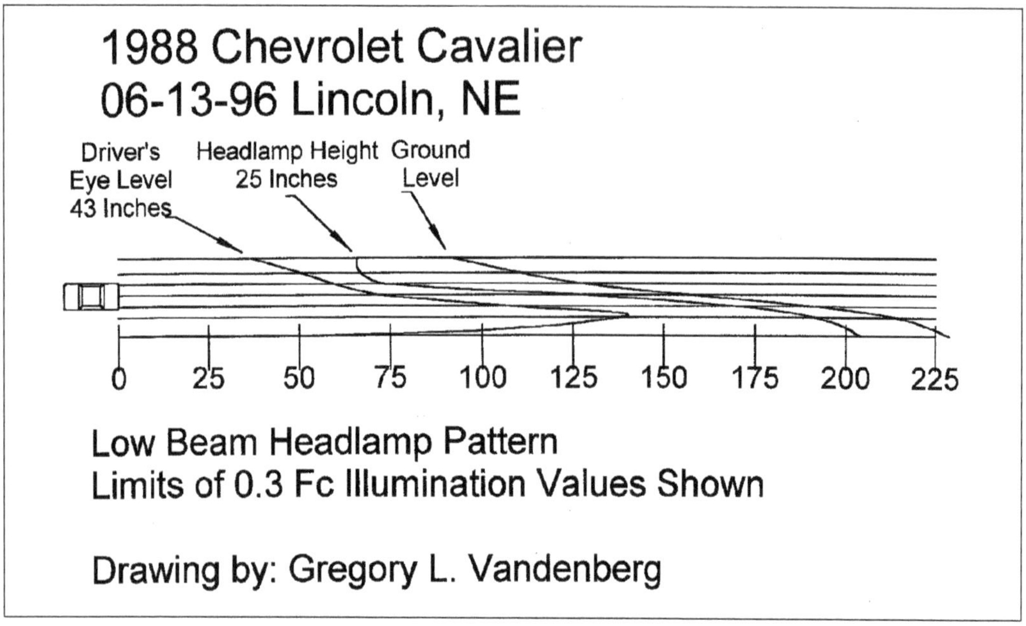


*Figure 12.7*

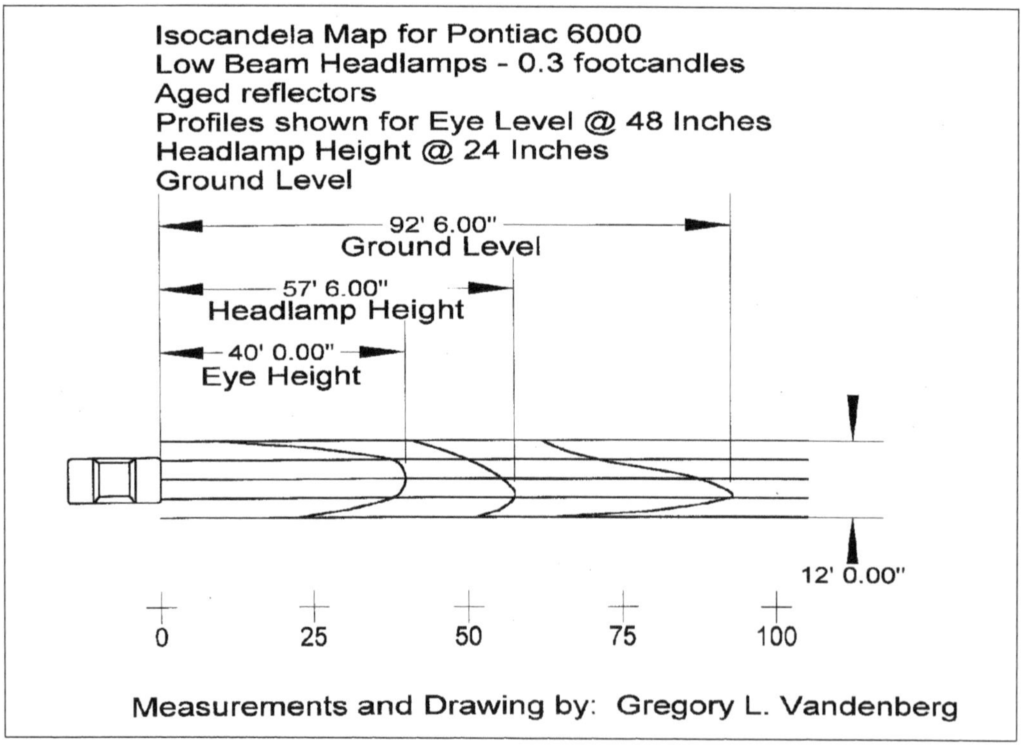


*Figure 12.8*

# Chapter 13

# Visibility Analysis 1: Physics

Marc Green, Ph.D.

*"It is a capital mistake to theorize before one has data."*
—Sir Arthur Conan Doyle

***Synopsis***



## 13.1 Introduction

This chapter and the next explain methodology for determining whether or not a target[1] were visibility. Recall that visibility refers strictly to the psychophysical task of detecting contrast, the difference between a target object and its background. It is not directly concerned with conspicuity, conscious perception or recognition. However, visibility is often the starting point for a visual accident reconstructionist since "Contrast detection is the basic task from which all other visual behaviors are derived" (p 3–15, Kaufman and Hayes, 1981).[2]

In most cases, expert analysis attempts to determine why a viewer failed to see a target. Since visibility sets the outer bound of what is humanly possible, it is the natural starting point. If the target were below threshold, then it is invisible, and the failure to see has been explained. If the target were above threshold, then the target was seeable, at least in theory. The analysis can then proceed to the issues of attention and conspicuity, etc. (Chapter 4).

The majority of psychophysical cases occur at night. In normal daylight, most targets are far above the contrast detection limit, so visibility *per se* is not an issue. Exceptions occur in adverse weather, when the target is very small and when viewer vision is impaired. In good daylight, however, contrast affects many perceptual judgments, such as speed, size, and distance.

A visibility analysis typically consists of four stages:

1. Determine whether a direct sightline existed;
2. Assess target and background luminance;
3. Compute the physical contrast of the target on the background; and
4. Estimate contrast threshold. Compare contrast threshold with physical contrast.

The ensuing discussion walks through these steps. Since psychophysics is physics plus psychology, the four steps divide neatly into the two categories. The initial stages, #1, #2, and #3, are the physics part while stage #4 is the psychology. This chapter explains the physics and the next chapter covers the psychology. Much of the discussion here builds on material covered in earlier chapters, especially Chapter 2. However, I repeat important points in order to make the visibility analysis as self-contained as possible. Lastly, these two chapters will be highly technical, and likely require some scientific, engineering, etc. background.

## 13.2 Step 1: Determine Whether a Direct Sightline Existed

The first step is the simplest—determine whether the viewer had an unobstructed sightline to the target. In most cases, it is easy to determine the sightline by visual inspection or by drawing a diagram of the objects in the environment. The role of some possible obstructions, such as vehicle roof pillars, however, may depend on small variation in eye position and may be more difficult to assess.

In some cases, the viewer may have a direct sightline but must look through a transparent surface such as a windshield or window. This adds two complications. First, it may affect the contrast calculation, as described below. Second, transparent surfaces can cause both accommodative and vergence errors, which degrade image clarity.

## 13.3 Step 2: Assess the Target and Background Luminance

Assuming a sightline exists, the next step is to assess the target and background luminance from the viewer's eye position on a line toward the target. Variation in eye position can produce error because parallax may change the background immediately behind the target. Further, reflectances may change with viewing angle for non-Lambertian surfaces.

A psychophysicist can determine luminance directly by measurement or indirectly by calculation or by some combination of methods. The most direct method uses a specialized instrument, a "luminance photometer." Indirect methods calculate luminance from illuminance and reflectance, which, in turn, may be either directly measured or indirectly estimated from tables and norms.

The methods for determining luminance and contrast vary in 'validity,' the extent that they capture actual conditions at the time of the event. Although the most accurate method is obviously the most desirable, cost and circumstance sometimes force the use of less precise methodology. The next sections discuss the methodologies for assessing luminance by measurement and by calculation.

## A. Direct Measurement of Luminance

### 1. General Methods

The simplest luminance measurement technique uses a "luminance photometer," preferably a "spot meter," such as the Minolta LS100. The user places the photometer at the eye location of the viewer. If the viewer were a driver, then the common methodology places an exemplar person of the same height in an exemplar vehicle in order to determine eye position. The reality, however, is that great eye-height precision is impossible. Different people of the same height have different upper and lower body proportions. Moreover, variables such as seat position and posture are typically impossible to specify. Fortunately, few cases require great precision. The target is relatively far from the viewer, so small shifts have little effect on parallax and viewing angle with respect to the target and the background.

Spot meters operate much like a camera. The user looks through an aperture, aims at the object or surface, and focuses (Figure 13.1).[3] Instead of taking a photograph, the user clicks a switch to see the luminance (in cd/m$^2$) in a readout. The value is an integration of luminance in the spot, most commonly 1° of visual angle. The ideal meter also has good stability and light sensitivity, measuring down to at least .001 cd/m$^2$, if required.

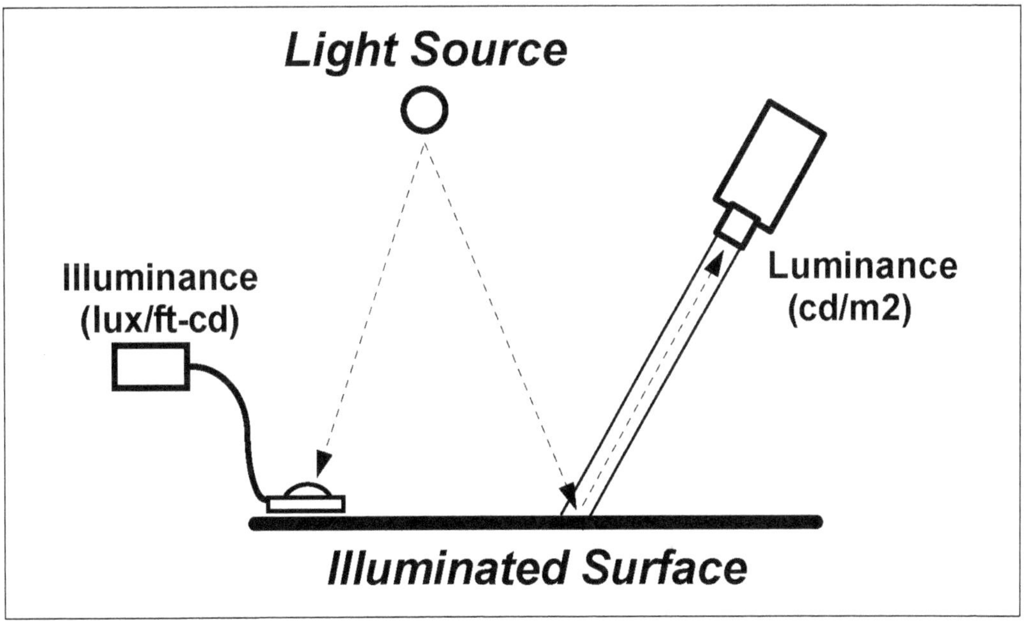


***Figure 13.1*** *Schematic representation of illuminance and luminance measurement.*

However, complications may arise. If the target is very small, then the meter's 1° aperture might include some of the background, making the reading an average of both. One solution is to use a meter with a smaller spot aperture, but there is a cost—smaller aperture photometers have less sensitivity and cannot measure the very low luminances that may occur at night. The simplest strategy is to move closer until the object fills the entire aperture. Recall that luminance does not change with distance. This might seem to violate the inverse square law, but it does not. The closer the sensor moves to the target, the less of the source falling in the aperture. The tradeoff between shorter distance (increased intensity) and smaller summation area is perfect and cancels out exactly. The only caveats are 1) in moving forward do not block any light sources and 2) be sure that the background does not change.

Lastly, the light measurements obtained with a luminance photometer may contain some inaccuracies in low light. Chapter 3 explained that scotopic and photopic vision have different luminous efficiencies, $V_\lambda$ and $V'_\lambda$. Photometers almost invariably use the photopic $V_\lambda$ function, which would be somewhat inaccurate in scotopic vision. Fortunately, real scotopic conditions occur rarely. However, urban or semi-urban environments create mesopic vision where both rods and cones operate. Despite attempts to develop a mesopic weighting function, none is generally accepted. Some have proposed curves based on performance measures or on a metric that weighs photopic and scotopic curves differently at different adaptation levels (Rea, Bullough, Freyssinier-Nova and Bierman, 2004).

It is probably impossible to have a single overall mesopic function for all visual field locations because the proportion of rods and cones varies with distance from the fovea. In mesopic foveal viewing, for example, cones dominate and the photopic curve is likely accurate. Laboratory research (e.g., Eloholma and Halonen, 1999) as well as studies of pedestrian visibility (Ketomäki, Eloholma, Orreveteläinen, and Halonen, 2003; Flannagan, 2007) confirm this expectation. In the periphery, however, rods become increasingly prevalent, and uncorrected photometer readings less accurate. Further, the relative importance of cones and rods changes as light level decreases within the mesopic range. At the top, vision is still mostly foveal and photopic. Near the bottom, vision is more scotopic and peripheral. Studies show, however, that the photopic curve, and hence photometer spectral sensitivity, is accurate for foveal viewing.

## 2. Measurement Scenarios

The ideal method accurately recreates the scene and obtains direct luminance measurements. Most accurate reconstruction generally requires at least 1) the original lighting and 2) the original target, clothing, vehicles, etc. If the readings must be taken outdoors, then the reconstruction requires 3) the same weather conditions and 4) the same time of day so that astronomical light sources, sun and moon, will be in the correct positions. Some departures from this ideal are important while others are relatively trivial.

*Lighting variations:* Following an accident in dim illumination, authorities frequently increase lighting as a remedial measure. They may add new lights or replace old bulbs/housings, etc. with new ones. Subsequent light readings will then be too high without some attempts to recreate original conditions. The obvious step is to mask or to filter the new lights to original levels. A less adequate alternative is to hood the target so that the increased lighting does not provide direct illumination. This still allows secondary reflection to affect light levels. Lastly, lamp outputs decrease with age, so a measurement taken years after an accident may be too low. The IESNA Handbook (2000) outlines a list of light loss factors that estimate the difference between new and old street lighting sources.

*Target, clothing, vehicle, etc. variations:* In some cases, the original objects (vehicle, person's clothes, etc.) may not be available. The best procedure is then to find substitutes that resemble the originals as closely as possible. For example, the scene recreation may require a pedestrian wearing similar clothing or a vehicle of the same make, model, color and year. Carefully chosen substitutes only minimally reduce measurement validity.

*Weather variations.* Measurements lose some validity if taken in different weather conditions than those existing at the time of the accident. If the variation is a difference in cloud cover, one strategy is to adjust measurements using the scale factors in United States Naval Observatory Circular No. 171.

*Date and time variations.* Date/time precision is not necessarily critical. Anniversary date/time can be reasonably simulated by equating for sun altitude. It isn't the clock that determines solar illumination but rather position in the sky or over the horizon. For example, suppose an accident occurred on November 1, 2004, at 5:40 p.m. in Pittsburgh. The sun altitude was -5.2° (5.2° below the horizon) and the azimuth (clockwise direction from north) was 255°. If the expert proposes to make measurements on October 1, 2007, then the best time would be slightly after 6:25 p.m. when the sun is at -5.1°. The azimuth will be 270°, but this likely creates a relatively small error, unless there is a large variation in the horizon height, i.e., the sun would move from a flat horizon to behind mountains. Large azimuth differences can be important, especially if the sun is just above or below the horizon.

Also, night is night. That is, if the accident occurs past the end of astronomical twilight, then exact time and sun position do not matter. The only complication arises from contributions by man-made light sources. If both 10:00 p.m. and 3:00 a.m. are nighttime, then solar illumination is the same. However, car headlamps and buildings may contribute significant light at 10:00 p.m. but not at 3:00 a.m..

Sun position also exhibits year-to-year variation, even on the anniversary date and time. According to the U.S. Naval Observatory, for example, on September 15, 2001, at 8:08 p.m. EDT in Pittsburgh, the sun altitude was -8.3° and azimuth was 280.8°. On the same date and time in 2004, the altitude was -8.4° and the azimuth was 280.7°. Measurement variations between these two conditions are lost in the noise.

Lastly, moonlight is a minor concern. The moon produces very little illumination and is usually an inconsequential light source unless the conditions are otherwise pitch black. The night sky also typically exhibits "sky glow," a general ambient light resulting from natural sources such as stars, and from man-made sources reflecting off the clouds or upper atmosphere. In comparison, even a full moon's contribution to illumination is likely small. For example, moonlight seldom exceeds .2 lux (United States Naval Observatory Circular No. 171), which equates about .03 cd/m$^2$ for a 50 percent reflectance object. The method for making this computation is the next topic.

## B. Indirect Luminance Determination

If direct measurement is not possible, then the indirect method calculates luminance by multiplying illumination and reflectance. The moonlight examples would be calculated:

$$\text{Luminance}(\text{cd}/\text{m}^2) = \frac{\text{Reflectance} \times \text{Illuminance}(\text{lux})}{\Pi} = \frac{0.5 \times 0.2}{3.1416} = .03$$

Both illumination and reflectance can be either directly measured or estimated from other data such as tables, light source specifications and astronomical positions. Each step away from direct luminance measurement, however, requires new assumptions that introduce uncertainty and lower validity. In order to explain both indirect methods and their limitations, I must digress back into light measurement theory and reflective surfaces, topics discussed earlier.

**Table 13.1**
**Typical illumination values (lux)**

| Lighting | Illuminance (lux) |
|---|---|
| Bright sun | 50,000–100,000 |
| Hazy day | 25,000–50,000 |
| Cloudy bright | 10,000–25,000 |
| Cloudy dull | 2,000–10,000 |
| Shop windows | 1,000–5,000 |
| Civil twilight | 3.3–333 |
| Office | 200–300 |
| Living rooms | 50–200 |
| Corridors | 50–100 |
| Good street light | 20 |
| Sunset | 1–100 |
| Full moon | 0.01–0.1 |
| Starlight | 0.0001–0.001 |

### 1. Luminance vs. Illuminance

Chapter 3 provided a general background in light measurement theory. The two most useful photometric units are illuminance and luminance, two concepts often confused. Luminance is the quantity of light reaching the eye from a given direction. It is normally measured in units of $cd/m^2$, although some books still use the antiquated term, "nits." Illumination is the amount of light falling on a surface. It is measured in units of lux (SI) or foot-candles (English), where 1 ft-cd = 10.76 lux.

There are both direct (making measurements) and indirect (normative data) methods for determining illumination. The direct method measures incident light by putting an "illuminance photometer" (also called an "illuminometer," "illuminance meter" or "lux meter.") up against the surface and reading the output (Figure 13.1). The meter may be parallel ("horizontal illuminance") or perpendicular ("vertical illuminance") to the ground. In measuring roadway lighting, vertical illuminance measurements are taken at a height of 4 feet or 1.5 meters above the road surface. Table 13.1 shows some typical illuminance readings.

While measuring the target illuminance is straightforward, measuring the background is more problematic at times. Suppose a viewer must detect a pedestrian or some other object against a distant background of sky, hills, etc. A vertical reading by an illuminometer pointed in the background direction measures light from all sources and locations. Some of these may be remote from the target and not part of the immediate background. The reading will only be useful if the background is essentially uniform.

Moreover, illumination, by itself, reveals little about the visual environment because it does not specify the amount of light actually reaching the eye:

> "Illuminance criteria have been proven to be inadequate predictors of the effectiveness of lighting systems. Although the visibility of targets is typically directly proportional to

illuminance (all other variables held constant), there are too many intervening variables that determine the visual stimulus and the efficiency with which that stimulus is processed by the visual system." (Staplin, Gish, Decina, Lococo, Harkey, Tawneh, Lyles, Mace and Garvey, 1997)

It is worth remembering this paragraph when evaluating illumination-based lighting regulations and guidelines. Illumination level criteria are at best a rough guide. They seldom consider reflectance or other environmental variables and usually assume young, normally sighted viewers. As a result of such considerations, standards should not be automatically accepted in forensic matters as realistic lighting guidelines. An analysis by Templer (1992), for example, suggests that lighting standards for stairs might be too low by a factor of four. Moreover, all lighting regulations and recommendations, as with most standards, are a compromise among many factors, including cost, light pollution, glare, etc.

Roadway lighting design has evolved beyond illumination criteria. Illuminance standards once governed roadway lighting, but these proved inadequate for reasons stated in the paragraph above. The next step in lighting design was luminance-based standards, since luminance more accurately reflects the quantity of light reaching the viewer's eye. Evidence (e.g., Janoff, 2002) suggested that even luminance-based standards are insufficient. Remember, people don't see light; they see contrast, so the newest design methods employ criteria that are psychophysical and based on a contrast detection measure VL, which is derived from the Adrian (1989) model discussed in the next chapter.

However, illuminance information can still be useful and can at least get you in the ballpark. Sometimes it is possible to estimate average reflectances. At other times, as in the Templer analysis and the "twilight envelope" in the next chapter, existing data roughly tie visual performance to illumination levels.

Illuminance can also serve as a step in the ultimate goal of determining luminance and eventually contrast, as the moonlight calculation shows. The next section discusses various methods for determining illuminance and reflectance.

## 2. Estimating Illuminance

An expert can either directly measure illuminance or estimate it from other data. The two most common scenarios requiring estimation are 1) outdoor accidents, where the sun is the main light source and 2) road accidents, where headlamps provide the primary lighting.

*Using astronomical data for outdoor accidents.* To estimate the solar contribution to illumination for an accident at a given date and time, first find the sun position, which is specified by elevation (angle above the horizon) and azimuth (clockwise horizontal angle from true north). Next, determine the amount of illumination provided from that position. Both steps can be accomplished computationally or by consulting tables.

The sun creates three main illumination components: direct, diffuse and reflected. The direct component is light that travels on a straight line from the sun to the surface. The amount of illumination falling on an outdoor surface is then highly related to sun position. On cloudy days there is no direct component. The sun still creates a diffuse component by means of atmospheric scatter. Surface orientation will, however, be less critical. Lastly, the sun can illuminate objects indirectly through reflection off of other surfaces, such as the ground.

Solar illumination variations are generally not critical when the sun is high in the sky. Contrast thresholds approximate Weber's Law in high daylight,[4] so sensitivity does not change with ambient illumination. (See Chapter 14.) Variation in sun position and its illumination is important only when the sun is near or over the horizon. In this case, ambient illumination, luminance and visibility vary greatly with sun position. Low sun altitude can also create glare, as discussed later.

Three landmark astronomical events occur as the sun rises/falls over the horizon. The first is sunrise/sunset, the time when the upper edge of the sun's disk is on the horizon. The second is twilight, the time when the sun is below the horizon but still providing illumination. Finally night begins at the end of twilight in the evening and ends at the beginning of twilight in the morning.

Twilight is a common time for outdoor accidents. Contrast sensitivity declines rapidly as the eye moves to mesopic and possibly to scotopic operation. The sun is still providing both foreground and background illumination, so artificial light sources, such as car headlamps are less effective at creating contrast. In addition, visual skills, such as reaction time, fall rapidly (Campbell, Rothwell and Perry, 1987).

Twilight divides into three different phases, which the U.S. Naval Observatory describes as:

> *Civil twilight:* "is defined to begin in the morning, and to end in the evening when the center of the Sun is geometrically 6 degrees below the horizon. This is the limit at which twilight illumination is sufficient, under good weather conditions, for *terrestrial objects to be clearly distinguished*; at the beginning of morning civil twilight, or end of evening civil twilight, the horizon is clearly defined and the brightest stars are visible under good atmospheric conditions in the absence of moonlight or other illumination. In the morning before the beginning of civil twilight and in the evening after the end of civil twilight, artificial illumination is normally required to carry on ordinary outdoor activities. Complete darkness, however, ends sometime prior to the beginning of morning civil twilight and begins sometime after the end of evening civil twilight;"
>
> *Nautical twilight:* "is defined to begin in the morning, and to end in the evening, when the center of the sun is geometrically 12 degrees below the horizon. At the beginning or end of nautical twilight, under good atmospheric conditions and in the absence of other illumination, *general outlines of ground objects may be distinguishable*, but detailed outdoor operations are not possible, and the horizon is indistinct;" and
>
> *Astronomical twilight:* "is defined to begin in the morning, and to end in the evening when the center of the Sun is geometrically 18 degrees below the horizon. Before the beginning of astronomical twilight in the morning and after the end of astronomical twilight in the evening the sun does not contribute to sky illumination; for a considerable interval after the beginning of morning twilight and before the end of evening twilight, *sky illumination is so faint that it is practically imperceptible.*"

In most U.S. latitudes, each twilight phase lasts roughly thirty minutes. Many available computer programs and tables specify twilight times as well as solar position. *The Explanatory Supplement To The Astronomical Ephemeris And The American Ephemeris And Nautical Almanac* (Seidelman, 1992) and the U.S. Naval Observatory (http://aa.usno.navy.mil/) provide times for sunset and various stages of twilight for any longitude and latitude over a wide range of days in the past and future. They also provide sun position at any time at any longitude or latitude. All of these sources, however, provide only approximations to sun (and moon) position. Originating from a naval observatory, the tables not surprisingly assume a perfectly flat horizon at sea level. Buildings, hills and other irregularities on the horizon can change estimates. In addition, local weather conditions cause refraction changes to the atmosphere that produce variations in sun locations near the horizon.

Several sources provide illuminance estimates as a function of sun position. *The Explanatory Supplement To The Astronomical Ephemeris And The American Ephemeris And Nautical Almanac* (Seidelman, 1992) also shows illumination estimates for sun positions. In addition, the United States Naval Observatory Circular No. 171 has hopelessly outdated Basic and Fortran computer programs for calculating astronomical events and resulting illuminances. These are of little use, but the document also provides handy figures showing illuminance for various sun and moon positions during daylight and twilight and under four different weather conditions, ranging from clear sky to heavy overcast.

*Estimating Illuminance From Headlamp Data.* The other common scenario is a road accident where headlamps are a prime light source. An expert may need to estimate headlamp illumination in order to determine road object contrast or to calculate viewer glare. The following steps permit estimation at any arbitrary point, such as the viewer's eye.

1. *Determine the horizontal and vertical angles between the left headlamp and the viewer's eye (or other point).* For example, if the oncoming vehicle's left headlamp is 5 feet to the viewer's left, then the lateral angle at 200 feet is arctan (5/200)=1.4°. If the viewer eye height is 42 inches and the lamp mounting height is 33 inches, then the vertical angle is arctan (.75/200)=.21°.
2. *Determine the number of candela being thrown by the light source to the viewer's eye at the specified angles.* Schoettle, Sivak and Flannagan (2002) provide a convenient reference source of headlamp outputs for low and high beam headlamps. Their tables show 25th, 50th and 75th percentile values for various angles left, right, up and down measured from sales-weighted samples of U.S. and European vehicles. For example, median (U.S.) low-beam output for a lateral angle of 1.4° left and .21° up would be about 987 candela.
3. *Calculate illuminance at the eye.* Apply the inverse-square law. Two hundred feet = 60.96m. At 200 feet, $987/(60.96)^2=987/(3716.12)=0.27$ lux.
4. *Sum the two headlamps.* Perform the first three steps for the oncoming vehicle's right headlamp and add it to the illuminance produced by the left.

The result is only approximate since it represents an "average headlamp." Moreover, it does not include variations due to lamp misalignment, wear, dirt, road grade or curvature, and lamp voltage.

### 3. Determining Reflectance

Chapter 3 discussed the surface variables, reflectance, texture and orientation. Dark objects reflect little of the incident light while lighter objects reflect most of the light falling on them. Reflection to the eye also varies with surface texture and orientation. Reflective surfaces fall into several classes: diffuse, specular, spread and retroreflective. Diffuse surfaces scatter incident light in many different directions. A "Lambertian" surface is a perfectly diffuse reflector that scatters light equally in all directions. Unless the surface is purely Lambertian, the viewer's eye position and angle with the surface affect the amount of light reaching the eye. Very smooth surfaces, such as a mirror, create "specular" reflection, which sends the light in only a narrow direction. The familiar "angle of incidence equals angle of reflection" rule applies. A "spread" surface resembles a specular surface, except that it reflects a cone of light rather than a single ray. Some surfaces are compound, meaning that they can exhibit diffuse, specular or spread reflection depending on the incidence angle. Lastly, retroreflective surfaces reflect light back in the direction from which it came regardless of incidence angle. It is the principle used to increase conspicuity of road signs and tractor-trailers at night.

There are three ways to determine reflectance. The first directly measures reflectance with a device called a "reflectometer," which sends a known intensity beam toward a surface and then measures the amount of light reflected back. Second, an expert can consult tables containing reflectances for common objects and surfaces. For example, the Illuminating Engineering Society of America Lighting Handbook (2000) classifies road surfaces and lists asphalt reflectance as 7 percent unless it is very smooth and lists Portland cement as 10 percent.

The third method compares luminance measurements of surfaces with known and unknown reflectance. A photometer measures the surface luminance and then measures the luminance of the standard reflector held at the same position. Assuming constant incident illumination and surface texture, the ratio of luminances is the ratio of reflectances. A readily available reference is the 18 percent[5] standard reflectance card used by photographers. If the surface luminance is half that of the card, for example, the surface has 9 percent reflectance.

Retroreflectors are an important method for increasing nighttime visibility on the roadway. If a sign surface were diffuse, much of the incident light would scatter, reflect in different directions and miss the viewer's eye. If the surface were specular, the reflected light would miss the viewer's eye unless the viewing and incidence angle were exactly 90°. In contrast, retroreflective surfaces return incident light striking a sign or strip of conspicuity tape back in the original direction, regardless of surface orientation. Studies show that retroreflection can dramatically increase visibility distance to both pedestrians (e.g., Shinar, 1985) and vehicles (e.g., Ziedman, Burger, Smith, Mullholland and Sharkey, 1981).

Retroreflector effectiveness depends on several variables, including:

- Coefficient of reflection. Some surfaces are more efficient light reflectors. The quantity "Specific Intensity per Unit Area" (SIA) in units of cd/lx/$m^2$ is a measure of the retroreflector's efficiency.
- Entrance angle: the angle at which the beam strikes the surface relative to the "surface normal," a line perpendicular to the reflector plane. The closer the entrance angle to the normal, the greater the effective SIA. Depending on the material (and observation angle), efficiency falls to about 35–50 percent for a 45° entrance angle.
- Observation angle: the angle between the viewer's eye and the entrance angle.[6] The observer sees less light as this angle grows, although the maximum is slightly off 0°. Variations in observation angle have more impact than variations in entrance angle. During tests, observation angles are .2° or .5°. Depending on material, observation angles as small as .7° can render retroreflective signs and tape invisible, making retroreflectors a mixed blessing.
- Color. Not surprisingly, the most efficient reflectors are white, followed by yellow, green and red. Research (Tansley, and Petrusic, 1994) has confirmed that white retroreflective tape is the most visible. However, the typical alternating white-red pattern presumably has better conspicuity. As discussed in Chapter 4, optimizing conspicuity is not synonymous with optimizing visibility.
- Age and dirt. Older and dirtier retroreflective material is less efficient.

- Grade. Retroreflective materials are categorized as Engineering Grades (ASTM Type I), Super Engineering Grade (ASTM Type II), High Intensity (ASTM Type III), and Micro-prismatic (ASTM Type IV, VII, VIII, IX and X). Each grade has its own values for the three main variables.

An example illustrates how these factors combine to determine visibility. Suppose a driver is traveling down a road that has been blocked ahead by a jackknifed tractor-trailer. The driver's headlamp beams strike the reflective tape along the trailer's side as well as the trailer itself. Will the driver see the trailer?

First, the retroreflective tape concentrates light and should be visible at a greater distance than the diffuse surface of a box trailer. If the trailer box is white, however, it will become visible sooner than if the box is painted a darker color. If the trailer is a flatbed, so that there is no upper surface, then the driver must rely exclusively on the retroreflective tape. It is hardly surprising then that retroreflective tape reduces accident rates most on flatbed trailers (Morgan 2001).

The tape's advantage depends on its retroreflective efficiency. Cleaner and newer tape has greater reflectance, and standard references provide data on efficiency of various grades. If the material is older, however, it may be desirable to measure the efficiency, a task most easily performed with a reflectometer. Measurement technique should follow the standard set of conditions of entrance and observation angles, etc.

Next, the driver's vehicle can influence observation angle. A truck driver sitting high above headlamp level, for example, has a greater observation angle than a driver in a small car, where eye and headlamp levels are closer together. On the other hand, the truck's higher mounted headlamps may throw more light farther, so the driver starts with more incident light.

Lastly, the angle of the tractor-trailer across the road affects the entrance angle. If the trailer is almost perpendicular to the roadway, the entrance angle is near optimum and retroreflective efficiency will be high. In many cases, however, the trailer is angled across the roadway. The entrance angle is large and efficiency drops. A similar vertical problem occurs if the driver approaches a tractor-trailer at the crest of a hill.

## 13.4 Step 3: Compute The Physical Contrast Of The Target On The Background

### A. Direct Looking

There are several different ways to calculate contrast. When reading a visibility paper, be sure to determine which calculation the author is using. Different methods give different results, and the relationship among different formulae can be confusing.

Older research sometimes calculated contrast as a simple ratio:

$$C = \frac{L_O}{L_B}$$

C is contrast, $L_O$ is the object luminance and $L_B$ is the background. This has become almost obsolete, and the most common calculation replaces $L_O$ with $L_O$-$L_B$, becoming the Weber contrast described in Chapter 2:

$$C = \frac{L_O - L_B}{L_B}$$

If the target is brighter than the background, then the contrast will be positive (light on dark). If the object is darker than the background, the contrast is negative (dark on light). This creates some calculation complications. Positive contrast can range from 0 to a very large number while negative contrast can range only from 0 to -1. Some prefer to multiple by negative contrast -100 in order to derive a percentage. In either case, positive and negative numbers are not directly comparable. One way to circumvent the problem is to calculate using the absolute value of ΔL:

$$C = \frac{|L_O - L_B|}{L_B}$$

This method avoids negative numbers. Further, equal size increments and decrements create equal contrast value. On a background of 10, for example, an increment of 1 and a decrement of -1 have the same contrast, .1. This is desirable because positive and negative contrasts are then directly comparable.

Anther calculation method is "Michelson contrast":

$$C = \frac{L_{max} - L_{min}}{L_{max} + L_{min}}$$

where $L_{max}$ and $L_{min}$ are the maximum and minimum luminances. Michelson contrast adds the target luminance to the denominator and produces a contrast range from 0 to 1. In negative contrast, the Michelson and Weber calculations give similar numbers if the target is dim and contrast is low. Generally, however, the two formulae give very different ranges of numbers and are not directly comparable.

Weber and Michelson are applicable in different circumstances. Weber contrast is the normal calculation for a small object on an approximately uniform background. For example, Weber contrast is appropriate for the visibility of a light or retroreflective tape against the uniform sky or a dark background at night. Michelson contrast has far less application, as it's primarily used in research with gratings composed of equal width light and dark stripes (e.g., Green, 1983). The IESNA Handbook (2000) notes that the formula is better termed "modulation" than "contrast."

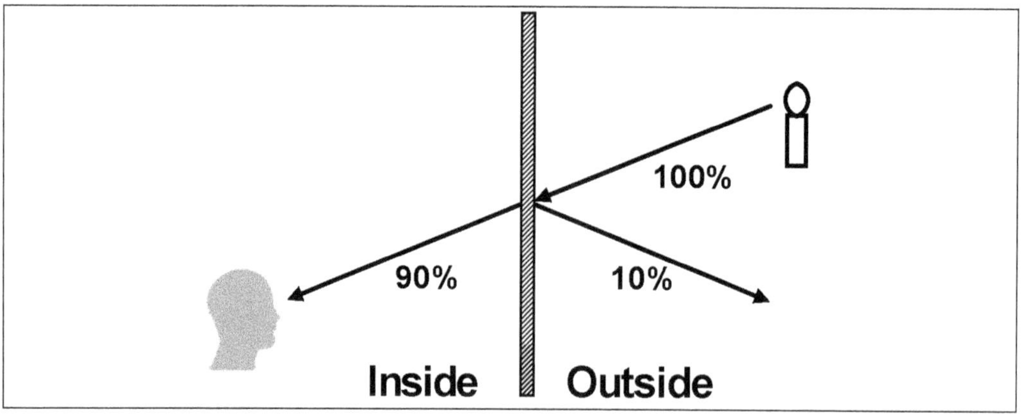


***Figure 13.2*** *Light rays for observer looking through a transparent surface. The picture ignores absorption and internal reflection.*

## B. Viewing Through A Transparent Surface

In some instances, the viewer has a sightline to the target but must look through a transparent surface such as a windshield, helmet visor or sheet of glass. Transparent surfaces can alter the physical contrast, create pattern masking and cause accommodative and vergence error.

Figure 13.2[7] shows the schematic of an observer looking through a transparent surface. In the example, assume that the viewer is looking at an object outside a window. Without the window, contrast calculations would proceed as described above. However, the window surface transmits 90 percent of the outside light, reflects 10 percent from the viewer and has negligible absorption. The window cuts the incoming light by 10 percent.[8]

$$C = .9\frac{(L_O - L_B)}{L_B}$$

However, the picture shows only one half of the story. The inside light is similarly striking the surface and is also being transmitted and reflected. The inside light reflection acts like a veil and lowers contrast, so it would be added to the denominator.

Ultimately, the importance of veiling depends on two factors. The first is the ratio of surface reflectance to transmission. High reflectance and low transmission create more veiling. The second is the ratio of inside and outside light intensity. If the outside light is much stronger, the veiling will have minimal effect. If the inside light is relatively high, as when a person inside a lighted room looks through a window out into the night, then the inside light might overwhelm the outside scene.

In addition to veiling, transparent surfaces may raise thresholds for other reasons. Pattern masking occurs when the inside light reflects a structured scene onto the surface and obscures the outside image. Unlike background camouflage effects, the pattern mask also covers the target, making it especially difficult to see. However, some structured reflection may be beneficial because it alerts the viewer to the surface's presence. In one case, a customer walked out of a dark bank vault into a bright office. She crashed into the vault's clear glass door because there was no inner reflection alerting her to the obstacle.

Lastly, a transparent surface can create accommodative and vergence error. The eye creates a sharp retinal image by accommodating focus to the viewing distance. If the viewer must see through a transparent surface, the accommodation tends to slip toward the surface's plane. This "Mandelbaum Effect" causes objects beyond the surface to appear out of focus. Similarly, the eyes tend to verge toward the plane of the transparency. Objects significantly nearer and farther are not fused.

## C. Glare Effects

Glare is a sensation created by a light source significantly brighter than the prevailing adaptation level. It is a complex phenomenon that is categorized along several dimensions, space, time and intensity. The simplest categorization distinguishes between discomfort and disability glare. Discomfort glare occurs when the glare source creates a feeling of annoyance or dislike, but no loss of contrast sensitivity. It is measured by the 9-point De Boer Scale, where 1 means unbearable glare and 9 means that it is just noticeable. "Disability glare" is similar, but causes a measurable visual loss. Disability glare further breaks down into subcategories: dazzle, scotomatic, flash-blindness, and veiling. Dazzle is light sufficiently intense to cause physical pain and produces protective responses, such as closing one eye. Scotomatic glare is something like an afterimage in that it reduces sensitivity to a particular portion of the retina after a flash. Flash blindness (essentially the transient adaptation described in Chapter 3) is a general loss of sensitivity following exposure to a flash. Finally, veiling glare (or "brightness glare") is the light scattered in the ocular media during a flash. The name is highly descriptive since the viewer is then effectively looking through a semi-transparent veil. The vast majority of glare research concerns veiling glare.

Veiling glare occurs when light entering the eye scatters in the optical media and creates stray light. The Weber contrast equation then becomes:

$$C = \frac{(L_O + L_v) - (L_B + L_v)}{L_B + L_v} = \frac{L_O - L_B}{L_B + L_v}$$

where $L_v$ is the equivalent veiling luminance, the luminance of a uniform area of light that would change contrast sensitivity by the same amount as the glare source.

There are several equations for calculating veiling glare. The Illuminating Society of North America Handbook (2000) uses:

$$L_v = 9.2 \sum_{i}^{n} \frac{E_i}{\theta_i(\theta_i + 1.5)}$$

Where $L_v$ is the equivalent veiling luminance in cd/m$^2$, $E_i$ = illuminance from the *i*th glare source at the eye in lux, and θi is the angle between the target and the *i*th glare source in degrees. From the equation, it is clear that glare increases with strength of the glare source and closeness to the sightline. If the visual field has multiple glare sources, then the total veil is the linear sum of the individual glares.

However, glare depends on the eye's optical quality, which decreases with age. The Holladay-Stiles equation for calculating veiling glare from a source 1°–30° in the periphery is:

$$L_{eq} = k \frac{E_{glare}}{\theta^2}$$

where k is an age-dependent constant.

## 1. Calculating k, Age Effects

Since aging degrades the optical media and increases scatter, glare effects are much greater in older viewers. Adrian (1989) has a simple age correction:

$$K = (.00752\ \text{Age} - 1.883)^2 + .92$$

By this calculation, glare effects double by about age seventy. However, age effects vary with glare angle. The CIE has several age-adjusted Holladay-Stiles equations, each applicable to a different range of glare angles.

For angles of 1°–30°, the equation is:

$$L_v = 10 \times \left[1 + \left(\frac{\text{Age}}{70}\right)^4\right] \times \frac{1}{\theta^2}$$

For angles going down from 30° to 0.1°:

$$L_v = \frac{10}{\theta^3} + \left[1 + \left(\frac{Age}{62.5}\right)^4\right] \times \frac{5}{\theta^2}$$

Finally, CIE has a more general equation for a broader angle range of 100°–0.1°:

$$L_V = \frac{10}{\theta^3} + \left[1 + \left(\frac{Age}{62.5}\right)^4\right] \times \left[\frac{5}{\theta^2} + 0.1p\right] + 0.025p$$

This equation adds a new variable, p, eye color, which becomes significant at larger angles. Brown eyes have a value of about 0.5 while light blue eyes might have a value of 1 or even 1.2.

## 2. Calculating E, Illuminance At The Eye

The final glare variable is $E_{glare}$, the glare illuminance at the eye. The most common forensic problem involves calculating this value for headlamps of oncoming cars. The method for estimating illuminance from vehicle headlamps was described above.

The recent advent of high intensity discharge (HID) headlamps has increased the likelihood that drivers will experience more disability glare on the roadways. Compared to normal headlamps, HID headlamps exhibit both higher luminous flux, that makes them appear brighter, and a shorter wavelength spectrum. They also have a wider beam pattern that illuminates areas farther from the roadway.

HID headlamps have several benefits. The increased brightness obviously allows a greater visual range and better contrast detection. The wider beam spread illuminates the roadside better and promotes detection of pedestrians at the curb. Further, the wider beams also produce a marginal improvement in steering performance. Lastly, HID headlamps last longer—as long as they aren't stolen off the car, a common occurrence.

On the other hand, the new technology increases glare due to the higher brightness and possibly due to the bluer spectrum, although evidence for this wavelength effect is weak. The increased glare can make pedestrians, turn signals, road signs, and other warnings less visible. HID headlamps will most seriously impair older drivers, who have high glare susceptibility. They will then most impair the segment of drivers who are already operating at a visual deficit. Since older people censor their driving based on their visual limitations, HID headlamps will likely force many older drivers off the road because they cannot contend with the increased glare.

## 3. Final Comments On Glare

In addition to veil intensity, several other factors affect glare's impact:

- Glare calculation should include all glare sources but are usually restricted to headlamps of oncoming vehicles. Other common glare sources include light from the reflection of the driver's own headlamps illumination on the road. Wet roads can create specular reflections that increase glare.
- Recovery time: Glare calculations only cover the time that the glare source illuminates the retina. However, driver vision is impaired for a period even after the glare source is gone. Not surprisingly, recovery time increases with longer exposure duration, high source intensity and low background luminance. Older people have longer recovery times.
- Temporal transients. Glare equations assume a steady glare to which the driver has adapted. Drivers may have contrast sensitivity disrupted more by transient than steady glare

(Bichao, Yager, and Meng, 1995). The loss is especially large in the first few seconds after glare removal, possibly because of the transient adaptation effect discussed in Chapter 3.

- Models assume that veiling glare equally affects the entire visual field. In fact, veiling is not necessarily uniform and may reduce visibility less for objects that are farther from the glare source.
- Optical imperfections can magnify glare effects. Scratched, abraded or dirty windshields or eyeglasses increase light scatter and glare.

## D. Atmospheric Effects

The viewer's sightline is always "obstructed" by both air molecules and "aerosols," very fine suspended particles such as dust. These atmospheric components can affect contrast calculation when the air is misty or foggy or when distance between an object and the eye is great. Atmospheric effects consist of two basic components. The first is scattering that puts additional veiling light ("air light") in the sightline between person and object. Second, light loses intensity as it travels through the medium. It is due to scattering, which occurs when a photon strikes an object and is reradiated in a new direction, and absorption, when the photon's energy is transferred to the object. The combined effect of scattering and absorption is called extinction, $\sigma$.

Extinction's magnitude depends on several factors including particle size and wavelength. Generally, very fine particles cause more scatter. However, scatter also maximizes when the particles/molecules and the light's wavelength are similar in size. The sky is blue because blue light scatters most—its wavelength is the same size as the diameter of air molecules. Aerosols come in various sizes and cause colored or gray veils, depending on their size distribution.

In calculating atmospheric effects on physical contrast, the important variables are $\sigma$ and $L_{sky}$, the sky brightness. The methods for determining the extinction coefficient are beyond the scope of this chapter but are readily available in some meteorology texts (e.g., Tricker, 1970). Models of sky luminance are available from sources such as the CIE. In cases where atmospheric extinction effects are important, visibility may be calculated in three different scenarios.

### 1. Standard Contrast Calculation

Contrast is calculated from luminance. The luminance of a distant object seen through an atmosphere of known extinction is:

$$L = \left\lfloor L_O e^{-x\sigma} \right\rfloor + \left\lfloor L_{sky}(1 - e^{x\sigma}) \right\rfloor$$

which gives the luminance of a target at distance *x*. The first term is the effect of extinction on an object whose luminance at 0 range is $L_o$, and the second is the effect of air light scatter between eye and object. To compute contrast for a distant object, use the luminances computed with this formula for object and background in the standard contrast equations. The same analytic method applies to contrast threshold determination in other situations, such as the ability to see through smoke in a building fire.

With a few caveats, contrast in heavy atmospheric conditions can be directly calculated as Koschmieder's relationship (1924):

$$C = C_o e^{-x\sigma}$$

where $C_o$ is contrast at distance 0.

### 2. Visual Range

In some cases, the visibility question is framed as maximum detection distance rather than in terms of contrast threshold. Here, the variable of interest is then "visual range," defined as the distance at which a black object is visible against the sky. The general equation is:

$$v = \frac{1}{\sigma}\log\frac{1}{\Delta}$$

where v is the visibility range and Δ is the (negative) contrast threshold. An assumed contrast threshold of .05 produces:

$$V = \frac{3}{\sigma}$$

However, .05 is an unrealistically low (or high) threshold in many situations. Middleton (1952) wisely dubbed this convention "meteorological range" since it may not represent visibility under real conditions.

### 3. Visibility of a Light

Lastly, the issue in some cases is the visibility distance at night of a self-luminous object, such as a warning light. According to Allard's Law, the illumination at the eye, *E*, produced by a point source of candela *I*, and distance *x* is simply the inverse square law modified to take extinction into account:

$$E = \frac{1}{x^2}e^{x\sigma}$$

The value, $E_t$, illumination threshold, can then be calculated for the visual range, *V*, as:

$$E_t = \frac{I}{V^2}e^{-V\sigma}$$

## E. Adverse Weather Effects

Fog, rain and snow impair many visual judgments. Most weather-related vision research has focused on visual range and only to a lesser extent on contrast detection. Adverse weather also impairs judgments of speed and distance.

Calculating visibility levels in poor weather is difficult. Multiple models exist for estimating visibility in just about any type of adverse weather. However, the models require values for weather variables that are difficult to estimate. Weather is local to time and place, and weather stations are seldom located exactly at accident sites. Fog swirls, drifts and changes height, so it is hard to know the variable values at the particular place and time of the accident. Moreover, stations do not record some of the required data. Variable values such as droplet size, snow concentration, etc. may not be readily available or easily computable. Further, nighttime visibility analysis is complicated by headlamp backscatter that further impairs vision.

The available research data are also sparse. The difficulty of experimentally producing and specifying the desired "weather" conditions has hampered research attempts to measure visibility as a function of environmental factors. The existing data are limited to a small subset of the possible variables and variable values, so generality is low. There are no studies that have manipulated target size, contrast, visual field location, driver age or any other important visual variables. However, the qualitative effects of adverse weather are readily predictable from research data. Given these caveats, here is a brief overview of the perceptual effects and some sample visibility models.

### 1. Fog

Fog decreases luminance and physical contrast and blurs edges. These conditions obviously contribute to road accidents by decreasing visibility distance and target detectability. In addition, fog has more subtle perceptual effects that are equally important. These include misjudgments of speed and distance and the narrowing of visual attention.

During the day, fog operates much like the atmospheric effects described above, lowering contrast through extinction. In this case, however, the particles are a suspension of very fine water droplets in the air. Extinction and contrast loss depend on the distance of the object and size and density of the moisture droplets suspended in the atmosphere. Visibility is a function of viewing distance, fog density, droplet size distribution, sun altitude and viewer orientation with respect to the sun. Since the droplets are bigger than wavelengths in the visible spectrum, there is no color selectivity.

At night, light beams, such as car headlamps, complicate fog effects. There are extinction and air light effects in both directions—when the light goes from source to object and then when it is reflected back to the eye. Fog weakens the headlamp's effectiveness by scattering the light forward on the outbound leg of its journey. Further, the fog causes some of the beam output to scatter back to the eye before reaching the target. This "backscatter" creates veiling, lowering contrast and possibly creating glare.

The amount of backscatter increases with beam intensity. It may seem natural to switch on high beams in order to see farther. In fact, the main effect is to scatter more light back to the eye and to decrease visibility. Fog lights minimize backscatter by sitting well below eye level, aiming straight ahead and minimizing direct reflection back to the driver's eye. They further illuminate fog near the ground, where density may be lower.

Fog and the resulting lowered physical contrast have several secondary effects on perception.

*Motion Perception.* First, fog lowers the apparent speed of other objects in the visual field. Low contrast objects appear to move slower (e.g., Anstis, 2003; Green, 1993; Snowden, Stimpson, and Ruddle, 1998; Stone and Thompson, 1992; Thompson, 1982), so discrimination between moving and stationary objects is more difficult. Imagine a person driving along a freeway and seeing a faint car. It will be very difficult to detect that it has stopped because the lower contrast impairs speed judgments. Moreover, the driver has an expectation that cars do not stop on freeways. The driver may then fail to realize that the car ahead is stopped until it is too late.

*Self Motion.* Fog can also cause a driver to underestimate his own speed. One way that drivers judge speed is by their movement relative to objects in the visual field. (It is easier to see clouds move by the edges of buildings than to see them move when they are merely suspended in the sky.) When driving fast, for example, telephone poles on the roadside zip by. In fog, perceived speed relative to other objects in the optic flow field is apparently lower, so a driver will likely underestimate his own speed. Objects can actually slow to a stop with sufficiently low contrast (Green, 1983) especially in the visual periphery which is the area most important for judging speed of self-motion. Moreover, Snowden, Stimpson, and Ruddle (1998) tested people in a driving simulator and found that drivers in low contrast conditions not only perceived slower motion of the scene but actually drove at higher speeds.

Denton (1980) illustrated the importance of having highly visible ground textures in judging speed. He tested drivers in a simulator where the "road" had a high density of markings or was more uniform. When there were many markings, the drivers adjusted their speed with good accuracy. When the road was more uniform, drivers underestimated the actual rate of motion. In fact, Denton concluded that artificially adding patterns to a roadway might be a good way to slow drivers, since they would feel as if they were moving faster than normal. Much recent research confirms that drivers use "edge rate," the number of objects passing a point in the visual field, as a means of judging speed. Fog has just the opposite effect: it removes scene pattern, slowing the apparent flow and causing drivers to believe that they are moving more slowly than their actual speed.

*Distance.* Fog also produces "aerial perspective," a visual effect that causes people to misjudge distance. People automatically perceive objects which are low contrast and indistinct as being farther away. The distance overestimation can cause accidents in several ways. The driver approaching the stopped car will judge it to be farther away than it really is and therefore underestimate the time and distance needed to stop. Further, one study (Cavallo, Colomb and Dore, 2001) suggests that drivers in fog also leave insufficient gaps with the car ahead.

*Attention.* In addition, the poor visibility causes people to concentrate their attention directly ahead in order to see where they are going. This decreases the probability of seeing pedestrians, signs, etc. in the peripheral field. A driver in theory could also judge speed by looking at the speedometer. However, drivers in fog are unlikely to risk looking at the speedometer, and away from the road, when visibility is low. Moreover, the driver is unaware that he is misperceiving his rate of motion and has no particular reason to confirm his speed with the speedometer.

Given these effects, it is hardly surprising that massive, chain-reaction crashes occur in foggy road conditions. Visibility distance is limited. Drivers are likely traveling faster than they realize while they keep their eyes glued to a lead vehicle which they are following too closely because they overestimate their distance. When the lead vehicle brakes, they have difficulty detecting the change in the angular velocity that signals a deceleration.

*Vehicle Control.* Lastly, fog and other poor visibility conditions impair steering performance. Drivers use two parts of the road to steer at high speeds. They monitor the near (lower visual field) part to maintain lane position and a distant (upper visual field) part to plan for future steering due to curves, etc. (Donges, 1978; Land and Horwood, 1995). Fog can restrict sight distance sufficiently to impair use of both the distant and near road information and produce erratic vehicle control (Harms, 1993).

## 2. Rain

Rain's effects on visibility are analogous to those of fog, but there is less scatter due to the larger particle size. Rain makes headlamps and other light sources less effective by filtering away some of their output and by reducing illumination on the road ahead. Backscatter from rain can also cause glare

However, rain introduces some new problems not present in fog. Passing cars may splash a film of dirty water on to the headlamps, further lowering headlamp effectiveness. Further, the raindrops act as lenses, distorting the light before it can reach the driver's eye and enhancing glare from oncoming vehicles. The clutter and movement caused by the raindrops falling on the windshield further draw attention and mask objects on the road. Windshield wipers do not completely solve the problem because they are never 100 percent efficient, typically leaving a smear of water across the windshield and cleaning only part of the visual field. Moreover, they periodically block vision.

Several authors have attempted to quantify visibility in rain. Bhise, Meldrum and Forbes (1981) tested driver visibility distance for detection of other vehicles in rain. They created a visibility distance model with input variables of rain rate, wiper speed and illumination. However, their model has limited practical application since it collapses data across a wide range of brightness and color contrasts.

Morris, Mounce, Button and Walton (1977) examined driver acuity and detection tasks. Results showed that acuity fell with increasing rain rate, but only at night. They calculated a simple model that specifies acuity loss as a function of rain rate and wiper speed.

$$V_a = 0.415r + 0.75559W_{25} + 0.59705W_{50} + 0.58486W_{75}$$

where $V_a$ is the visual acuity loss in minarc and r is the rain rate. If the windshield wipers were operating, then the model uses the W term for the correct speed, 25, 50 or 75 cycle/min. However, this model is limited as the authors also concluded that drop size is an important variable at night and confounds the relationship between visibility and rain rate. Windshield rake angle may also be a factor.

Rain also affects visibility by changing the amount of light reflected from the road back to the driver's eye. A normal road has a rough surface, which causes some of the headlight beam to reflect back to the driver's eye. Rainwater fills in the rough irregularities and creates a smooth specular finish on the road. The headlamp beams then strike the road, and instead of scattering, reflects almost entirely forward. The road appears darker and therefore it becomes harder to see pedestrians who are wearing dark clothes. The mirror-finish of the road also increases the chance of glare from any available source, streetlamps, business signs or headlamps of other cars. On the other hand, headlamps hit the more reflective road and bounce forward, giving them effectiveness at a greater distance. Lastly, water can reduce the reflectivity of most materials, such as clothing. Dark pedestrians become darker.

### 3. Snow

Snow also lowers visibility, especially in windy conditions. The key variable is Mf, the mass of snow passing through an area per unit time. Mf is in turn a function of both wind speed and snow concentration, which can be difficult to estimate. Given a known Mf, however, Matsuzawa, Kajiya, and Takeuchi (2002) estimated that visibility distance is related to Mf by:

$$\log(Vis) = 0.773\log(Mf) + 2.845$$

Lastly, color is also an important factor for visibility in snow and other types of bad weather. Ironically, the colors that enhance vehicle conspicuity in normal conditions can decrease their visibility in snow. Yonas and Zimmer (2006), for example, found that the orange color that makes snowplows conspicuous, creates low visibility in snow. Orange has moderately high brightness on the spectral luminosity curve and does not create much luminance contrast with the white snow. Construction vehicles are often painted yellow, which should be even less detectable because of higher brightness.

## 13.5 Conclusion

This chapter has outlined the initial steps required to perform a visibility analysis. It has examined the "physics" part of psychophysics—light measurement and methods for calculating physical contrast under a variety of conditions. Further, it has described some non-visibility effects of environmental variables on perception of speed and distance. This has been the easy part of the visibility analysis. The next chapter examines the more difficult "psycho" part of psychophysics—estimation of contrast thresholds.

## References

Adrian, W. 1989. Visibility of targets: model for calculation. *Lighting Research And Technology* 21, 181-188.

Anstis, S., 2003. Moving objects appear to slow down at low contrasts. *Neural Networks 16*, 933-938.

Bhise, V. D., J. F. Meldrum, L. M. and Forbes. 1981. Predicting driver seeing distances in natural rainfall. *Human Factors* 23, 667-682.

Bichao, I. C., D. Yager, and T. Meng. 1995. Disability glare: effects of temporal characteristics of the glare source and of the visual-field location of the test stimulus. *Journal of the Optical Society of America* A 12, 2252-2258.

Blackwell, H. R. 1946. Contrast thresholds of the human eye. *Journal of the Optical Society of America* 36, 624-643.

Bullough, J. D., Z. Fu, and J. Van Derlofske. 2002. "Discomfort and Disability Glare from Halogen and HID Headlamp Systems (Report No. SAE 2002-01-0010)." *Society of Automotive Engineers World Congress & Exhibition 2002* (SP-1668, pp. 1–5). Warrendale, PA: Society of Automotive Engineers.

Campbell, F., S. Rothwell, and M. Perry. 1987. Bad light stops play. *Ophthalmic and Physiological Optics* 72, 165-167.

Cavallo, V., M. Colomb, and J. Dore. 2001. Distance perception of vehicle rear lights in fog. Human Factors 43, 442-51.

Denton, G. 1980. The influence of visual patter on perceived speed. *Perception*, 9, 393-402.

Donges, E. 1978. A two-level model of driver steering behavior. *Human Factors* 20, 691-707.

Eloholma, M., and L. Halonen. 1999. Vision in mesopic lighting levels – The effect of spectrum and luminance levels, CIE Proceedings, Publication CIE 133.

Flannagan, M. 2007. Vision in night driving, the roles of cone and rod photoreceptors. 4th International Driving Symposium on Human Factors in Driver Assessment, Training, and Vehicle Design Skamania Lodge Stevenson, Washington, 25-31.

Green, M. 1993. Contrast detection and direction discrimination of drifting gratings. Vision Research 23, 281-289.

Harms, L. 1993. The Influence of Sight Distance on Subjects' Lateral Control: A Study of Simulated Driving in Fog. In A. G. Gale, I. D. Brown, C. M. Haslegrave, H. W. Kruysse, and S. P. Taylor (eds.), *Vision in Vehicles IV* (109–116). Amsterdam, the Netherlands: Elsevier Science.

Janoff, M. 2002. Visibility under roadway lighting. In R. Dewar and P. Olson *Human Factors In Traffic Safety*. Tucson, AZ: Lawyers & Judges Publishing Company, Inc.

Kaufman, J., and H. Haynes. 1981. IES Lighting Handbook. New York: Illuminating Engineering Society of North America.

Ketomäki, J., M. Eloholma, P. Orreveteläinen, and L. Halonen. 2003. Mesopic lighting conditions and pedestrian visibility. Ingineria Illuminatului No 11, Summer, 29-40.

Koschmieder, H. 1924. Theorie der Horizontalen Sichtweite. *Beitraege zur Physik der Atmos—phare*, vol. 12, pp. 33-53, 171-181.

Land, M., and J. Horwood. 1995. Which parts of the road guide steering. *Nature* 377, 339-340.

Leibowitz, H., and D. A. Owens. 1991. Can normal outdoor activities be carried out during civil twilight? *Applied Optics* 30, 3501-3503.

Matsuzawa, M., Y. Kajiya, and M. Takeuchi. 2002. Estimating Visibility in Blowing Snow by Wind Velocity and Snowfall Intensity. *Monthly Report of Civil Engineering Research Institute* 593, 20-27.

Middleton, W. E. K. 1952. *Vision Through The Atmosphere*. University of Toronto Press: Toronto.

Morgan, C. 2001. Effectiveness of retroreflective tape on heavy trailers. NHTSA Report DOT HS 809 222.

Morris, R. S., J. M. Mounce, J. W. Button, and N. E. Walton. 1977. Visual performance of drivers during rainfall. Transportation Research Record 628:19-25.

Rea, M. 2000. The Illuminating Engineering Society of America lighting Handbook. New York: Illuminating Engineering Society of America lighting Handbook.

Rea, M., J. Bullough, J. Freyssinier-Nova, and A. Bierman. 2004. A proposed unified system of photometry. *Lighting Research and Technology*, 36, 85-111.

Schoettle, B., M. Sivak, and M. Flannagan. 2001. High-Beam and Low-Beam Headlighting Patterns in the U.S. and Europe at the Turn of the Millennium. Report UMTRI-2001-19.

Seidelman, P., 1992. Explanatory Supplement To The Astronomical Ephemeris And The American Ephemeris And Nautical Almanac (Herndon, Va.: University Science Press).

Shinar, D. 1985. The effects of expectancy, clothing reflectance, and detection criterion on nighttime pedestrian visibility, *Human Factors* 27, 327-333.

Snowden, R., N. Stimpson, and S. Ruddle. 1998. Speed perception fogs up as visibility drops. *Nature* 392, 450.

Staplin, L., K. Gish, L. Decina, K. Lococo, D. Harkey, M. Tarawneh, R. Lyles, D. Mace, and P. Garvey. 1997. Synthesis of human factors research on older drivers and highway safety. Volume II: Human Factors and Highway Safety Research Synthesis. FHWA-RD-97-095.

Stone, L., and Thompson, P. 1992. Human speed perception is contrast dependent. *Vision Research*, 32:1535–1549.

Tansley, B. W., and W. Petrusic. 1994. The perceptual basis of heavy vehicle conspicuity and the role of retroreflective materials in increasing driver decision sight distances. Technical report for Transport Canada, Road Safety.

Templer, J. 1992. The staircase: studies of hazards, falls and safer design. The MIT Press Massachusetts Institute of Technology, Cambridge: Massachusetts.

Thompson, P. 1982. Perceived rate of movement depends on contrast. *Vision Res.* 22, 377–380.

Tricker, R. A. R. 1970. Introduction to Meteorological Optics. Mills & Boon, London.

Yonas, A., and L. Zimmerman. 2004. Improving the ability of drivers to avoid collisions with snowplows in fog and snow. Minnesota Depart Of Transportation Report MN/RC-2006-29.

Ziedman, K., W. J. Burger, L. R. Smith, M. U. Mullholland, and T. Sharkey. 1981. Improved Commercial Vehicle Conspicuity and Signaling Systems: Task II Analysis Experiments and Design Recommendations. Washington, D.C: U.S. Department of Transportation, National Highway Transportation Administration.

## Endnotes

1. The terminology of "target" has unfortunate connotations, but it is standard in visual science.

2. The discussion covers only brightness (really luminance) contrast, which is by far the most important type. In some situations, however, color, texture or even motion contrast may be relevant.

3. The focusing is not needed to sharpen the image. Rather, it properly aligns the viewer's sightline with the photo-sensitive element. That is, it ensures the meter is really reading where the viewer is looking.

4. Remember that Weber's Law may not apply to very small objects, even in daylight.

5. The 18 percent standard is based on a misunderstanding of an old Kodak study which found that average reflectance of objects is 13 percent.

6. The discussion covers only flat surfaces. Curved surfaces require more complicated calculations.

7. The figure ignores some effects, such as internal reflection and scattering. The image is also slightly displaced.

8. In the Weber's Law range, contrast sensitivity would be unaffected. In the DeVries-Rose Law range, it would be slightly lower.

# Chapter 14

# Visibility Analysis 2: Contrast Thresholds

Marc Green, Ph.D.

*"We prefer seeing to everything else. The reason is that this, most of all the senses, makes us know and brings to light many differences between things."*

—Aristotle

***Synopsis***



## 14.1 Introduction

The previous chapter outlined methods for assessing luminance and for calculating physical contrast. This chapter covers the final stage of forensic visibility analysis: determining contrast threshold and comparing the threshold to physical contrast.

Threshold determination is far more complex than contrast calculation. The expert faces two problems. First, psychology is more complex than physics but not because it is inherently any less scientific. Rather, the number of variables is greater, the variables can be difficult to quantify or even to specify, and they interact nonlinearly. *The Engineering Data Compendium* (Boff and Lincoln, 1988), for example, lists fifteen variables affecting contrast detection, and the list is far from complete. No single research study could measure all possible variable combinations, and no single data set includes more than a few variables. The state-of-the-art models that combine data sets by mathematical means, still cover only a small subset of relevant variables. Many other variables that are not part of any model can have significant effects on threshold. Second, research data often use a 50 percent detection level, which may be too low for real-world application. Moreover, most threshold data originate from laboratory conditions, which are far simpler and more favorable for detection than those of the real world. The laboratory-based thresholds must be adjusted upward.

This chapter explains how a visibility analysis solves these problems to determine a contrast threshold. Much of the initial discussion focuses on the Adrian (1989) contrast detection model, which is widely used. The subsequent section discusses variables not included in the model but which may be important in determining threshold. The discussion then addresses contrast multipliers, factors used to convert laboratory-based thresholds to more realistic values. The chapter concludes by briefly describing alternative analyses, acuity and the twilight envelope, for assessing visibility.

## 14.2 Step 4: Determine Contrast Threshold

### A. Using Data And Models

The ultimate goal is a contrast threshold for viewing conditions at the time of the accident. This threshold is likely to be a function of numerous variables. No single research study could possibly manipulate more than a few at a time, so there is no single graph or table that incorporates all the needed variable values.[1] The only solution is a combination of data from different sources.

There are two possible methods for combining data. The first is manual adjustment of one data set based on a second. For example, Blackwell (1946) has sets of contrast threshold data as a function of background luminance and size. However, the study did not parametrically vary viewing duration. Another research paper might have varied viewing duration for a specific background luminance and size. The duration data in the second paper could be used to adjust threshold values from the first. This same process would then be repeated on other major variables.

The other method calculates thresholds using a model that has already combined data from various sources. In essence, the model has done the job described above, only mathematically rather than manually. However, even the most ambitious models still contain only a relatively small number of variables, albeit the most important ones.

One problem with models is that they are opaque to jurors. Humans think causally, not quantitatively, so it can be difficult to explain a model's operation and that it is simply mathematical functions fitted to sets of data. The functions themselves have no meaning. They are just numbers that work, i.e., they describe the data and allow interpolation between points.

A simplified example clarifies how models work. Suppose someone performs an experiment to measure contrast threshold as a function of viewing time. The data might look like those portrayed in Figure 14.1.

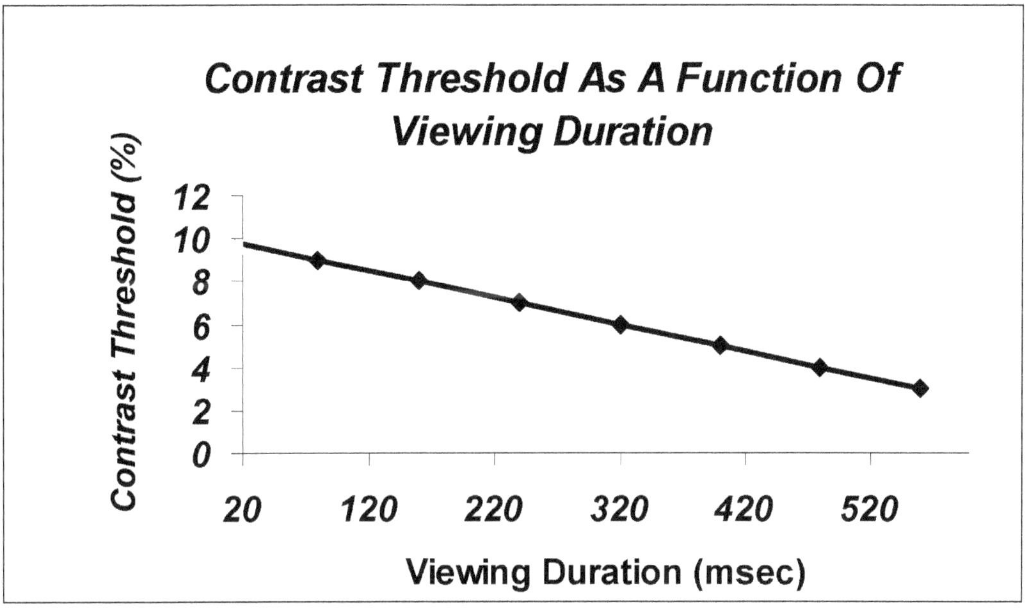


***Figure 14.1*** *Hypothetical contrast vs. duration curve.*

The line is a "best-fitting" function through the data points and has the equation:

$$\text{Contrast Threshold} = (-0.0129 \times \text{duration}) + 10.068$$

The numbers -0.0129 and 10.068 have no meaning outside the equation, but they are useful for determining threshold. Suppose viewing duration were 200 msec, a time which has no data point. I could estimate the correct value with the equation: =7.8 percent.

This is how contrast models work, except that rather than using a single variable, such as duration, the curves have been simultaneously fitted to many variables from different research studies. Instead of the simple linear model shown here, contrast models are far more complex because variables operate nonlinearly and interact with each other. For example, size interacts with adaptation level. Threshold falls with increasing size, but the decline magnitude depends on adaptation level. As a result, there is no single threshold-size function that is applicable in all situations.

Several authors (e.g., Akerman and Kinzly, 1979; Hills, 1976; Farber, 1988; Farber and Matle, 1989; Adrian, 1989; Matchko and Gerhart, 2001) have proposed contrast detection models. The Adrian (1989) model is the only one in wide use. The "Small Target Visibility" (STV) model (ANSI/IESNA, 2000) has adopted the Adrian (1989) model as its method of computing contrast thresholds. The calculation method appears in the original source Adrian (1989), but the "American National Standard Practice For Roadway Lighting" document RP-8-00 has a far more readable version. To use the model, write a computer program or simply create an Excel spreadsheet. Enter the variable values for the viewing conditions and read the output, which is an increment/decrement threshold, ΔL. The Weber contrast threshold is simply $\Delta L/L_B$.

The Adrian model has several advantages over its competitors. It includes more important variables. Moreover, it has the best pedigree. When asked in a Daubert challenge whether the theory and technique is generally accepted by the relevant scientific community, an expert using the Adrian model can then confidently exclaim "Yes" and pull out RP-8-00.

Several studies have found that the model predictions agree reasonably well with viewer estimates of suprathreshold visibility on actual roads (e.g., Menard and Cariou 1994; Güler, Onaygil, 2003). However, it has some limitations. First, it makes predictions not entirely borne out by research data. Second, it does not include many variables, most notably retinal location. As a result, the model's output may require modification. The following section discusses the key variables included in the Adrian model. It is important to understand how these variables operate to avoid using mere cookbook science and to appreciate where and why the Adrian model sometimes needs adjustment.

## B. Adrian Model Variables

### 1. Background Luminance

The fundamental relationship between background luminance and threshold is the well-known Weber's Law described in Chapter 2:

$$k = \frac{\Delta L}{L_B}$$

where k is the contrast threshold or "Weber fraction." The most important implication of Weber's Law is that increasing ambient illumination has no effect on visibility. To see why, suppose that the detection threshold occurs when the target reflects 30 percent of the incident light and the background reflects 25 percent. When the incident light is 100, then

$$\frac{.3(100) - .25(100)}{.25(100)} = \frac{30 - 25}{25} = 0.2$$

and k, the contrast threshold, is .2. Doubling the ambient light to 200 produces:

$$\frac{.3(200) - .25(200)}{.25(200)} = \frac{60 - 50}{50} = 0.2$$

The contrast threshold is still .2. The Weber ratio is a constant, so altering ambient lighting has no effect unless the change differentially illuminates target and background. At mesopic levels, however, the DeVries-Rose Law operates. Increasing headlamp intensity does not change contrast but produces modest improvements in visibility (Roper and Howard, 1938; Sivak, Shoettle, Minoda and Flannagan, (2006).

### 2. Size

Larger targets usually have lower thresholds. As area increases, the threshold falls in three stages: complete, partial and no spatial summation. As shown in Figure 14. 2, small objects have a perfect tradeoff between area increments and contrast—doubling area halves contrast threshold. Spatial summation is then complete ("Ricco's Law"). Increasing area further decreases threshold, but the tradeoff is no longer perfect, so there is only partial summation. In some cases, the threshold may fall with the square of the area ("Piper's Law"). Eventually size increases have no further effect.

As happens in many cases, however, it is impossible to specify an exact value or even general function for areas of complete, partial and no summation. The transition points depend on many variables, most importantly, luminance, visual field location, and duration. For foveal viewing, however, significant summation usually ceases after an object reaches about 1° of visual angle in photopic vision and extended duration. In peripheral vision, further increases improve detection. (See discussion below on "cortical magnification.")

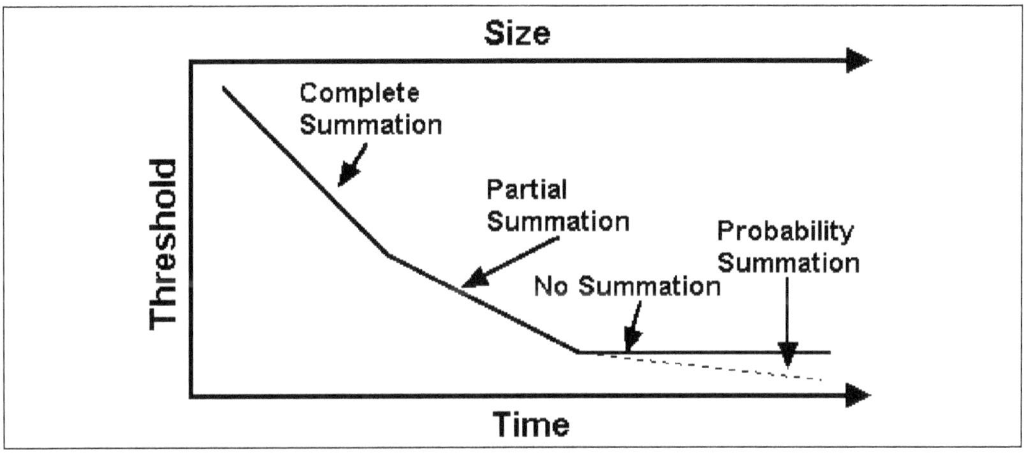


***Figure 14.2*** *Spatial/temporal summation and Ricco's/Bloch's Law.*

### 3. Duration

The viewing duration-threshold relationship is similar to the size-contrast function; there is a period of complete temporal summation ("Bloch's Law"), followed by a period of partial temporal summation and finally a limit of no further summation. The period of complete summation depends on viewing conditions, most notably becoming shorter for higher luminance. Temporal summation asymptotes at about 0.5–1.0 second or less under most conditions.

The Blondel-Rey Law is sometimes used to approximate brightness of warning lights as:

$$\Delta IT = \Delta I_{\infty}(T + a)$$

where $\Delta I$ is the JND, T = viewing duration, $\Delta I_{\infty}$ is the JND for a light of infinite duration, and a is a constant (~.2 sec).

The relationship between duration and visibility, however, is not so simple. Although it seems counterintuitive to many, briefer exposures (0.1–0.2 second) can be more visible than longer ones (the "Broca-Sulzer Effect"). This is why lights flashing at 2.5–5 Hz are the usually the most detectable and appear the brightest. The effect is more pronounced for large targets.

Many contrast detection studies use durations of 0.2–0.25 second (usually specified as 200–250 msec) for threshold estimation because it is roughly the dwell time for an eye in the midst of a series of saccades. However, this is just a rough estimate; the viewer may be keeping the eyes steady and dwell times are typically longer for poor visibility and in some other circumstances. There is no doubt, however, that the biggest duration effect occurs within those first 200–250 msec when temporal summation is large.

Lastly, temporal summation effects fall into two categories. One is "neural summation," the temporal addition of activity in the lower part of the visual system. A second type of summation, "probability summation," is analogous to the effect that occurs when you buy two lottery tickets rather than one. The more chances you have, the more likely that you will win. Similarly, the longer a viewer looks, the more likely he is to see the target. Based on neural summation alone, a viewer who looks for 3 seconds rather than for 1 second is unlikely to have a lower detection threshold. However, there is a given probability of detection for each 1 second look. With "three looks" and three chances of detection, threshold falls.

### 4. Polarity

Contrast has two polarities: positive (increments over the background) and negative (decrements from the background). In general, negative contrast is more detectable. The Adrian model contains a polarity adjustment factor than can make negative contrast more than twice as detectable as positive contrast.

While the greater detectability of decrements is a common finding, the ratio of negative/positive thresholds varies across studies. Many find negative advantages smaller than those suggested by the Adrian model. For example, Legge and Kersten (1983) found only a 9 percent advantage overall but a 22 percent advantage for sharply focused targets. Bowen, Pokorny and Smith (1989) found a 26 percent advantage. However, Patel and Jones (1968) found up to a 220 percent advantage, and Short (1966) obtained up to a 250 percent advantage.

Two factors likely affect the decrement/increment ratio. First, the effect is larger at low adaptation levels. This follows directly from the compressive psychometric function for brightness (Figure 2.8). At any point on the curve, an equal luminance step has a greater effect on brightness in the negative direction than in the positive direction. As a result, decrements will have a greater visual effect. However, the curve also predicts that the difference will largely disappear at high luminances where the curve flattens and runs nearly perpendicular to the Y ($\Psi$) axis. Several studies (e.g., Blackwell, 1946; Short, 1966) have confirmed that decrements lose their advantage at higher luminances. However, Legge and Kersten (1983) still found that decrements are more detectable at 340 cd/m$^2$. Second, decrements should lose some of their advantage with very small targets. Light scattered from the brighter surround "fills in" decrements, effectively reducing contrast and size.

### 5. Age

As people age, most visual functions decline. Measurable contrast sensitivity losses start appearing as early as the forties (Green, Huang, and Odom, 2004) and become significant by about age sixty to sixty-five. The eye's optics lose clarity, becoming cloudy and yellow and cataracts develop. Image quality declines and glare susceptibility increases as light entering the eye scatters and veils. Yellowing impairs color perception and affects contrast perception of blue targets. The pupil also shrinks, allowing less light to enter the eye. By age sixty, the amount of light reaching the retina declines to 1/3, the level of the twenty year old's eye. By the late seventies, retinal illumination falls to 1/8. As a result, older viewers show especially large losses in dim light. Lastly, cognitive and attentional decline further impair the ability to process sensory input.

Given the rapid increase of the older population, aging vision and cognition will soon become very common issues in many accident cases. If the viewer is over forty to forty-five, then any calculation of contrast sensitivity should incorporate an age factor. The common approach is to use Blackwell's data or other norms. There are several published formulas giving age corrections. Adrian (1989) has a correction formula, based largely on physiological data, which breaks the age factor down into ranges:

$$\text{If Age} \leq 64 \text{ Then} = \frac{(\text{Age} - 19)^2}{2160} + 0.99$$

$$\text{If Age} > 64 \text{ Then} = \frac{(\text{Age} - 56.5)^2}{113.6} + 1.43$$

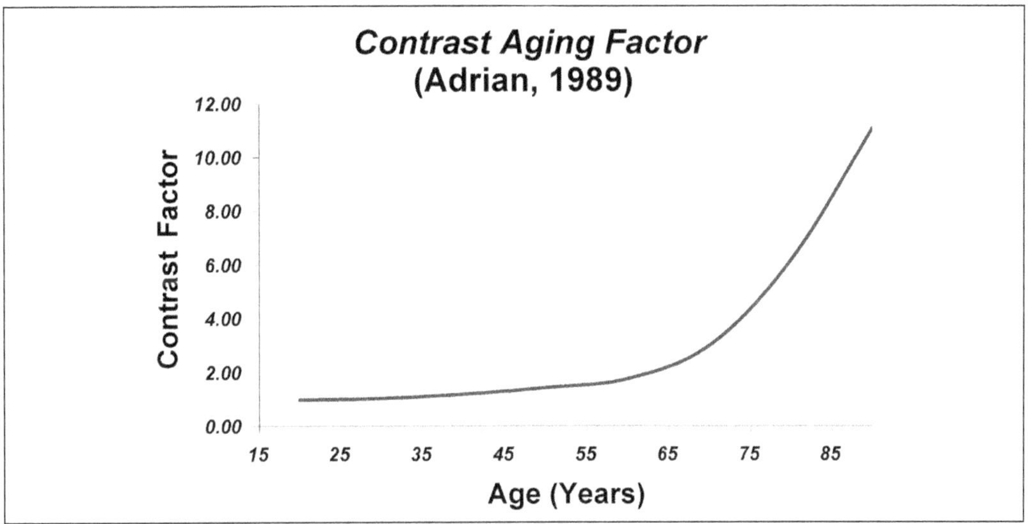


***Figure 14.3*** *Increase in contrast threshold as a function of age calculated from Adrian.*

This formula is context-independent, meaning that it is unaffected by other visual variables. However, research (e.g., Blackwell and Blackwell, 1971; Sloane, Owsley and Alvarez, 1988) shows that older viewers exhibit a greater loss of contrast sensitivity at lower adaptation levels and with smaller targets (Sloane, Owsley and Alvarez, 1988). The aging formula likely requires adjustment to take these factors into account.

Aging also impairs many other aspects of vision. It reduces the "useful field of view." Elderly people are far less likely to see objects if they lie off the direct sight-line in peripheral vision. They have a narrower 'attentional spotlight,' a concept that is discussed in Chapter 4. They also have reduced attentional capacity and are more likely impaired by distractions and divided attention. Older viewers suffer greater loss from both pattern and light masking. Older viewers also dark-adapt slowly, so they exhibit poorer vision when moving between light levels of different intensities. In one accident, for example, an elderly man tripped on the edge of a handicapped ramp after walking from a brightly illuminated parking lot to a street corner with no streetlamp. The accident occurred because of both low physical contrast and the impaired recovery from the higher light level in the parking lot. See Chapter 9 for more discussion of visual aging.

## C. Additional Visual Variables

The basic variables described above form the core of the Adrian and other models. However, they do not exhaust the list of variables that can influence contrast detection. The next section describes some of the additional variables. Each is a large topic which could easily consume an entire chapter or even an entire book. The discussion is a whirlwind tour that provides only a broad overview.

### 1. Visual Field Location

Visual field location is the most important variable not included by Adrian or many other models. In photopic vision, the sparser photoreceptor spacing causes contrast sensitivity declines with increasing distance from the fovea. In scotopic vision, photoreceptors are denser in the periphery and contrast sensitivity remains relatively stable in the central 20–40° of the visual field. In mesopic vision, as might be expected, the results are mixed; sensitivity is still greatest at the fovea, but the peripheral decline is not as steep. As light levels fall, sensitivity across the retina becomes increasingly flat to resemble scotopic vision.

*Photopic Vision.* One way to estimate peripheral thresholds is through "cortical magnification" or "m-scaling" (Rovamo, Virsu, and Naesaenen, 1978). The underlying concept relies on physiological data[2], but it has been confirmed in psychophysical experiments. At heart, it is a simple idea: peripheral targets are simply minified versions of foveal targets. For example, suppose a peripheral target of 40 minarc images 5° from the fovea. If the cortical magnification were 2, then it is merely a magnified version of a 20 minarc foveal target and should have the same threshold. In order to find threshold for the 40 minarc peripheral target at 5°, merely find the foveal threshold for a 20 minarc target. This idea could be applied to any data or model that specifies foveal thresholds.

The m-scaling function specifies the required amount of magnification. Within the central 1°, there is little change in scale. Beyond 1° eccentricity, the function is approximately linear. Virsu and Hari (1996), for example, proposed:

$$M^{-1} = 0.0685 + (4.32 \times \sin(E))$$

where $M^{-1}$ is magnification and E is retinal eccentricity in degrees. Several studies (e.g., Wright and Johnson, 1983) have confirmed the m-scaling prediction that contrast sensitivity falls linearly with foveal distance.

M-scaling can provide a useful estimation, but this approach has limits. M-scaling functions only exist for photopic vision. Further, spherical aberration in the periphery may cause optical degradation that also lowers sensitivity. In addition, m-scaling functions arise mostly from data points along the horizontal meridian. Other data (e.g., Regan and Beverly, 1983) suggest that contrast sensitivity drops faster for locations off the horizontal meridian. Lastly, m-scaling fails to capture perceptual aspects of peripheral vision. At greater eccentricities, the photoreceptor mosaic is less regular as well as sparser. Viewers perform more poorly on tasks such as recognition and localization than would be expected from m-scaling alone. Peripheral vision also exhibits increased "crowding effects," where contours near the target create masking.

*Scotopic Vision.* Riopelle and Bevan (1953) found that scotopic and photopic visual fields differ significantly. Scotopic sensitivity is lowest at the fovea where there are no rods. Sensitivity then increases slightly out to about 12–20° eccentricity and holds roughly steady before rising again in the far periphery. Riopelle and Bevan (1953) further found greater sensitivity in the upper and the nasal than in the lower and temporal visual fields.

*Mesopic Vision.* Mesopic peripheral sensitivity is more difficult to assess because both rods and cones are operating. Moreover, the ratio of rods and cones changes with retinal location. Blackwell (1959) found that sensitivity fell by a factor of four at a location of 2° in the periphery. However, steepness of peripheral decline changes with both target size and with adapting luminance. Larger peripheral targets will begin to intrude on the retina, i.e., a 1° target centered at 2° from the fovea will have its left edge only 1.5° from the optical axis. However, the greater spatial summation in peripheral vision also slows the sensitivity loss in more eccentric locations. For example, one study of mesopic vision (Plainis, Chauhan, Murray and Charman, 1999) found that viewers detecting a 3° target did not experience a sensitivity loss of 4 until targets were about 40° from the fovea. The study also found great cross-viewer variability, which is typical of peripheral vision experiments. Peripheral data would then need a higher detection level multiplier. (See below.)

## 2. Color

Color *per se* has little effect on luminance contrast threshold. The visual system consists of two subdivisions: the achromatic system, which processes brightness, and the chromatic system, which processes color. To a first approximation, the retinal image is decomposed and processed independently by each system. The chromatic system has relatively poor contrast sensitivity, so the more-sensitive achromatic system generally determines threshold. However, color cannot be ignored entirely because different colors have different brightnesses. The relationship between color and brightness is shown by the spectral efficiency curves (Figure 3.12). Colors from the center of the spectrum (e.g., yellow and green) are brighter than colors from the extremes (e.g., red and blue).

Best detection occurs when bright and dark colors appear together. Among chromatic colors, black/yellow and blue/yellow produce best contrast. Conversely, green/orange produce low brightness contrast since they have similar brightness values. Lastly, the luminosity curve only represents spectral colors. Brightness can always be increased by desaturation—adding white.

As usual, however, there are a few caveats. First, chromatic aberration can cause blue objects to be slightly less detectable. Short-wavelengths refract at a sharper angle than long and middle wavelengths, so it is impossible to bring all wavelengths into sharp focus simultaneously. The eye usually focuses the long and middle wavelengths, leaving some blue blur at borders.[3] Second, color can attract attention, as discussed in Chapter 4. Lastly, color can affect contrast sensitivity for people with impaired color vision. Aging causes the eye's optics to yellow and makes blues appear darker. An older person viewing a blue object on a dark background will see lower contrast. Conversely, a blue target on a bright background will be more visible. Some colorblind people (protanopes, people missing the long-wavelength pigment) have little sensitivity to 'red' light, which then produces less contrast on a dark background and more contrast on a bright one.

## 3. Temporal Transients

Flicker and motion can both raise and lower contrast thresholds. Slow motion has little effect on contrast sensitivity or acuity ("dynamic visual acuity"), but more rapid motion and flicker impair detection of fine detail. When viewing a moving object, such as an automobile, a person may be able to see the overall shape but will lose the ability to discern details, such as the driver's face. If the motion duration is sufficiently long, however, the viewer can restore sensitivity with smooth-pursuit eye movements. When objects are large, motion has little effect on detection. In fact, motion and flicker can actually enhance detection of large objects if they are blurred or have indistinct edges.

## 4. Masking

Contrast thresholds increase when the background masks the target. Traditionally, masking falls into two basic types. "Masking by form" ("pattern masking") occurs when the background is textured or cluttered. "Masking by light" occurs when the background is uniform but flashing (e.g., Green, 1984). A flashed, structured mask produces both.

Masking by light (also called "transient light adaptation"' or the "Crawford Effect" [Crawford, 1947]; See Chapter 3) is a short-term effect lasting a second or so and should not be confused with normal light adaptation. Masking by light occurs, for example, when a driver enters a tunnel and there is a transition from light to dark or when a driver's eye passes through the headlamp beams of an oncoming vehicle.

Form masking might occur when a target appears in front of a highly structured street scene containing lights, signs, etc. or when a traffic signal is surrounded by other lights and signs (e.g., Boersma, Zwaga and Adams, 1989; Boersma and Zwaga, 2000). Paulmier (2001) measured detection of objects on patterned backgrounds and concluded that the required visibility levels rose by a factor of 10–25 for detection. This result demonstrates the potential magnitude of masking effects but has no generality and cannot be applied as a rule to forensic analysis.

Masking also divides into three categories: forward, simultaneous and backward, depending on whether the mask occurred before, during or after the viewer sees the target. Lastly, there are also many specialized forms of masking, such as metacontrast masking, peripheral masking and the "far out jerk effect." Some masking effects are psychophysical, some cognitive and some are both.

Because of the great variety of masks and masking conditions, there is no easy way to quantify their effects on threshold. The phenomenon is too complex and too situation-specific to find a general estimate that can be applied across a wide range of conditions. Moreover, Boersma and Zwaga (2000) note that the effect of masking "never depends merely on the characteristics of the visual stimulus." It is always affected by attentional set and other cognitive factors. If this were a hypertext document, there would be a link back to Chapter 4.

### 5. Adaptation State

In examining visibility, the viewer's immediate history may be important. Whenever a person moves between environments of high and low luminance, vision is temporarily impaired. People see best when they are adapted to the prevailing light level. For example, viewers are almost blind when they enter a movie theater on a bright day. After an initial period of poor vision, sensitivity then increases rapidly with time in the dark. Conversely, a person walking out of the theater into much brighter light suffers light adaptation which also impairs vision. However, recovery in light adaptation is far quicker than in dark adaptation. In both cases, the sensitivity loss will be bigger when the difference between the prior and current luminance level is greater and/or the time for adapting to the new level is shorter. In some cases, sensitivity loss is also a function of adapting field size and duration. Lastly, an exception occurs at very low luminances, where adaptation effects disappear entirely.

Misadaptation is a frequent contributor to accidents. In one, a driver failed to see a road worker under an overpass, striking and killing him. The shadow cast by the overpass lowered light levels in the work area. In another, a man leaving a brightly illuminated house failed to see a step because a broken light left the porch very dim. Such accidents are particularly common in older people because they are unable to quickly compensate for rapid light adaptation changes and are effectively blind to deeply shadowed areas. Proper design should create smooth transitions from light to dark. For example, building entrances and tunnels now often incorporate a zone of middle light level between the dark night outside and the bright interior lighting. This smoother transition reduces adaptation effects and permits better vision.

In fact, misadaptation is the rule, not the exception. Laboratory studies typically use viewers who have had time to fully adapt to the background level. Real scenes have areas of light and dark. Viewers move their eyes around, so each retinal location samples these light and dark areas over time and achieves an adaptation state that is some weighted average of the samples. As a result, real viewers are usually somewhat misadapted and laboratory experiments overestimate contrast sensitivity.

### 6. Binocularity

Brady (1992) noted that "There's certainly nothing better than a human eye. Except perhaps, two of them." He is correct, as viewers with one eye operate under several disadvantages. The reduced visual field is obvious, but they also lose stereopsis and have lower contrast sensitivity.

Viewers using both eyes are "binocular," while those with only one functioning eye are "monocular" and exhibit several forms of visual impairment. First, they have poorer contrast sensitivity. Their thresholds are 1.44 ($\sqrt{2}$) higher for stationary targets and about 1.7 higher for large, moving or flickering ones. Second, they lose stereopsis, which can be a useful cue for perceiving shape, for performing figure-ground segregation and for detecting motion directly towards or away from the eyes. Third, monocular viewers lose about 30–40° of the far contralateral (opposite side) visual field. Some countries ban monocular viewers from driving large commercial vehicles.

The effect of monocularity on driver accident probability is unclear. One study (Keeny, Garvey, and Brunker, 1981) found that monocular drivers had twice the accident rate of binocular drivers as well as more reckless driving citations. However, their sample was small. Moreover, the study contained a classic form of sampling bias. The authors used only monocular drivers who had been in accidents and who might represent the worst monocular drivers. The authors then presumed to extrapolate their results to all monocular drivers, including those who had never been in an accident. This is a highly questionable method that is unfortunately common in epidemiological research.

McKnight, Shinar and Hilburn (1991) tested the performance of monocular and binocular truck drivers. The monocular drivers exhibited some performance decrements in specific tasks, but showed little impairment of normal driving. Another study (Wood and Troutbeck, 1994) created monocular drivers by putting goggles on normals and again found minor effects on driving performance. Of course, neither study evaluated performance in emergency situations with impending collisions. In most cases, drivers maintain a large margin for error that masks impairment (Gibson and Crooks, 1938).

In assessing the impact of the monocular driver's field loss, remember that all drivers effectively lose a large portion of both temporal visual fields. Movement through the environment smears the outer portion of the optic flow field. The visual field reduces with increased speed, shrinking to as little as the central 45° when traveling at 60 mph. Further, monocular viewers generally scan the visual field more in order to partially compensate for the visual field loss. Functionally, the monocular driver may not always be operating at a visual field deficit relative to the binocular driver.

### 7. Eye Disease And Optical Correction

Visual impairment can decrease contrast sensitivity. Optical impairments, myopia and hyperopia, are common. Poor optical correction creates blur, which by itself impairs detection. Most other diseases are due to retinal damage. Common examples include glaucoma, age-related macular degeneration (ARMD), diabetic retinopathy, and retinitis pigmentosa. Since these diseases are associated with aging and the elderly population is booming, increasing numbers of forensic cases will involve viewers with impaired vision.

Eye disorders can create complications for nonmedical experts, as opposing attorneys will try to cast them as being unqualified to discuss such issues. However, it is not necessary to be a medical expert to estimate contrast thresholds for people with visual impairment, if there are contrast sensitivity data for patients. In theory, a well-versed psychophysical expert can take a medical diagnosis, find the relevant data and use it to adjust the "normal" contrast threshold. The procedure is the same as incorporating "normal" aging effects.

Optical correction can also affect contrast sensitivity. Obviously, a viewer failing to wear optical correction may have lower contrast sensitivity. Less obviously, optical correction can change retinal image size. A person wearing negative lenses experiences a minification while a viewer wearing positive correction experiences a magnification. The effect of correction on retinal image size for objects at infinity is calculated as:

$$m = \frac{1}{1 - hF}$$

where *m* is magnification, *h* is the distance of the lens from the sensor (or retina) and F is the lens power in diopters. The *h* for the eye is about 17 mm (Westheimer, 1986) from the entrance pupil to the retina. Changing focal length alters magnification. A 6 diopter lens changes retinal image size by about 10 percent. For purposes of contrast threshold calculation, a 30 minarc object for a person without spectacles would be equivalent to a 33 minarc object for a person with 6 diopters of plus spectacle correction, giving him superior contrast sensitivity. Conversely, a person with 6 diopters of minus correction has an equivalent object size of 27 percent. The effects of contact lenses are smaller.

### 8. Arousal Level

Viewers in most research studies are highly alerted, tested during normal business hours, etc. However, real drivers may exhibit low arousal due to fatigue, boredom, or drugs/alcohol. Even small alcohol doses within the legal limit for driving can affect threshold and reaction time. However, it is unclear whether these smaller effects impact accident likelihood because the effects of alcohol depend on several variables. The largest effect occurs during divided attention, but if a driver is simply traveling without distraction along an easy roadway and has excess attentional capacity, then even large alcohol doses may have relatively small effects. Factors such as previous drinking history, amount recently eaten, body weight, and so forth are also important.

It may seem that drivers should be blamed for the lowered arousal and subsequent performance impairment, but this is not always the case. Even a normal driver at 2 a.m. is likely to have a higher contrast threshold and longer reaction time (e.g., Colquhoun, Blake and Edwards, 1868; Lenne, Triggs and Redman, 1997) than a normal driver in a research study, but not because he has done anything wrong. Real-world drivers may suffer from low arousal due to variations in circadian rhythms and from the boredom inherent in long monotonous drives with little to see. Unfortunately, most studies confound fatigue and these other factors, so it can be difficult to separate the specific causes of low arousal. However, a large-scale study of truck drivers (Wylie, Shultz, Miller, Mitler, and Mackie, 1996) found that simple time of day, not hours of sleep, was the best predictor of accidents.

### 9. Uncertainty And Expectation

Any source of uncertainty in location, size, shape, time of appearance, etc. can increase detection threshold. Blackwell (1959) performed experiments which suggested that thresholds should be increased by a factor of 1.31 for location uncertainty, 1.1 for temporal uncertainty and 1.4 for advanced warning. None of these values has much significance outside the particular tasks that he tested.

Location uncertainty effects can be much greater than those suggested by Blackwell (1959). One study (Cohn and Wardlaw, 1985) of spatial uncertainty compared detection of a target that appeared in a known location to one that could appear in one of 140 different locations, all within the fovea. The threshold under uncertainty was 10 times higher than under certainty. Large uncertainty effects occur when pilots sometimes operate under "see and avoid rules" and must keep separation from other planes visually. Alerted pilots are 8 times more likely to see the other plane than unalerted pilots (Transportation Safety Board of Canada, 1995).

Threshold also increases with uncertainty about spatial frequency (Davis, Kramer, and Graham, 1983) and with combinations of temporal, location and shape uncertainty (e.g., Roper and Howard,1938). Lastly, reaction times become much slower when the responder has no advanced warning. As discussed in Chapter 17, advanced warning can halve driver reaction times.

The scale of uncertainty effects likely depends on several factors. First, highly conspicuous targets attract attention and are less affected by uncertainty. For example, large flashing objects stimulate the transient system (magnocellular pathways) and should suffer less from spatial, location and temporal uncertainty. Conversely, small objects stimulate sustained system (parvocellular pathways) and are less conspicuous. Second, uncertainty effects are greater when the target violates a strong expectation.

### 10. Other Target Variables

Research studies (e.g., Blackwell, 1946) typically use sharply focused round targets. Real targets are far more variable and have additional properties which affect detectability:

- Blur. Targets with sharp edges are more detectable than those with blurred edges (Ogle, 1960). There are a few notable exceptions, however, such as large objects that are viewed very briefly or are moving (e.g., Green, Corwin and Schor, 1981);
- Orientation. Contrast thresholds are lower for horizontal and vertical edges than for diagonals, a phenomenon called "oblique effect" or "retinal anisotropy" (e.g., Apelle, 1972). Verticals are also very slightly more detectable than horizontals;
- Shape. Thresholds are lower for elongated targets than would be expected from their area alone. A ratio of about 3:1 is optimal (e.g., Polat and Tyler, 1997).

## D. Contrast Multipliers

The visibility analysis next multiplies laboratory thresholds by two factors in order to obtain a more realistic value. First, laboratory thresholds represent a 50 percent detection level. Some prefer to multiply the 50 percent threshold to achieve a 99+ percent "commonsense" detection level,[4] representing almost certain detection. Second, both psychophysical and cognitive factors cause real-world thresholds to be higher than those obtained in the laboratory. Research subjects know when and where the target will appear, they know what it will look like, practice the same task extensively, are not performing a concurrent driving task, encounter no background masking, etc. An additional "field multiplier" increases threshold to compensate for these differences.[5] The final threshold value is the laboratory threshold multiplied by detection level and psychological "field" factors:

$$\text{Threshold}_{\text{Final}} = \text{Threshold}_{\text{Lab}} * \text{Multiplier}_{\text{DL}} * \text{Multiplier}_{\text{F}}$$

Note that field multipliers blur the distinction between psychophysics and cognition, so they take the analysis beyond the realm of strict visibility and into perception.

### 1. Detection Level Multipliers

The 50 percent laboratory threshold is too low for practical application, so most models use a multiplier to bring the threshold to a 99 percent+ detection level. The multiplier's size depends on data variability. Lower variability creates steeper psychometric functions and hence less distance along the X axis (contrast) between any two detection levels. To see this, look at Figure 2.4 and imagine a steeper curve.

Data sets with different variability will require different multipliers. Blackwell (1959) suggested a number in the low 2's to reach 99 percent detection while Hills (1976) required a multiplier of four. The Adrian model provides a 99.93 percent detection level by incorporating a built-in 2.6 multiplier.

Since the size of the variability changes with circumstances, the multiplier, in theory, also changes. Blackwell (1959) found that the multiplier was lower with shorter viewing durations, which is not surprising because briefer durations produce lower variability. On the other hand, variability increases with higher viewer age, peripheral location and some other factors. Moreover, controlled laboratory conditions are likely to produce far less variability than exists in the real world. There are no models which capture this need to modify detection level multipliers with conditions.

Lastly, some simply avoid the problem by using tasks which inherently require 100 percent detection. For example, Blackwell and Blackwell (1970) used method-of-adjustment, a task where viewers set contrast to the point where it is just perceptible. In good agreement with Adrian, Blackwell and Blackwell found that method-of-adjustment thresholds were 2.5 times higher than 50 percent forced-choice thresholds. Similarly, Gallagher, Koth and Freedman (1975) determined thresholds by recording the point at which unsuspecting drivers avoided sudden road obstacles. This represents 100 percent detection, since logically only viewers who saw the obstacles responded.

### 2. Field Multipliers

The second multiplier compensates for differences between the laboratory and road conditions. These multipliers go under different names, including "field factor," "visibility level" and "visibility index." Although conceptually similar, they differ slightly in meaning.

Blackwell (1959) first suggested the "field factor" multiplier to capture the effect of variables differing between laboratory thresholds and the real world. He performed laboratory experiments in order to determine multipliers for specific psychophysical and "psychological" effects. By combining the individual multipliers, Blackwell concluded that an overall field factor of 15, which included his detection level adjustment, would be correct. However, this number has no generality. For example, he applied a field factor of four in order to expand the detection area from the fovea to 2° eccentricity. He based this on data (Blackwell and Moldauer, 1958) showing that threshold for a 1 minarc spot was four times higher at 2° from the fovea. As discussed above, the falloff with eccentricity is much slower with larger targets and lower adapting luminances, so the field factor would be much lower. Further, his psychological field factors are based on specific laboratory tests and are not necessarily applicable to any real-world task. Lastly, Blackwell himself noted that there is no known way to combine the effects of the individual field factors.[6]

Visibility level (VL) is essentially the inverse of the field factor. In simplest terms, it is the physical contrast divided by the threshold.[7] If the contrast is .3 and threshold is .1, then VL=.3/.1=3. VL levels are widely used to calculate putative visibility for road design. As noted above, suprathreshold visibility estimates agree reasonably well with VL. Rather than attempting to determine field factors for individual variables, Adrian (1987) analyzed driver data and proposed a global VL of 15-20.

Gallagher, Koth and Freedman (1975) suggested the concept of "visibility index" (VI) which closely resembles Adrian's VL. They determined the relationship between VI and their dependent measure, time to target, for drivers encountering unexpected objects in the roadway. Gallagher, Koth and Freedman found that the relationship was curvilinear. Performance improved rapidly with initial VI increases and more slowly with subsequent increases. The curve began to asymptote at a VI of about 10–12. The data then skip to VI of 50, where there was a marginal improvement of perhaps 5–10 percent. Moreover, there is considerable overlap in the data ranges for VI 10–12 and VI 50.

Adrian's (1987) estimate of 15–20 was also apparently based on the Gallagher, Koth and Freedman (1975) data. His VL estimate of 15-20 represented optimum performance. In fact, his calculations agree with Gallagher, Koth and Freedman (1975), showing that VL 10–12 produced about 90 percent of peak performance and that the further increases produced at most another 10 percent benefit. Note that the 10–12 estimate derives from drivers who successfully avoided the unexpected objects in their paths. The actual "threshold" VL must be somewhat lower.

Janoff, Kroth, McCunney, Freedman, Duerk, and Berkovitz (1977) attacked the problem from another angle by looking at unsuccessful avoidances; they examined the relationship between VI and accident rates. The data showed a slightly lower VI where the relationship more clearly asymptoted at about 10.

Lastly, two other authors estimated the visibility difference between drivers who were alerted to look for a particular pedestrian in a particular place and drivers who are unalerted. Hills (1976) put the visibility factor at seven while Olson (2003) estimated five. These multipliers are likely smaller because they compare unalerted drivers to alerted drivers rather than to laboratory data. It may be a coincidence, but Hill's multipliers of four for detection criterion and seven for field factors multiply to a total value of 28, while Adrian's numbers of 2.6 and 10–12 multiply to similar values, 26-31.

Taken together, the data suggest that multiplying increasing visibility up to 5-6 times threshold greatly enhances driver performance. Additional increases up to 10-12 produce further improvement but at a slower rate, and the relationship approaches an asymptote at 10-12. Higher visibility levels produce small, but measurable improvement. Lack of data, however, makes estimation of the true asymptote point problematic. Overall, however, research suggests that a multiplier of 10-12 is somewhat analogous to the 85th percentile driver in roadway design, i.e., a level that includes most but not all drivers.

### 3. Limitations of Multipliers

The analysis compares physical contrast to the contrast threshold resulting from the multiplication of laboratory-based thresholds by detection criterion and field multipliers. If physical contrast were higher, then the target was visible. This all sounds very cut and dry, but it is not.

It is naïve to believe that a single multiplication number can possibly capture the full complexity of psychophysics and of cognition. At the same time he proposed field factors, Blackwell (1959) warned that the applicable multipliers might vary considerably depending on circumstances and proposed a range of 5–20. For example, a driver has higher expectation of pedestrians in a crosswalk, at an intersection and in an urban area than on a rural road. There is much more spatial uncertainty for a pedestrian, who can appear from anywhere on either side of the road, than for other vehicles that can only appear directly ahead or from side streets. A pedestrian on a dark road will appear in positive contrast against a uniform dark background. A pedestrian in the city, however, may appear against an illuminated background that creates masking. How can there be one multiplier to account for all of these situations?

Further, multipliers are incomplete. They fail to include many of the additional variables listed above. They also blur the distinction between sensation and perception, giving the illusion of fully compensating for cognitive factors. For example, they make no allowance for attentional set, goals, payoffs, cognitive blindness and many of the factors discussed in Chapter 4. This, like any other (e.g., Hyzer, 2007) attempt to use multipliers without a real understanding of underlying visual processing, is naïve cookbook science.

We all love our "magic bullets," simple solutions that kill complex problems. Life would be easier if we could always apply a single number to all situations. It would be nice if driver reaction time were always 1.5 seconds and if the contrast multiplier were always ten, etc. Then there would be no need to understand the complexities of reaction time, psychophysics and cognition and no need to spend years learning the basic science. Unfortunately, magic bullets do not exist because vision and other aspects of behavior are too complex and context-dependent to be characterized by single numbers. At best, numbers such as multipliers are like landmarks on a map. They are not your final destination but may help guide you to your final destination.

In sum, multipliers are not a substitute for genuine understanding of psychophysics and cognition. Multipliers were developed to guide roadway design and not to perform forensic analysis. Roadway design requires a generalized solution that will be applicable to average (or 85th percentile) drivers. There is no desire or need to understand individuals or individual situations in detail. In contrast, forensic analysis examines a specific person in a specific context. This requires a much closer level of analysis.

## 14.3 Alternatives To Contrast Thresholds

### A. Acuity

Some readers will be surprised that I have not yet mentioned "visual acuity," the ability to resolve fine detail of a highly visible target. The reason is simple: with the exception of clinical vision, contrast sensitivity has become the dominant dependent measure for characterizing spatial vision.

Acuity reigned as the prime measure of spatial vision and detection for many years. The reason is largely pragmatic. Acuity measurement is simple and easy and requires no complicated equipment. Acuity tests use only a single contrast level, the highest achievable,[8] and, best of all, provide a simple result. There is a single dependent variable, size of the finest resolvable detail. Measuring contrast sensitivity is much more arduous and requires much more time and effort as well as highly specialized equipment. Unlike acuity, however, contrast sensitivity provides a measure of visual performance for objects of any size or shape. Moreover, contrast detection better reflects the tasks that viewers actually perform in the real world. Viewers are generally detecting the contrast of larger objects against a background and not resolving details of highly visible objects.[9] Since the introduction of computers and CRT screens made measurement far easier, contrast threshold has become increasingly accepted as the cornerstone of spatial vision. Acuity's last stronghold is the medical world, where the speed, ease and succinctness still outweigh the limitations.[10] (See Rosenthal, 2006, for the medical perspective on acuity vs. contrast.)

#### 1. Types Of Acuity

Visual acuity not so simple a topic as it appears at first glance. Acuity is not a single task but rather an umbrella term for several distinct tasks, each producing a different threshold and each likely reflecting a different aspect of spatial vision. Further, acuity may be expressed by several different measures. Figure 14.4 shows the basic types with examples.

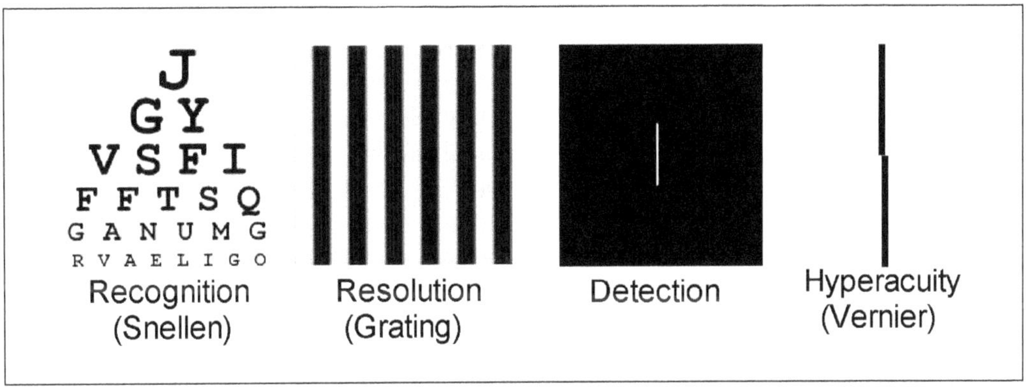


***Figure 14.4*** *Four basic types of acuity with an example of each.*

*Recognition Acuity*: the ability to recognize some object. Snellen acuity, ability to read letters from a chart, is the most familiar type. Snellen acuity is expressed as a ratio of distances, such as 20/20. The numerator is the typical testing distance of 20 feet, the size of the average eye exam room. The denominator is the distance at which a normal viewer can resolve the detail. A viewer who is 20/40, for example, can only resolve the same size detail at 20 feet that would be perceptible to a normal viewer at 40 feet. While 20/20 (or 6/6 in meters) is considered normal, many viewers reach 15/20 or even better in good viewing conditions. In order to obtain a driver's license, most U.S. states require at least binocular 20/40[11] acuity with correction. (No states have a contrast sensitivity criterion for drivers.) A person is legally blind when corrected acuity is 20/200 or worse.

Snellen is popular in medical domains because it is a good, quick-and-dirty measure of spatial vision. In most testing, the examiner measures acuity for each eye separately (monocular) and for the eyes together (binocular). Charts show the left eye as "LE" or "OS" (oculus sinister), the right eye as "RE" or "OD" (oculus dexter) and binocular as "BE" or "OU" (oculus uterque). There may be two sets of acuities, one with and the other without optical correction. If the results are normal, the chart may show "WNL" (within normal limits). Lastly, an examiner may test a viewer for "pin-hole acuity" if the acuity score is low. The viewer sees the chart through a very small aperture, which minimizes the optical blurring of light rays reaching the retina. If pin-hole acuity is better than corrected acuity, then the viewer needs new spectacles.[12]

*Resolution Acuity (Minimum Separable Acuity):* the ability to resolve a gap or separation between two objects. There are many types of resolution acuity tests. Figure 14.4 shows "grating acuity," where the viewer must distinguish the light and dark bars. Other common methods are "minimum separable angle," the size of a gap between two bars, and "Landolt C," the size of a bite taken out of a ring. Outside the medical world, resolution acuity is the most commonly used type of acuity. If a visual scientist uses the term "acuity" without a qualifier, he is almost certainly referring to resolution acuity. Recognition and resolution are closely related and typically give similar results although resolution acuities are typically expressed in minarc, the size of the smallest resolvable detail. Alternatively, they may be expressed as decimal acuity, the inverse of the smallest resolvable detail. If the smallest resolvable detail were 5 minarc, then decimal acuity would be 1/5 or .2. This is convenient because "normal" acuity is 1.

*Detection Acuity (Minimum Visible Acuity)*: the ability to detect a small object on a background of the opposite polarity, i.e., a light object on a dark background or a dark object on a bright background. If the dependent measure is size, then the threshold is expressed in minarc or in decimal acuity. However, this is contrast detection and not resolution or recognition acuity in the ordinary sense. See below.

*Hyperacuity*: a collection of acuities that share only one property—they have threshold values far lower than those of the recognition or resolution acuities. One example is vernier acuity, the detection of a small offset. Another example is stereoacuity, the detection of offset in depth due to image disparities between the two eyes.

*Dynamic Visual Acuity*: While the target remains stationary in standard acuity tests, dynamic visual acuity measures acuity for a moving recognition or resolution target. Some regard this as a more realistic test, since real-world targets are often moving, e.g., a pedestrian crossing the road or an approaching car. Results typically show that acuity remains near optimum up to a surprisingly high range of velocities. With fast motion, however, acuity declines.

### 2. Optimal Acuities

The "normal" values for the various tasks vary greatly (Table 14.1). Resolution acuity is 1 minarc, which translates to a Snellen score of about 20/20. In optimal laboratory conditions, however, thresholds can be significantly lower, perhaps .6 minarc and 15/20 or even 10/20. Optimal hyperacuities are far finer, at about 2–5 arcsec. Detection acuity can be the best, with thresholds as small as 0.5 arcsec (1 inch at 6.5 miles!), depending on line length.

However, detection acuity is not really acuity. A viewer can readily see an object with sufficient intensity even if it is far smaller than the typical .6–1 minarc resolution limit of normal acuity. For very small targets, viewers readily confuse brightness, size and distance. If a bright light of 1 minarc target shrinks, the viewer cannot perceive a size change because it is below the resolution limit. Instead, the viewer sees the brightness decrease due to smaller summation area—but he can still see it. However, the viewer implicitly interprets the lower brightness in terms of the inverse square law (Chapter 3) and infers that the object lies at a greater distance. For example, suppose a driver sees a dim light far ahead. If the headlight is dirty or dimmed by a headlamp cover, the driver will perceive it as being farther away.

Acuity has fewer applications than contrast sensitivity, but it is still useful in some circumstances. If an object is very distant or consists of very fine details, acuity may be a simpler variable. It may also be easier to relate visibility to medical records, which express spatial vision as an acuity score. However, contrast detection and resolution acuity are different tasks and may produce results that are not directly comparable.

## B. The Twilight Envelope

During civil twilight, ground illuminance in good weather declines by a factor of about 100, from roughly 330 lux to 3.3 lux. Assuming a 20 percent average reflectance, the illumination present at the beginning of civil twilight supports near maximum photopic visibility while the luminance level at the end is well into the mesopic range (Leibowitz and Owens, 1991). At the same time, the U.S. Naval Observatory describes civil twilight as a time for "terrestrial objects to be clearly distinguished," an assertion supported by performance data on tasks such as acuity, contrast sensitivity and reaction time.

**Table 14.1**
**Acuity thresholds under optimized conditions**

| Acuity Type | Best Thresholds |
|---|---|
| Recognition (Snellen) | ~20/15 |
| Resolution | ~.6 minarc |
| Detection | 0.5+ arcseconds |
| Hyperacuity | ~3-5 arcseconds |

Owens, Francis and Leibowitz (1989) have proposed the visibility concept of "twilight envelope," which suggests that an illumination of 3.3 lux, the level at the end of civil twilight, can act as a rough lower bound for adequate headlamp illumination. Drivers should have reasonably good foveal vision in the area illuminated above 3.3 lux but relatively poor foveal vision when illuminance falls below this twilight envelope. The "twilight distance" is the point down the road where illumination falls below 3.3 lux and the envelope ends. Owens, Francis and Leibowitz (1989) estimated different twilight distances at different heights above the roadway. For headlamps mounted 27 inches high, for example, they estimated distances of 260 feet at the roadway, twilight distances of 175 feet at headlamp level, and only 80 feet at a driver eye height of 42 inches.

This twilight envelope approach is limited, most notably because detection is a direct function of luminance and only an indirect function of illuminance. Objects of different reflectances may vary greatly in their physical contrast with the background and exhibit different detectability. Still, the twilight envelope can be a useful tool for visibility experts because it defines a performance border where vision declines sharply. A good heuristic may be the best solution when a problem is too ill-defined or too complex for detailed analysis. The mathematically inclined have a temptation to err by overspecifying a problem—attempting complex mathematical analysis when the needed data are not available. While pages of fancy mathematics may look meaningful and impress a jury, they do not automatically ensure insight that trumps a good heuristic. In many cases, it is good to remember the old adage: *"When formality*[13] *comes in the door, reality goes out the window."*

## 14.4 Conclusion

This chapter has reviewed the general methodology for determining contrast threshold. The task is complex because of the large number of variables which interact nonlinearly. However, existing data on thresholds for key variables—background luminance, target size, age and viewing duration—provide a good starting point. Data can be combined manually or by means of a model, with Adrian's (1989) being the most likely candidate. It may be necessary to tweak this original value to account for many other psychophysical and cognitive variables. The final step increases the laboratory-based thresholds by detection level and field multipliers. Do not be misled, however, by the apparent orderliness of this description; it cannot be done by cookbook science. Ten is a nice field multiplier number, but it will only apply in some cases.

Finally, what does this threshold number actually represent? It defines the limits of the human ability to see. If a target is below detection threshold, then the viewer cannot see and respond to it. If the target is above detection threshold, then it is detectable. This does not necessarily mean that the viewer *should* see and respond to the target. Viewers may fail to see even highly visible objects for perfectly good psychological reasons. Seeing involves attention and the other cognitive processes. The next chapter should probably be "Attention And Conspicuity Analysis," but since these issue are covered in Chapter 4 the next chapter skips to a specific scenario, the pedestrian crossing accident.

## References


Adrian, W. 1987. Visibility levels under nighttime driving conditions. *Journal of the Illuminating Engineering Society*, 16, 3-12.

Adrian, W. 1989. Visibility of Targets. *Lighting Research Technology* 21, 181-188.

Akerman, A., and R. Kinzly. 1979. Predicting aircraft detectability. *Human Factors* 21, 277-291.

ANSI/IESNA. 2000. *American National Standard Practice for Roadway Lighting*. Illuminating Engineering Society, New York RP-8-00.

Appelle, S. 1972. Perception and discrimination as a function of stimulus orientation: The 'oblique effect.' *Psychological Bulletin* 78, 266-278.

Blackwell, H. R. 1946. Contrast thresholds of the human eye. *Journal of the Optical Society of America* 36, 624-643.

Blackwell, H. R. 1959. Development and use of quantitative method for specification of interior illumination levels on the basis of performance data. *Illuminating Engineering*. 54, 317-53.

Blackwell, O., and H. R. Blackwell. 1971. Visual performance data for 156 normal observers of various ages. *Illuminating Engineering Society Journal*, October, 3-13.

Blackwell, H., and A. Moldauer. 1958. Detection Thresholds For point Sources in The Near Periphery. ERI Project 2455. Bureau Of Ships, Department of The Navy.

Boersma, T., and H. Zwaga. 2000. Visual conspicuity of objects in complex scenes. SPIE Vol. 3959, p. 548-558, *Human Vision and Electronic Imaging V*, Bernice E. Rogowitz, Thrasyvoulos N. Pappas (eds.)

Boersma, T., H. J. Zwaga, and A. Adams. 1989. Conspicuity in realistic scenes: An eye-movement measure. *Applied Ergonomics* 20, 267-273.

Bowen, R., J. Pokorny, and V. Smith. 1989. Sawtooth contrast sensitivity. Vision Research 29, 1501-1509.

Brady, F. 1992. *The Singular View: The Art of Seeing With One Eye. Canadian Edition*. Edgemore Enterprises: Toronto.

Cobb, P., and F. K. Moss. 1928. Four fundamental factors in vision. Transactions of the Illuminating Engineering Society 23, 496-506.

Cobb, P., and F. K. Moss. 1928. Four variables of visual threshold. *Journal of the Franklin Institute*. 205, 831-847.

Cohn, T. E., and J. Wardlaw. 1985. Effect of large spatial uncertainty of foveal luminance increment detectability. *Journal of the Optical Society of America A2*, 820-825.

Colquhoun, W., M. Blake, and R. Edwards. 1968. Experimental studies of shift-work I: A comparison of 'rotating' and 'stabilized' 4-hour shift systems. *Ergonomics* 11, 437-453.

Connor, J., and R. Ganoung. 1935. An experimental determination of visual thresholds. *Journal of the Optical Society of America* 36, 287-294.

Davis, E. T., P. Kramer, and N. Graham. 1983. Uncertainty about spatial frequency, spatial position, or contrast of visual patterns. *Perception & Psychophysics 33*, 20-28.

Farber, E. 1988. *Revising the DETECT seeing distance model.* SAE Technical Paper Series #880716.

Farber, E., and C. Matle. 1989. *PCDETECT: A Revised Version of the Detect Seeing Distance Model*, Transportation Research Record 1213.

Gallagher, V., B. Koth, and M. Freedman. 1975. The Specification of Streetlighting Needs. Philadelphia. Report FHWA-RD-76-17.

Gibson, J. J., and L. Crooks. 1938. A theoretical field analysis of automobile-driving. *American Journal of psychology*, 51, 453-471.

Green, M., T. Corwin, and C. Schor. 1981. Spatiotemporal variations in the square/sine ratio: evidence of independent channels at low spatial frequencies. *Vision Research* 21, 423-5.

Green, M., W. Huang, and J. V. Odom. 2004. Aging vision in visual clutter. Human Factors and Ergonomics Society Meeting.

Güler, Ö., and S. Onaygil. 2003. Evaluation of Visibility Level Formula in Road Lighting with Field Measurements, Third International Conference on Electrical and Electronics Engineering, 245-249, Bursa.

Hills, B. 1976. Visibility under night driving conditions. Part 3. *Lighting Research and Technology* 8, 11-26.

Hyzer, B. 2007. Visibility reconstruction of nighttime collisions: Correcting for investigator bias. *Proceedings of the American Academy of Forensic Sciences.* 159.

Janoff, M. 2002. Visibility under roadway lighting. In R. Dewar and P. Olson (eds.) *Human Factors In Traffic Safety*. Tucson, AZ: Lawyers & Judges Publishing.

Janoff, M., B. Kroth, W. McCunney, M. Freedman, C. Duerk, and M. Berkovitz. 1977. Effectiveness Of Highway Arterial Lighting. Report FHWA-RD77-37.

Keeney, S. A., J. Garvey, and G. Bunker. 1981. Current experience with the monocular drivers of Kentucky. *American Association for Automotive Medicine Proceedings*, 215-220.

Koschmieder, H. 1924. Theorie der Horizontalen Sichtweite. *Beitraege zur Physik der Atmos—phare* 12, pp. 33-53, 171-181.

Legge, G., and D. Kersten. 1983. Light and dark bars: Contrast discrimination. *Vision Research* 23, 473-483.

Lenne, M., T. Triggs, and J. Redman. 1997.Time of day variations in driving performance. *Accident Analysis and Prevention* 29, 431–437.

Matchko, R., and G. Gerhert. 2001. ABC's of foveal vision. *Optical Engineering* 40, 2735-2745.

McKnight, A., D. Shinar, and B. Hilburn. 1991. The visual and driving performance of monocular and binocular heavy-duty truck drivers. *Accident Analysis and Prevention* 2, 225-237.

Menard, J., and J. Cariou. 1994. Road lighting: An assessment of an installation based on the contrast of a standard target. *Lighting Research and Technology* 26, 19-22.

Ogle, K. 1960. Blurring of the retinal image and contrast thresholds in the fovea. *Journal of the Optical Society of America* 50, 307-315.

Olson, P. 2003. Lighting sources other than headlamps. In (Olsen, P. and E. Farber, eds.) *Forensic Aspects of Driver Perception And Response.* Tucson, AZ: Lawyers & Judges Publishing.

Owens, D. A., E. L. Francis, and H. W. Leibowitz. 1989. Visibility distance with headlights: A functional approach. SAE Technical Paper Series, #890684, Warrendale, PA: Society of Automotive Engineers.

Patel, A., and R. Jones. 1968. Increment and decrement visual thresholds. *Journal of the Optical Society of America* 58, 696-699.

Paulmier, G. 2001. The influence of visual complexity on the detection of targets investigated by computer generated images. *Lighting Research and Technology* 33, 197-205.

Phillips, E., T. Khatua, G. Kost, and R. Pizali. 1990. *Vision and visibility in vehicular accident reconstruction.* SAE Technical Paper Series #900369.

Plainis, S., K. Chauhan, I. Murray, and W. Charman. 1999. Retinal adaptation under night-time driving conditions. In Vision in Vehicles VII. Edited by A.G. Gale, I.D. Brown, C.M. Haslegrave, and S.P. Taylor, Elsevier, Amsterdam.

Polat, U., and C. W. Tyler. 1997. What pattern does the eye see best? *Investigative Ophthalmology and Visual Science* 38, S1. Suppl.

Regan, M., and K. Beverly. 1983. Visual fields described by contrast sensitivity, by acuity, and by relative sensitivity to different orientations. *Investigative Ophthalmology & Visual Science* 24, 754-759.

Riopelle, A., and W. Bevan. 1953. The distribution of scotopic sensitivity in human vision. *American Journal of Psychology* 66, 73-80.

Roper, V., and E. Howard. 1938. Seeing with Motor Car Headlamps, *Transactions of the Illuminating Engineering Society* 33, 417-438.

Rovamo, J., V. Virsu, and R. Nasanen. 1978. Cortical magnification factor. predicts the photopic contrast sensitivity across the visual field. *Nature* 271, 54-56.

Rosenthal, B. 2006. Visual Acuity vs. Contrast Sensitivity. *Optometric Management*, March.

Schoettle, B., M. Sivak, and M. Flannagan. 2001. High-Beam and Low-Beam Headlighting Patterns in the U.S. and Europe at the Turn of the Millennium. Report UMTRI-2001-19.

Short, A. 1966. Decremental and incremental visual thresholds. *Journal of Physiology* 185, 646-654.

Sivak, M., B. Shoettle, T. Minoda, and M. Flanagan. 2006. Potential Visibility Gains on Straight and Curved Roads from Proportional Increases in Low-Beam Headlamp, *Lighting Research and Technology* 38, 259-266.

Sloane, M. E., C. Owsley, and S. Alvarez. 1988. Aging, senile meiosis and spatial contrast sensitivity at low luminance. *Vision Research* 28, 1235-1246.

Transportation Safety Board of Canada 1995. *Aviation Occurrence Report A95H0008*, sections 1.9.3 and 1.9.8.

Virsu, V., and R. Hari. 1996. Cortical magnification, scale invariance, and visual ecology. *Vision Research* 36, 2971–2977.

Westheimer, G. 1986. The eye as an optical instrument. In K.R. Boff, L. Kaufman, and J.P. Thomas, eds., *Handbook of Perception and Human Performance*. New York: John Wiley.

Wood, J., and R. Troutbeck. 1994. Effects of visual impairment on driving. *Human Factors* 36, 476-487.

Wright, M., and A. Johnson. 1983. Spatiotemporal Contrast Sensitivity and Visual Field Locus. *Vision Research* 23, 983-989.

Wylie, C., T. Shultz, J. Miller, M. Mitler, and R. Mackie. 1996. Commercial Motor Vehicle Driver Fatigue and Alertness Study: Project Report (FHWA-MC-97-002). Washington, D.C.: Federal Highway Administration.

## Endnotes

1. The number of possible variable values required by such a lookup table would be $n^m$, where m is the number of variables and n is the number of values that each can take. If there are 15 variables, each taking 5 values, the hypothetical lookup table would have $5^{15}$ entries.

2. Each square mm of retina projects an area on the surface of the cortex. With increasing distance from the fovea, the area of cortex devoted to each mm of retina shrinks. M-scaling attempts to increase image size with increasing distance from the fovea so that the amount of cortex analyzing the area remains constant at every location.

3. The blur is not normally noticeable unless it is large. The sharper edges created by the other wavelengths mask the blur. This is but one of many de-blurring mechanisms that the eye uses to produce clear vision.

4. The psychometric function never reaches 0 percent or 100 percent, so there is no statistical means for determining 100 percent detection.

5. Some use a multiplier for glare. The alternative is to treat glare as a contributor to physical contrast as in the previous chapter.

6. It is important to understand Blackwell's overall strategy in order to evaluate his conclusions. He realized that he had tackled a very large and complex problem, a characterization of everyday vision that included both psychophysics and cognition. Further, he wanted a system that could be practically applied to predict vision in the real world. In order to achieve his goals, he greatly oversimplified many issues. Combining individual field factors into a global number is an example. Even while doing it, however, he said that it is unfounded. Second, when in doubt, he generally took the most conservative route and estimated the highest possibility visibility requirement. Using a 1' target to determine field factor of 4 for a 2° retinal eccentricity is an example. Larger targets surely lower this number, as he must have known. Blackwell is upfront about these compromises. Anyone reading Blackwell must be impressed with his thoroughness, his clarity of analysis and, perhaps most of all, his forthrightness. However, his conclusions should not be blindly accepted. Moreover, much of the current knowledge about cognition was not available in his day.

7. In the Small Target (STV) ANSI/IESNA (2000) model, VL has a more specific meaning. It is a composite visibility for a set of measured points. Here, VL is simply the ratio of available contrast to threshold contrast.

8. There are few acuity studies that have varied contrast, e.g., Cobb and Moss, 1928 and Connor and Ganoung, 1935.

9. Reading small print is a notable exception.

10. However, there are now plates, analogous to Snellen charts, that allow clinicians to perform relatively fast contrast sensitivity measurements. Their use, however, is not yet routine.

11. Since acuity declines with dim light, a driver with even 20/20 acuity during the day is likely to have acuity lower than 20/40 at night. In other words, if potential drivers were tested at nighttime luminance levels, no one would pass!

12. Pinhole viewing restricts the light entering the eye to rays traveling close to the optical axis, where little refraction, i.e., optical correction, is necessary. In fact, if you forget reading glasses and want to read small print, simply take a sheet of paper and puncture it with a pen to create a small hole. You can then read the print through the hole.

13. Formality refers to formal system, i.e., mathematics, logic, etc. Most people naively believe that such formal systems inherently contain absolute truth. In fact, they are highly arbitrary and rest on untested assumptions. Also never forget, "Garbage in, garbage out."

# Chapter 15

# Pedestrian Accident Analysis

Marc Green, Ph.D.

*"[T]he excessive speed of automobiles costs the lives of many persons; and that scarcely a week, sometimes scarcely a day passes without chronicling from one to a dozen deaths occasioned by the reckless driving of these machines. Fortunately, the chauffeur and his guests are the usual sufferers, and in their misfortunes as law-breakers, the general public do not much concern themselves. Our sympathies are rather reserved for...the bystander who is run down and crushed by the enormous weight of these engines."*

—Brown, H. B. 1908. The status of the automobile. *Yale Law Journal* 17, 223-231.

***Synopsis***



## 15.1 Introduction

Pedestrian fatalities constitute about 14 percent of roadway deaths (Campbell, Zeeger, Huang and Cynecki, 2004).[1] These David vs. Goliath confrontations between man and machine generate both sympathy for the pedestrian and blame for the driver. After all, no sane person walks in front of a moving vehicle. Moreover, the driver might imply his own guilt by meekly confiding that he didn't see the pedestrian until the moment of impact. Obviously, the driver was inattentive.

However, courts frequently misplace both sympathy and blame. Of course, drivers cause accidents by speeding, by engaging in distracting behavior, by ignoring signs and signals, etc. However, police reports (e.g., Preusse, Wells, Williams and Weinstein, 2002) of road accidents attribute greater blame to pedestrians than to drivers. This finding might seem surprising and counterintuitive when viewed through the lens of victim sympathy, but scientific data tell a different story. Pedestrians are difficult to see at night, when most severe accidents occur (Campbell, Zeeger, Huang and Cynecki, 2004). The driver must see the pedestrian far ahead of the collision because reaction time and vehicle stopping physics consume distance. Vehicle headlamps have limited effectiveness. Pedestrians frequently exhibit behaviors that contribute to their own accidents.

Below, I explain how these factors conspire to cause vehicle-pedestrian collisions. The discussion has three parts. The first explains that driver ability to avoid pedestrians is limited by three constraints: perception-reaction time, the physics governing vehicle stopping distance and difficulties of contrast detection. The discussion centers on nighttime pedestrian accidents and explains the low effectiveness of vehicle headlamps in providing illumination. A brief review of some research data then reveals that pedestrians only become visible to drivers at astonishingly short distances. Next, I analyze a specific collision to show why drivers often have little chance of avoiding a pedestrian. Simple calculations demonstrate that pedestrians will be difficult to detect at a distance sufficient for avoidance response. The last section explains how adult and child behavior often further contribute to pedestrian accidents.

The chapter focuses on the common case where a driver collides at night with a pedestrian crossing the road in front of the vehicle. It will draw on the discussion of contrast detection from previous chapters and, as the prototypical right-angle collision scenario, will provide groundwork for the next chapter on collision analysis. Other accidents may occur in good daylight visibility or when the pedestrian is stopped or moving parallel to the roadway. These situations are somewhat different but the general factors outlined below still apply.

## 15.2 Constraints On Pedestrian Avoidance

Pedestrian avoidance is limited by both psychology and physics. The driver must see the pedestrian and perform an avoidance response. The vehicle must then respond by slowing or by changing direction.

### A. Perception-reaction time

The time required for seeing and responding is "perception-reaction time," which involves not just contrast detection, but also a series of mental processes. As explained in Chapter 1, drivers must first detect contrast, the difference in brightness between an object and its background. When there is sufficient contrast for detection, then the object is at "contrast threshold" and is "visible." Contrast detection is a very low level mental process that does not result in conscious awareness. In order to be consciously perceived, the object must engage attention ("There is an object in the road"). Next, the viewer must recognize the object ("The object is a pedestrian") and then gain "situational awareness" by analyzing the situation and extrapolating into the future ("I am on a collision course and will hit the pedestrian unless I do something"). The driver must then select and mentally program a response ("I will brake as hard as possible"). Lastly, the driver moves his muscles. All of this processing takes time and consumes distance.

"Experts" commonly cite some textbook or accident reconstruction course and state that normal perception-reaction time for these events is 1.5 seconds. However, a large number of research studies have shown that driver response varies greatly with circumstances. As Chapter 17 explains, the 1.5 seconds value applies, at most, to a 1) young driver 2) with good eyesight, 3) braking 4) to an unexpected, 5) lane incursion by a vehicle or pedestrian cutting across the driver's path, 6) in daytime, 7) with good visibility and 8) no external distractions. Perception-reaction time may vary with changes in any of these factors. Moreover, variability is about half a second. If expected reaction time is 1.5 seconds, then a reasonable response time falls roughly between 1–2 seconds.

The perception-reaction sets a lower limit on the visibility distance needed for pedestrian avoidance. A vehicle traveling 45 mph (66 ft/sec) will have moved 66–132 feet closer to the pedestrian in the time between contrast detection and response initiation.

The 1–2 seconds, however, represent data from studies conducted in good daylight visibility. At night, the lower visibility likely inflates perception-reaction time. A reasonable estimate, depending on visibility, would be 2–3 seconds and possibly longer. In this time, the vehicle has traveled 132–198 feet before the driver responds.

These estimates will often be optimistic. Chapter 1 mentioned that drivers sometimes operate under low arousal due to fatigue, circadian rhythms and/or vigilance decrement. Tiredness slows reaction time, but even rested people experience circadian rhythms, a 24-hour cycle in their arousal level and performance. For people on a normal wake-sleep cycle, there is a significant low point between midnight and 6 AM. One study (Wylie, Schultz, Miller, Mittler, and Mackie, 1996) for example, found that time of day, but not number of hours slept, correlated highly with accidents. Regardless of time of day, people performing a routine, dull task can suffer "vigilance decrement," a loss of arousal and performance that can occur in as little as 20–30 minutes. Lastly, normal behaviors such as checking mirrors and viewing traffic controls can further slow perception-reaction time.

## B. Stopping distance

Reaction time is sometimes defined as "the interval of time between the application of a stimulus and the first indication of a response." The perception-reaction time then only covers the period from detection to initial response—just touching the brakes.[2] Many accident reconstructions overlook the additional time required to actually depress the brake pedal and to engage the brakes fully. This time is difficult to quantify because drivers use different braking strategies. Of course, some braking occurs during this period, but for simplicity sake, I just assume a brake lag of 0.3 second with 0 braking. This adds 20 more feet, making the distance 152–218 feet and the time 2.3–3.3 seconds. Heinrich, Allin, Bowler, and Siegmund (2004) provide data for more precise estimates of pre-skid distances. (See Chapter 16 for a further discussion of braking.)

Lastly, vehicles do not stop instantaneously. Physical forces must act on the vehicle to change its speed or direction. For example, a vehicle traveling 45 mph will require about 90 feet and 2.7 seconds to stop.[3] In sum, the nighttime detection-to-stopping distance at 45 mph is about 242–308 ft. and stopping time is about 5–6 seconds. Of course, this estimate will vary with circumstances.

## C. Contrast Detection

Contrast detection of clothing is a key factor in most pedestrian accidents. Intuitively, light clothing reflects more luminance back to the driver's eye and should create better visibility. Similarly, commonsense suggests that the more light that headlamps and streetlamps throw on the pedestrian, the greater the visibility. However, contrast detection is not so simple and, surprisingly, light clothing and increased amounts of illumination can actually decrease pedestrian visibility.

### 1. Contrast Polarity

This apparent paradox is due to "contrast polarity," a phenomenon depicted in Figure 15.1. Positive polarity occurs when a light object has a dark background. Negative polarity occurs when a dark object lies on a brighter background. Depending on circumstances, a driver may see a pedestrian in positive, negative or even both types of contrast. Moreover, factors that promote one type of contrast polarity weaken the other. Imagine a car on a dark rural road at night. The driver will likely see a pedestrian in positive contrast because the light from the headlamps reflects off of the clothing back to the eye and because the background is dark. In this case, pedestrian clothing is an important factor in visibility. If wearing light clothes, then much of the headlamp illumination reflects back to the driver's eye. Visibility will be far lower for pedestrians wearing dark clothes, which reflect less light.

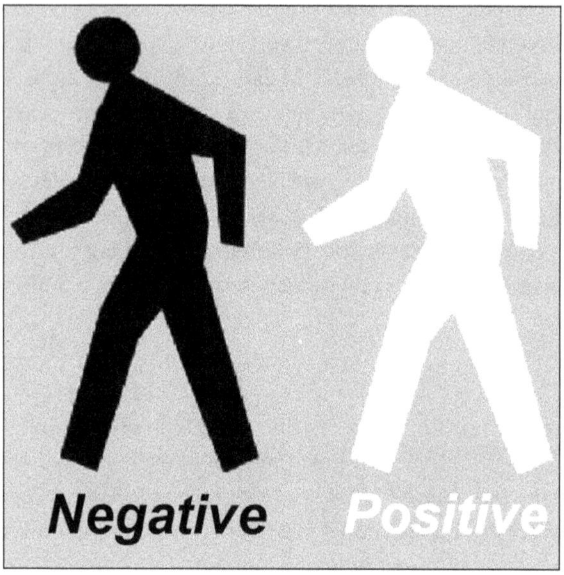


***Figure 15.1*** *Positive and negative contrast.*

Negative contrast occurs when the prevailing light originates behind the pedestrian. If there is backlighting from streetlamps, stores, sky glow, moonlight, oncoming headlamps, etc., pedestrians appear as a silhouette against the lighted backdrop. In this case, the pedestrian's outline is black regardless of clothing, so light clothing provides no special advantage. On the contrary, the lighter clothing decreases negative contrast by better reflecting any ambient front-light to the driver's eye. With negative contrast, dark clothing actually creates better visibility. However, it creates poorer recognition (Green, 2005).

Complications arise, however, because positive and negative contrast can cancel one another, and the pedestrian can change from positive to negative at different distances. Since car low-beam headlamps provide very limited visibility, only shorter distances promote positive contrast. At longer distances, visibility favors negative contrast if there is much backlighting.

As the car approaches, front lighting from headlights begins to increase positive illumination, and the pedestrian can switch from negative to positive contrast. The car headlamps are trying to create positive contrast and make the pedestrian brighter than the background. Meanwhile, street lighting behind the pedestrian is trying to create negative contrast by making a silhouette against a brighter background. There must be a point where the two cancel out and the pedestrian is invisible. Increased backlighting can further reduce visibility by illuminating background clutter that masks detection. It can also make different parts of the visual scene vary in brightness, so the driver changes dark adaptation state with scans of the scene.

Pedestrian contrast polarity typically depends greatly on the type of street lighting, which can be classified as bidirectional, direct or counterbeam. Bidirectional typically used in two way streets sends light in both directions of traffic and does not favor one type of polarity over another. Direct lighting aims in the direction of traffic. It acts something like super-headlamps because it illuminates the road in the direction that the driver is heading. Like headlamps, it creates positive polarity. Counterbeam light faces traffic and backlights the scene creating negative contrast.

Lastly, the headlamp beam partially destroys driver dark adaptation. Drivers on a dark road will typically look at the end of their headlamp beam because they are watching for obstacles in the road ahead and because there isn't enough ambient light to see much else. The driver will then be adapted to the relatively bright beam and be less able to see pedestrians emerging from darkness.

In sum, the messages here are simple: 1) direction of lighting is just as, or even more, important than the amount of lighting and 2) the effect of clothing depends on the direction of the light. Perhaps the worst situation occurs when the pedestrian wears mixed light and dark clothing, i.e., a light shirt and dark pants. The clothing then decomposes the human form into two smaller and less visible and less conspicuous pieces, one favoring positive contrast and the other favoring negative contrast.

### 2. Limited Headlamp Effectiveness

Much of the pedestrian detection problem lies in the limited effectiveness of vehicle headlamps. Intuitively, highly intense headlamps might seem desirable since the driver could see farther. However, large increases in beam intensity produce only modest improvements of visibility distance (see below). Moreover, headlamp design must trade off increased visibility against the danger of creating glare in the eye of oncoming drivers. Headlamp design balances these contradictory demands both by limiting headlamp output and by aiming the beam slightly downward and to the right. The beam is concentrated so that illumination falls rapidly outside the travel lane. In short, the beam primarily illuminates the road directly ahead. As will become clear, the driver must detect the contrast long before the pedestrian is in the road and being illuminated by the beam's core.

The downward and rightward aim of headlamps has important consequences. The downward aim causes headlamps to illuminate pedestrians in the worst possible location, near the ground. To see why, consider where the light from car headlamps hits the pedestrian and background (Figure 15.2). In an ideal world, headlights would maximize positive contrast by illuminating the pedestrian but not the background. Headlight illumination falls with distance, so the farther the background from the pedestrian, the less light it receives and reflects and the closer the approximation to the ideal background.

Figure 15.2 shows that the ideal is better approximated higher in the visual field. Point A, the pedestrian's leg, is only slightly in front of point B, the road just behind the leg. The headlamps illuminate the background almost as well as the pedestrian's lower body. Visibility then depends on the difference in reflectance between the pedestrian's pants and the roadway because they receive similar intensity light.

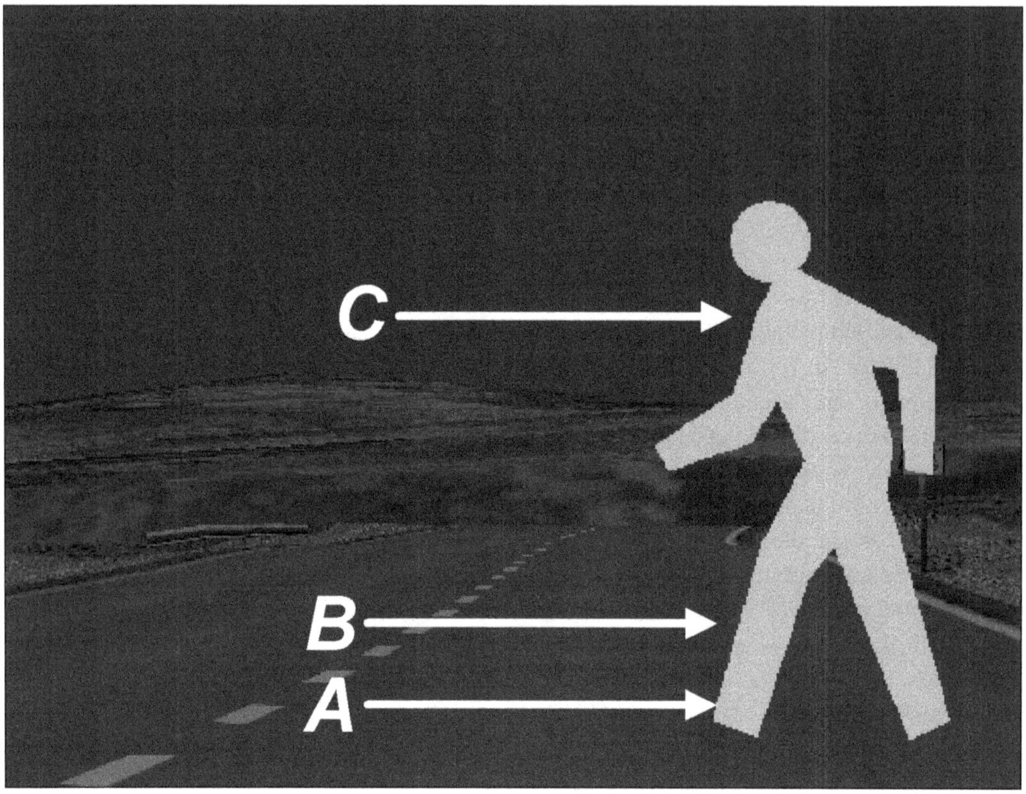


***Figure 15.2*** *Pedestrian on a dark road.*

Now look at point C high up on the pedestrian's body. Less light reaches the upper body because the headlights point down. On the other hand, the background is far away. It does not reflect any illumination back to the driver's eye, so positive contrast maximizes. In sum, the downward pointing headlights illuminate the most where it does the least good—where the distance between pedestrian and background is small—and illuminates the least where it does the most good—where the distance between pedestrian and background is large.

This explains why increases in headlamp output produce modest changes in visibility distance. More intense headlamps put more light on both the pedestrian and the roadway immediately behind the pedestrian. There is more illumination but little contrast change. Remember, people don't see light; they see contrast.

The downward aim also suggests that drivers will have difficulty detecting child pedestrians, who are already low visibility due to small size. They are closer to the ground, so they must be detected where the headlights illuminate both pedestrian and roadway. When the driver first sees the child, moreover, it will be judged as being farther away because of "size-distance constancy," a phenomenon that causes smaller objects to be perceived as farther away.

### 3. Pedestrian Visibility Distance Is Short

Pedestrian visibility distance is a central issue in analysis of pedestrian accidents. Some sources mistakenly assume that visibility distance is the same as the effective range of low-beam headlamps, roughly 300 feet. Actual research on pedestrian visibility typically finds far shorter distances.

The rightward headlamp aim also suggests that visibility distances will depend on whether the pedestrian is approaching from the right or left. As might be expected from the beams' rightward angle, pedestrians approaching from the left are more difficult to detect. Research studies have confirmed that pedestrians to the vehicle's left have shorter visibility distance. One study (Olson and M. Sivak, 1983), for example, found that young drivers could detect dark-clad pedestrians standing to the vehicle's right at 165 feet but that visibility distance for pedestrians to the left was about half, 88 ft. The visibility advantage of pedestrians approaching from the right is largely offset, however, by the speed with which the accident unfolds. For example, less than a second passes from the time that pedestrian steps off the right-hand curb and into the path of a vehicle traveling the curb lane. Pedestrians coming from the left are less visible, but they are in the roadway for a much longer time prior to collision. Lastly, this and many other studies (Flannigan, Sivak, Traube and Aoki, 1995; Chrysler, Danielson and Kirby, 1996; Wood, Tyrrell and Carberry, 2005) have found that older drivers detect pedestrians at drastically shorter seeing distances.

While these studies demonstrate surprisingly short visibility distances for pedestrians, they may still overestimate visibility in realistic conditions. First, the drivers in these studies had optimized positive contrast because the study took place on a completely dark road with no background light to reduce contrast or reveal masking clutter. Second, the pedestrians were on or near the road and hence near the intense portion of the headlamp beams. A pedestrian crossing the road emerges from left or right where the headlamp beam is far weaker, as I discuss below. Third, and perhaps most importantly, the drivers in all of the cited studies knew in advance that pedestrians would be present and knew at least roughly where they would be located. Real drivers do not know where a pedestrian will be located and when a pedestrian will appear. They do not get the opportunity to practice the response over and over again. Moreover, drivers in the study are in the high state of arousal because they know that they are in a research study and that they are being closely monitored.

Most forensic analyses compensate for these differences between research subjects and real drivers by cutting visibility distance 50 percent, based on the results from the classic Roper and Howard (1938) study. After applying this factor to cited data, visibility distances become an astonishingly short 82 feet to the right and 44 feet to the left. However, the 50 percent reduction is not universally applicable and may change with lighting conditions, likelihood of pedestrian activity, etc. (Mortimer, 1996).

Although the research data provide a base for estimating pedestrian visibility, there can be no single distance estimate. A large number of variables influence visibility distances: driver factors (age, eyesight, expectation and arousal), pedestrian factors (age, location, speed and clothing), background factors (masking clutter), headlamp factors (alignment, mounting height, aim and cleanliness), vehicle factors (speed), road factors (type of surface and dryness) and environmental factors (weather and atmospherics conditions).

Visibility also depends on the location and brightness of other light sources. In some cases, as already explained, more light can create less visibility. In the extreme, other light sources, such as oncoming vehicle headlamps, can cause glare and can drastically reduce visibility. Glare problems grow dramatically with age and are a major difficulty for older drivers (and pedestrians). The new HID headlamps are especially prone to create glare in elderly drivers.

### 4. Anticipating Pedestrian Behavior

In order to avoid collision, drivers must often detect pedestrians before they actually enter the roadway. However, not all pedestrians on the sidewalk pose a threat and require a reaction. The driver then faces the task of picking out cues that allow prediction of future pedestrian behavior.

Larsson (2005) has investigated this task using the "safe field of travel," a concept that Gibson and Crooks (1938) proposed as a general model of driver collision avoidance. The "safe field of travel" is the area of possible paths that a driver may take without encountering any objects of "negative valence," i.e., obstacles. It is a cocoon surrounding the driver that moves with him and describes the acceptable margin of error.

The field's shape, however, may change from moment to moment due to environmental circumstances, such as other traffic, rain, and poor visibility. In this view, driving consists primarily of steering a middle path through the field of safe travel while considering the safe field of other drivers and attempting to avoid overlap. Conversely, sudden field contraction induces a steering or braking response.

The driver must consider the sidewalk when defining his safe field. Cues from the pedestrians still on the sidewalk determine whether they have negative valence. If so, then the safe field contracts in that location and the driver must react. Larsson's (2005) study found that drivers reacted to several pedestrian cues, including location in the road, proximity to the road, paths obviously toward the road and even slowing by pedestrians walking parallel to the road. Drivers also reacted more frequently to multiple pedestrians than to isolated ones.

More importantly, however, drivers did not react to pedestrians, regardless of other cues, until distance was 150 feet (45 meters) or less. Depending on vehicle speed, this may already be too close to avoid collision. The likely explanation is that drivers depend on pedestrians to avoid collisions, since pedestrians can start, stop and change direction much more readily than vehicles.

## 15.3 Analysis of A Pedestrian Collision

### A. Basic Analysis

I have explained the difficulties that drivers face in attempting to detect pedestrian contrast and that even the most optimistic research finds very short visibility distances. Combined with the limitations of perception-reaction time and vehicle stopping distance, drivers often face a formidable task that may be outside of human capability. An example will illustrate the point.

Recall that for a vehicle traveling 45 mph, the total stopping distance is about 242–308 feet in 5–6 seconds. Assume that the pedestrian approaches from the left at a steady rate of 4.5 ft/sec, a typical walking speed (e.g., Eubanks, Malmsburym, Schmunk, Beck and Casteel, 2008), and eventually collides with the vehicle's left headlamp.

The analysis starts by calculating the location of driver and the pedestrian at various times prior to collision (Table 15.1). The columns show 1) time prior to impact, 2) pedestrian location to the left of the impact point, and 3) the vehicle distance from the impact point.

Table 15.1 shows that when the driver is 242–308 feet from impact, the pedestrian is about 16 feet to the vehicle's left and far outside any useful headlamp illumination. A typical roadway might consist of two 10-foot wide lanes, so the pedestrian had not even stepped off the curb in the opposite lane. Further, recall from Chapter 4 that viewers tune spatial attention to different distances. Drivers usually look down the road for obstacles and tune their attention accordingly. They are less likely to notice and object that appears in peripheral vision at a short distance. *It is ironic when an "expert" report blames a driver for "not looking where he is going." In fact, he probably was looking where he was going, but that's not where the pedestrian was located until less than a second before impact.*

**Table 15.1**
**Analysis of vehicle pedestrian accidents**

| | | Vehicle = 45 mph | | Vehicle = 30 mph | |
|---|---|---|---|---|---|
| Time To Impact (sec) | Ped To Impact (ft) | Vehicle To Impact (ft) | Visual Angle (deg) | Vehicle To Impact (ft) | Visual Angle (deg) |
| 0.0 | 0.0 | 0 | - | 0 | - |
| 0.5 | 2.3 | 33.1 | 3.9 | 22.1 | 5.8 |
| 1.0 | 4.5 | 66.2 | 3.9 | 44.1 | 5.8 |
| 1.5 | 6.8 | 99.2 | 3.9 | 66.2 | 5.8 |
| 2.0 | 9.0 | 132.3 | 3.9 | 88.2 | 5.8 |
| 2.5 | 11.3 | 165.4 | 3.9 | 110.3 | 5.8 |
| 3.0 | 13.5 | 198.5 | 3.9 | 132.3 | 5.8 |
| 3.5 | 15.8 | 231.5 | 3.9 | 154.4 | 5.8 |
| 4.0 | 18.0 | 264.6 | 3.9 | 176.4 | 5.8 |
| 4.5 | 20.3 | 297.7 | 3.9 | 198.5 | 5.8 |
| 5.0 | 22.5 | 330.8 | 3.9 | 220.5 | 5.8 |

The pedestrian is also located in peripheral vision at 3.9°. Perhaps more importantly, note that the angle between the pedestrian and the driver's eye does not change. The pedestrian's image remains at a fixed location on the driver's retina. This deviation may not seem like much, but it is enough to cause significantly higher contrast thresholds, especially in mesopic vision. (See Chapter 14.) As the driver approaches, however, the pedestrian's retinal image grows and eventually intrudes into the fovea when distance is very short. This is likely why so many drivers say that they didn't see the pedestrian until the moment of collision.

Further, there is no overall motion cue to improve conspicuity. Recall that the fundamental perceptual process is figure-ground segregation. Motion is very helpful in segregating foreground objects from the background. For example, pedestrians are more detectable if they swing their arms than if they walk with their arms straight down.

One way to improve both figure-ground segregation and identification may be the use of "biological motion."[4] Johansson (1973) attached lights to a few key points, such as the head and joints, of people in various activities. Subjects then saw the lights but not the rest of the body. From the few key points, the viewers could tell not only what the actors were doing, but could identify other characteristics such as age and gender. As soon as the actors stopped and motion ceased, however, the viewers saw only a meaningless random pattern. This has led some (Owens, Antonoff, and Francis, 1994) to suggest that attaching lights or reflectors to pedestrian joints would greatly enhance safety.

The rightmost columns show a similar analysis, except the car is traveling only 30 mph. Intuitively, the driver should have a better opportunity to avoid the pedestrian because stopping distance is shorter. However, there is visibility loss that at least partially cancels this advantage. With a slower vehicle, visual angle grows to 5.8° between the pedestrian and the driver's eye and vehicle headlamp beams; pedestrians fall further into peripheral vision and become more dimly illuminated. In general, the faster the pedestrian moves relative to vehicle speed, the more difficult the task that the driver faces in detecting the pedestrian. If the pedestrian were walking briskly at 7 ft/sec, for example, the angle would be 9°. In vehicle-vehicle accidents discussed in Chapter 16, the angle can easily be 60°.

However, the driver does not have to completely stop the vehicle in order to avoid collision. The vehicle need only slow sufficiently to arrive at the collision point after the pedestrian has passed, perhaps slightly over 1 second (a 6-foot wide vehicle and a walking speed of 4.5 seconds) However, note that at 2 seconds prior to collision, a minimum reaction time, the pedestrian is still 132 feet away and 9 feet to the left. At 3 seconds, the driver is 198 feet away and the pedestrian 13.5 feet to the left. Since these distances exceed even optimistic visibility estimates for pedestrian detection, the driver won't see the pedestrian in time to take any action. Moreover, this analysis includes neither the time required to depress the brakes nor for the vehicle to slow sufficiently to gain the needed time/distance.

The calculations show the difficulty in seeing a pedestrian crossing the road at night. Of course, other factors may be operating to improve detection. Streetlamps may provide added useful illumination, pedestrians may wear lighter clothing, or drivers may simply make fortunate eye movements in the pedestrian's direction. Further, a driver approaching an intersection is more likely to scan for other objects outside the immediate travel lane. Conversely, the situation is worse if the pedestrian darts suddenly into the road, fails to wait for a sufficiently large traffic gap or crosses at an unexpected location. In fact, pedestrian behavior often contributes significantly to accidents.

## B. Sensory and Cognitive Analysis

The calculations in the previous section demonstrate the difficulty of pedestrian avoidance. However, there is more to analyzing a pedestrian collision. Depending on circumstances, an analysis might examine a large number of perceptual and cognitive factors. The following example illustrates how a more complete analysis might work. It first examines sensory factors in contrast detection and then moves to an information-processing examination of cognition, attention, recognition, etc.

### 1. Facts and Overview

Mr. X, age sixty-five, is driving down a rural road, Hobart St., at 9:00 p.m. in an unfamiliar part of town. He is late because he promised to pick up his wife at 8:45. Mr. X is listening to a hockey game on the car radio while he looks for Front St., where his wife said to turn in order to reach his destination. Ms. Y, wearing a dark blue coat and white hat, stepped from the left hand shoulder into the middle of Hobart St. without looking. Mr. X does not see Ms. Y until the last moment and strikes her with his car. Police arrive and question Mr. X, who says that he never saw the pedestrian. Mr. X admits that he has had a few beers but his blood alcohol content is .06, within the legal limit. The police do not charge him with DWI.

In the hypothetical situation described above, the accident would not have occurred if everything had worked properly. Following the information processing sequence, the ideal driver would take the actions noted in Table 15.2.

Perfect performance by the ideal driver, does not guarantee that he could actually avoid the pedestrian. The factors of perception-reaction and stopping distance always limit what a driver can do. For now, however, I will temporarily ignore these issues and examine how the situation departed from the ideal.

**Table 15.2**
**Information processing for a pedestrian**

| Processing | Steps In Avoidance |
|---|---|
| 1. Search and Vigilance | Look down road. |
| 2. Detection and Visibility | Detect Ms. Y's blue coat or white hat as a blob in the visual periphery at a sufficient distance. |
| 3. Attention and Conspicuity | Turn eyes toward her to define the shape. |
| 4. Recognition | Retrieve the necessary information from memory to identify the shape as a person. |
| 5. Situation Awareness | Realize that a collision is imminent. |
| 6. Response Selection | Select a braking response. |
| 7. Response | Brake. |

### 2. Sensation

The starting point of any analysis is the question: Could Mr. X have detected Ms. Y? After all, if the conditions had made Ms. Y undetectable at the sensory level (contrast too low), then no further information processing would have been possible and the collision was unavoidable.

An object's visibility is determined not by its absolute brightness or color, but by the relative intensity (and sometimes color) between the object and its background. The analytical first step is to determine whether the actual contrast were sufficiently high for object detection. This is not straightforward, however, since many factors affect the minimum contrast necessary to see an object in a given set of circumstances (Chapters 2, 4 and 14).

A rough initial examination reveals that Ms. Y was wearing a dark blue coat, which would have little contrast against the dark background existing at 9:00 PM. The white hat had higher reflectance and would produce better contrast but not necessarily better visibility. It is small compared to the coat, so that it might be less visible. Of course, if the background were bright, say a brightly illuminated shopping strip, then the dark coat might be highly visible and the white hat relatively hard to see. The shopping strip might also have created a masking background, which is absent on a dark rural road.

Mr. X would initially detect Ms. Y first in the low-resolution peripheral field some time after she stepped off the left shoulder. If he were looking straight down the road, the eccentricity could be calculated as above. However, Mr. X was searching for a street sign, so the eccentricity might have been greater and the contrast threshold accordingly higher. Her approach from the left further reduced detectability because car headlights point down and to the right. Any other car headlights, neon signs, etc. causing glare would further increase contrast threshold.

Mr. X is sixty-five years old, so he likely has a moderate age loss of contrast sensitivity. More over, he had had a few beers, so his blood alcohol level (BAC) was .06. Although this is below legal limit, .06 is a high enough BAC to impair contrast detection. Other issues are: Was he wearing optical correction? Was the correction correct? Does he have any eye disorders? He probably had some degree of night myopia.

At this point, analysis could proceed in one of two ways. One method performs the required light measurements and/or calculations on the pedestrian's clothing (or exemplars) and the background and then estimates size and distance in order to calculate exact values. The expert would ideally take measurements at the same date and time and under the same weather conditions as the actual accident. If impossible or not feasible, then the analysis would have to use other sources of data to estimate contrast (Chapter 13). The alternative method estimates visibility distance from the large number of research studies that have examined the effects of visibility variables on pedestrian detection. In many cases, this is more practical and just as valid. Perceptual/cognitive factors, however, may modify conclusions based on either approach.

### 3. Perception

Let's assume that Ms. Y's contrast level were above detection threshold. The next step is to assess the likely operation of information processing and cognition (Chapter 4). The analysis would look at all sources of information processing input and examine any factors that might affect attention, recognition or situation awareness or that might shift his psychometric function (Chapter 2). In theory, sensation and perception are different processes and analyses. In practice, they overlap. Lastly, response selection factors, such as swerving left/right options, may be relevant.

Mr. X was driving on a dark, unfamiliar street with low visibility and looking for the Front St. sign. He was trying to recall his wife's directions and listening to the radio. If it was an important hockey game involving his favorite team, then he might be spending more concentration on it. Since he was late, he may have been driving fast.

All of these factors would combine to overload attention. Under ideal conditions of good visibility, low traffic, simple roads, no distraction, etc., drivers may have much spare attentional capacity. However, both the low visibility and the number of information sources (visual, radio, recall) stressed Mr. X's age-reduced attentional capacity. If he were traveling fast, the increased flow of new visual input would further stress the attentional filter. However, older people are likely to risk compensate by traveling at lower speed. Moreover, the flow of new visual information is relatively low on a dark road with few visible objects.

Mr. X's visual attentional beam (Chapter 4) would undoubtedly become very narrow. Older viewers typically have a reduced useful-field-of-view (UFOV, Chapter 9) in even benign conditions, but here he was looking for a small street sign in low visibility in an unfamiliar environment. He was further stressed because he was late. Regardless of contrast factors, he would have a very difficult time seeing objects in the peripheral field.

Factors lowering Mr. X's attentional capacity compounded the problems of attentional overload and reduced UFOV. At sixty-five, he likely had age-related attention loss. The .06 BAC also likely also lowered his overall attentional capacity.

Mr. X's expectations would also lower probability of detection and notice. He knew that pedestrians probably cross at intersections and that pedestrians are rare on dark rural roads at night. His criterion would be high (SDT, see Chapter 2), so his contrast threshold would be increased. If Mr. X had frequently driven down the same stretch of highway and frequently seen crossing pedestrians, then his expectations would be greater that a pedestrian might appear. Moreover, he did not expect pedestrians to step into the road late at night and in front of his car.

Even if he had detected Ms. Y, he must recognize her as a person and gain situational awareness that he might strike a pedestrian. The low probability of pedestrians in that context reduced likelihood of both correct recognition and situation awareness. If only her hat had exceeded contrast threshold, he would not readily recognize the light source as a pedestrian. Suppose that both hat and coat were visible. The hat might have caused "overshadowing," where more visible and conspicuous objects draw attention away from less visible and conspicuous ones. Mr. X would fixate the hat and not notice the pedestrian shape. In either case, the low visibility and uncertainty would greatly increase perception-reaction time.

### 4. Conclusion

Many factors contributed to the collision: low visibility conditions, pedestrian approach from the left, the driver's hurry, age, attention being shared across several inputs (radio, road and recall), moderate blood alcohol level, uncertainty about the directions and unfamiliarity with the street. Ms. Y's low visibility clothing was also a contributing factor by making her less conspicuous. Lastly, she crossed the street at an unexpected location, further making detection and perception difficult.

This list of factors still leaves the central question in forensic analysis. Was the collision avoidable by a normal, prudent driver? To answer this question, the analysis initially considers what the normal (i.e., young, properly corrected) driver, focusing on the road with no distraction, no glare etc. could do. If even the ideal driver could not avoid the collision, then Mr. X's age, BAC, search for the street sign, etc. are irrelevant. If an ideal driver could have avoided the accident, then the analysis examines these other factors in search of an explanation for the accident. Some additional factors may lie in pedestrian rather than in driver behavior.

## 15.4 Pedestrian Behavior Often Causes An Accident

While drivers are usually the focus of attention, research suggests that pedestrian-vehicle accidents are more often due to the pedestrian than to the driver. Police reports (Preusse, Wells, Williams and Weinstein, 2002) blame pedestrians for 50 percent of collision, drivers for 39 percent, and the remainder to both. Campbell, Zeeger, Huang and Cynecki (2004) concluded that pedestrians are responsible for 43 percent and drivers for 35 percent. However, fault attribution changed with circumstances. Police blamed pedestrians primarily for midblock accidents and cases where the pedestrian darted out at an intersection. Drivers received more blame during turns, when driver attention is most heavily taxed, especially on turns to the left. More recent research (Spainhour, Wootton, Sobanjo, Brady, 2006) found that pedestrian behavior contributed to 75 percent of accidents, although factors such as low illumination were also important. Such statistics have led to the opinion that, "Pedestrians often consider themselves outside the law" (Dewar, 2002 ).

### A. Violate Driver Expectation

Pedestrians can contribute to accidents in several ways. They often violate driver expectation, crossing midblock or appearing from behind an obstruction. They tend to wear dark clothes and overestimate their visibility. Moreover, pedestrians are subject to the same faults that afflict drivers: they are often distracted and impaired by alcohol or drugs.

Expectation is a major determinant of visibility and conspicuity. Drivers develop expectations as to where pedestrians are likely to appear. Several studies demonstrate that the majority of vehicle-pedestrian collisions occur outside crosswalks and away from intersections. One study (Cycnecki, 1980), for example, found that only 25 percent of pedestrian accidents occurred within an intersection.

### B. Overconfidence

Pedestrians implicitly assume that because the oncoming vehicle is highly visible to them that they must be highly visible to the oncoming driver. Various research studies (E.g., Allen, Hazlett, Tacker and Graham, 1970; Shinar, 1984; Tyrrell, Brooks, Wood and Carberry, 2004) have found that this overestimation can range from 40 percent to as much as 200 percent. The pedestrians then mistakenly believe that even if they are on a collision course with a vehicle that the driver will have enough time to slow or to stop.

Several studies (Herms, 1972; Zeeger, Stewart, Huang and Lagerway, 2005) suggest another form of overconfidence. Pedestrian accident rates are higher at unsignalized midblock locations when a marked crosswalk is present than when there is no marked crosswalk. One explanation is that pedestrians become overconfident, assuming that the crosswalk is as visible to the driver as it is them and that the driver will certainly give way. The pedestrians would then fail to perform sufficient visual search. Another study (Bungum, Day and Henry, 2005) found that only 13.5 percent of pedestrians looked both left and right as they entered a crosswalk at signalized locations.

## C. Distraction

While driver distraction is a major focus of attention, recent research shows that pedestrian distraction is also becoming a potential accident cause. Pedestrians are often distracted by cell phones (Hatfield and Murphy, 2006; Bungum, Day, and Henry, 2005; Nasar, Hecht, and Wener, in Press) and other electronic devices. The problem has become so severe, that some localities are considering banning pedestrian use of cell phones as well as mp3 players, Blackberries, video games, etc., in crosswalks.

## D. Drugs and Alcohol

Lastly, many studies show injured and killed pedestrians frequently had high blood alcohol levels and/or were on drugs. Here is very brief sampling of studies:

- Drinking pedestrians constitute half of all adult fatalities and that 1/3 had blood alcohol levels over 0.15 (Leaf, 1997);
- 35 percent of pedestrians in fatal accidents had blood alcohol levels exceeding 0.10 (Dickman, 1992);
- Blood alcohol level exceeded 0.08 in 38 percent (Holubowycz, 1994) and 33 percent (Holubowycz, Kloeden and McLean,1994) of pedestrian accident victims;
- 16 percent of pedestrian accident victims had been using drugs (Holubowycz, Kloeden and McLean, 1994);
- 34 percent of all pedestrians and 46 percent of pedestrians aged twenty-one to twenty-four in fatal accidents had a BAC of 0.08 or higher (National Highway Transportation Safety Administration, 2006).

The rates are probably much higher for some demographic groups. Elderly victims were almost never under the influence of alcohol or drugs, so the rates of young and middle-aged victims must be much higher.

A Department of Transportation (Shankar, 2001) analysis suggests the most startling and counterintuitive fact of all. Only 7 percent of fatal accidents occurred when the pedestrian was sober and the driver was impaired. When the situation was reversed with the driver sober and the pedestrian inebriated, the percentage tripled to 25 percent. Drunken walking may be more dangerous than drunken driving.

## E. Child Behavior and Accidents

Pedestrian accidents constitute the leading cause of child fatalities in industrialized countries. The highest incidence occurs at about ages 5–9 (e.g., Assilly, 1997), the age range where children have developed both sufficient motor skills and independence to put themselves in harm's way but have not yet developed full adult abilities.

The exact cause for the high rate of child pedestrian accidents is a frequent topic of research and speculation, but no clear-cut answer has emerged. Various authors have suggested that the cause lies in situational variables, child behavior and/or driver behavior.

The same situational factors that plague avoidance of adult pedestrians also affect avoidance of child pedestrians, i.e., low visibility, peripheral location, headlamp ineffectiveness, etc. These effects should be even greater with child pedestrians. Their small size lowers their detectability, and increases their apparent distance and time-to-collision from looming.

Many accidents are certainly due to the child's behavior (Hoffrage, Hertwig, Weber, and Chase, 2003). Sensory explanations suggest that children have lower contrast sensitivity. In this account, children are simply poorer at seeing the oncoming vehicle. Contrast sensitivity is low at birth and improves with age. In unpublished research, I found that children do not reach adult foveal contrast sensitivity until about the age of eight. However, the improvement from about five to eight is relatively small, so low foveal contrast sensitivity is unlikely to be a major factor. A similar explanation suggests that children have reduced peripheral contrast sensitivity. However, research (David, Chapman, Foot, and Sheehy, 1986) shows that children have adult levels of peripheral vision.

A different theory says that children see the oncoming traffic but are unable to correctly judge safe crossing gaps. Somewhat surprisingly, most research (e.g., Demetre, Lee, Pitcairn, Grieve, Thomson, Ampofo-Boateng, 1992) has found that children were actually more cautious than adults. Another study (Plumert, Kearney, and Cremer, 2004) confirmed that children (bicycle riders) exhibited adult abilities in gap acceptance but that they left themselves a smaller margin for error by starting across the road later. However, Connely, Conaglen, Parsonson, and Isler (1998) systematically varied traffic speed and found children judge gaps based on traffic distance and do not sufficiently consider speed. If so, then they will more likely have an accident if the oncoming car travels unusually fast. The underlying reason for the faulty strategy is unclear, but perhaps children are unable to judge looming properly.

A third class of explanations suggest that some children lack impulse control. Hoffrage, Hertwig, Weber, and Chase (2003) concluded that children make fast decisions and exhibit less tolerance for delay. Children are then presumably more likely to dart out into traffic without waiting for a safe gap. Their conclusion seemingly conflicts with the studies showing greater caution in children than in adults. The paradox is only apparent because Hoffrage, Hertwig, Weber, and Chase (2003) suggest that only a subset of children exhibit the failed impulse control.

Perhaps the most frequently proposed explanation is lack of attention. Presumably, the problem is simply that children don't notice oncoming traffic rather than an inability to detect it or properly judge gaps. While this has some face validity, and some suggestive research support, it is still speculative. One study supporting the attentional explanation (Determete and Gaffin, 1994) found that given the choice of crossing at locations where parked cars obstructed the view of oncoming traffic and where the view was clear, six year olds showed no preference. As age increased, children more frequently chose the unobstructed location.

Finally, driver behavior also contributes to some child pedestrian accidents. Thompson, Fraser and Howarth (1985) is one of several studies which found that drivers insufficiently slow or respond to child pedestrians. Drivers normally rely on pedestrians to control their own movements, so they do not prepare for the unpredictability of child behavior. Howarth (1988) further found that although drivers' subjectivity rate the risk of striking a child pedestrian as high, their actual behavior is governed by the learned objective rate, which is low. This harkens back to the Chapter 2 discussion that the societal perspective on safety emphasizes payoffs more than probabilities while the individual perspective may differ.

## 15.5 Conclusion

Natural victim sympathy creates a pervasive bias against drivers, which is obvious in many ways. Drivers are the almost exclusive target of both accident reduction programs and the media. While driver blood alcohol tests are common, some localities have laws against testing pedestrian blood alcohol level. There is no such organization as MAPP: Mothers Against Polluted Pedestrians.

Here's the reality. Successful pedestrian avoidance requires a relatively long visibility distance. Both driver perception-reaction time and the physical forces required to stop a vehicle limit the time/distance available. Moreover, seeing pedestrians at night is a highly difficult task due to the low contrast, the weak intensity and eccentric aim of headlamp beams, and the visual angle between the pedestrian and the driver's eye. Lastly, pedestrians frequently compound visibility problems by their behavior. The number of accidents attributed to pedestrians would likely increase if police and courts were aware of these factors.

In many, if not most, nighttime crossing situations, the pedestrian will have the better chance of avoiding collision. Vehicles are far more visible and conspicuous than pedestrians. Vehicle location is generally far more predictable—a pedestrian knows to look left in near lane(s) and right in far lane(s). Moreover, pedestrians are far more maneuverable, being able to stop, start and turn more quickly than any vehicle.

This discussion has explained the scientific factors that provide a rational basis for assigning blame for vehicle-pedestrian accidents. The purpose is *not* to play "blame the victim" or to let drivers off the hook. Nothing I've said totally excuses a driver who is distracted, who speeds, or who runs through a STOP sign or red light. Pedestrians, like drivers, rely on others to act normally and predictably and to obey traffic regulations. Moreover, judging approach speed and distance of an oncoming vehicle can be a difficult task. For example, pedestrians may overestimate vehicle distance for many "normal" reasons such as size-distance constancy; smaller cars with closer set headlamps will appear farther away. Other distortions include "aerial perspective" (mist or fog makes objects appear more distant), "height in the visual field" (vehicle approaching from a top of a rise may seem farther away), and dim headlamps, which may confound the use of brightness as a distance cue. All of these effects can magnify the pedestrian tendency to overconfidence.

## References

Allen, M., R. Hazlett, H. Tacker, and B. Graham. 1970. Actual pedestrian visibility and the pedestrian's estimate of his own visibility, *American Journal of Optometry and the Archives American Academy of Optometry*, 44-49.

Assilly, J. 1997. Characterization and prevention of child pedestrian accidents: An overview. *Journal of Experimental Child Psychology* 18, 257-262.

Bungam, T., C. Day, and J. Henry. 2005. The association of distraction and caution displayed by pedestrians at a lighted crosswalk. *Journal of Community Health* 30, 269-279.

Campbell, B., C. Zegeer, H. Huang, and M. Cynecki. 2004. A *Review of Pedestrian Safety Research in the United States and Abroad* (FHWA-RD-03-042). Washington, DC: U.S. Department of Transportation, Federal Highway Administration.

Chrysler, S., S. Danielson, and V. Kirby. 1996. Age differences in visual abilities in nighttime driving field conditions. Proceedings of the Human Factors and Ergonomics Society 40th Annual Meeting, Philadelphia. 923.

Connely, M., H. Conaglen, B. Parsonson, and R. Isler. 1998. Child pedestrians' crossing gap thresholds. *Accident Analysis & Prevention* 30, 443-453.

Cycnecki, M. 1980. Development of a Conflicts' Analysis Technique for Pedestrian Crossings, Transportation Research Record 743.

David, S., A. Chapman, H. Foot, and N. Sheehy. 1986. Peripheral vision and child pedestrian accidents. *British Journal of Psychology* 77 (Pt 4), 433–450.

Demetre, J., and S. Gaffin. 1994. The salience of occluding vehicles to child pedestrians. *British Journal of Educational Psychology*, 64, 243-251.

Demetre, J., D. Lee, T. Pitcairn, R. Grieve, J. Thomson, and K. Ampofo-Boateng. 1992. Errors in young children's decisions about traffic gaps: Experiments with roadside simulations. *British Journal of Psychology* 83, 189-202.

Dewar, R. 2002. Pedestrian and bicyclists. In R. Dewar and P. Olson (eds.) *Human Factors In Highway Safety*. Tucson, AZ: Lawyers & Judges Publishing.

Dickman, F., and W. Cope. 1992. Drug Related Pedestrian And Bicycle Crash Injuries, *Transportation Research Circular* 397, 5-6.

Downing, P., D. Bray, J. Rogers, and C. Childs. 2004. Bodies capture attention when nothing is expected. *Cognition* 93, B27-B38.

Eubanks, E., R. Malmsburym, G. Schmunk, R. Beck, and D. Casteel. 1998. *Pedestrian Accident Reconstruction and Litigation*. Tucson, AZ: Lawyers & Judges Publishing Company.

Flannigan, M., M. Sivak, E. Traube, and M. Aoki. 1995. Effects of Foreground illumination, Wet Pavement, and Driver Age on Pedestrian Detection Distance, Report No. UMTRI-9523 University of Michigan Transportation Research Institute.

Gibson, J. J., and L. Crooks. 1938. A theoretical field analysis of automobile-driving. *American Journal of Psychology* 51, 453-471.

Green, M. 2005. Is It A Gun? Or Is It A Wallet?" Perceptual Factors In Police Shootings of Unarmed Suspects, *Police Marksman* July/August 52-58.

Hatfield, J., and S. Murphy. 2006. The Effects of Mobile Phone Use On Pedestrian Crossing Behaviour at Signalised and Unsignalised Intersections, *Accident Analysis and Prevention* 197-205.

Heinrich, B., B. Allin, J. Bowler, and G. Siegmund. 2004. Vehicle speed affects both braking kinematics and average tire/road friction. *Accident Analysis and Prevention* 36, 839-840.

Herms, B. 1972. Pedestrian crosswalk study. *Highway Research Record*, 406, 1-13.

Hoffrage, U., R. Hertwig, A. Weber, and V. Chase. 2003. How to keep children safe in traffic: find the daredevils early. *Journal of Experimental Psychology: Applied* 9, 249-260.

Holubowycz, O. 1994. Age, Sex, And blood alcohol Concentration Of Killed And Injured Drivers, Riders, And Their Passengers, *Accident Analysis and Prevention 26*, 483-492.

Holubowycz, O., C. Kloeden, and A. McLean. 1994. Usual Drinking And Drink-Driving Behaviour Of Injured Male Drivers and Riders: A Comparison Between Those With Zero And High Blood Alcohol Concentration" in D. South and A. Cavallo (eds.), *Australasian Drink-Drive Conference Proceedings*; 1993 Nov 22–23, Melbourne.

Howarth, I. 1988. The relationship between objective risk, subjective risk and behaviour. *Ergonomics* 31, 527-535.

Larsson, A. 2005. Pedestrian detection and driver attention: cues needed to determine risky pedestrian behaviour in traffic. Unpublished Master's Thesis, Linköping University.

Leaf, W. and D. Presusser. 1997. Identification of Alcohol Related Crash Problems Among Selected Racial/Ethnic Groups, Report DOT HS 808 641, 1997.

Mortimer, R. 1996. The effect of expectancy on visibility in night driving. *Proceedings of the Human Factors And Ergonomic Society* 40, 506-510.

Nasar, J., P. Hecht, and R. Wener. In Press. Mobile telephones, distracted attention, and pedestrian safety. *Accident Analysis and Prevention.*

National Highway Transportation Safety Administration. 2006. Traffic Accident Facts. Washington, D. C.: National Highway Transportation Safety Administration.

Olson, P., and M. Sivak. 2003. Improved Low-Beam Photometrics, Report UMTRI-83-9, University of Michigan Transportation Research Institute, Ann Arbor, MI.

Owens, D. A., R. A. Antonoff, and E. Francis. 1994. Biological motion and nighttime pedestrian conspicuity. *Human Factors* 36, 718-732.

Plumert, J., J. Kearney, and J. Cremer. 2004. Children's perception of gap affordances: Bicycling across traffic filled intersections in an immersive virtual environment. *Child Development* 75, 1243-1253.

Preusse, D., J. Wells, A. Williams, and H. Weinstein. 2002. Pedestrian Crashes In Washington, DC and Baltimore. *Accident Analysis and Prevention* 703.

Ro, T., C. Russell, and N. Lavie. 2001. Changing faces: a detection advantage in the flicker paradigm. *Psychological Science* 12, 94-99.

Roper, V., and E. Howard. 1938. Seeing with Motor Car Headlamps, *Transactions of the Illuminating Engineering Society* 33, 417-438.

Shankar, U. 2001. Pedestrian roadway fatalities, Department of Transportation Technical Report HS 809 456.

Shinar, D. 1984. Actual versus estimated night-time pedestrian visibility, *Ergonomics* 27, 863-871.

Spainhour, L., I. Wootton, J. Sobanjo, and P. Brady. 2006. Causative Factors and Trends in Florida Pedestrian Crashes. Transportation Research Record 1982, 90-98.

Thompson, S., E. Fraser, and C. Howarth. 1985. Driver behaviour in the presence of child and adult pedestrians. *Ergonomics* 28, 1469-1474.

Tyrrell, R., J. Brooks, J. Wood, and T. Carberry. 2004. Nighttime Conspicuity from the Pedestrian's perspective Transportation Research Board Annual Meeting CD.

Wood, J., R. Tyrrell, and T. Carberry. 2005. Limitations Drivers' Ability to Recognize Pedestrians at Night, *Human Factors* 47, 644-653.

Wylie, C., T. Schultz, J. Miller, M. Mittler, and R. Mackie. 1996. Driver Fatigue and Alertness Study. U.S. Department of Transportation, Federal Highway Administration and Transport Canada – Transportation Development Centre report TP1287E.

Zeeger, C., R. Stewart, H. Huang, and P. Lagerway. 2005. Safety effects of marked vs. unmarked crosswalks at uncontrolled locations: Analysis of Pedestrian crashes in 30 cities. *Transportation Research Record* 1773, 56-68.

## Endnotes

1. Down from 42 percent! in 1927.

2. Strictly speaking, reaction time is a purely mental event. However, it could not be measured without a physical response, so "contamination" by some motor component is unavoidable. In basic research, the motor component is minimized as much as possible. Brain wave studies often show a spike in mental activity about 100 or more msec prior to actual muscle movement.

3. Assuming a straight, level road and a 0.75 coefficient of friction.

4. See http://www.michaelbach.de/ot/mot_biomot/index.html for an online demonstration of biological motion.

# Chapter 16

# Collision Analysis

Marc Green, Ph.D.

*"Carriages without horses shall go,*
*And accidents fill the world with woe."*
—Mother Shipton (circa 1530)

***Synopsis***



## 16.1 Introduction

Vision is invariably a factor in determining whether a driver can avoid an impending collision. The visual analysis of collisions follows roughly the same path as visual analysis of contrast detection. First, determine amount of sensory information available to the driver. Next, determine threshold. Lastly, adjust the laboratory data to reflect real-world conditions.

However, collision analysis differs somewhat from a purely visibility analysis. Although contrast can play a role, the critical sensory information is motion, and the threshold of interest is motion detection. Further, the driver must make suprathreshold sensory judgments of path/time/distance to collision. The driver must then gain situational awareness of whether action is necessary. Collision avoidance further requires both response selection and execution. Lastly, the vehicle responds to the driver input.

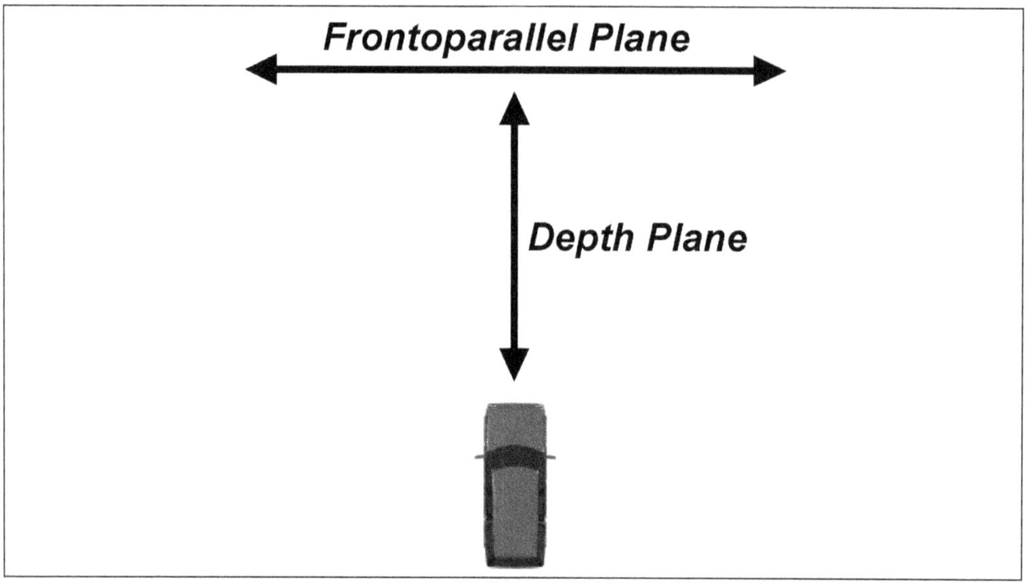


***Figure 16.1*** *Frontoparallel and depth planes.*

This chapter explains methodology for performing a collision analysis. I divide the chapter into two sections based on the collision angle. Right-angle collisions occur when the vehicle meets another object moving on an orthogonal path across the "frontoparallel plane." (See Figure 16.1.) Zero-angle collisions occur when the objects are moving along the same depth plane at different speeds. The vehicles may meet head-on (180°), head-rear (0°) or side-swipe.

Of course, other collisions fall between the zero and right-angle cases, but for simplicity sake I consider only these extremes. Further, this chapter focuses on zero-angle collisions. The previous chapter covered right-angle vehicle-pedestrian collisions. Since the analysis is similar for other right-angle collisions (vehicle-vehicle, vehicle-train, etc.) this chapter only adds a few new points. Of zero-angle collisions, the chapter concentrates on head-rear (rear-end) collisions, which constituted roughly 30 percent of all road accidents in 2004 (Fatal Accident Report System).

## 16.2 Zero-Angle Collisions

### A. Rear-End Collision

Rear-end collisions typically fall into one of two scenarios. First, the lead car decelerates but continues moving while the following car continues at the same speed. The following car then eventually overtakes and collides with the lead car. Second, a moving vehicle collides with a stopped vehicle, the scenario in about two-thirds of all rear-end collisions (Knipling, Hendricks, Koziol, Allen, Tijerina, and Wilson, 1992).

In order to avoid a rear-end collision, a driver must perform the steps described above: motion detection, "time-to-collision" (TTC) estimation, and response. Performing these steps is difficult for two reasons. First, drivers expect other vehicles to travel at about the same speed as they travel. Second, judging the motion of objects heading straight toward or away from the eye is difficult. The explanation lies in optics, as a quick calculation demonstrates. Suppose a 6-foot wide object at 200 feet moves a distance of 20 feet along the frontoparallel plane in one second. The distance moved is arctan(20/200) or 5.8°, so the angular velocity is 5.8°/sec. If the same object moves 20 feet in the depth plane toward the observer in one second, its image grows by .2° (arctan(6/200) = 1.7° to arctan(6/180)=1.9°). Since the object dilates symmetrically, each edge moves only half of the distance. The actual average motion is 0.1°/sec., or about 2.0 percent as fast as the equivalent frontoparallel plane motion.

Viewers can detect motion in depth using indirect or direct perception. The indirect method mentally "calculates" motion from perceived speed and distance. On the roadway, for example, drivers may use the indirect method to estimate "headway," the change in lead vehicle distance as a function of time. As I will explain, the indirect method has the advantage of being available at long distances but the disadvantage of being slow and imprecise.

The alternate method extracts motion directly from optical transformations of the visual array. Gibson (1969) noted that as viewers move through the world, the visual scene undergoes predictable optical transformations. According to Gibson's (1969, 1977) theory of "direct perception," viewers can use this optical information to guide action without the need to infer motion indirectly from mental calculations of speed and distance. Lee (1976) later developed an explicit theory describing how a driver could use optical motion to decide when to swerve/brake. The centerpiece of his theory is the optical variable $\tau$ ("tau"), which gives the time-to-collision (TTC) and whose temporal derivative $\dot{\tau}$ ("tau dot") specifies the required deceleration rates. In theory, $\tau$ has two advantages over headway. It is perceived rapidly, being directly extracted from the optic array, and it provides very precise TTC information. On the negative side, it is available only when the following driver is relatively close to the lead vehicle.

Lee's theory has been among the most heavily examined topics in perception and motor control of both humans and animals. The physics part, the possibility of deriving TTC from purely optical information, is doubtless correct. The psychology part, whether drivers actually use this information exclusively or even partially, is less certain. Much as scientists and engineers like simple and elegant theories such as $\tau$, real behavior is seldom so straightforward. Vision is a highly opportunistic enterprise, and viewers guide action with any available and useful information. Moreover, they do it unconsciously, so discovering how people perform tasks such as driving is extremely difficult.

Still, optical information likely plays a critical role in collision avoidance, especially in situations where the driver is heading toward another vehicle in an impending rear-end or head-on collision. In these cases, forensic collision analysis starts by determining detection threshold for the critical motion in the optic array. Next, the analysis goes through the stages of interpretation and action that are outlined in Chapter 1.

This focus on optical motions further highlights both the importance of distinguishing between distal and proximal events and the critical role of optics in vision. The distal event may be a car stopped in the roadway ahead. However, the only information available to the driver lies in the retinal image of the car. We can speak of seeing a car coming down the street, but the driver never directly sees the car. Instead, he sees only the image that the car casts on the retina. As the driver approaches, this retinal image transforms, and it is this transformation that provides the information needed to see and to avoid the impending collision. In sum, vision depends on the retinal image, so that's where the analysis should start. After first briefly discussing headway, the majority of the chapter discusses retinal image transformations and their role in collision avoidance.

## 1. Headway

In headway determination, the driver notes the amount of roadway to the lead vehicle and then observes how that distance changes with time. Studies (e.g., Mortimer, 1971) suggest that the JND/

Weber fraction (Chapter 2) for headway change is about .12 before the gap decrease is noticeable. For example, assume that a driver turns on to a road where a car has stopped 1000 feet ahead. The driver should notice when the gap has dropped to 880 feet (12 percent of 1000 is 120 and 1000-120=880). If the driver were traveling at 55 mph (80.8 ft/sec), it would take him about 1.5 seconds to cover the needed distance. If the lead vehicle were moving, then the driver would require more time to reach the .12 threshold.

In real situations, however, detection of headway change may be poorer. If the viewer looks away from the road momentarily, the change may not be readily detectable. However, drivers generally use headway at such a great distance that such variations are not often critical.

The more important problem is that headway cues provide limited rate information. The driver may perceive that he is closing on the lead vehicle, but he cannot accurately estimate the *rate* of closing and time to collision. This is an important fact because Evans (1991) suggests that violation of strong expectations about normal traffic flow is the major cause of rear-end collisions. Drivers assume that other vehicles will be moving at about the same speed. It is not unusual to close somewhat on a lead vehicle, so the simple fact of closing is not sufficient to require response or even close attention. The driver may perceive the closing distance but not necessarily perceive that the rate of change is high and that the lead vehicle is stopped or decelerating rapidly. Drivers need readily detectable and accurate rate (TTC) information that can overcome the strong expectation. Optical transformation in the visual array can provide this information.

### 2. Looming—Theory

In "The Black Cloud" (1957), science fiction writer Fred Hoyle posed the following problem: suppose a "black cloud" were heading straight toward the earth. Would it be possible to determine the time before impact when actual speed and distance were unknown? He discovered that the TTC could be derived directly from the object's rate of image growth.

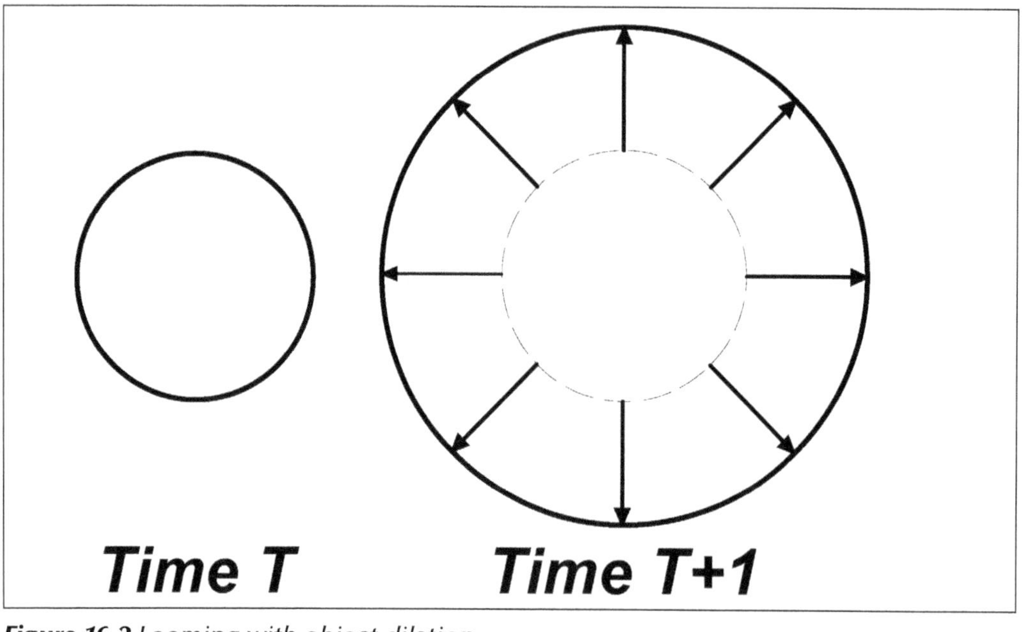


***Figure 16.2*** *Looming with object dilation.*

Drivers approaching a stopped or decelerating vehicle face a similar problem (Lee, 1976). In theory, a driver can use the rate of retinal image growth and angular velocity to precisely determine the TTC. The driver need have no knowledge of the distal information—lead vehicle's size, distance or the actual approach velocity.

The approach of an object is called "looming," and Figure 16.2 illustrates the concept. Suppose someone throws a ball directly at your eye. At time T, it projects an image onto the retina. As the ball moves closer at time T+1, its retinal image grows symmetrically and the edges move outward. The rate of outward motion is the angular velocity. The faster the ball approaches, the faster the edges move outward and the shorter the time until the ball fills the entire visual field and hits the eye.

Mathematically, the time-to-collision (TTC) is approximately the retinal image size, θ, divided by the rate of retinal image growth (the derivative of image growth with respect to time). TTC is then:

$$\tau = \frac{\theta}{\left(\frac{d\theta}{dt}\right)}$$

where variable $\tau$ ("tau."),[1] is the TTC in seconds. The numerator is just the visual angle[2] while the denominator is the instantaneous angular velocity or "looming rate," which can be readily calculated from size, distance and approach velocity. Using the small angle approximation (Chapter 3), a vehicle of width W and distance D has a visual angle of:

$$\theta = \frac{W}{D}$$

As the following driver approaches with relative velocity V, the angular velocity of the lead vehicle in radian/second is:

$$\frac{d\theta}{dt} = \frac{WV}{D^2}$$

Table 16.1 shows how looming allows TTC estimation. In this example, a vehicle is traveling 55 mph (80.8 ft/sec) and is approaching a stopped vehicle that is 6 feet wide. The first four columns show distance, relative velocity, car width and visual angle in radians. The "Looming" column shows the angular velocity in radian/sec. TTC is the distance remaining divided by velocity. The final column shows $\tau$, which is TTC calculated from the purely optical information, the visual angle divided by the looming rate. TTC and $\tau$ methods give the same answer. As Hoyle required, the driver need not know the actual distance, speed or object size to determine TTC. However, this does not preclude that driver's use of such information.

While $\tau$ theoretically allows a viewer to directly perceive TTC, its strict applicability to the real world is still debated. Shelves of research papers argue over whether viewers in the laboratory and in the real-world actually use $\tau$, whether they use it exclusively, whether they use it in combination with other variables (e.g., Smith, Flach, Dittman, and Stanard 2001), or whether they use some other related optical variable. For now, I will just say that viewers likely use $\tau$, or some closely related variable, but that they likely use other visual information as well.

The one issue on which there is no debate, however, is that viewers cannot use $\tau$ to estimate TTC if the angular velocity, $d\theta/dt$, is below motion detection threshold. The driver must first perceive the outward motion of the approaching object. The looming threshold plays the same role in collision analysis as contrast threshold does in visibility analysis; it specifies the point at which the driver theoretically has sufficient direct sensory information to begin reacting. Of course, the driver may use brake lights or other non-optical information, but I will put that on hold until later.

The looming calculation, $d\theta/dt=(WV)/D^2$, shows that the variables size, relative velocity and distance determine looming rate. First, larger size creates higher angular velocity. A driver can more easily detect that he is closing on a stopped 8-foot wide tractor-trailer than on a 5.5-foot wide sports car. Second, high relative speed also increases looming rate. This is hardly surprising, but the inherent tradeoff between speed and perception-reaction time is not so obvious. A driver who is traveling fast will hit a stopped vehicle sooner and have less time to react than one who is traveling slowly. However, the faster driver will detect looming at a greater distance, which provides more time to react. This tradeoff between speed and looming detection distance means that vehicle speed may have little effect on the time available to respond. Of course, faster speed means longer physical braking distance, so the driver's opportunity to avoid may be lower.

Note also that velocity refers to the *relative* velocity between the driver and lead vehicle. There is no theoretical difference between a driver traveling 30 mph approaching a stopped lead vehicle and a driver traveling 60 mph approaching a lead vehicle traveling 30 mph. The relative velocity is 30 mph in both cases. However, driver speed is not totally irrelevant. A driver traveling in a faster vehicle likely has somewhat less acute vision. In addition, driver speed may affect braking strategy, as discussed below.

Third, viewing distance has a strong influence on looming rate. Table 16.1 shows the key fact that looming rate does not grow linearly but rather hyperbolically as the driver approaches the object. Figure 16.3 shows this relationship more clearly. When an object is far away, the angular velocity is so slow that the driver cannot detect the expansion and cannot perceive the rate of closure. In fact, the lead vehicle appears stationary if there are no other motion cues. As the driver approaches, the expansion rate remains low but then suddenly explodes when distance is short. The message from Figure 16.3 is clear: drivers will not readily detect looming until they come relatively close to the lead vehicle when TTC is short. At that point, the impending collision will suddenly become very obvious. The exact distance at which the driver detects looming and the impending collision depends on human motion detection threshold. The next section discusses research on this threshold.

**Table 16.1**
**Comparison of looming thresholds and time to collision**

| Distance | Velocity | Size | Vis Ang | Looming | TTC | $\tau$ |
|---|---|---|---|---|---|---|
| feet | Ft/sec | Feet | $\theta$ | $d\theta/dt$ | d/v | $\theta/(d\theta/dt)$ |
| 50 | 80.8 | 6 | 0.1194 | 0.1939 | 0.62 | 0.62 |
| 100 | 80.8 | 6 | 0.0599 | 0.0485 | 1.24 | 1.24 |
| 150 | 80.8 | 6 | 0.0400 | 0.0215 | 1.86 | 1.86 |
| 200 | 80.8 | 6 | 0.0300 | 0.0121 | 2.48 | 2.48 |
| 250 | 80.8 | 6 | 0.0240 | 0.0078 | 3.09 | 3.09 |
| 300 | 80.8 | 6 | 0.0200 | 0.0054 | 3.71 | 3.71 |
| 350 | 80.8 | 6 | 0.0171 | 0.0040 | 4.33 | 4.33 |
| 400 | 80.8 | 6 | 0.0150 | 0.0030 | 4.95 | 4.95 |
| 450 | 80.8 | 6 | 0.0133 | 0.0024 | 5.57 | 5.57 |
| 500 | 80.8 | 6 | 0.0120 | 0.0019 | 6.19 | 6.19 |
| 550 | 80.8 | 6 | 0.0109 | 0.0016 | 6.81 | 6.81 |

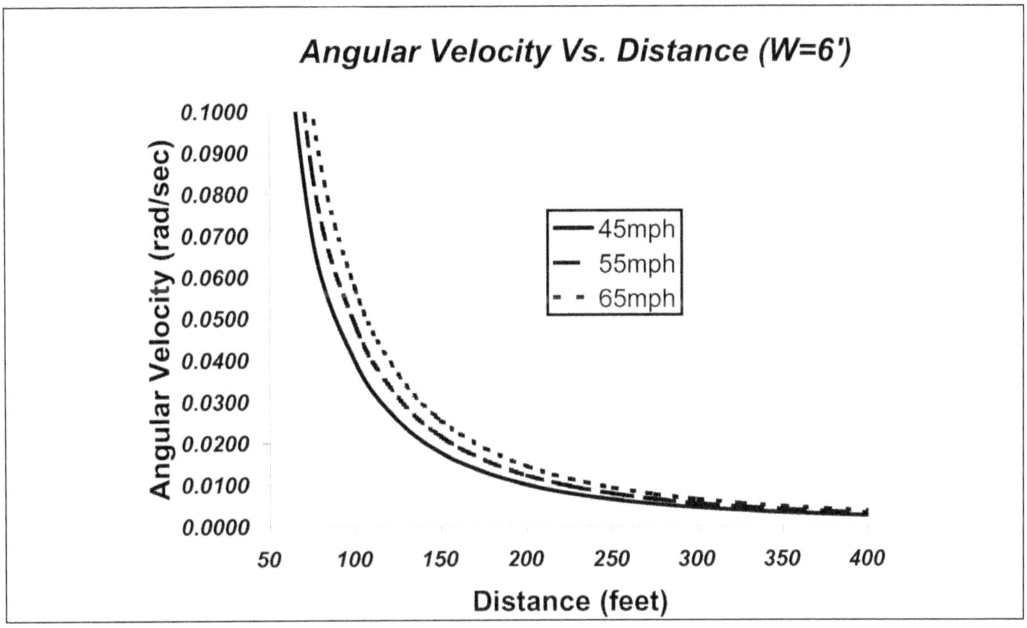


***Figure 16.3*** *Angular velocity ("looming rate") as a function of distance approaching a stopped 6-foot wide car.*

### 3. Looming—Data and Thresholds

Rear-end collision analysis frequently begins with estimation of this looming threshold. Although many studies have examined viewer judgments of TTC from $\tau$, very few have measured angular velocity thresholds and even fewer are translatable to actual road conditions.

In most forensic analyses, experts cite Mortimer (1990) and proclaim that angular velocity threshold is .0030–.0035 radian/sec. However, Mortimer (1990) gives no specific data, so there is no reason to accept this value out-of-hand. Moreover, Mortimer (1990) doesn't say whether this is an experimental threshold or one that could be directly applied to actual collisions. As the discussion of contrast threshold showed, there is a big difference between the thresholds of research subjects and the expected thresholds of real-world drivers. Lastly, Mortimer (1990) makes no mention of normal variability.

Let's look at the data. Table 16.2 shows the results from the few experimental studies that determined an angular velocity threshold for "drivers." Surprisingly, only two published studies have actually tested driver response on the road. Most have used indirect methods.

The most common indirect method has "drivers" judge the speed of approaching vehicles in film clips. The experimenters placed a camera in a vehicle and filmed while approaching a lead vehicle at various speeds. Subjects then viewed the film clips and judged TTC. The researchers then inferred threshold by determining the minimum angular velocity needed before the "driver" could make reliable TTC judgments. The technique relied on the assumption that viewers could not make judgments until the angular velocity had just reached threshold. For practical purposes, this is exactly what we want to know—when can the driver make reliable TTC judgments.[3]

Hoffman (1994) concluded that the threshold was around .002 radian/sec while Hoffman and Mortimer (1996) obtained thresholds ranging from .0021 to .0052. Further, they also reexamined an older study, Farber and Silver (1967), and concluded that it provided evidence for a .003 radian/sec threshold. Hoffman (1968) used an older study (Bierly, 1963) to produce another data point of .00315 radian/sec.

**Table 16.2**
**Looming threshold studies**

| Author | Year | Thresh | Method | Comment |
|---|---|---|---|---|
| Hoffman | 1994 | 0.0020 | Infer | |
| Hoffman and Mortimer | 1996 | 0.0052 | Infer | Scaling problem? |
| Hoffman and Mortimer | 1996 | 0.0030 | Infer | |
| Hoffman and Mortimer | 1996 | 0.0021 | Infer | |
| Hoffman and Mortimer | 1996 | 0.0022 | Infer | |
| Hoffman and Mortimer | 1996 | 0.0052 | Infer | |
| Farber and Silver | 1967 | 0.0030 | Infer | See Hoffman et al. (1996) |
| Bierley | 1963 | 0.0032 | Road Test? | See Hoffman (1968) |
| Baker and Steedman | 1961b | 0.0035 | Lab Experiment | Subjects stationary |
| Summala et al | 1998 | 0.0020 | Road Test | At 60 m following |
| Lamble et al. | 1999 | 0.0038 | Road Test | At 20 m following |
| Lamble et al. | 1999 | 0.0022 | Road Test | At 40 m following |
| Mean | | 0.003 | | |
| Standard Error | | 0.0010 | | |
| Brown et al. | 1989 | 0.0014 | "Road" Test | Stationary observer |
| Brown et al. | 1989 | 0.0015 | "Road" Test | Stationary observer |
| Brown et al. | 1989 | 0.0014 | "Road" Test | Stationary observer |
| Plotkin | 1984 | 0.0275 | Statistical Analysis | Used accident data |

In a more direct test, Baker and Steedman (1961b) performed a laboratory study of viewers detecting looming of an actual light. They obtained a .0035 radian/sec threshold. However, their observers were stationary, which likely lowered threshold, as explained below.

Two studies measured angular velocity threshold by having drivers respond to decelerations of a lead vehicle. Summala, Lamble and Laasko (1998) recorded thresholds of .002 while Lamble, Laasko and Summala (1999) obtained thresholds of .00215 and .0377 radian/sec. Evans and Rotherty (1973), however, note that subjects in such research can learn to detect the lead vehicle pitching up or down slightly in response to deceleration. If so, then real thresholds, especially for a stopped vehicle, might be higher.

Fiske, Obenski and Olson (1989) used a semi-realistic paradigm. An observer sat on the roof of a truck and responded when he could perceive the motion of an approaching or receding vehicle. I recalculated their data from their graphs to estimate the angular velocity thresholds. Their thresholds in looming experiments were .0014 and .0015 radian/sec. They were independent of closing speed and lower than those found in the other studies.[4]

The Fiske et al. thresholds were low for several reasons. First, subjects sat up high, so the approaching car did not head straight for the eye. The retinal image then deformed and may have provided additional cues. Second, and more importantly, the observers were stationary. As a driver moves through the environment, he sees the optical flow field of outward moving points. He must then disentangle the optical motion of flow field from the outward motion of the looming object, an extra task which impairs performance (Probst, Krafczyk, and Brandt, 1984).[5] This is also why Baker and Steedman's threshold is also artificially low. While the Brown et al. thresholds are not directly applicable to moving drivers, the data are likely closer to an expected threshold for a stationary pedestrian or a stopped driver looking down the road to find a suitable gap.

Lastly, Plotkin (1984) examined accident data, performed calculations and concluded that the angular expansion threshold was .0275 radian/sec, an estimate higher than others by almost a factor of ten. Mortimer (1990) correctly noted, however, that this represents only the very worst drivers—those who crashed, and says little about the population in general. In other words, Plotkin did not include data for drivers who did not crash. Moreover, Plotkin did not know the exact circumstances of the crashes. For example, some of the drivers may have been looking away from the road until the last moment, etc. Plotkin also assumed an unreasonably low reaction time. However, part of the discrepancy between Mortimer's and Plotkin's estimates is that Mortimer's .003–.0035 radian/sec is a laboratory value while expected real-world values would be higher.

To derive a single threshold number, I averaged the data from the top half of Table 16.2, excluding Brown and Fiske and Plotkin for reasons already described. The mean value was .003 radian/sec and the median was also .003 radian/sec, agreeing well with the Mortimer (1990) estimate. Determining variability is more problematic. However, standard error produces lower variability estimates than standard deviation. For at least one set of experiments (Hoffman, 1974, which is apparently the data source of his later papers), the standard deviations across various size viewer groups were .0013, .0007, .0009, .0004, .0007. This averages out to .0008 radian/sec. If weighted by the number of subjects in each group, the standard deviation is .0083 radian/sec. Roughly speaking, a "normal" variability of about, .001, or about one standard error, seems reasonable. The normal range for an alerted, prepared, practiced test-subject driver is then about .002–.004 radian/sec.

### 4. Looming—Threshold Field Factors

Looming thresholds, like contrast thresholds, must increase by a field factor in order to account for differences between experimental subjects and real drivers. Most of the same differences apply. Real drivers did not know for certain that the lead vehicle would decelerate. On the contrary, the normal expectation is that vehicles travel in the same direction at about the same speed. Moreover, a stopped vehicle on a roadway, especially a limited access highway, is an extremely rare and unexpected event. This violated expectation would doubtless push thresholds higher. As noted in the Signal Detection Theory discussion of Chapter 2, low probability biases response toward "No" and misses.

Real drivers do not necessarily fixate the exact middle of the lead vehicle at every moment. Although drivers spend most of their time looking directly ahead, they also move their eyes around to sample parts of the road, check their mirrors, etc. If the driver's gaze is away from the midpoint of the lead vehicle, then looming thresholds increase because fixating anywhere else puts some of the motion in peripheral vision where motion detection is poorer (Green, 1981). Lamble et al. (1999), for example, found that looming threshold increased by a factor of three at a viewing angle of 45°.

Further, drivers, especially late at night, are less aroused, than their experimental counterparts, who are alerted and highly aroused from being in a research study. (See the Langham quote near the end of Chapter 1.) Lastly, experimental subjects get to practice and their data are the results of numerous trials in which they learn to perform the identical task over and over. This also creates artificially low variability.

In other perceptual roadway judgments, field factor estimates have ranged from the Roper and Howard's (1938) factor of two for pedestrian visibility distance to numbers as high as 15–20 (Blackwell, 1959; Adrian, 1987) for contrast detection in general. The high field factors used in contrast thresholds probably do not apply because there is less uncertainty. Instead, it is tempting to simply apply the Roper and Howard (1938) rule of thumb that visual performance will be half as good when there is no expectation as when there is foreknowledge. This would make the "real-world" threshold .006 radian/sec for the average driver. With a .001 normal variability, the normal range is .005 to .007 radian/sec. Variability often increases proportionally with the mean, so variability also doubles to .002 and the final and best estimate for a normal range is .004 to .008 radian/sec. However, it is unclear whether the doubling rule can simply be applied, so a field factor of two would be a very rough estimate. In some cases, the multiplier may be even higher. Like any multiplier, the best value depends on circumstances. A driver on a freeway has less expectation of approaching a stopped vehicle than a driver approaching a signaled intersection.

Data from a recent study (Muttart, Messerschmidt and Gillen, 2005) are at least consistent with this threshold range. Subjects viewed a highly schematized computer graphic of a road scene and had to respond to pedestrians and to the sudden stopping of a leading "truck" traveling directly ahead. It is difficult to compare the results to other studies since it inferred thresholds from ranges of reaction time and used several model-based corrections. However, the study did find that reaction times for alerted drivers asymptoted at about .0065 radian/sec.

### 5. Looming—Example Threshold Analysis

Suppose that a driver traveling on a clear day encounters a vehicle unexpectedly stopped on the roadway. Can the driver avoid a collision? The initial analysis would include calculations of looming rates and TTC, as shown in Table 16.1. The next step would be an examination of the time and distance that a driver would require to perform each possible avoidance response. This step requires some physics and selection of parameter values. The example will use the typical value of 0.75 for braking coefficient of friction and 0.3 for lateral acceleration.[6] Finally, the analysis compares time/distance available to time/distance required.[7]

The driver can avoid collision by either braking to a stop or swerving around the lead vehicle. Table 16.3 shows an analysis of braking and two possible swerving responses. One is a simple miss where the driver swerves to avoid the stopped vehicle. The second is a lane change, where the driver swerves and then reverses steering to come parallel to the original heading but in a different lane.

The first four columns are similar to those shown in Table 16.1. "Looming" is angular velocity[8] at each distance while TTC shows time-to-collision. The first new column is TTC-PRT, the time-to-collision minus an assumed perception reaction time of 1.5 seconds. During this time, the vehicle travels 1.5 × 80.8 feet or 121.3 feet. The next column, $TTC\text{-}D_{PRT}$ shows the distance to collision remaining after the 121.3 feet is subtracted. For example, when the driver's car is 225 feet from collision, the perception-reaction time eats up 121.3 feet leaving only 103.7 for the vehicle to brake or to swerve.

**Table 16.3**
**Collision Analysis**

| Distance | VA | Looming | TTC | TTC-PRT | TTC-Dprt | Stop D | Swerve | Parallel |
|---|---|---|---|---|---|---|---|---|
| ft | θ | dθ/dt | d/v | sec | | 134 ft | 90 ft | 127 ft |
| 0 | | | 0.0 | -1.5 | -121.3 | -255.3 | -211.28 | -248.28 |
| 25 | 0.24 | 0.7762 | 0.3 | -1.2 | -96.3 | -230.3 | -186.3 | -223.28 |
| 50 | 0.12 | 0.1940 | 0.6 | -0.9 | -71.3 | -205.3 | -161.3 | -198.28 |
| 75 | 0.08 | 0.0862 | 0.9 | -0.6 | -46.3 | -180.3 | -136.3 | -173.28 |
| 100 | 0.06 | 0.0485 | 1.2 | -0.3 | -21.3 | -155.3 | -111.3 | -148.28 |
| 125 | 0.05 | 0.0310 | 1.5 | 0.0 | 3.7 | -130.3 | -86.3 | -123.28 |
| 150 | 0.04 | 0.0216 | 1.9 | 0.4 | 28.7 | -105.3 | -61.3 | -98.28 |
| 175 | 0.03 | 0.0158 | 2.2 | 0.7 | 53.7 | -80.3 | -36.3 | -73.28 |
| 200 | 0.03 | 0.0121 | 2.5 | 1.0 | 78.7 | -55.3 | -11.3 | -48.28 |
| 225 | 0.03 | 0.0096 | 2.8 | 1.3 | 103.7 | -30.3 | 13.7 | -23.28 |
| 250 | 0.02 | 0.0078 | 3.1 | 1.6 | 128.7 | -5.3 | 38.7 | 1.73 |
| 275 | 0.02 | 0.0064 | 3.4 | 1.9 | 153.7 | 19.7 | 63.7 | 26.73 |
| 300 | 0.02 | 0.0054 | 3.7 | 2.2 | 178.7 | 44.7 | 88.7 | 51.73 |
| 325 | 0.02 | 0.0046 | 4.0 | 2.5 | 203.7 | 69.7 | 113.7 | 76.73 |
| 350 | 0.02 | 0.0040 | 4.3 | 2.8 | 228.7 | 94.7 | 138.7 | 101.73 |
| 375 | 0.02 | 0.0034 | 4.6 | 3.1 | 253.7 | 119.7 | 163.7 | 126.73 |
| 400 | 0.01 | 0.0030 | 4.9 | 3.4 | 278.7 | 144.7 | 188.7 | 151.73 |
| 425 | 0.01 | 0.0027 | 5.3 | 3.8 | 303.7 | 169.7 | 213.7 | 176.73 |
| 450 | 0.01 | 0.0024 | 5.6 | 4.1 | 328.7 | 194.7 | 238.7 | 201.73 |
| 475 | 0.01 | 0.0022 | 5.9 | 4.4 | 353.7 | 219.7 | 263.7 | 226.73 |
| 500 | 0.01 | 0.0019 | 6.2 | 4.7 | 378.7 | 244.7 | 288.7 | 251.73 |

The next three columns show the outcomes for the three responses. The total distance required for braking avoidance is the sum of two factors, the distance traveled during perception-reaction time and the distance required by frictional forces to slow the vehicle to 0. The distance traveled during a perception-reaction time of 1.5 seconds is the 121.3 feet. Stopping distance is about 134 feet, so the total distance needed is 255 feet. At that point, the looming rate is about .0078 radian/sec, the upper end of the .004–.008 radian/sec threshold range. Most normal drivers will avoid collision, but a few will not. At this point, however, we are just talking theory and not practice.

The next two columns show the outcome of a driver who attempts to swerve around the stopped vehicle. A driver must move laterally by enough distance to bypass the lead vehicle. The required lateral distance depends on widths of both following and lead vehicles. The table assumes a driver in a 6-foot wide car trying to avoid a lead vehicle that is also 6 feet wide. If the vehicles are aligned center-to-center in the lane, the driver of a standard 6-foot wide car approaching another 6-foot wide car would have to move 6 feet laterally in order to just avoid the collision. If the lead vehicle were an 8-foot wide tractor-trailer, then the required lateral distance would be 7 feet. If both vehicles were 8-feet wide tractor-trailers, then the lateral movement must be 8 feet.

While the driver is swerving laterally, his car is moving down the road. The critical question is how far the car moves down the road (the X direction) in the time required to move the 6, 7 or 8 feet laterally (the Y direction). Following Bonnet's (2001) calculation method, the X distance required for the driver of a 6-foot wide car to move laterally and to just miss another 6-foot wide car is about 90 feet. That is, the car moves forward 90 feet in the time required to move left 6 feet and to just miss the stopped vehicle ahead. Added to the 121.3 feet of reaction-time distance, the driver requires 211.3 feet. At this distance, the looming rate is .011 radian/sec. In this scenario, the collision is theoretically avoidable.

There is a problem, however, in using the "just miss" criterion. A driver who just misses at full lateral acceleration may find himself in a ditch or hitting a median before he can straighten his vehicle out. Malaterre, Ferrandez, Fleury, and Lechner (1988), in fact, found that drivers in emergencies often swerve so severely that they cannot recover. The driver could attempt the safer maneuver of a lane change—swerve in one direction to avoid collision and then steer back in the opposite direction to regain control.

On a typical freeway, the driver would move 12 feet laterally to perform a full lane change. The required X distance is 180 feet of roadway, double the 6 feet "just miss" distance. In a sense, this represents the other extreme, the maximum amount of roadway required. However, it is an overestimate because the driver does not need to move the entire 12 feet to avoid collision. The real distance lies somewhere in between the swerve to just miss (6 feet) and the full lane change (12 feet).

Partial lane changes (see "parallel" column in Table 16.3) are intermediate cases. Instead of a full lane change, assume that the driver swerves and comes parallel as close as possible to the stopped vehicle's lane position. In this case, the lateral "lane change" is 6 feet rather than 12, a maneuver that requires 127 feet along the X direction. The final column shows the total distance required to successfully execute this swerving avoidance—250 feet from impact when the looming rate is about .0078 radian/sec.

This analysis overlooks some fine points. First, a 6-foot lane change is a bare minimum, and a driver should be allotted a margin for error. A 7-, 8- or 9-foot "lane change" is more realistic than 6. Further, these calculations of distance required for a lane change are unrealistically optimistic. They assume that the vehicle reverses direction instantaneously. In a real situation, there will be a driver steering reaction time and a vehicle response time to the steering input.

Conversely, the estimates ignore some factors that help the driver. First, the swerving adds length to the path—the driver moves sideways while traveling down the road in the X direction. A driver in a 12-foot lane change does not quite need the entire 180 feet of straight roadway. Second, the driver may brake, which slows the vehicle and buys some extra distance.

Lastly, even when swerving is the better, or even the only effective avoidance response, drivers clearly prefer braking (e.g., Prynne and Martin, 1995). The psychological reasons are unclear, but braking is simpler, more direct and depends on brute force of response with no planning. Swerving requires the driver to look ahead, make a decision as to which way to swerve and then to plot a new course. It also creates new risks of running off the roadway or colliding with an oncoming vehicle. Moreover, braking slows the car, bringing it under more control while swerving sharply at high speed risks a control loss. Whatever the reason, drivers will not necessarily swerve even if it is theoretically the only viable avoidance option.

### 6. Looming In Low Visibility

The discussion so far has concerned looming during daylight and good visibility when the driver can clearly see the vehicle in front of him. At night, a driver might see only the stopped vehicle's retroreflective tape and/or a set of taillights. In other cases, the vehicle might be parked with no taillights and no retroreflective tape so that it first appears as a low contrast blur.

In theory, looming thresholds under nighttime conditions should be exactly the same as during the day. If an 8-foot wide tractor-trailer has an 8-foot wide strip of retroreflective tape across the back, then the strip contains the same angular velocity information as the entire trailer. Similarly, if the taillights are at the outermost part of the trailer so that their outer edges span 8-feet, then the rate at which two taillights move apart ($\tau$ type 1) is the same as the rate at which the entire vehicle image dilates[9] ($\tau$ type 2).

However, there are no data to support the theory or to demonstrate that looming thresholds are the same for reflective strips and for taillights as for an entire vehicle. On the contrary, there are both theoretical considerations and some indirect research evidence to suggest that looming detection at night is more difficult.

A discussed in Chapter 14, psychophysical thresholds often exhibit a phenomenon called "probability summation." Simply put, you have a better chance of winning the lottery if you buy two tickets rather than one. If there are independent probabilities of detecting each of N objects, then the probability of detecting 2N objects is greater because there are twice as many detection opportunities. A viewer approaching a fully visible trailer sees all the edges moving outward. In contrast, a driver approaching a strip of disembodied retroreflective tape or set of taillights sees very little outward edge motion. The smaller the amount of information available to the driver, the lower the probability of detection. Hence, looming will be more difficult to detect from taillights and a strip of retroreflective tape alone than from an entire vehicle. Further, some of the non-looming cues that drivers use (see below) are likely less effective at night.

Another possible problem is lack of background. People are generally better at seeing relative than absolute motion (Leibowitz, 1955). That is, people can see the motion of an object better when there are other, stationary objects and textures in the background. For example, an airplane in the sky appears faster when it moves past clouds than when the background is clear sky. This has obvious implications for looming detection in day vs. night. During the day, the looming vehicle has a visible background that will make the outward edge motion more detectable. At night, the background is likely black or less distinct, so relative motion is less perceptible and motion thresholds higher. One study (Cavallo, Mestre and Berthelon, 1997) apparently confirms this hypothesis by finding that drivers underestimate TTC in environments with fewer visual cues in the environment. However, other evidence is less supportive.

Empirical evidence also suggests that thresholds will be higher with single strips of reflective material and with taillights. Olson, Campbell, Massie, Battle, Taub, Aoki, Sato, and Pettis (1992) compared response times to looming of various retroreflective "taping patterns," which were actually images on a CRT screen. Subjects responded faster to a full rectangle than to a single horizontal line of the same width.

Other evidence suggests that looming thresholds will be higher in bad weather or other conditions where contrast is low. Chapter 13 discussed how fog lowers contrast and slows perceived motion, sometimes to the point of making moving objects appear stationary. This loss of motion sensitivity will likely impair looming detection and lead to more rear-end collisions.

### 7. Looming and Brake Lights

In the case of collision with a decelerating lead vehicle, brake lights normally signal slowing. However, brake light onset says nothing about closing rate, so it is a somewhat ambiguous cue. In some cases, the driver is following closely and has looming information to supplement the brake light. (Liebermann, Ben-David, Schweitzer, Apter and Parush, 1995). When following very closely, drivers have learned that brake lights signal deceleration and that a response may be required to prevent closing too rapidly on the lead vehicle. Normally, drivers following closely respond rapidly and automatically to brake lights because it is a highly overlearned response that readily attracts attention through its meaningfulness. In some cases, the driver seems to respond even before becoming consciously aware that the brake lights have appeared. However, when the driver is following at close distances, then looming rate will be high and may be contributing to the rapid response.

Many studies have attempted to determine the human perception-reaction to the sudden onset of brake lights (Chapter 17). However, the expected reaction time depends on several factors. Most studies have only measured the response of healthy males aged twenty to fifty in daylight and have not used truly urgent conditions. Older drivers and females may respond more slowly. Conversely, high urgency reduces reaction time. Weather and visibility conditions also influence reaction time. Brake lights may be less visible in fog or rain or when there is significant sun glare. "Poorer" visibility conditions at night, however, can actually improve reaction time because signal lights are more obvious against a dark background. For example, flashing railroad lights produce faster reaction time at night than during the day. However, if it is so dark that the driver cannot clearly see the car ahead, then the brake lamps become disembodied points of light. This will slow reaction time if the driver must exert cognitive effort to correctly interpret the points as brake lights. The slowing at night would be more pronounced if the light configuration is unusual or if some of the lights are inoperative.

In other cases, the driver sees the brake lights relatively far down the road before looming rate is perceptible. The brake lights signal only that braking *may* be necessary. This situation is more uncertain and requires more extensive situation analysis. Drivers do not need to decelerate to every brake light 500 feet down the road, so they must decide whether to decelerate based on the available information. Without looming rate, the driver will likely rely heavily on other information. For example, drivers respond faster when encountering conditions where lead vehicle deceleration is likely. Drivers may even increase headway in anticipation of lead vehicle deceleration (van der Hulst, Meijman, and Rothengatter, 1999). Further, drivers may know that traffic often slows severely at a given location or they may find a sea of brake lights indicating a traffic jam with very slow traffic. A single set of vehicle lights is far more ambiguous.

Lastly, the lead vehicle may have four-way flashers operating. Flashing masks motion (e.g., Green, 1981) and causes the outward looming motion to become jerky and irregular, degrading perception. From a purely psychophysical standpoint, this will further impair looming detection and cause threshold to rise. Hecht, Kaiser, Savelsbergh, Van Der Kamp (2002), for example, found that viewers judged TTC as being longer when objects flashed while looming. On the other hand, a driver is likely to interpret the flashing lights as a cue for caution. The total effect is likely to raise looming threshold but decrease reaction time and even possibly cause the driver to slow before he reaches looming detection distance.

### 8. Assess Time/Distance to Collision

Even after a driver detects that he is closing on a lead vehicle, he must still decide whether a response is necessary. If the response is braking, the driver must also determine how much force to apply. These decisions require an estimate of closing time, which the driver can determine two ways, from headway change or from $\tau$. The direct method is presumably better because it requires no mental calculation and is faster.

For many years, research data apparently showed that viewers greatly underestimated TTC, and presumably $\tau$, by as much as 20–40 percent. If true, people would be making very cautious TTC judgments, perhaps due to some innate notion of safe behavior. However, this finding is probably due to a procedural artifact.[10] When the artifact is removed, viewers cease systematically underestimating TTC (e.g., Gray and Thornton, 2001).

However, other studies have revealed several non-$\tau$ variables that affect TTC judgments.

*Monocular distance cues.* These are variables that affect perceived size and distance, suggesting that drivers combine direct and indirect methods for TTC estimation. Any cue that makes an object appear farther away will make TTC seem longer. Research finds, for example, that viewers judge TTC to small objects, which appear farther, as being longer than to large objects. Horswill, Helman, Ardiles, and Wann (2001) have suggested that this influence of size on TTC could be responsible for some car-motorcycle accidents. Drivers are more likely to leave an insufficient gap for the motorcycles since their smaller size makes them appear farther away and the time gap to be greater (Caird and Hancock, 1994). Similarly, viewers judge objects that are higher in the visual field or are occluded, and hence perceived as farther away, as having a longer TTC (DeLucia, Kaiser, Bush, Meyer and Sweet, 2003).

*"Familiar size."* Viewers have learned that certain familiar objects appear a specific size at specific distances. A car that is a block away creates a smaller retinal image than one that is 10 feet away. Yet, the viewer does not perceive that car down the block as a tiny car. The viewer takes two factors into account when judging size. One is the perceived distance. The viewer implicitly knows that objects at a distance create smaller retinal images. Somehow, the mind performs a "size-distance tradeoff" to arrive at a proper perceived size. This tradeoff is abetted by the "familiar" size of the car. That is, the viewer has learned through experience that cars have a typical real-world (distal) size regardless of the retinal image (proximal) size that they create.

One theory suggests that "size-distance tradeoff" causes accidents with children (Stewart, Cudworth and Lishman, 1993). The familiar size cue will suggest that the children are normal-sized adults viewed at a greater distance so that TTC is longer. Similarly, familiar size explains why drivers follow closer behind small cars (Herman Lam and Rothery, 1973) and why small cars are more often rear-ended (Eberts and Macmillan, 1985). However, drivers may use other depth cues to overcome the effect (Wann, Rushton and Caldwell, 1999). In general, familiar size effects should always be considered when extrapolating laboratory data based on arbitrary shapes to real-world objects that the viewer knows.

*Motion adaptation.* Viewing an expanding visual optic flow lowers motion sensitivity for drivers (Gray and Regan, 1999) and raises looming thresholds and also TTC estimates. As shown in Figure 16.2, looming perception derives from detection of edges moving outward in the expanding retinal image. This motion perception results from activation of neurons in the brain. These neurons, however, become fatigued if overworked (e.g., Green, 1991), which is exactly what happens when a person has been on the road for an extended period. Chapter 3 described how drivers moving through the world experience an optic flow field of points moving outward from a focus of expansion. Prolonged viewing of outward flow adapts motion-detecting neurons, causing them to fatigue and to become less sensitive. Subsequently viewed motion in the same direction then looks slower or even stopped (Thomson, 1981). The loss of motion sensitivity will impair the driver's ability to detect the edge expansion on looming objects, such as a vehicle on the road ahead. It is also likely one reason that drivers begin to "velocitate," lose track of their speeds and to judge themselves traveling slower than their actual rates.

*Acceleration.* The looming analysis assumes that the driver moves toward the obstacle at a constant velocity, as when a driver approaches a stopped vehicle. If the following driver approaches a lead vehicle that has begun to brake, then the rate of approach will not be constant. The lead vehicle's gradual braking effectively creates an acceleration toward the constant-velocity approaching driver. Research (Trewhella, Edwards, and Ibbotson, 2003) suggests that drivers are very poor at perceiving the acceleration of looming objects. The driver may then underestimate the TTC as the braking lead vehicle "accelerates" toward him.

*Age.* Older viewers (e.g., Kennedy, Jentsch, and Smither, 2001) have higher looming thresholds, especially in dim light. See Chapter 9 for more discussion.

*Disparity.* In addition to looming, approaching objects create a second source of TTC information, relative disparity change (Regan and Beverly, 1979). Recall that a fixated object casts images on the retina of each eye. These images may fall at corresponding or at noncorresponding points creating disparity and the perception of depth. As an object approaches, disparity changes and provides a method for judging TTC:

$$\mathrm{TTC} = \frac{I}{D \times d\delta / dt}$$

where $I$ is interpupillary distance, D is object distance and $d\delta/dt$ is the rate of relative disparity change. Drivers combine this disparity change with looming to judge TTC. Research (e.g., Baker and Steedman, 1961a) has confirmed that monocular drivers have higher looming thresholds. The disparity cue grows in importance as object size decreases and may even dominate looming at very small sizes.

In sum, drivers may estimate TTC using $\tau$ or some similar optical variable, but they also likely use disparity and indirect non-$\tau$ information, such as pictorial distance cues. Further, driver looming judgments are affected by their own speed (Cavallo, Laya and Laurent, 1986) and distance from the lead vehicle (Liebermann, Ben-David, Schweitzer, Apter and Parush, 1995). Lastly, motion adaptation may raise looming thresholds and increase TTC estimates.

## B. Head-On Collisions While Overtaking

The other common class of zero-angle accidents is the head-on collision that occurs when a driver attempts to overtake a lead vehicle and crashes into oncoming traffic. These accidents are less common than rear-end collisions, but the high speed differential causes dire consequences more frequently. One estimate (Clark, Ward and Jones, 1998), for example, claimed that overtaking collisions constitute 10 percent of fatal accidents. The high rate is especially striking since overtaking is a relatively rare driving maneuver. Research (e.g., Jones and Heimstra, 1964; Clarke, Ward and Jones, 1999) suggests that drivers are simply poor at making the required judgments for safe overtaking.

The overtake maneuver requires a series of perceptual judgments. Most notably, 1) the driver must judge the TTC of oncoming traffic and 2) judge the time required to pull out into the oncoming lane and then back in front of the lead vehicle. In assessing TTC, the approach speeds are high so the driver must make the judgment far in advance when looming rate is low and possibly imperceptible. Moreover, motion adaptation (Gray and Regan, 1999) likely leads to overestimates of TTC. Headway, the other obvious candidate for judging TTC, is very crude. The driver must correctly judge distance and velocity of the oncoming traffic in order to mentally calculate TTC=d/v. Velocity is difficult to perceive, so drivers may just assume that oncoming vehicles are traveling at the speed limit (Farber and Silver, 1967). Distance is also difficult to judge. Drivers may overestimate distance due to various depth cues: aerial perspective (e.g., fog or haze), small size (e.g., motorcycle), or height in the visual field (e.g., it is coming down a hill). At night, drivers may judge distance based on separation and brightness of oncoming car headlamps. Vehicles with smaller inter-headlamp distance or with headlamps dimmed by dirt, misalignment or covers appear farther away. In judging the time required to perform the overtake, the driver must further estimate his own speed. Research (e.g., Denton, 1976) shows that unless they look at their speedometers, drivers are poor at estimating their own speed. They may have also velocitated.

The overtaking driver must also avoid collision with the lead vehicle as well as with oncoming traffic. In fact, collision with the lead vehicle constitutes 37 percent (Clarke, Ward and Jones, 1999) of overtaking accidents. The driver must decide how close to come to the lead vehicle before beginning to overtake. Drivers often judge closeness by "temporal headway," the time before the front bumper of his car reaches the current position of the lead vehicle's rear bumper. Accidents often occur because the temporal headway is very short, the driver starts to move out, but is forced back into his lane by unexpected traffic and cannot avoid collision. The problem is magnified by the driver's need to switch attention to the oncoming traffic. Once he decides to pull out, he loses track of his proximity to the lead vehicle.

Drivers are prone to approach the lead vehicle too closely because it permits faster and "safer" overtaking with less time spent in the oncoming traffic lane. It also allows the driver to accept a shorter TTC gap for the oncoming traffic. When oncoming traffic is heavy, drivers frequently tailgate the lead vehicle because they expect short TTC gaps and must perform the overtake very quickly.

# 16.3 Right-Angle Collision

As in zero-angle approaches, drivers can judge the likelihood of crossing collisions by either indirect or direct means. The indirect methods require: 1) judging the approaching vehicle's speed in the frontoparallel plane, its distance to the path intersection, and its time of arrival, 2) judging the driver's own time to arrive at the intersection and 3) comparing the two times. In the direct method, the viewer judges the sign of retinal image motion.

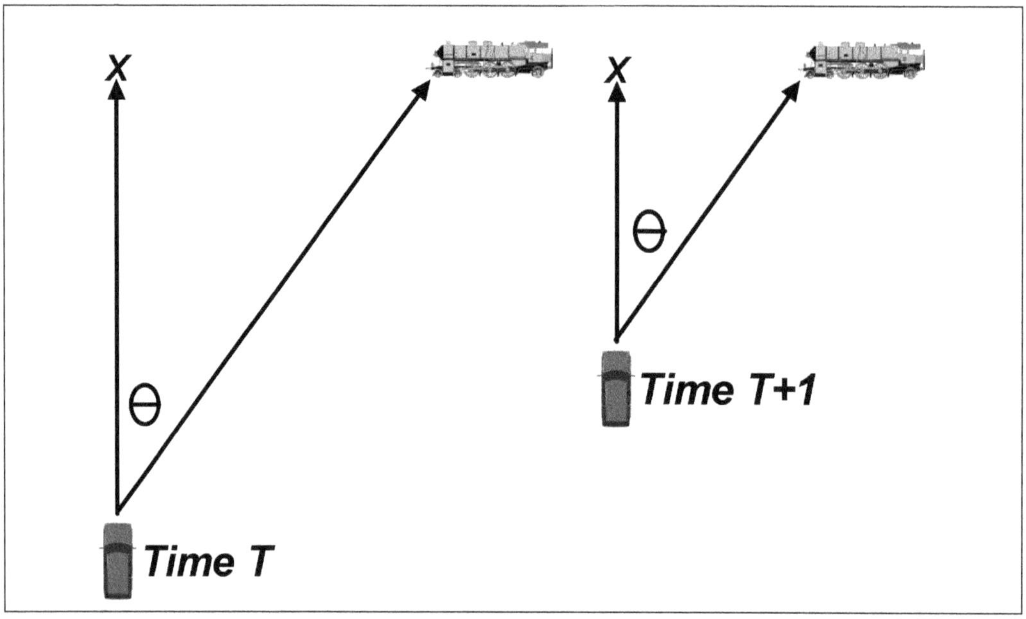


***Figure 16.4*** *Optical changes as objects approach toward a right-angle collision.*

## A. Judging Time To Arrival

Figure 16.4 illustrates a potential right-angle collision between a car and a train. At time T, the angle between the driver's eye and the train is θ. The train continues moving leftward at some speed. The driver moves forward, however, with optic flow simultaneously pushing the train in the opposite direction—rightward away from the focus of expansion. The driver can use the optical sign of the retinal image motion (or change in θ) as a cue. As the car and train approach the point of intersection at constant velocity, θ can change in one of three ways.

1. The θ increases, and the retinal image moves farther rightward into the periphery. The driver will arrive at the intersection point before the train.
2. The θ decreases, and the retinal image moves leftward toward the fovea and the focus of expansion. The train will arrive before the driver.[11]
3. The θ remains constant, as shown in Figure 16.4 at time T+1. The driver and the train arrive at the same moment. The train's motion and the effects of optic flow exactly cancel. There is no retinal image motion ("retinal slip"), and hence no motion conspicuity. In aviation, instructors warn students to watch out for the flyspeck on the windshield that doesn't move but just keeps growing. It's another airplane on a collision course.

Research (i.e., Schiff and Oldak, 1990; Berthelon and Mestre, 1993) has shown that drivers are relatively good, but not perfect, at judging whether an approaching vehicle is on a right-angle collision course. Stationary reference points improve accuracy (Berthelon and Mestre, 1993), probably because motion judgments are generally "object relative." Viewers judge motion by perceiving the relative displacement of one object relative to another (Leibowitz, 1955). Other research (Runeson, 1974, 1975), however, found that people make systematic errors in judging frontoparallel plane speed and predicting collisions. Viewers do not perceive constant velocity as constant. Rather, they exhibit a form of motion adaptation; the longer viewers watch, the slower the motion appears. This misjudgment would lead to underestimation of arrival time possibly to collision.

This analysis assumes that the objects travel in a straight line at a constant velocity toward their meeting. Some common scenarios do not exactly fit these constraints.

Scenario 1. A driver approaches a stationary object, such as a pedestrian standing on a curb. As the driver approaches, the visual angle θ grows, as in case 1 above. The pedestrian recedes further into the periphery as the car approaches. The movement into the visual periphery decreases detectability, but the growth of image size should increase detectability. One theory suggests that these two detectability effects exactly cancel out. Presumably, people have evolved this constancy mechanism in order to keep the world stable as we move forward through the environment. Cole and Hughes (1984) found, however, that in practice the two effects do not cancel perfectly and that proximity to the sightline is more important than size and even reflectivity. Their results suggest the highly unintuitive conclusion that drivers are more likely to detect a roadside object when it is far away and near the sightline than when it is close but in the periphery. Once the pedestrian starts moving across the driver's path, then the above analysis applies.

Scenario 2. A vehicle pulls out from a STOP sign ahead of a car or a train. The driver must perceive that the vehicle has moved from the STOP sign in order to avoid collision. However, a vehicle leaving a STOP sign on the driver's left is not traveling at constant velocity but rather accelerating. The initial slow motion toward the focus of expansion may be canceled by the outward optic flow, so the driver fails to detect the motion. By the time the vehicle has accelerated to a perceptible speed, the driver finds it too late to avoid the collision. Runeson (1974) also found that viewers judged accelerated motion as appearing to be constant velocity, which could also lead to arrival time underestimation.

Scenario 3. The road approaching the intersection is curved. All of the above analysis has assumed that the driver is traveling straight toward the intersection point. A curved path, however, changes the optic flow information in complex ways. I'll just roughly summarize the effects by saying that if the road curves leftward, image points to the right move outward faster than those to the left. This further slows the apparent approach of vehicles coming from the right (Berthelon and Mestre, 1993).

Lastly, many of the same factors that affect looming perception can cause drivers to underestimate the time at which another vehicle will cross its path.

*Size.* People generally perceive larger objects as moving slower (Leibowitz, 1985), so a driver racing a train might underestimate its arrival time at the crossing.

*Contrast.* Low contrast objects appear to move slower. Similarly, fog, rain and mist can produce low contrast that slows apparent motion.

*Flashing.* Flashing lights slow apparent motion for frontoparallel movement just as they do for motion in depth. Theoretically, the drivers could underestimate the speed of emergency vehicles with overhead flashing lights.

*Motion Adaptation.* Adaptation to the outward optic flow away from the fovea impairs detection of motion toward the fovea (Gray and Regan, 1999).

*Age.* Older people perceive motion as slower (e.g., Lakshminarayanan, and Raghuram 2004), especially at low contrast. See Chapter 9 for more discussion.

## B. Peripheral Detection

Before judging motion, the viewer must first detect the approaching vehicle's presence. In research studies (e.g., Berthelon and Mestre, 1993) the viewers knew where to look for the approaching vehicle, so detection was not an issue. Real drivers face a more difficult task because they do not know for certain where to look and they must detect the approaching object in the far visual periphery. Further, a variety of possible obstructions may block the driver's sightline.

### 1. Visual Fields and Detection

I have already explained that a converging object remains at a constant θ in the driver's visual field. Chapter 15 mentioned that this θ changes with relative speed of driver and pedestrian. However, the θ with pedestrians is relatively small because they move slowly compared to vehicles. The θ between a driver and another fast-moving vehicle or a train will be much greater. For example, if the two vehicles are moving at the same speed, then the angle will be 45°. If a driver traveling 40 mph approaches the track of a train going 60 mph, the visual angle is 56.3°. The driver will have difficulty seeing the train at these eccentricities. First, contrast sensitivity is very low in such remote retinal locations. Second, vehicle headlamps are ineffective at such extreme angles. Third, the driver must detect the train far in advance when the retinal image is small. As calculated in Chapter 15, it takes a car traveling at 45 mph about 242–308 feet and 5–6 seconds to stop prior to point of collision. Fourth, there are no motion cues to aid conspicuity. The image remains at a constant location with no retinal slip and there is no biological motion or human form to help conspicuity. Fifth, the entire visual field shrinks when drivers travel faster. Hamilton and Thurstone (1937) summarized the effects of speed on visual fields in a set of propositions:

- *As speed increases, concentration increases.* Since the driver travels farther per second, objects at increasing distance become closer in time. The driver has more potential hazards and less time to react.
- *As speed increases, point of concentration recedes.* Drivers must look farther down the road in order to have time to react to these more distant obstacles.
- *As speed increases, peripheral vision diminishes.* The increased concentration causes tunnel vision. According to Hamilton and Thurstone (1937), a driver's field of view is only 65° at 45 mph and 40° at speeds above 60 mph. The driver would not see objects lying at even moderate retinal eccentricities (Hamilton and Thurstone failed to note another effect—objects in the peripheral flow field move faster and become less perceptible).
- *As speed increases, foreground detail begins to fade.* Near objects move too rapidly for clear vision. For example, they conclude that drivers traveling 40 mph will not clearly see objects closer than 80 feet away.
- *As speed increases, space perception becomes impaired.* Drivers become "velocitated," adapting and underestimating their own speed. They then overestimate the time to arrival at objects down the roadway.

### 2. Obstructions

Obstructions may further impair peripheral detection. Drivers have an internal "obstruction" in the blind spot, the location where the optic nerve leaves the retina and where there are no photoreceptors. Its exact location varies across individuals but is generally about 15–20° from the fovea near the horizontal meridian in the temporal visual field. Size also varies around 2.5–3°, increasing with age. In addition, various eye diseases such as glaucoma create blind spots (scotomas). Viewers do not notice blind spots because the brain, like nature, abhors a vacuum and somehow fills in the blank area.

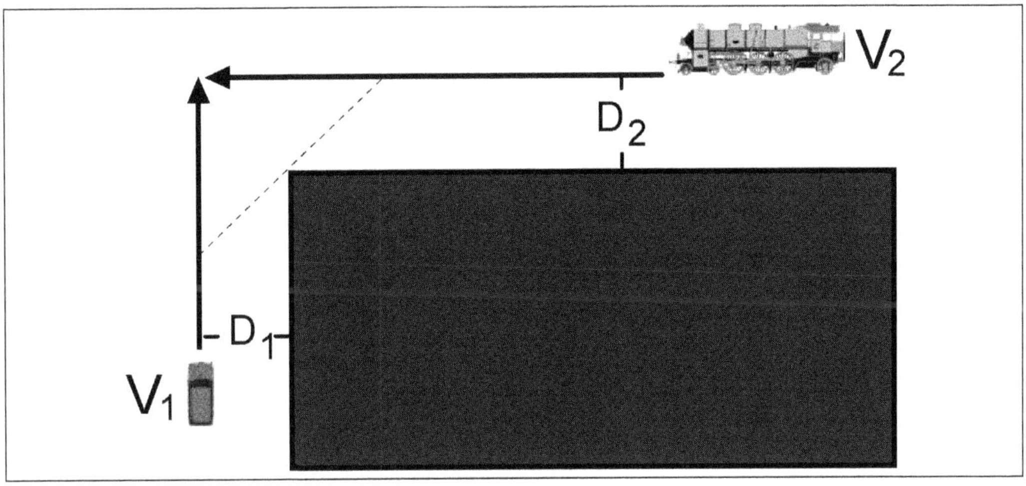


***Figure 16.5*** *Sight distance with an obstruction.*

External obstructions include the vehicle features, such as roof support pillars and side mirrors, as well as environmental features such as buildings, signs, foliage and grades. Environmental obstructions are especially common factors in vehicle-rail crossing accidents because the high speed of trains puts them in the driver's far periphery. Figure 16.5 depicts a typical situation.

The train approaches from the right but is blocked from the driver's view by buildings and/or by bushes and foliage. $D_1$ (in feet) is the distance of the obstruction from the driver's path, and $D_2$ is the distance of the train's path from the obstruction. The TTC (in seconds) at which the driver and train engineer have unobstructed sightlines to each other is (Limpert, 1994):

$$TTC = \frac{D_2}{V_1} + \frac{D_1}{V_2}$$

This calculation is crucial in determining whether a driver can avoid the collision. Suppose that a car traveling 45 mph (66 ft/sec) and a train traveling 65 mph (96 ft/sec) are on a collision course. Further, the train is running 12 feet from a row of trees and buildings which ends 300 feet to the driver's right. As calculated in Chapter 15, a driver would require 242–308 feet. and about 5–6 seconds to stop, assuming a reaction time of 2–3 seconds. Can the driver stop in time? Table 16.4 provides the answer. The driver could see the train 3.3 seconds prior to collision and likely could not stop before reaching the crossing. Of course, the 3.3 seconds represent only the earliest possible point when the driver can see the train. At grade crossings, drivers must search left and right as well as ahead before proceeding. This additional search can inflate the overall response time. Moreover, the train might appear in the driver's far peripheral field, as described above. The calculation also is made from driver eye position, not from the front bumper, which is closer to the track. Lastly, the same analysis applies to other cases of obstruction, such as a pedestrian darting out from behind a parked car.

## C. Braking and Swerving

Liebermann, Ben-David, Schweitzer, Apter and Parush (1995) note that braking has two components. The first is "triggering," where the driver decides on the need to brake. The second is "modulation," where the driver decides on the strength of response. $\tau$ theory specifies not just the TTC needed for triggering but also modulation of braking deceleration. The derivative of $\tau$ with respect to time, $\dot{\tau}$ ("tau dot"), supplies the information required to brake without collision (Lee, 1976).

**Table 16.4**
**TTC for unobstructed view**

| $D_1$ | $D_2$ | $V_1$ | $V_2$ | TTC |
|---|---|---|---|---|
| **50** | 12 | 66 | 96 | 0.7 |
| **100** | 12 | 66 | 96 | 1.2 |
| **150** | 12 | 66 | 96 | 1.7 |
| **200** | 12 | 66 | 96 | 2.3 |
| **250** | 12 | 66 | 96 | 2.8 |
| **300** | 12 | 66 | 96 | 3.3 |
| **350** | 12 | 66 | 96 | 3.8 |
| **400** | 12 | 66 | 96 | 4.3 |
| **450** | 12 | 66 | 96 | 4.9 |
| **500** | 12 | 66 | 96 | 5.4 |

While $\tau$ tells the driver the time before collision, $\dot{\tau}$ tells the driver how hard he will hit the lead vehicle. If a driver could perceive and maintain its value at -0.5 during deceleration, he would stop just at the lead vehicle. If $\dot{\tau} > -0.5$, then he would stop short of the collision while $\dot{\tau} < -0.5$ would lead to collision. The ability of drivers to perceive and to use $\dot{\tau}$ is heavily debated. Some research (e.g., Treffner, Barrett and Petersen, 2002) found that braking drivers maintain the ideal -0.5. In contrast, other research concluded that drivers use additional information (e.g., Andersen, Cisneros, and Atchley, 1999) or that drivers did not use $\dot{\tau}$ at all (Rock, Harris, Yates, 2006). Moreover, the theory of constant $\dot{\tau}$ conflicts with the common finding of two-stage braking where drivers pause during deceleration before going to open-loop behavior and locking up the brakes. (See below.) Even if drivers use $\dot{\tau}$ on some occasions, there is little evidence that they use it during emergencies.

This underscores a critical point: the difference between a driver in a research test and one in a real emergency is likely great. In some analyses presented above, I have estimated the time/distance available to a driver for performing a swerving or braking avoidance. This is a common exercise in forensic matters, since the ultimate question is whether a person acted "reasonably." In real emergencies, however, it is often difficult to characterize "reasonable" response.

Drivers acting in emergency situations will likely perform more poorly than those tested in controlled studies with their expected targets, low stress, practiced responses, etc. To some extent, field multipliers align real and research visual thresholds. However, multipliers do not completely compensate for the effects of emergencies on smooth performance of sensory-motor behavior. Even in research with "contrived" emergency tests, drivers virtually never employ the full braking capability that is theoretically available.

For example, drivers have a strong tendency to brake in two stages (Prynne and Martin, 1995; Kiesewetter, Klinkner, Reichelt, and Steiner, 1999). The driver has an initial stage of about 1/3 brake pressure (Prynne and Martin, 1995), then stops to evaluate the situation (closed-loop behavior) before slamming on the brakes (open-loop behavior). The overall brake depression time can range as a high as a second (Barrett, Kobayashi, and Fox, 1968) in non-urgent situations. The hesitation is also more pronounced in complex and low visibility situations, such as fog and rain. Uncertainty is the enemy of quick response. Further, research (e.g., Reed and Keskin, 1989; Goudie,

Bowler, Brown, Heinrichs, and G. Siegmund 2000; Heinrich, Allin, Bowler, and Siegmund, 2004) found that even a full out brake application is likely to take roughly .3 seconds or more from touching the pedal to brake lockup and skid.

Further, most drivers have little or no experience with life-threatening emergencies. They don't have practiced and well-rehearsed responses available. Taking the time to reason through the situation while hurtling toward collision risks fatal delay. Should I rely on braking? Should I swerve left or right? Is it worth taking the risk of going left into oncoming traffic or right into a ditch. Tick, tick, tick. Drivers are hesitant and uncomfortable at suddenly swerving sharply and braking completely at high speeds when they may lose control of the vehicle. They must also weigh the severity of response against the loss of control. Tick, tick, tick.

The psychology of response conflict would say that drivers often must make an "avoidance-avoidance" decision, a situation where the actor must decide between two aversive alternatives. This contrasts with "approach-approach" conflicts, where there are two desirable outcomes, and "approach-avoidance," where there is one positive and one negative.[12] Avoidance-avoidance conflicts are the most difficult to resolve and create very long reaction times. The person simply freezes between the alternatives, which is doubtless why so many drivers in underride accidents never respond at all.

Alternatively, the driver can fall back on practiced, but inappropriate, responses that they used in previous non-emergencies (hence the initial stage of moderate braking). By the time the driver realizes that normal response is inadequate, it may be too late.

Intense stress and emotional arousal reduce driver ability to think and disrupt coordinated motor control. It might be asked why drivers do not rely more on swerving than braking since swerving generally requires less time and distance. However, a driver heading straight for the side of a tractor-trailer across the road perceptually narrows and does not think about all available options. He is too aroused to perform a finely tuned swerve and must decide on an all-or-none open-loop response that entails high risk. Malaterre, Fernandez, Fleury and Lechner (1988) conclude that:

> If one adds considerations such as the effects of stress and temporal constraints, one might assume that people do not rely on refined perceptual judgements for taking collision avoidance decisions, but tend to follow simplified strategies, resorting to braking as their initial reaction, except when the obstacle is very close and positioned laterally to their trajectory. (p. 653)

Lastly, it is impossible to leave the topic of stress and arousal without mentioning the best known "law" of behavior, the Yerkes-Dodson (1908) Law. It says that 1) behavior is an inverted U-shape function of arousal—behavior is best when arousal is neither too low nor too high—and 2) optimal stress level is a function of task complexity. This law is probably as valid as any that rests on a single study that measured learning in a handful of mutant mice. On the other hand, stress and arousal are complex and multifaceted and cannot be collapsed into a single variable (Hockey and Hamilton, 1983).

However, some relationships between stress and performance are clear. First, the more complex the task, the more likely that stress will impair performance. Complex tasks require more information processing, but stress causes perceptual narrowing. The performer is then less able to process the required information. This is precisely why good design is important in emergencies. Users can't be expected to think too much, so the design must fit the strong innate predispositions discussed in Chapter 1. Second, training and experience likely decrease the effects of stress. In highly trained tasks, the users require less cognitive processing. They may have preprogrammed motor schema that need only be triggered. On the other hand, triggering the wrong motor schema can be disastrous. A good example occurs when a jet-ski rider sees an object coming from the side on a collision course. His motor-schema says to brake and swerve, so he quits accelerating to slow. Since continued forward motion is needed for steering, however, the jet-ski driver loses steering control and cannot avoid the collision.

In sum, there is a gulf between a theoretical analysis based on controlled research studies and what real drivers actually do. It is difficult and dangerous to put people in real emergencies so there are few data on real emergency behavior. The limited research so far suggests that real drivers perform more poorly than those in controlled research. It is difficult to say how much worse, however, because driver behavior in emergencies is so variable and difficult to predict (e.g., Malaterre, Ferrandez, Fleury, and Lechner, 1988).

## 16.4 Conclusion

This chapter has discussed road collisions and their analyses. As always, the first question is whether the viewer had sufficient sensory information to perform the task. In most collisions, the critical sensory information is motion, which may be determined directly from optical information or indirectly by calculating from distance and time. Either way, humans have severely limited abilities.

Analyses of human avoidance capabilities must further appreciate the difference between controlled research and real-world conditions. Experts frequently use Mortimer's .003 radian/sec looming threshold in forensic analyses. This is just as unrealistic as judging visibility using Blackwell's (1946) data. In both cases, the research thresholds should be multiplied to take into account realistic detection levels, variability and differences between expectations, practice levels, age, visibility conditions, uncertainty, etc. of test subjects and of real drivers. This fact is well understood by those who opine on visibility but apparently not by those who testify on rear-end collisions and who haven't examined the original studies. Lastly, any analysis must consider the effect of emergency conditions on driver arousal level, cognition and sensory motor response.

Although the discussion has emphasized the causal role of limited human perception, drivers may also cause accidents by making poor decisions. Drivers may become distracted by non-driving activities such as cell phone use. In some cases, the distraction increases reaction time, so a driver will respond more slowly to lead vehicle behavior. One study (Stutts, Huang and Hunter, 2002) claims that cell phone use doubles the probability of rear-end collision. However, the study was merely a small sample telephone survey, which makes the data highly unreliable due to responder self selection, memory error, and other problems associated with such techniques (e.g., Green, 2001).

Drivers may also follow too closely, so that there is little time to react to the behavior of a lead vehicle. One study (Wasielewki, 1979) found that the average temporal headway was only 1.32 seconds. Drivers likely learn to maintain such short headways because they seldom have negative consequences. Drivers can also anticipate the likelihood of lead car deceleration from road conditions, heavy traffic, upcoming intersection, etc., so reaction times are shorter if deceleration does occur. Drivers may also look through the lead vehicle windows to see conditions further down the road. This is why SUV's may promote rear-end collision—they block driver view and preview (Harb, Radwan, Yan and Abdel-Aty, 2007). Further, the driver and lead car travel at about the same speed, so there is no sense of relative speed or risk. Lastly, drivers may learn that leaving a large temporal headway is futile. In today's heavy road traffic, a driver leaving a large temporal headway will often be cut off by another vehicle. The end result of leaving a large gap is then a small gap. This is likely why typical temporal headways have shrunk over the last twenty years (Taieb-Maimon and Shinar, 2001).

## References

Baker, C., and W. Steedman. 1961a. Perceived movement in depth as function of object luminance, *Science* 133, 1356-1357.

Baker, C., and W. Steedman. 1961b. Perceived movement in depth as a function of luminance and velocity. *Human Factors* 3, 166-173.

Barrett, G., M. Kobayashi, and B. Fox. 1968. Feasibility of studying driver reaction to sudden pedestrian emergencies in an automobile simulator, *Human Factors* 10, 19-26.

Bertheln, C., and D. Mestre. 1993. Curvlinear approach to an intersection and visual detection of collision. *Human Factors* 35, 521-534.

Blackwell, H. R. 1946. Contrast thresholds of the human eye. *Journal of the Optical Society of America* 36, 624-643.

Blackwell, H. R. 1959. Development and use of a quantitative method for specification of interior illumination levels on the basis of performance data. *Illuminating Engineering* 54, 317-353.

Bonnett, G. 2001. The problem with turns. Retrieved from www.rec-tec.com/turns.htm 3 Aug 04.

Caird, K., and P. Hancock. 1994. The perception of arrival time for different oncoming vehicles at an intersection, *Ecological Psychology* 6, 83–109.

Cavallo, V., O. Laya, and M. Laurent. 1986. The estimation of time-to-collision as a function of visual stimulation. In A. G. Gale, M. H. Freeman, C. M. Haslegrave, P. Smith, and S. P. Taylor (eds.), Vision in Vehicles (pp. 179-183). Amsterdam: Elsevier Science Publishers.

Cavallo, V., D. Mestre, and C. Berthelon. 1997. Time-to-Collision Judgments: Visual and Spatio-Temporal Factors. In T. Rothengatter and E. C. Vaya (Eds.) *Traffic and Transport Psychology: Theory and Application*. 97-111, New York: Elsevier Science.

Clarke, D., P. Ward, and J. Jones. 1998. Overtaking road accidents: differences in maneuver as a function of driver age. *Accident Analysis & Prevention* 14, 179-185.

Clarke, D., P. Ward, and J. Jones. 1999. Processes and countermeasures in overtaking road-accidents. *Ergonomics* 42, 846-867.

DeLucia, P., M. Kaiser, J. Bush, L. Meyer, and B. Sweet. 2003. Information integration in judgments of time to contact, *Quarterly Journal of Experimental Psychology* 57A, 1165-1189.

Denton, G. 1976. The influence of adaptation on subjective velocity for an observer in simulated rectilinear motion. *Ergonomics* 19, 409-430.

Eberts, R. E., and A. MacMillan. 1985. Misperception of Small Cars. In R. E. Eberts and C. G. Eberts (eds.) *Trends in Ergonomics/Human Factors II*. North-Holland: Elsevier Science Publishers.

Evans, L. 1991. *Traffic Safety And The Driver*. New York: Van Norstrand Rheinhold.

Evans, L., and R. Rothery. 1973. Experimental measurements of perceptual thresholds in car-following. *Highway Research Record* 464, 13-29.

Farber, E., and C. Silver. 1967. (Report No. 1-193-11). The Franklin Institute Research Laboratories.

Fiske, J., K. Obenski, and T. Osborn. 1989. *Forensic Engineering Reconstruction of Accidents*. Springfield, Ill.: Charles C. Thomas.

Gibson, J. J. 1966. *The Senses Considered As Perceptual System*. Boston: Houghtom Miifflin.

Gibson, J. J. 1979. *Ecological Approach to Visual Perception*. Hillsdale: Lawrence Erlbaum Associates Publishers.

Goudie, D., J. Bowler, C. Brown, B. Heinrichs, and G. Siegmund. 2000. Tire friction during locked wheel braking. In Accident Reconstruction: Analysis, Simulation, and Visualization, 479-490. Warrendale: Society of Automtove Engineers.

Gray, R., and D. Regan. 1999. Adapting to expansion increases perceived time to collision. *Vision Research* 39, 2602-2607.

Gray, R., and I. Thornton. 2001. Exploring the link between time-to-collision and representational momentum. *Perception 30*, 1007-1022.

Green, M. 1983. Contrast Detection and Direction Discrimination of Drifting Gratings. *Vision Research*, 23, 281-289.

Green, M. 2001. Lies, damned lies and...controls," *Risk Management* November, 8–9.

Hamilton, J., and L. Thurstone. 1937. *Safe Driving: Human Limitations In Automobile Driving*. Doubleday Doran, New York. Cited in C. Tunnard and B. Pushkarev, 1963. *Man-Made America: Chaos or Control?: An Inquiry into Selected Problems of Design in the Urbanized Landscape*, New Haven: Yale University Press.

Harb, R., E. Radwan, X. Yan, and M. Abdel-Aty. 2007. Light truck vehicles (LTVs) contribution to rear-end collisions. *Accident Analysis and Prevention* 39, 1026-36.

Hecht, H., M. Kaiser, G. Savelsbergh, and J. Van Der Kamp. 2002. The impact of spatio-temporal sampling on time-to-contact judgments, *Perception & Psychophysics* 64, 650-666.

Heinrich, B., B. Allin, J. Bowler, and G. Siegmund. 2004. Vehicle speed affects both braking kinematics and average tire/road friction. *Accident Analysis and Prevention* 36, 839-840.

Herman, R., T. Lam, and R. Rothery. 1973. An experiment on car size effects in traffic. *Traffic Engineering and Control* 15, 90-93, 99.

Hockey, G., and P. Hamilton. 1983. The cognitive patterning of stress. In: G. Hockey (Ed.). *Stress and fatigue in human performance*. 331-362. New York: Wiley.

Hoffman, E. 1974. Perception of relative velocity. In *Studies of Automobile And Truck Rear Lighting And Signaling Systems* Report NO. UM-HSRI-HF-74-25. Ann Arbor: University of Michigan Transportation Research Institute.

Hoffman, E. 1994. Estimation of time to arrival—effects of age on use of available information. *Perception*, 23, 947-995.

Hoffman, E., and R. Mortimer. 1996. Scaling of relative velocity between vehicles. *Accident Prevention and Analysis*, 28, 415-421.

Horswill, M., S. Helman, P. Ardiles, and J. Wann. 2001. Motorcycle accident risk could be inflated by a time to arrival illusion. *Optometry and Vision Science* 82, 740-746.

Hoyle, F. 1957. *The Black Cloud*. New York: Signet.

Jones, H. V., and N. Heimstra. 1964. Ability of drivers to make critical passing judgements. *Journal of Engineering Psychology* 3, 117-122.

Kennedy, R., F. Jentsch, and J. Smither. 2001. Looming detection among drivers of different ages. *Proceedings of the Human Factors and Ergonomics Society*, 240-244.

Kiesewetter, W., W. Klinkner, W. Reichelt, and M. Steiner. 1999. The new brake assist of Mercedes-Benz: Active driver support in emergency braking situations, In *Vehicle performance : understanding human monitoring and assessment information*, 67-83. J. Pauwelussen (ed.) Lisse: Swets and Zeitlinger.

Knipling, R., D. Hendricks, J. Koziol, J. Allen, L. Tijerina, and C. Wilson. 1992. A Front-End Analysis of Rear-End Crashes. *Proceedings of the IVHS America 1992 Annual Meeting* 733-745.

Lakshminarayanan, V., and A. Raghuram. 2004. Aging and Estimation of time to collision. *Vision Sciences Society Meeting*, Sarasota, Florida.

Lamble, D., M. Laasko, and H. Summala. 1999. Detection thresholds in car following situations and peripheral vision: implications for positioning of visually demanding in-car displays. *Ergonomics* 42, 807-815.

Lee, D. 1976. A theory of visual control of braking based on information about time-to-collision. *Perception*, 5, 437-459.

Leibowitz, H. 1955. Effect of reference lines on the discrimination of movement. *Journal of the Optical Society of America* 45, 829-830.

Leibowitz, H. W. 1985. Grade Crossing Accidents and Human Factors Engineering. *American Scientist* 73, 534-540.

Liebermann, D., G. Ben-David, N. Schweitzer, Y. Apter, and A. Parush. 1995. A field study on braking responses during driving. I. Triggering and modulation. *Ergonomics* 38, 1894-1902.

Limpert, R. 1994. *Motor Vehicle Accident Reconstruction and Cause Analysis, 4th edition.* Mitchie: Charlottesville, Va.

Malaterre, G., F. Ferrandez, D. Fleury, and D. Lechner. 1988. Decision making in emergency situations. *Ergonomics* 31, 643-655.

Mortimer, R. 1971. The value of an accelerator release signal. *Human Factors* 13, 481-486.

Mortimer, R. 1990. Perceptual factors in rear-end collisions. *Proceedings of the Human Factors Society Meeting* 34, 591-594.

Muttart, J., W. Messerschmidt, and L. Gillen. 2005. Relationship between relative velocity detection and driver response times in vehicle following situations. *Society of Automotive Engineers* 2005-01-0427.

Olson, P., K. Campbell, D. Massie, S. Battle, E. Taub, T. Aoki, T. Sato, and L. Pettis. 1992. Performance Requirements for Large Truck Conspicuity Enhancements, Report No. DOT HS 807 815. National Highway Traffic Safety Administration, U.S. Department of Transportation, Washington, DC. Transportation Research Institute, University of Michigan, Ann Arbor, Michigan.

Plotkin, S. 1984. Multiple Causation. *Automotive Engineering and Litigation* 1, 215–228. New York: Garland Law Publishing.

Probst, T., S. Krafczyk, and T. Brandt. 1984. Interaction between perceived self-motion and object-motion impairs vehicle guidance. *Science* 225, 536-538.

Prynne, K., and P. Martin. 1995. Braking behavior in emergencies. *SAE Technical Paper* 950969.

Reed, W. and A. Keskin. 1989. Vehicular deceleration and its relationship to friction. SAE Technical Paper 890736.

Regan, M., and N. Beverly. 1979. Monocular and binocular stimuli for motion in depth: changing-disparity and changing-size inputs feed the same motion-in-depth stage. *Vision Research* 19, 1331-1342.

Rock, P., M. Harris, and T. Yates. 2006. *A Test of the Tau-Dot Hypothesis of Braking Control in the Real World. Journal of Experimental Psychology: Human Perception and Performance* 32, 1479-1484.

Runeson, S. 1974. Constant velocity – not perceived as such. *Psychological Research* 37, 3-23.

Runeson, S. 1975. Visual prediction of collision with natural and nonnatural motion functions. *Perception & Psychophysics* 18, 261-266.

Schiff, W., and R. Oldak. 1990. Accuracy of judging time to arrival: Effects of modality, trajectory, and gender. *Journal of Experimental Psychology: Human Perception and Performance* 16, 303-316.

Smith, M. R., J. M. Flach, S. M. Dittman, and T. Stanard. 2001. Monocular optical constraints on collision control. *Journal of Experimental Psychology: Human Perception and Performance* 27, 395–410.

Stewart, D., C. J. Cudworth, and J. Lishman. 1993. Misperception of time-to-collision by drivers in pedestrian accidents. *Perception* 22, 1227-1244.

Stutts, J., H. Huang, and W. Hunter. 2002. *Cell Phone Use While Driving in North Carolina: 2002 Update Report*. The University of North Carolina, Highway Safety Research Center, Chapel Hill, NC.

Summala, H., D. Lamble, and M. Laasko. 1998. Driving experience and perception of the lead car's braking when looking at in-car targets. *Accident Analysis and Prevention*, 30, 401-407.

Taieb-Maimon, M., and D. Shinar. 2001. Minimum and comfortable driving headways: Reality versus perception," *Human Factors* 43, 159-172.

Thompson, P. 1981. Velocity after-effects: the effects of adaptation to moving stimuli on the perception of subsequently seen moving stimuli. *Vision Research* 21, 337-345.

Tijerina, L., F. Barickman, and E. Mazzae. 2004. Driver Eye Glance Behavior During Car Following. National Highway Traffic Safety Administration.

Treffner, P., R. Barrett, and A. Petersen. 2002. Stability and skill in driving. *Human Movement Science* 21, 749-84.

Trewhella, J., M. Edwards, and M. Ibbotson. 2003. Sensitivity to the acceleration of looming stimuli. *Clinical and Experimental Ophthalmology* 31, 258-261.

van der Hulst, M., T. Meijman, and T. Rothengatter. 1999. Anticipation and the adaptive control of safety margins in driving. *Ergonomics* 42, 336-345.

Wann, J., S. Rushton, and C. Caldwell. 1999. Why do cars hit children? Dismissing the role of relative size in driver judgements of depth. Applied Vision Association Meeting 17th Meeting.

Wasielski, P. 1979. Car following headways on freeways interpreted by the semi-Poisson headway distribution model. *Transportation Science* 13, 36-55.

Yerkes, R. M., and J. Dodson. 1908. The relation of strength of stimulus to rapidity of habit-formation. *Journal of Comparative Neurology and Psychology* 18, 459-482.

## Endnotes

1. A few details about $\tau$: First, $\tau$ has several definitions. The major distinction is between global $\tau$ and local $\tau$ which further divides in type 1 and type 2. This chapter is only concerned with

local $\tau$, primarily with type 2, the dilation of a solid object and to a lesser extent with type 1, the spreading of single points. Second, in the strictest sense, local $\tau$ reveals time-to-collision only under a limited set of circumstances. Most importantly 1) the object must be heading straight toward the viewer's eye, 2) it must expand uniformly and without rotation (unless it is spherical) and 3) its approach velocity must be constant.

2. Some have suggested that drivers might simply use the visual angle $\theta$ to detect headway. As distance decreases, $\theta$ increases linearly. The driver might then detect closure by seeing change in $\theta$ over time.

3. However, film clips provide no relative disparity information.

4. They also measured threshold for detecting a vehicle moving away from the observer and found even lower thresholds, .007 and .008 radian/sec. The likely explanation is their method was essentially descending method of limits, which gives lower thresholds as explained in Chapter 2.

5. This point does not apply to the film clip studies even though the experimental subjects were actually stationary. They saw images taken from the perspective of a moving driver.

6. 0.3 represents the maximum lateral acceleration that drivers like to use under "normal" conditions. In emergencies, drivers can chose a much higher acceleration rate.

7. To simplify the example analysis, I have ignored three factors. First, the analysis does not include the time required for brake pedal depression, as explained in Chapter 16. Second, perception-reaction time for steering is about .2 seconds faster than for braking (Chapter 17.) If the PRT for braking is 1.5 seconds, then the PRT for steering should be 1.3 seconds. Third, the viewer's eye is several feet behind his front bumper, so there is a slight discrepancy between viewing distance and vehicle distance.

8. I have been using the terms "velocity" and "speed" interchangeably, although strictly speaking they are different concepts. Velocity is a vector with magnitude and direction. Speed does not have a directional component. For practical purposes, however, they are identical on straight paths.

9. The information contained in dilation and in the spread of two taillights is not always equivalent. For the current discussion, the difference is irrelevant.

10. The artifact in question is "representational momentum," a perceptual tendency to mislocate the stopping point of a moving object as farther forward in the direction of movement. That is, if a driver sees a pedestrian move left to right in front of him before stopping, the driver will remember the pedestrian as stopping farther right (the direction of motion) than the actual location.

11. People are better at judging motion toward the fovea than away from it, presumably because evolution has provided a useful survival mechanism to help us detect and avoid objects coming toward the face.

12. Response conflicts can be more complicated. For example, there can be "double approach-avoidance," where each outcome has both positive and negative consequences.

# Chapter 17

# "How Long Does It Take to Stop?": Methodological Analysis of Driver Perception-Brake Times

Marc Green, Ph.D.

Human perception-brake reaction time (RT) studies have reported a wide variety of results. By analyzing a large number of data sets, however, it is possible to estimate times under specific conditions. The most important variable is driver expectation, which affects RTs by a factor of 2. When fully aware of the time and location of the brake signal, drivers can detect a signal and move the foot from accelerator to brake pedal in about 0.70 to 0.75 sec. Response to unexpected, but common signals, such as a lead car's brake lights, is about 1.25 sec, whereas RTs for surprise events, such as an object suddenly moving into the driver's path, is roughly 1.5 sec. These times are modulated somewhat by other factors, including driver age and gender, cognitive load, and urgency.

Driver RT has important consequences for both the design of safe roads and for the assessment of liability in court. Although standards organizations have established norms, 2.5 sec in the United States and 2.0 sec in Europe, these values have sometimes been criticized (e.g., Hooper & McGee, 1983a, 1983b). Many researchers have therefore continued to seek a canonical brake RT value and to investigate the variables that affect it.

The literature has reported braking time estimates that differ by a factor of almost 4. Results vary greatly because investigators have used many different signals, responses, and testing conditions. Because it is impossible to derive a single, all-purpose number, the better strategy is to analyze the studies and to determine expected brake RT for specific situations.

There are several ways to tease out the important variables. One is to blindly code studies by type, to plug them into a mathematical formula and then to perform a factor analysis. This approach is liable to produce rather odd conclusions, such as the notion (Sohn & Stepleman, 1998) that the major RT variable is the country where the RT took place! Moreover, authors (e.g., Sens, Cheng, Weichel, & Guenther, 1989; Sohn & Stepleman, 1998) of previous surveys have tended to accept research results at face value, paying little attention to methodological flaws, limitations, and variations (although see Olson, 1989).

TRANSPORTATION HUMAN FACTORS, *2*(3), 195–216

## Overview

My primary goal is to determine typical brake RT values for different driving conditions. The method is to review a large number of brake RT studies—far more than have been examined in any previous analysis—and to analyze and to critique the methods and variables used. In addition, I will connect the applied braking and basic RT literature. By understanding the factors underlying RT in general, it will be easier to reconcile differences across studies and to generalize results. Last, it is time for an updated review, because the last comprehensive overview is more than 10 years old.

In the ensuing discussion, I first provide a brief background on the basic concepts of RT analysis. In the subsequent section, I describe and critique the methodologies that have been used to measure driver braking times. Next, I examine effects of the principal variables—expectation, urgency, age and gender, and cognitive load—on brake times. I very briefly describe data on steering RTs and then make a few concluding remarks.

Before starting, a few disclaimers are in order. First, I only considered data for good conditions—daylight (with one exception), good weather, clear visibility, and so forth. In fact, data on brake RTs in less favorable conditions are rare. Second, I do not claim that the results included here constitute a complete summary of all brake RT studies. I excluded some commonly cited data due to large methodological flaws (e.g., Grime, 1952, which allowed anticipatory responses), and I was simply unable to obtain others (e.g., Allen Corporation, 1978.) My goal was merely to gather enough data to see the general trends. Third, in the analysis, I focus on expected values and pay cursory attention to population variability. Although important for practical purposes, analyzing variability would add complexity to the already difficult task of combining diverse data sets.

Last, in order to integrate data from such a large number of studies and variables, in the discussion, I gloss over some smaller methodological details. Table 1 summarizes the braking time results. In order to make general trends visible at a glance, I have sometimes collapsed data across less important variables. During the discussion, however, I drill down on these variables.

## Background

In order to interpret and generalize the brake RT studies following, it is important to understand the fundamental concepts from basic RT and information-processing research. In the following, I very briefly outline the basic theory necessary to analyze brake RTs. For fuller details, see Boff and Lincoln (1988).

### Response Components

When a human responds to a sensory input, the total RT can be decomposed into a sequence of components:

1. Mental processing time is the time it takes for the responder to perceive that a signal has occurred and to decide on a response. For example, it is the time required to detect that a person is running across the roadway directly ahead and that the brakes should be applied. Mental processing time can be further decomposed into subcomponents:
    a. *Sensation* is the time it takes to detect an object in the roadway. ("There is a shape in the road.") All things being equal, RT decreases with greater signal intensity (brightness, contrast, size, loudness, etc.), foveal viewing, and better visibility conditions. Best RTs are also faster for auditory signals than for visual ones.

b. *Perception* is the time needed to recognize the meaning of the sensation. ("The shape is a person.") Time increases with low signal probability, uncertainty (signal location, time or form), and surprise. "Choice" RT, when there are multiple possible signals and responses, is generally much slower than simple RTs, which occurs when there is only one possible signal or response pair, or both.

c. *Response selection and programming* is the time necessary to decide which, if any, response to make and to mentally program the movement. ("I should steer left instead of braking.") Response selection slows under choice RT when there are multiple possible responses. Conversely, practice decreases the required time. Strictly speaking, mental processing time should not be called *perception time* because it reflects mental response preparation as well as perception.

2. *Movement time* is the time it takes the responder's muscles to perform the programmed movement. For example, it is the time required to lift the foot from the accelerator and then to touch the brake pedal. In general, the more complex the movement, the longer the movement time. Increased arousal level and practice decreased movement time.

3. *Device response time* is the time it takes the physical device to perform its response. For example, it may be measured as the time it takes to bring a car to a halt after brake engagement.

In the truest sense of the term, *RT* should refer only to the first component—the mental processing time. However, this quantity is internal and cannot be directly and objectively measured without a physical response. Most basic RT studies use finger responses, such as the release of a spring-loaded telegraph key, which minimize the movement and device response components. However, movement times cannot be completely eliminated and always affect reaction time measurement.

Unfortunately, terms are used inconsistently in the literature. *RT*, for example, has been used to mean mental processing time alone and has sometimes combined with movement time. A few authors even included the device response time.

To avoid confusion, I follow the technically incorrect convention of referring to mental processing time as *perception time*. The combined perception and movement time will be called *brake reaction time*. *Stopping time* is brake RT plus device response time.

**Human Information Processing and Speed of Response**

Humans operate under two information-processing modes. The first, often called *automatic response* (Schneider & Schiffrin, 1977), occurs under two conditions. One is when there is a strong, innate stimulus–response compatibility. For example, humans will tend to move in the direction opposite that of an object on a collision trajectory. The second situation occurs when making highly practiced responses to common signals. Automatic mode is fast because there is no requirement for conscious decision making. The response seems almost a reflex, as if signal processing goes straight from sensation to movement without the need for perception or for response selection and programming. The visual search and attention literature (e.g., Green, 1991, 1992; Green & Senders, 1998) sometimes calls this *preattentive mode* because it doesn't appear to require focal attention and seems often to have no capacity limitation.

Hitting the brake pedal in response to the flashed brake lights of the car ahead is an example of learned, automatic response. This seemingly occurs automatically and without volition. Drivers often have the feeling that they responded before they became consciously aware of the brake light, especially if their attention was directed elsewhere when it flashed.

TABLE 1
Brake Reaction Times

| Study | Variables | PT | MT | TT | N | Distance to Collision | Speed | Paradigm | Signal | Response |
|---|---|---|---|---|---|---|---|---|---|---|
| Expected | | | | | | | | | | |
| Norman (1952) | | | | | 53 | 700 | High | Road exp | "Brillant light" | Touch brake pedal |
| | | | | 0.73 | | | | | | |
| Olson and Sivak (1986) | Age<br>Alertness | 0.50 y[a]<br>0.50 o[a] | 0.20 y[a]<br>0.22 o[a] | 0.70 y[a] | 49 | 46 m/3–4 sec | 27 mph | Road exp | Yellow foam | PT: release accelerator<br>MT = depress brake |
| Sivak, Post, Olson, and Donohue (1981a) | Light location<br>Speed<br>Distance | | | 0.73 | 12 | | | Road exp | Brake light | Push button |
| Dureman and Boden (1972) | Fatigue<br>Shock | | | 0.7 | 8 | | | Simulator | Tone | Press pedal |
| Johansson and Rumar (1971) | Alertness | | | 0.66[a] | 321 | | | Road exp | Sound-klaxon | Brake light |
| Korteling (1990) | Age<br>Road difficulty | | | 0.620 y<br>0.709 o | 40 | 15 m | 100/80 kph | Road exp | Brake light | "Brake pedal response" |
| Nagler and Nagler (1973) | Many | | | | 225 | | | Simulator | Stop sign on panel | Move foot from accelerator to brake "depressed" |
| | | | | 0.63 | | | | | | |
| Lisper, Laurell, and Stening (1973) | Fatigue | | | 0.65 | 10 | | | Road exp | Tone | Vocal |
| Olson and Sivak (1986) | Age<br>Alertness | 0.40 y[a]<br>0.48 o[a] | 0.19 y[a]<br>0.20 o[a] | 0.59 y[a]<br>0.68 o[a] | 49 | | | Road exp | Red light | PT: release accelerator<br>MT = depress brake |
| Lings (1991) | Practice<br>Disability<br>Age<br>Gender | 0.318[a] | 0.27 o[a] | 0.588[a] | 109 | | | Simulator | Red traffic signal | PT: release accelerator |
| Schweitzer, Apter, Ben-David, Lieberman, and Parush (1995) | Distance<br>Speed<br>Alertness | | | 0.535[b] | 45 | 6/12 m | 60/80 kph | Road exp | Brake lights | Apply brakes |
| Greenshields (1936) | Age | | | | 1461 | | | Simulator | Red on mock traffic signal | From accelerator to "pressure on brake" |
| | | | | 0.496 | | | | | | |
| Scott, Chandler, and Li (1996) | Seat position<br>Driver height | 0.247[b] | 0.218[b] | 0.465[b] | 84 | | | Simulator | Green light turns red | Release accelerator, depress brake |
| Wright and Shephard (1978) | Age<br>Carbon monoxide<br>Gender | 0.25 | 0.17 | 0.42 | 348 | | | Simulator | Light | PT: release accelerator<br>MT = depress brake |
| Davies and Watts (1969) | Pedal height | | 0.149<br>0.309 | | 10 | | | Simulator | Light | From accelerator to "pressure on brake" |

*(Continued)*

TABLE 1
*(Continued)*

| *Study* | *Variables* | *PT* | *MT* | *TT* | *N* | *Distance to Collision* | *Speed* | *Paradigm* | *Signal* | *Response* |
|---|---|---|---|---|---|---|---|---|---|---|
| Unexpected | | | | | | | | | | |
| Triggs (1987) | Day | | | | | | | Naturalistic | Railroad signal–day | Brake light |
| | | | | 1.77 | | | | | | |
| Sivak et al. (1981a) | Brake light location | | | 1.38 | 277 | | | Naturalistic | Brake light | Brake light |
| van Winsum and Brouwer (1997) | | | | 1.35 | 1 | | | Simulator | Brake lights | Press brake pedal |
| Chang, Messer, and Santiago (1985) | Speed<br>Distance | | | $1.3^{b}$ | 1614 | | 25–55 mph | Naturalistic | Yellow light | Brake light |
| Mortimer (1969) | | | | 1.3 | 80 | | | | Brake light | Press brake pedal |
| Sivak, Olson, and Farmer (1982) | Speed<br>Distance | | | 1.21 | 1644 | 1 2/3–5 lengths | 32–40<br>56–72 kph | Naturalistic | Brake light | Radar response |
| Triggs (1987) | Night Time | | | $1.16^{b}$ | | | | Naturalistic | Railroad signal–night | Brake light |
| Gazis, Herman, and Maradudin (1960) | | | | 1.14 | | | | Naturalistic | Yellow traffic signal | Brake light |
| Alm and Nilsson (1994) | Cell phone<br>Road difficulty | | | 1.13 | 40 | | 100 kph | Simulator | Red square | Depress brake 10 mm |
| Triggs (1987) | | | | 0.92 | | | | Naturalistic | Brake light | Brake light |
| Nilsson and Alm (1991) | Age<br>Cell phone use | | | 0.92 y<br>1.32 o | 40 | | 105 kph | Simulator | Red square | Depress brake 10 mm |
| Johansson and Rumar (1971) | Alertness | | | $0.9^{a}$ | 5 | | | Road exp | Sound-buzz | Apply brake |
| Schweitzer et al. (1995) | Distance<br>Speed<br>Alertness | | | $0.606^{b}$ | 45 | 6/12 m | 60/80 kph | Road exp | Brake lights | Apply brakes |

| | | | | | | | | | | |
|---|---|---|---|---|---|---|---|---|---|---|
| Lieberman et al. (1995) | Distance<br>Speed | 0.399 | 0.24 | 0.638[b] | 45 | 6/12 m | 60/80 kph | Road exp | Brake lights | Apply brakes |
| Schweitzer et al. (1995) | Distance<br>Speed<br>Alertness | | | 0.606[b] | 45 | 6/12 m | 60/80 kph | Road exp | Brake lights | Apply brakes |
| Unexpected | | | | | | | | | | |
| Summala and Koivisto (1990) | Time-collision<br>Age | | | 1.75 y<br>1.95 o | | 0–6 sec | | Naturalistic | Policeman stop | Deceleration (radar) |
| McGehee, Mazzae, and Bladwin (2000) | Track versus simulator | 1.28-t | | (1.58-t)[d] | 192-t | | 45 mph[d] | Simulator and | "Intersection incursion"[e] | Release brake |
| | | 0.96-s | | (1.26-s)[c] | 120-s | | 45-55 mph[c] | Road exp | Blow up foam vehicle[d] | |
| Hankey (1996) | Time-collision<br>Gender | 1.23 | 0.324 | 1.55[b] | 48 | 2.85–4.35 sec | 55 mph | Road exp | Car | PT: release accelerator<br>MT = depress brake |
| Lerner (1994) | Age | | | 1.5 | 116 | 200 ft | 40 mph | Road exp | Trash barrel | Touch brake |
| Broen and Chang (1996) | Pedal configuration<br>Age<br>Gender | 1.16 | 0.17 | 1.33 | 100 | | 25 mph | Simulator | "Obstacle" | No specified |
| Arbuthnott (1980) | Field dependence<br>Sound | 0.904[b] | 0.313[b] | 1.27[b] | 100 | | | Simulator | Car pulling out | PT: release accelerator<br>MT = depress brake |
| Olson and Sivak (1986) | Age<br>Alertness | 0.70 y[a]<br>0.75 o[a] | 0.40 y[a]<br>0.35 o[a] | 1.1 y[a]<br>1.1 o[a] | 49 | 46 m/3–4 sec | 27 mph | Road exp | Yellow foam | PT: release accelerator<br>MT = depress brake |
| Barrett and Thornton (1968) | | | | 1.05 | 19 | 76.5 ft | 25 mph | Simulator | Dummie from shed | "Began to depress pedal" |
| Barrett, Kobayashi, and Fox (1968) | Field dependence | | | 1.02 | 10 | 82.5 ft | 25 mph | Simulator | Dummie from shed | "Began to depress brake" |
| Triggs (1987) | | | | 0.97 | | | | Naturalistic | Tire road shoulder | Brake light |

*Note.* PT = Perception time; MT = Motor time; TT = Total time; Exp = Experiment; Y = Young; O = Old.
[a]Value is a median. [b]Data collapsed over several variables. [c]Estimated. [d]Track. [e]Simulator.

The second mode of processing mode is termed *attentive* or *controlled* and requires thought. It generally occurs when there are novel events that require extra processing time both in perception (more sensory input and more memory retrieval to interpret) and decision (more time required to assess significance and to decide what, if any, response is warranted.) Attentive processing occurs, for example, when a driver sees an unexpected shape in the road, especially at night and other situations where visibility is poor.

In sum, understanding the driver's dominant information processing mode is important for predicting and analyzing RTs. Attention is a graded function, so the two modes represent a graded continuum rather than a dichotomy (e.g., Schneider and Detweiler, 1988). Drivers operating in the more automatic mode will response faster, whereas drivers forced to move toward the controlled end of the continuum will respond more slowly and likely with greater error (Kay, 1971).

## Brake RT Studies

Table 1 shows total brake RT from a wide range of studies. Where available, I provide separate columns for perception and movement times. In several cases, studies failed to report means or medians, so I read data off of graphs. (Several authors showed only analysis of variance, correlations, and so forth, but not actual data. For example, van Winsum and Brouwer, 1997, only showed actual data for a single driver.) Means for young (y) and old (o) drivers are noted separately.

Each line also shows other significant properties: method, number of subjects, signal, response, distance from hazard at trial onset, and traveling speed. Blank cells indicate that the variable did not apply to the study or that it was not stated.

Before discussing research results in detail, however, I outline common methodological techniques. It is important to keep methodology in mind in order to assess ecological validity to uncover factors that might bias results up or down and to aid in reconciling different brake RT results.

### Methodology

*Paradigms*

Studies have employed one of three basic paradigms: simulator studies, controlled road studies, or naturalistic observation.

*Simulator studies.* Off-road (in the lab or at a public gathering such as a fair) studies were performed in a car mock-up or in the cabin of a real vehicle. In older studies, "drivers" typically braked in response to an actual traffic light placed in front of the simulator, although a few studies used film loops for more authenticity. Modern studies used computer graphics to produce more realistic visual scenes.

*Controlled road studies.* The participant drove public or private roads or a track while a researcher sat in the passenger seat. The participant usually knew that she or he was being tested, but the investigator may or may not have revealed the real purpose of the study. Investigators often measured RT to "unexpected" events.

*Naturalistic observation.* The researchers set up recording equipment and measured the response of drivers who were unaware of being monitored. The typical study recorded the interval between a yellow traffic signal, brake lights of a leading car (possibly driven by a researcher), and so forth, and onset of the naive driver's brake lights.

**Paradigm Comparison and Evaluation**

Each paradigm has significant limitations in ecological validity, the degree to which results generalize to normal driving conditions. For example, there are obviously large differences between simulators and the roadway. Compared to the roadway, simulators present simplified visuals, loss of small texture cues, smaller field of view, no depth from stereopsis, and so forth. There are usually no nonvisual cues, which may play an important role in motion perception (e.g., Ohita & Komatsu, 1991). Moreover, there are fewer distractions, cognitive load is small, and the driver likely makes fewer eye movements to investigate objects in the peripheral field. There is no rear-view mirror to check. McGehee, Mazzae, and Bladwin (2000) attempted a direct comparison and concluded that simulators produce brake RTs that are 0.3 sec faster. However, they found steering times similar.

In controlled road studies, drivers are also more alert than they would be during normal driving. Moreover, some road experiments, as well as naturalistic observation studies, also suffer from the problem that not all drivers perform the expected response. Studies often found that some drivers avoided the obstacle by steering rather than by braking or performed both responses. The obtained braking RT estimate is then a biased sample. It might be hypothesized, for example, that people who are the slowest brakers have learned to avoid the obstacle by steering when possible. If so, then their times were unmeasured, and the results underestimate brake RT for the general population. On the other hand, the data might overestimate brake RT because the drivers were considering alternative responses, and choice RT is slower than simple RT. There is no evidence whether either of these hypotheses is true, but they demonstrate the potential bias sources introduced by allowing participants to make alternate responses.

In addition, most simulator and controlled road studies created large practice effects. With a few exceptions, the researchers collected data for many trials on each driver. Participants became highly practiced, which would reduce times compared to those likely in actual driving conditions. Lings (1991), for example, found that the first brake response in a series was always slower.

Naturalistic observation has the merit of high ecological validity. Normal driving is largely an automatic information-processing task, but simulator and controlled road studies put drivers on alert and probably switch them to a more conscious and controlled mode. It has been hypothesized (Kay, 1971) that accidents most commonly occur when a person is forced to suddenly switch from automatic to controlled processing. Only naturalistic observation can capture this switch. In addition, naturalistic studies generally measured times for a very large number of drivers.

However, the naturalistic method is limited because the researchers cannot easily test effects of independent variables, place drivers in emergency or even urgent situations, or measure perception and movement times separately. Last, they are unable to record data about driver demographics, so sample bias is always possible.

A quick glance at Table 1 reveals some paradigm trends in overall speed estimates. The table organizes studies first by driver expectation (which is the most important variable—see the following) and then by mean brake RT. Although not an overwhelming trend, simulator times are generally faster than those found on the road, at least in expected and unexpected conditions. Although there are few relevant studies, the data show no clear difference between road and naturalistic studies for the unexpected condition, the only category they share. (As discussed following, I discount the anomalous Schweitzer, Apter, Ben- David, Liebermann, & Parush, 1995, and Liebermann, Ben-David, Schweitzer, Apter, & Parush, 1995, studies.)

**Signals and Responses**

*Braking signals.* Studies have used a wide range of signals to induce braking. The most common are brake lights of a leading car and traffic signals (either in the simulator or on the road). Other studies have used unexpected incursions by another vehicle, an object such as a trash can, or even a dummy pedestrian. A few studies used auditory signals, and one simulator study used an arbitrary computer graphic—a red square. Finally, there are several studies that used the slowing of a lead car with an inoperative brake light. The test driver responded to change in velocity, which is much more difficult to detect than the onset of a light or the sudden appearance of an object. I have excluded these studies from the table because they produce a much higher range of RTs than those found using other signals. However, I will mention some of the results where relevant.

There are several sources of potential variability inherent in the sensory detection of this wide variety of signals. First, RT will be faster when the signal is foveally viewed than when it is seen in the visual periphery. Response times to incursions from the side of the road should be slower than from objects viewed immediately ahead. Some incorrectly believe that motion is more salient in the visual periphery so that objects approaching from the side will more readily grab attention. In fact, research (e.g., Green, 1983) demonstrates that viewers are much poorer at detecting motion in the periphery. Brake and traffic lights have their slow rise time, effects which, in part, cancel out the slower detection of peripheral objects.

Last, auditory signals generally produce faster RTs. Humans, like other animals, probably have an innate tendency to interpret sounds as warnings. Moreover, auditory transduction is mechanical, whereas visual transduction requires a relatively slow, biochemical process.

*Response.* Some studies recorded only a single total braking RT, some measured perception and movement time separately, and some examined only movement time. In almost all cases, perception time was measured from the onset of the signal to the release of the accelerator and movement time was the period from release of the accelerator until brake application.

Researchers measured response times either by directly recording brake depression with a microswitch attached to the pedal or by observing onset of the driver's brake lights. However, standard brake lights have a slow rise time and do not become visible until 0.05 to 0.1 sec or more after activation. RT estimates obtained by viewing brake light onset should therefore be slightly slower than times obtained from pedal microswitches. In fact, the finding (Sivak, Flannagan, Sato, Traube, & Aoki, 1994) that special fast-rise brake lights could decrease reaction times by over 0.15 sec suggests a significant difference between the two measurement methods. Last, braking responses have also been measured by means of radar, which detects deceleration. These RTs should also be faster than times measured from brake lights.

However, use of microswitches also has problems because it takes appreciable time to fully depress a brake pedal. Studies using a microswitch, unfortunately, are often vague as to what was actually recorded. Many authors simply have said that they stopped the reaction timer when there was pressure on the brake (Davies &Watts, 1969) or there was brake pedal response, (Korteling, 1990), and so forth. This is probably one reason that brake RT data are so variable—the more depression required to close the microswitch, the longer the resulting RT. Different studies may have used different pedal depression criteria.

A few studies measured the complete braking response, from initial pedal activation to complete depression. Because estimates (Barrett, Kobayashi, & Fox, 1968; Hankey, 1996; van Winsum & Brouwer, 1997; McGehee et al., 2000), range upward from 0.5 sec, it is important for studies to be precise in explaining exactly how much pedal depression constituted a response. Moreover,

Barrett et al. found a relation between speed of initial and full brake pedal depression. The fastest responders (about 0.8 sec) slammed on the brakes, going from initial to full depression in approximately 0.5 sec. Slower responders, however, took much longer to fully depress the pedal. Those with perception times of 1 sec, for example, took 0.8 to 1.0 sec for full depression, and the slowest responders never reached full depression at all.

This result is important for estimating stopping distances. At 55 mph, a driver is traveling 81 ft/sec, so the difference in stopping distance for a 0.2 sec delay would be calculated as 16 ft. Because slower initial brake RTs mean slower pedal depression, the deceleration is slower, and stopping time and distance are greater. Most studies only measure initial brake response. Therefore, taking their brake RTs at face value may underestimate stopping distances and times for the slower responders.

**Data Analysis**

Most brake RT studies report means, which produce high expected RTs. When values of a random variable approximate a normal distribution, then mean, median, and mode produce similar estimates of expected value. However, RT data are almost always skewed toward longer values (Figure 1). A relatively very few long RTs in the distribution tail usually inflate mean values. For example, Chang, Messer, and Santiago (1985), one of the few studies that reported both, found that medians were 0.2 sec lower than means.

Similarly, standard deviations will be misleading because they combine the smaller variance of the fast responders with the larger variance of the slowpokes. (See Summala & Koivisto, 1990, for a graphic depiction of the slow brakers' greater variance.) As a result, there will be more slow responders than the data variance suggest.

Some investigators (e.g., Schweitzer et al., 1995) seemed aware of these problems and cut off the RT distribution's tail at longish RTs. The mean and median then moved closer together, but the question remains whether arbitrarily dropping the long values biases the outcome and misrepresents the population. It may be supposed that these very long times represent driver errors or gross lack of attention, but there is no way to ensure that tail cutting does not compromise ecological validity.

**Results**

In the following, I discuss brake reaction as a function of several driving-related variables. In the first section I focus on expectancy, because it is the most important determinant. I then examine demographics (age and gender), urgency (time to collision) and cognitive load (distraction). In the final section I compare responses for braking and for steering.

**Expectancy**

Brake RT studies can be divided into those that investigate RT with the driver alerted and expecting a signal to brake and those that use unexpected signals. The first group is interested determining the upper bound for behavior under ideal circumstances, whereas the second aims to measure RTs under more natural conditions.

However, the terms *expected* and *unexpected* are used inconsistently across studies. For example, most authors term a condition as *expected* when the driver is explicitly told that a brake response must be made. Johansson and Rumar (1971), however, had a condition in which the driver is told to respond to a buzzer, yet the authors called this *unexpected.*Moreover, a simple dichotomy does not fully capture the full gamut of driver readiness gradations. Some signals are truly unexpected, whereas others are fairly common and only have some temporal uncertainty. For didactic purposes, I crudely decompose expectation level into three categories: expected, unexpected, and surprise.

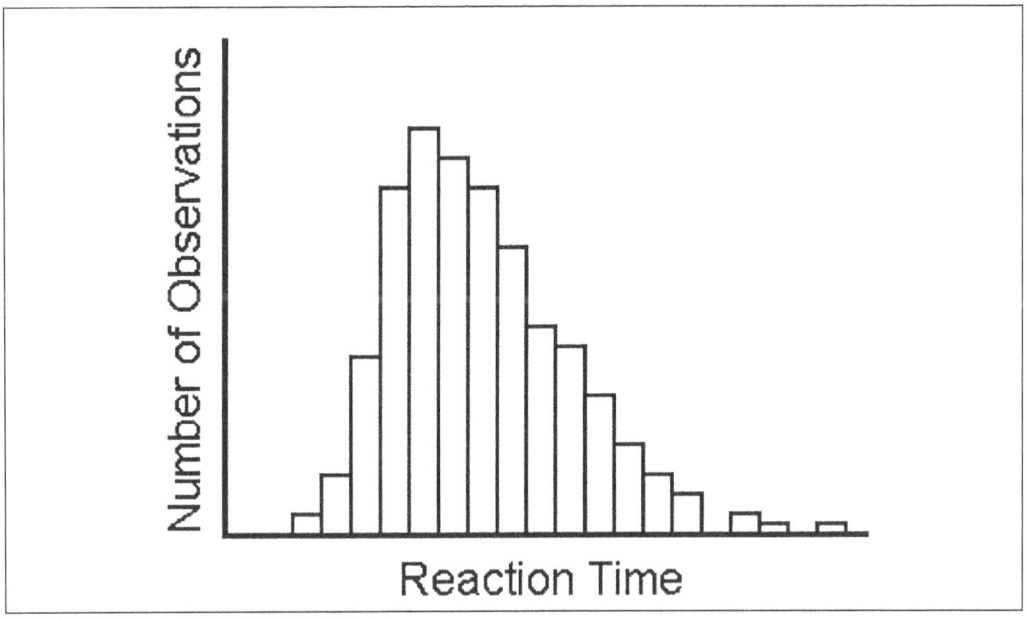


***Figure 1** Hypothetical Reaction Time Distribution.*

*Expected.* RT studies must always employ a degree of signal uncertainty in order to prevent anticipatory responses. However, RT increases with uncertainty of signal onset (Boff & Lincoln, 1988). In some cases, investigators have minimized uncertainty in order to determine best possible braking performance or to conveniently study the effects of some variable (drugs, brake pedal separation, etc.). Participants knew that they were to make the brake response, and temporal uncertainty was usually no more than fractions of a second or a few seconds at most. Moreover, there was little spatial uncertainty, because the signal was fixed in position. This is an important type of study, because it constrains the universe of possible brake RTs by determining the boundary condition.

Norman (1952) performed perhaps the clearest road study of braking under low uncertainty. Drivers traveled an aircraft taxiway at "high speeds" and braked on seeing an expected "brilliant light" 700 feet ahead. The mean brake RT was 0.73 sec and the 95th percentile was at 0.89 sec. Norman's values are consistent with data from the expected conditions of several other road studies (Olson & Sivak, 1986, for obstacle; Sivak, Post, Olson, & Donohue, 1981b), although their variability was much higher. Olson and Sivak (1986) also found a slightly lower RT for a light signal attached to the hood of the car. The value is likely lower because of lessened spatial uncertainty, and because the table value is for the median rather than the mean. Finally, Summala, Lamble, and Laakso (1998) reported RTs of roughly 0.5 sec to brake lights of a leading car. However, drivers started with the foot already on the brake, which would likely subtract 0.2+ sec movement time from the normally measured total brake RT.

Although Norman's (1952) conditions might seem designed to produce the fastest RTs possible on the roadway, Table 1 shows that several studies report even faster total brake RTs. The oft-cited Johansson and Rumar (1971) study found median RTs of 0.66 sec under expected conditions. The lower estimate is not surprising for several reasons. First, Norman used only one run per driver, so there was no practice effect. As another study has shown (Lings, 1991), brake RTs decreased markedly from the first to subsequent trials even under conditions of minimal uncertainty.

Johansson and Rumar (1971) also used an auditory signal (a Klaxon™), which produces faster optimal RTs than those obtained with a visual signal. The use of an auditory signal likely also explains the slightly lower RTs reported by two other studies, Dureman and Boden (1972) and Lisper, Laurell, and Stening (1973), which also had large practice effects. Last, Johansson and Rumar also reported medians rather than means. Korteling (1990) found his younger participants responding in 0.620 sec, whereas older drivers required a mean of 0.709 sec. (I averaged his low and high cognitive load conditions.) However, he discarded RTs greater than 2.0 sec. All things considered, there are many studies that agree that a mean brake RT of about 0.70 to 0.75 sec is the best that can be expected on the road.

Companion papers by Schweitzer et al. (1995) and Liebermann et al. (1995), however, reported anomalously fast RTs compared to those of other studies using similar methodology. There are several possible reasons for their fast estimates. First, they also truncated the data, throwing away RTs greater than 1.7 sec. Second, their participants were in an unusually heightened state of arousal. The lead car performed a series of "alternative misleading emergency maneuvers." Surely, the participants must have been highly alert and primed for fast response.

Third, there were likely large practice effects. The investigators collected times in three successive conditions: (a) naive, drivers told nothing; (b) drivers told to expect to brake; and (c) drivers told to brake in response to brake light. There were 48 trials in all, but it is unclear how many were in the naive condition. In any event, there were surely practice effects. By the time the expected condition occurred, the viewers were highly experienced in the task.

Last, simulators studies (Greenshields, 1936; Lings, 1991; Scott, Chandler, & Li, 1996; Wright & Shephard, 1978) in primitive mock-ups—drivers viewed a simple traffic light or panel rather than film or computer graphic—found the fastest brake RTs ranging from 0.4 to 0.5 sec. In all of these studies, the driver responded to a light onset at a predetermined location, therefore, spatial and temporal uncertainty as well as cognitive load were very low. The relevance of these brake RTs to actual driving conditions is questionable. Both simulator and road studies (Olson & Sivak, 1986) that measured a separate movement time found that drivers required slightly over 0.2 sec to take the foot off of the accelerator and move it to the brake pedal.

In sum, the Norman (1952) estimate is probably the most ecologically valid result for the braking time under favorable conditions—low uncertainty, intense visual, foveally viewed signal, but no recent practice. The best expected brake RT is about 0.7 to 0.75 sec, which consists of about 0.5 to 0.55 perception time and 0.2 sec movement time. Authors of a previous review (DeSilva & Forbes, 1937) reached a similar conclusion.

*Unexpected.* A very common method tested driver RT to onset of brake lights or of a traffic light in the naturalistic observation paradigm. Authors always described these conditions as reaction times to an unexpected event because the driver is not explicitly told that the need to brake is imminent. However, the term *unexpected* is inappropriate. One of the problems with such studies is that they view drivers as a tabula rasa, as if they knew nothing and started with no expectations. In fact, drivers have many expectations based on their years of driving. They expected something unusual to happen because there is a stranger sitting in the passenger seat. They expect cars to sometimes brake ahead of them requiring an immediate brake response. They expect traffic lights to change periodically, and so forth. Such events are never totally unexpected. At most, they are temporally uncertain.

Studies of expected reaction times produced results varying over a 2:1 range. One set of studies (Chang et al., 1985; Mortimer, 1969; Sivak et al., 1981b; van Winsum & Brouwer, 1997) agree with an expected brake RT in the range of 1.3 to 1.4 sec (The Chang et al. estimate is actually the slowest because it is a median.) Another set (Gazis, Herman, & Maradudin, 1960; Sivak, Olson, & Farmer, 1982; Triggs, 1987, for railroad signal night) bunch closely at 1.14 to 1.21 sec. Alm and Nilsson (1994) also found a mean reaction time of about 1.13 (the mean of their easy and hard conditions.)

There is a third cluster of results (Alm & Nilsson, 1994, easy condition; Johansson & Rumar, 1971; Triggs, 1987, for brake lights) at 0.9 sec. The Johansson and Rumar result is undoubtedly low because the reported value is a median, the signal was auditory (a buzzer), and the drivers were explicitly instructed to brake when the buzzer sounded—it was not exactly an unexpected condition. It is unclear why Triggs's mean times for response to lead car brake lights should be so much faster than those found by Sivak et al. (1981a), van Winsum and Brouwer (1997), and Sivak et al. (1982).

Finally, there are a few anomalous findings. The Schweitzer et al. (1995) and Liebermann et al. (1995) studies again have the fastest estimates, ranging from 0.605 to 0.678. I have already suggested possible reasons for their anomalously fast times. The authors claimed that they were recording RTs to unexpected events, brake lights in a lead car. However, recall that the lead car performed a series of "alternative misleading emergency maneuvers." The need for braking could hardly be called *unexpected.* Moreover, long reaction times were discarded from the data.

There is also an anomalously slow estimate by Triggs (1987) for drivers responding to a railroad crossing during the day. Interestingly, he found that brake RT to railroad signals was much faster at night, when times agree with other studies, than during the day. Triggs attributed the difference to low signal discriminability, but the validity of this explanation is unproven.

In sum, the data vary, but the best guess is that brake RT to common, but uncertain signals lies between 1.2 and 1.35 sec. Standard deviations of results vary widely across studies, but 0.6 seems a good estimate. Therefore, the American Association of State Highway and Transportation Officials norm of a 2.5 sec brake reaction is a reasonable guess for time achievable from 90 percent to 95 percent of the general population. However, this estimate is only valid for a specific set of conditions: brake response to "normal" road events in good weather with high visibility.

*Surprise intrusion.* A few studies tested RT for truly unexpected, low probability signals. Most of these studies fit into the category of the *intrusion* (or *incursion*) paradigm, in which an object suddenly moves into the driver's path from off the road. (Of course, each participant provides only one trial in order to maintain the surprise.) Although such events do happen in normal driving, they have very low probability and drivers have not had sufficient experience to develop automatic response.

Surprise incursions produce slow brake RTs. Hankey (1996) performed the best study, in which the driver traveled a country road at 55 mph when another vehicle suddenly cut across an intersection immediately ahead. He found that brake RTs ranged from 1.55 to 1.80 sec depending on time-to collision. RT for steering was about 0.3 sec faster, roughly the extra time it takes to move the foot from accelerator to brake pedal. Summala and Koivisto (1990) measured brake RTs for the surprise intrusion of a policeman holding up his hand to stop traffic. They also found the brake RTs depended on time-to-collision, and the estimate (reading from their graph) of 1.7 sec at a 3-sec time-to-collision agrees well with Hankey's 1.8 sec under a similar time constraint. However, the studies differed greatly in the effects on urgency at other times-to-collision, perhaps because of different bases for their contact time estimates (see later). Lerner (1994) reported a similar mean time of 1.5 sec for a road study where a trash barrel on a chain rolled out into the road. Finally,

McGehee et al. (2000) reported a perception time of 1.28 sec for drivers on a track. Adding the 0.3-sec movement time brings the total to an estimated 1.58 sec. Times for a simulator study 0.3 sec faster. Regardless of the differences, these surprise intrusion studies report the longest brake RT in the literature.

There were slightly lower values reported by several simulator studies: Arbuthnott (1980) (1.27 sec, no noise condition) and Broen and Chiang (1996, 1.33 sec.) Barrett (Barrett et al., 1968; Barrett & Thornton, 1968) published two simulator studies with slower brake RT of 1.05 and 1.02 sec. (These data may have been from the same experiment). I have already suggested reasons that simulator studies should produce faster times—lower cognitive load and lower uncertainty. However, there is no obvious reason for Barrett's relatively fast times.

Olson and Sivak (1986), one of the most frequently cited brake RT studies, fits best in this class. Drivers traveled over a rise, found an object (yellow foam) in the road and braked. Although there was no intrusion from the side of the road, discovery of an obstacle in the roadway was presumably a genuinely unexpected event.

Olson and Sivak (1986) found that the RT for this unexpected condition was 1.1 sec, about a half second faster than time reported by Lerner (1994) and Hankey (1996) and Summala and Koivisto (1990). There are several likely explanations for the difference. First, the 1.1 sec estimate is a median, which should be lower than the mean. Another reason for the faster brake RT was the location of the obstacle in the middle of the road. Its appearance in the central visual field would cause fast detection. Intrusions from the side, on the other hand, would be detected by the less-sensitive visual periphery.

Moreover, the Olson and Sivak (1986) unexpected condition was hardly that. There was no direct measurement of the drivers' perception time. Instead, the authors determined perception RT by having the participants redrive the route and call out when they saw the foam. By then, of course, drivers knew that there was an obstacle in the road ahead, so this was an expected not an unexpected condition.

The only other anomalously low estimate is 0.97 sec by Triggs (1987). However, this was a minor intrusion, someone changing a tire by the side of the road. The lane was not blocked as in the other intrusion studies, and urgency was low.

In sum, the data clearly show that the surprised driver takes longer to brake. Overall, it takes the average driver roughly twice as long, 1.5 sec or more, to respond to an intrusion compared to a completely expected event, which requires only about 0.75 sec.

Intrusion probably slows reaction at all three mental-processing stages of human RT. Detection is slower due to the need to use the peripheral retina; perception is slower because the event is unusual and requires time to interpret; and response selection is slower because the driver must weight braking versus steering.

Moreover, data show that movement time is also slower when the driver is surprised. Most studies also found movement times over 0.3 sec, a 50 percent increment over those obtained under expected conditions. The difference might reflect the slower brake RTs that occur when participants have no chance to practice (Lings, 1991) or possibly uncertainty over response selection. In any event, for real-world estimates, 0.3 sec is probably more accurate than the 0.2 sec times sometimes suggested by authoritative sources (e.g., Shinar, 1977).

### Age

Basic RT studies generally find a slowing with increased age (e.g., Welford & Birren, 1965.) Surprisingly, brake RT studies have produced mixed results. Older drivers responded more slowly in some cases (Broen & Chiang, 1996; Greenshields, 1936; Lings, 1991; Nilsson & Alm, 1991; Sivak et al., 1981b, for pushing a button; Summala & Koivisto, 1990). However, other studies (Korteling, 1990; Lerner, 1994; Olson & Sivak, 1986; Wright & Shephard, 1978; see also Kloeppel, Peters, James, Fox, & Alicandri, 1994) found no slowing with age.

There are several possible explanations for the absence of a robust age effect. One is sample bias. Older people who are in better health are more likely to drive and therefore to be participants in driving studies. Another explanation is experience. Olson and Sivak (1986) suggested that older drivers are more practiced, which compensates for any slowing of perception or movement. Arbuthnott (1980) supported this conclusion by finding that older drivers more quickly recognized dangerous situations. Last, the definition of *older driver* varies with each study. A common definition is 56 years of age in driving studies, but most basic research uses an much higher definition of older, usually at least 60 or 65.

However, part of the answer may also lie in methodology. Researchers using simulators tend to find age effects, whereas road studies do not (with the exception of Summala & Koivisto, 1990). Even when found, the effect is only 100 msec at most. Age effects are likely small relative to other factors and are easily lost in the noise. Moreover, aging affects people very differently, making older drivers an inherently heterogenous population and their data accordingly noisier. The effect may only reveal itself in the more carefully controlled simulator studies that generally employ more participants and record more trials per participant.

Another difficulty is that the effects of aging on brake RT may depend on other, often uncontrolled, variables. One factor that may encourage an age effect is cognitive load. Alm and Nilsson (1995) found that cellular phone use caused a greater slowing of RT in older drivers than in younger drivers (see also, McKnight & McKnight, 1993; Wolffsohn, McBrien, Edgar, & Stout, 1998.) However, an earlier study (Nilsson & Alm, 1991) reported that a cell phone task had similar effect on all age groups.

Korteling's (1990) road study captures the difficulties in demonstrating an effect of age on brake RT. He concluded that there was no age effect, although older drivers had a mean brake RT 0.05 sec slower than that of young participants. Moreover, driving conditions that increased cognitive load doubled the young–old difference to 0.1 sec, yet the difference again failed to reach statistical significance.

In conclusion, although the data from driving studies are mixed, it is difficult to ignore the significant slowing demonstrated in many basic research studies. Moreover, there are enough positive driving results (e.g., Summala & Koivisto, 1990, reported a 0.3 sec slowing) to suspect that an aging effect exists in brake RT. The magnitude of the effect likely grows with increased information-processing demands and task complexity, but exact magnitude is uncertain. Alm and Nilsson (1995), for example, found a 1.5 sec difference between young and old drivers with cognitive loading, but this study used a very difficult signal to detect. Moreover, all of the studies described here used high visibility conditions. Normal aging produces major vision losses, so brake response would likely slow significantly at night and in poor weather. However, even if braking slows with age, it may not constitute a major problem. Older drivers apparently compensate for their poorer braking, at least in part, by driving more slowly (e.g., Summala & Koivisto, 1990).

### Gender

The research data are mixed. Some studies found faster response by men (Lings, 1991; Sivak et al., 1981b, for pushing a button; Wright & Shephard, 1978; see also American Automobile Association, 1952), although others found no difference (Hankey, 1996; Nagler & Nagler, 1973). None have found that women are faster.

**Urgency**

Many investigators hypothesized that drivers would respond faster under greater *urgency*, by which they invariably meant shorter time-to-collision. A priori, one might guess that greater urgency produces faster RT because of the greater arousal—the Yerkes-Dodson law (Yerkes & Dodson, 1908). Results, however, suggest that brake RT is a U-shaped function, decreasing with greater urgency but then paradoxically becoming very long when time-to-collision is short.

Studies have manipulated time-to-collision by varying speed, distance, or both. Chang et al. (1985) found that reaction time to a yellow light decreased a half second as speed increased from 25 mph to 40 mph, whereas further increases in speed up to 55 mph produced no additional effect. Liebermann et al. (1995) and Schweitzer et al. (1995) tested effects of both speed and following distance on brake RT. They found no speed effect, but the negative result may have been due to the comparison of very similar speeds, 60 kph and 80 kph. On the other hand, shorter following distances (6 m vs. 12 m) produced faster response in both studies. Sivak, Post, Olson, and Donohue (1981a) measured push-button responses rather than actual braking and also found that drivers responded faster to a combination of higher speed and shorter following distance. However, the following distance effects may not be one of urgency but rather of probability. Drivers know from experience that when they are trailing the next car by a substantial distance there will be little need to brake in order to avoid collision. As the distance diminishes, the need for braking increases so that it becomes a more probable response.

Summala and Koivisto (1990) measured RT as a function "subjective urgency" (p. 681), time-to-collision based on a formula that combined preferred speed, stopping distance, and deceleration. They concluded that RT decreased by almost 1 sec as time-to-collision decreased from 6 sec and approached 0.

In contrast, Hankey (1996) found that brake RT increased 0.4 sec as time-to-collision grew shorter, from 4.35 to 2.85 sec. As time-to-collision decreases, probability of steering increases relative to braking (Malaterre, Fernandez, Fleury, & Lechner, 1988). A very short time-to-collision likely forced the driver to decide whether there was sufficient time to brake or whether steering was the only possible action. This introduced mental-processing time for response selection. Moreover, the driver had to weigh the risk of steering into the oncoming lane, possibly check traffic there first, and then to fight the highly learned tendency to avoid traveling in the "wrong" lane. Often, drivers both braked and steered, which might take more mental response programming and slow both.

Although both Summala and Koivisto (1990) and Hankey (1996) used a surprise intrusion paradigm, the opposing conclusions are likely due to methodological differences. First, the authors figured time-to-collision differently. The Summala and Koivisto estimate included the time required for the car to brake to a halt, whereas Hankey estimated the contact time for a driver maintaining full speed of 55 mph. It is also worth noting that Summala and Koivisto showed a data point at a negative time-to-collision, so the validity of the formula must be questioned. Another possibility is that Hankey's participants were driving much faster. Summala and Koivisto did not state the speed of their drivers, but it seems reasonable to guess that the test took place in the city, where speeds would be much lower than the 55 mph used by Hankey's drivers on an empty rural road. Moreover, although Hankey's drivers had a response alternative, it seems unlikely that any of Summala and Koivisto's drivers would have considered simply steering around the policeman rather than obeying the "stop" command. Hence, there was no response competition. Last, drivers seeing a car cut them off at an intersection often expect it to stop (van Elslande & Faucher-Alberton, 1997), creating a slight hesitation and a longer RT.

Overall, the evidence suggests that drivers will respond faster under shorter time-to-collision, at least until time becomes very brief and there is the opportunity for alternative responses. When confronted with severe emergency, drivers probably slow response to increase time required for assessing the situation and to check feasibility of other escape actions.

**Cognitive Load**

Several investigators predicted that high cognitive load would slow RT. Attention is a limited resource, so any factor that draws from the resource pool will distract the driver from detecting the brake signal and slow RTs.

One method for increasing cognitive load is to complicate the driver's path. Presumably, following turns in a winding road requires more attention than simply steering a straightaway. Results support this assumption. Korteling (1990) found slower brake RTs when a lead car varied speed and the road had more turns. Alm and Nilsson (1994) found longer times for a simulated road that contained sharper turns.

Another source of cognitive load is use of in-car devices. Summala et al. (1998) found slower response when drivers viewed in-car displays. However, looking at objects inside the car forces the driver to view the road through the peripheral visual field and to accommodate to a near distance, so slowing might be an effect of poorer vision as well as cognitive load.

One recent hot topic in cognitive loading is the potential danger posed by cellular phone use. Although it would be expected that attentional allocation to nondriving tasks should slow response, visual tasks are much less impaired by a concurrent auditory task, such as listening, than by a second visual task. A priori, it is therefore not clear whether cellular phone use would be a significant hazard.

Epidemiological studies (e.g., Redelmeier & Tibshirani, 1997; Violanti, 1998; Violanti & Marshall, 1996), however, have concluded that accident likelihood increases dramatically during cell phone use. Moreover, studies found the same results for telephones with and without hand controls, suggesting that the effect is due to loss of attention and not to interference of motor control. Of course, epidemiological studies cannot determine whether such relations are cause and effect.

Several experimental road (Brookhuis & deWaard, 1994; Lamble, Kauranen, Laakso, & Summala, 1999; McKnight &McKnight, 1993) and simulator (Alm & Nilsson, 1995) studies attempted to demonstrate the cause–effect relation by testing drivers during cellular phone use. All found that cellular phones increased RTs by about 0.5 sec.

These results may exaggerate the hazard. In the studies cited earlier, the signal was acceleration –deceleration of a lead car, and, except for Alm & Nilsson (1995), there was no discrete signal, such as brake lights, a traffic signal, or even a roadway hazard. Instead, the drivers had to detect a much subtler cue, such as change in size, distance, and so forth, a notion confirmed by the unusually long control RTs. Discrete signals, such as the onset of a light, are more likely to break through attention, especially if they suggest a highly practiced response. For example, Summala et al. (1998) found that brake RTs were 1 to 2 sec slower when the lead car does not have operating brake lights.

Nilsson and Alm (1991) performed a better simulator study in which the brake signal was the sudden appearance of a red square on the "roadside." The concurrent use of a cell phone lengthened RTs by about 0.4 sec.

Moreover, not all studies have found a negative effect of cellular phone use. Alm and Nilsson (1994) paradoxically found drivers speaking on a cellular phone may decrease RT when road conditions are tricky. From a strict cognitive load viewpoint, this should have produced the slowest

RTs of all. One guess is that the drivers may have been aware that they were engaging in risky behavior and actually became more attentive to the road. Often, drivers confound theoretical expectation by taking risk-compensatory precautions.

In sum, there is empirical research showing that drivers who are using cellular phones have slower brake RTs. Studies (e.g., Briem & Hedman, 1995; Lamble et al., 1999) of other driving behaviors also found performance deterioration during cellular phone use. However, the extent of the danger and the conditions that modulate it are uncertain. Even authors of recent epidemiological studies (e.g., Min & Redelmeier, 1998) have begun to back off the extreme conclusions from earlier analyses. The issue is still open, and there is clearly a need for more research under more varied conditions.

**Responses: Braking Versus Steering**

Whereas most driver RT studies have examined braking responses, a few have measured steering times. Hankey (1996) found that drivers could make initial steering response about 0.3 sec faster than initial braking. This makes sense, because the movement time should be far less than the 0.3 sec needed to move the foot from the accelerator to the brake pedal. Summala, Leino, and Vierimaa (1981) measured steering RTs using a minor intrusion, a car door opening into the driver's lane. They claimed that RT was 1.5 sec, which would agree nicely with Hankey's results. However, his graphs clearly show that initial course correction had begun somewhat earlier, at about 1 sec. In sum, it seems likely that initial steering response is a few tenths of a second faster than initial braking.

**Summary of Brake RT Results**

There is no single "best-guess" value for brake RT. However, there is sufficient convergence among studies of similar methodology to enable reasonable estimates for specific situations. Overall, the literature demonstrates that expectancy has the greatest effect. With high expectancy and little uncertainty, the best driver response time is about 0.70 to .075 sec, of which 0.2 sec is movement time. With normal, but common, signals such as brake lights, expected times are about 1.25 sec. Last, the most ecologically valid driver response time for surprise intrusions is about 1.5 sec, including a 0.3 sec movement time. These are all mean values, so subtract roughly 0.1 sec to estimate the median.

Urgency is another important variable. Drivers respond faster when highly aroused by shorter time-to-collision. The size of this effect varies greatly across studies from a hundredths of a second to a full second, so it is difficult to set a single normal value or even a reasonable range of values. However, extreme emergency may actually produce longer RTs, especially if there is competition among response alternatives.

The data on age are conflicting, but it seems likely that older people respond 0.1 to 0.3 sec more slowly in many cases. However, older drivers probably compensate with lower speeds. This lower urgency may be part of the reason that they respond more slowly. Data on gender effects are also unclear. There is probably some effect, however, because men are sometimes faster than women, but no study shows women being faster than men.

Drivers are also likely to respond more slowly when there is high cognitive load, either from driving (complex roadway) or nondriving (cellular phones) factors. It is impossible, however, to precisely quantify the effect due to the wide variation in results. If the brake signal is common and meaningful and likely to break through the attentional filter (a brake light flash ahead), the effect is probably a few tenths of a second at most. When the brake signal is subtle (such as acceleration–deceleration), the effect may be upwards of half a second. However, drivers might compensate for the risk by attending to the road more, not less, than under normal conditions.

All of these conclusions are admittedly based on a rough mental combination across diverse studies mixed with some general trends in the basic RT literature. Unfortunately, there can be no other way. No single study can reproduce the full complexity of human behavior and its sensitivity to environmental variables. Moreover, studies cannot be quantitatively combined because no mathematical formalism can capture the subtle effects of methodology and variable interaction or incorporate general knowledge from the basic science literature on RT, perception, and cognition. For the time being, RT estimation remains part science and part intuition, that is, part application of a general knowledge about human factors.

## Acknowledgments

I thank Dr. John Senders for helpful discussion and Dr. John Hankey for providing the data from his dissertation.

## References

Allen Corporation. (1978). *Field validation of taillights—Report on phase 1: Pilot testing* (Rep. No. DOT HS 70156).

Alm, H., & Nilsson, L. (1994). Changes in driver behaviour as a function of handsfree mobile phones—A simulator study. *Accident Analysis and Prevention, 26*, 441–451.

Alm, H., & Nilsson, L. (1995). The effects of a mobile telephone task on driver behaviour in a car following situation. *Accident Analysis and Prevention, 27*, 707–715.

American Automobile Association. (1952). Age and complex reaction time. *Traffic Engineering and Safety Department*. (Rep. No. 41).

Arbuthnott, D. (1980). Effects of noise and perceptual style on reaction to a simulated driving emergency. *Canadian Journal of Behavioural Science, 12*, 78–85.

Barrett, G., Kobayashi, M., & Fox, B. (1968). Feasibility of studying driver reaction to sudden pedestrian emergencies in an automobile simulator. *Human Factors, 10*, 19–26.

Barrett, G., & Thornton, C. (1968). Relationship between perceptual style and driver reaction to an emergency situation. *Journal of Applied Psychology, 52*, 169–178.

Boff, K., & Lincoln, J. (1988). *Engineering data compendium: Human perception and performance*. Wright- Patterson Air Force Base, OH: Armstrong Medical Research Laboratory.

Briem, V., & Hedman, L. (1995). Behavioural effects of mobile telephone use during simulated driving. *Ergonomics, 38*, 2536–2562.

Broen, N., & Chiang, D. (1996). Braking response times for 100 drivers in the avoidance of an unexpected obstacle as measured in a driving simulator. *Proceedings of the Human Factors and Ergonomics Society, 40*, 900–904.

Brookhuis, K., & de Waard, D. (1994). Measuring driving performance by car-following in traffic. *Ergonomics, 37*, 427–434.

Chang, M., Messer, C., & Santiago, A. (1985). Timing traffic signal change intervals based on driver behavior. *Transportation Research Record, 1027*, 20–32.

Davies, B. T., & Watts, J. M., Jr. (1969). Preliminary investigation of movement time between brake and accelerator pedals in automobiles. *Human Factors, 11*, 407–409.

DeSilva, H., & Forbes, T. (1937). *Driver testing results*. Cambridge, MA: Harvard Traffic Bureau.

Dureman, E., & Boden, C. (1972). Fatigue in simulated car driving. *Ergonomics, 15*, 299–308.

Gazis, R., Herman, R., & Maradudin, A. (1960). The problem of the amber signal light in traffic flow. *Operations Research, 8*, 112–130.

Green, M. (1983). Contrast detection and direction discrimination of drifting gratings. *Vision Research, 23*, 281–289.

Green, M. (1991). Visual search, visual streams and visual architectures. *Perception and Psychophysics, 50*, 388–403.

Green, M. (1992). Visual search: Detection, identification and localization. *Perception, 21*, 765–777.

Green, M., & Senders, J. (1998). *Human error in road accidents*. Retrieved January 8, 2000 from the World Wide Web: http://www.ergogero.com/pages/roadaccidents.html

Greenshields, B. (1936). Reaction time in automobile driving. *Journal of Applied Psychology, 20*, 353–357.

Grime, G. (1952). Traffic and road safety research at the Road Research Laboratory. *Proceedings of the Highway Research Board*, 466–486.

Hankey, J. (1996). *Unalerted emergency avoidance at an intersection and possible implications for ABS implementation*. Ames: University of Iowa.

Hooper, K., & McGee, H. (1983a). Correction to driver characteristic specifications and standard formulations for intersection sight distance. *Transportation Research Record, 904*, 30–32.

Hooper, K., & McGee, H. (1983b). Driver perception-reaction time: Are revisions to current specification values in order? *Transportation Research Record, 904*, 21–30.

Johansson, G., & Rumar, K. (1971). Drivers' brake reaction times. *Human Factors, 13*, 23–27.

Kay, H. (1971). Accidents: Some facts and theories. In P. Warr (Ed.), *Psychology at work* (pp. 121–145). Baltimore: Penguin.

Kloeppel, E., Peters, R., James, C., Fox, J., & Alicandri, E. (1994). Comparison of older and younger driver responses to emergency driving events. *Proceedings of the Human Factors and Ergonomics Society, 38*, 986.

Korteling, J. E. (1990). Perception–response speed and driving capabilities of brain-damaged and older drivers. *Human Factors, 32*, 95–108.

Lamble, D., Kauranen, T., Laakso, M., & Summala, H. (1999). Cognitive load and detection thresholds in car following situations: Safety implications for using mobile (cellular) telephones while driving. *Accident Analysis and Prevention, 31*, 617–623.

Lerner, N. (1994). Brake perception–reaction times of older and younger drivers. *Proceedings of the Human Factors and Ergonomics Society, 38*, 206–209.

Liebermann, D., Ben-David, G., Schweitzer, N., Apter, Y., & Parush, A. (1995). A field study on braking responses during driving I. Triggering and modulation. *Ergonomics, 38*, 1894–1902.

Lings, S. (1991). Assessing driving capability: A method for individual testing. *Applied Ergonomics, 22*, 75–84.

Lisper, H.-O., Laurell, H., & Stening, G. (1973). Effects of experience of the driver on heart-rate, respiration rate, and subsidiary reaction time in a three hours continuous driving task. *Ergonomics, 16*, 501–506.

Malaterre, G., Fernandez, F., Fleury, D., & Lechner, D. (1988). Decision making in emergency situations. *Ergonomics, 31*, 643–655.

McGehee, D., Mazzae, E., & Bladwin, G. (2000). Driver reaction time in crash avoidance research: Validation of a driving simulator study on a test track. *Proceedings of the International Ergonomics Association 2000 Conference.*

McKnight, A. J., & McKnight, A. S. (1993). The effect of cellular phone use upon driver attention. *Accident Analysis and Prevention, 25*, 259–265.

Min, S. T., & Redelmeier, D. A. (1998). Car phones and car crashes: An ecologic analysis. *Canadian Journal of Public Health, 89*, 157–161.

Mortimer, R. (1969). *Dynamic evaluation of automobile rear lighting configurations.* Ann Arbor: University of Michigan, Highway Safety Research Institute.

Nagler, C. A., & Nagler, W. M. (1973). Reaction time measurements. *Forensic Science, 2*, 261–274.

Nilsson, L., & Alm, H. (1991). *Safety and mobility in older drivers. Strategic highway research program and traffic safety on two continents.* Gothenburg: Sweden.

Norman, O. (1952). Braking distance of vehicles from high speed. *Public Roads, 27*, 159–169.

Ohita, H., & Komatsu, H. (1991). Speed perception in driving—comparison with TV observation. In G. Gale (Ed.), *Vision in vehicles* (Vol. III). Amsterdam: Elsevier.

Olson, P. (1989). Driver perception response times. In *Motor vehicle accident reconstruction: review and update* (pp. 67–77). Warrendale, PA: Society of Automotive Engineers.

Olson, P., & Sivak, M. (1986). Perception–response time to unexpected roadway hazards. *Human Factors, 28*, 91–96.

Redelmeier, D. A., & Tibshirani, R. J. (1997). Association between cellular-telephone calls and motor vehicle collisions. *New England Journal of Medicine, 336*, 453–458.

Schneider, W., & Detweiler, M. (1988). The role of practice in dual-task performance: Toward workload modeling in a connectionist/control architecture. *Human Factors, 30*, 539–566.

Schneider, W., & Schiffrin, R. (1977). Controlled and automatic human information processing I: Detection, search and attention. *Psychological Review, 84*, 1–66.

Schweitzer, N., Apter, Y., Ben-David, G., Liebermann, D., & Parush, A. (1995). A field study on braking responses during driving II. Minimum driver braking times. *Ergonomics, 38*, 1903–1910.

Scott, P., Chandler, J., & Li, J. (1996). Response times in motor vehicle drivers. *Applied Ergonomics, 27*, 411–416.

Sens, M., Cheng, P., Weichel, J., & Guenther, D. (1989). *Perception/reaction time values for accident reconstruction* (Society of Automotive Engineers Paper No. 890732).

Shinar, D. (1977). *Psychology on the road. The human factor in traffic safety.* Toronto, Canada: Wiley.

Sivak, M., Flannagan, M. J., Sato, T., Traube, E. C., & Aoki, M. (1994). Reaction times to neon, LED, and fast incandescent brake lamps. *Ergonomics, 37*, 989–994.

Sivak, M., Olson, P., & Farmer, K. (1982). Radar-measured reaction times of unalerted drivers to brake signals. *Perceptual and Motor Skills, 55*, 594.

Sivak, M., Post, D., Olson, P., & Donohue, R. (1981a). Automobile rear lights: Effect of the number, mounting height, and lateral position on reaction times of following drivers. *Perceptual and Motor Skills, 52*, 795–802.

Sivak, M., Post, D., Olson, P., & Donohue, R. (1981b). Driver responses to high-mounted brake lights in actual traffic. *Human Factors, 23*, 231–235.

Sohn, S. Y., & Stepleman, R. (1998). Meta-analysis on total braking time. *Ergonomics, 41*, 1129–1140.

Summala, H., & Koivisto, I. (1990). Unalerted drivers' brake reaction times: Older drivers compensate their slower reaction times by driving more slowly. In T. Benjamin (Ed.), *Driving behaviour in a social context* (pp. 680–683). Caen, France: Paradigme.

Summala, H., Lamble, D., & Laakso, M. (1998). Driving experience and perception of the lead car's braking when looking at in-car targets. *Accident Analysis and Prevention, 30*, 401–407.

Summala, H., Leino, M., & Vierimaa, J. (1981). Drivers' steering behavior when meeting another car: The case of perceptual tropism revisited. *Human Factors, 23*, 185–189.

Triggs, T. J. (1987). Driver brake reaction times: Unobtrusive measurement on public roads. *Public Health Review, 15*, 275–290.

van Elslande, P., & Faucher-Alberton, L. (1997). When expectancies become certainties: A potential adverse effect of experience. In T. Rothengatter & E. Vanya (Eds.), *Traffic and transport psychology* Tarrytown, NY: Pergamon.

van Winsum, W., & Brouwer, W. (1997). Time headway in car following and operational performance during unexpected braking. *Perceptual and Motor Skills, 84*, 1247–1257.

Violanti, J. M. (1998). Cellular phones and fatal traffic collisions. *Accident Analysis and Prevention, 30*, 519–524.

Violanti, J. M., & Marshall, J. R. (1996). Cellular phones and traffic accidents: An epidemiological approach. *Accident Analysis and Prevention, 28*, 265–270.

Welford, A., & Birren, J. (1965). *Behavior, aging, and the nervous system: Biological determinants of speed of behavior and its changes with age*. Springfield, IL: Thomas.

Wolffsohn, J. S., McBrien, N. A., Edgar, G. K., & Stout, T. (1998). The influence of cognition and age on accommodation, detection rate and response times when using a car head-up display (HUD). *Ophthalmic Physiological Optics, 18*, 243–253.

Wright, G. R., & Shephard, R. J. (1978). Brake reaction time—effects of age, sex, and carbon monoxide. *Archives of Environmental Health, 33*, 141–150.

Yerkes, R., & Dodson, J. (1908). The relative strength of stimulus to rapidity of habit-formation. *Journal of Comparative and Neurological Psychology, 18*, 459–482.

# Addendum: Reaction Time Supplement

Marc Green, Ph.D.

*"Any man who afflicts the human race with ideas must be prepared to see them misunderstood."*
—H. L. Mencken

The preceding perception-reaction time article is eight years old. Little has changed in the meantime, but some supplementary comments are in order. Some arise from reactions that the article has elicited during the intervening time. Others come from simply re-reading the article and wishing that I had been clearer on some points and emphasized others more strongly.

Like most authors, I am often amazed at the interpretations and misinterpretations people make of my writing. Recently, for example, I testified in a case where a pedestrian stepped off the curb into the path of an oncoming vehicle. I opined that a pedestrian could stop or turn away from a vehicle with a perception-reaction time of .5–.75 second. A human factors "expert" claimed that I was contradicting myself because the article said that perception-reaction time is 1.25-1.5. She then assigned the same 1.25 seconds value to both driver and pedestrian.

She apparently failed to grasp the simplest and most important fact about reaction time: *different tasks have different reaction times.* Braking or swerving a vehicle to avoid a pedestrian is a different task from stopping or turning your body to avoid a vehicle. Instead of using a cookbook number, she should have searched the research literature for data on the correct task. I based my opinion on research (e.g., Cao, Schultz, Ashton-Miller Alexander, 1998) which found that the perception-reaction time for pedestrians to stop and to turn was .4–.5 second. I increased the time to compensate some for circumstantial variables.

Moreover, there isn't even one reaction time for a given task across all situations. The cookbook value of 1.5 seconds perception-reaction time applies only in a very restricted set of circumstances:

1. *A young driver...* If visibility is good and the situation simple, then older drivers will exhibit little slowing of reaction. Older drivers will slow considerably when more cognitive processing is required, i.e., complex situations, such as low visibility, high traffic, and complex roadways. Like drivers who are on cell phones or under the influence of drugs or alcohol, major impairments only reveal themselves when cognitive processing is stressed and attentional capacity is taxed. Chapter 9 discusses this issue in more detail.
2. *With good eyesight...* Visual impairments such as lower contrast sensitivity, reduced visual field, etc. are likely to raise perception-reaction times.

3. *Who is braking*...Swerving reaction time is about .2 second faster than braking. (See article.)
4. *To an unexpected obstacle*...Perception-reaction time is slower to unexpected events. (See article.)
5. *Making a lane incursion*...Perception reaction-time is slower to peripheral targets because sensitivity is lower and the attentional spotlight is weaker. Moreover, the driver must make a saccade toward the target. A vehicle pulling out of a driveway or a pedestrian stepping off the curve is first seen in the driver's peripheral field, so perception reaction times are relatively long. The 1.5 seconds value arises primarily from studies using this type of lane incursion. If the obstacle is directly ahead, then the driver first sees it foveally where attention is centered, and perception-reaction time should be at least faster. For example, the driver comes over a rise and sees a truck stopped in the middle of the road.
6. *In daytime*...The 1.5 seconds value is not necessarily applicable at night, where visibility is lower. Viewers respond more slowly to low contrast targets, especially if they are small. Low light level alone is sufficient to increase reaction times. The fewer the quanta entering the eye, the longer the time required for neurons to reach threshold to create action potentials that initiate visual processing. Moreover, viewers are slower to identify objects and subsequently to gain situational awareness in dim light. Exceptions can occur. For example, the contrast of an illuminated signal light, such as at a railroad crossing, is higher against a dark background at night than against a brighter background during the day.
7. *With good visibility and*...Even in daytime, fog and other weather factors can impair visibility and recognition and increase reaction time. Cluttered backgrounds and glare or any other visibility factor can affect reaction time.
8. *No external distractions.* Reaction time in most tasks slows with sufficient attention-consuming distraction.

Lastly, a few additional points and some clarification:

*Urgency.* Although noted in the article, I failed to sufficiently underscore the importance of urgency. Some lane incursion studies simulate urgent conditions, but they are usually not real emergencies. Studies of response to normal but unexpected signals such brake lights and traffic signals seldom employed even moderately urgent conditions. As a result, the 1.25 seconds value suggested in the article is probably too long for drivers facing the urgent situation. For example, a driver closely following a lead vehicle can likely respond in under a second to the sudden onset of rear brake lights. On the other hand, emergencies with no clear correct avoidance response (avoidance-avoidance conditions) can create very long reaction times. Further, behavior in extreme urgency can be difficult to predict (e.g., Malaterre, Ferrandez, Fleury and Lechner, 1988; see also Chapter 16).

*Mean vs. median.* Perception-reaction time distributions are invariably skewed toward long values. As a result, the median is a better reaction time statistic than the mean. Research (see article) suggests that means are .1 to .2 seconds lower. However, such a small difference is likely lost in the noise of variability and context factors. Besides, very few studies report medians; estimating variability is problematic.

*Variability.* The original article ignored variability, but it is an important practical issue. Research suggests that driver perception-reaction time distributions with a mean of 1.5 seconds will have a standard deviation of about .45 second. Roughly speaking, normal variability is then 1–2 seconds. However, data variability typically increases with the mean. The longer reaction times in night driving will also exhibit greater standard deviations.

*Stages of Mental Processing.* The review article divides mental processing into three stages, sensation, perception and response selection, and programming. A more sophisticated decomposition has four components, created by dividing perception into two stages: recognition and situational awareness. This provides a more detailed account of psychological factors controlling response. However, attempts to assign specific times to each stage and to derive an overall perception-reaction time by summing stages is probably futile. The data simply do not exist and the assumption that each stage is independent of the others is likely incorrect.

*Response Bias.* The Signal Detection Theory discussion in Chapter 2 explained how probabilities and payoffs affect viewer placement of his yes-no criterion. The placement also affects perception-reaction time. Viewers who have a low criterion (high signal probability, high payoff for hits, high penalty for misses) respond faster than those with a high criterion.

## References

Cao, C., A. Schultz, J. Ashton-Miller, and N. Alexander. 1998. Sudden turns and stops while walking: kinematic sources of age and gender differences. *Gait & Posture* 7, 45-52.

Malaterre, G., F. Ferrandez, D. Fleury, and D. Lechner. 1988. Decision making in emergency situations. *Ergonomics* 31, 643-655.

# Chapter 18

# Visual Analysis of Pictorial Evidence

Marc Green, Ph.D.

*"All photographs of any kind are always distorted relative to reality."*
—Evans (1976)

***Synopsis***

## 18.1 Introduction

Confucius summarized the power of images by saying, "One picture is worth a thousand words." Graham (1982) more recently noted that a picture "provides the trier of fact with an opportunity to draw a relevant first hand sense impression." Litigants have long sought to capitalize on these notions by presenting photographs and other pictorial images as evidence in court.

This chapter focuses on one particular type of pictorial evidence—the use of pictures to represent what a viewer would/could have seen. Typically, the litigant introduces the picture to prove that a viewer should have seen some particular object. For example, a plaintiff might introduce the picture of a nighttime roadway scene to prove that a driver was not attentive because he should easily have seen the pedestrian or the stopped truck. The presumed justification of introducing pictures is that jurors can see for themselves and make an informed opinion about whether the original viewer acted reasonably. In this case, "a photograph can be seen as testifying to the reality of the situation it records" (Messaris, 1997).

However, courts should fully understand the limitations and potentially harmful effects of such pictures. People generally accept that "seeing is believing" and succumb to naïve realism. Pictorial evidence creates a "gut" impression by acting directly through the senses rather than through rational or logical thought. Our species relied on direct visual impression to know the world long before we developed speech and other higher cognitive processes. However, pictures have no more inherent credibility than witness statements or any other evidence and should undergo the same scrutiny and critique. Unfortunately, pictures far too frequently escape close examination. Courts operate in a largely verbal tradition and, being subject to naïve realism like everyone else, are often not even aware that there is anything to question. The legal literature contains some critics, such as Dellinger (1997), who notes that pictures "elude the skepticism with which written opinions are generally reviewed." Dellinger and others, however, are not perception experts and do not fully understand the issues. Moreover, even experts who present pictorial evidence are seldom knowledgeable about the perceptual and cognitive issues that pictures raise.

Courts may base admission of pictorial evidence on whether it is "substantially similar" to the actual scene. The courts must then use some criteria to determine whether the picture meets the similarity burden. This chapter discusses the proper criteria and makes several points about them. First, the criteria should be based on science rather than on commonsense and on casual introspection alone. Mere inspection is insufficient to determine whether a picture properly depicts a scene. Second, the criteria are not restricted to the image but rather include psychological factors. Viewers cannot see a picture without filtering it through their interpretive, cognitive processes. Third, the criteria depend on the picture's intended purpose. The criteria for representing scene layout are different from those for representing visibility and conspicuity. However, viewers may not use pictures for the intended purpose.

The visual evidence analysis takes the discussion full circle back to Chapter 1. Recall that vision occurs when an external stimulus (a scene or a picture) creates a retinal image of sufficient magnitude to produce sensation. The attentional filter passes only a small subset of the sensation to higher cognitive processing, which involves application of memory and decision making. In short, vision is then a function of two components, the physical retinal image and the viewer's psychological responses of sensation and perception. Each forms a criterion for judging similarity. I will call these criteria "image fidelity"[1] and "psychophysical and perceptual fidelity."

Image fidelity is the degree of match between the retinal images created by the scene and the picture. The retinal image is the proximal stimulus for vision, so ideally a juror looking at the picture receives the same retinal image as the original viewer looking at the original scene. Three sets of factors determine image fidelity:

- *Optical factors: perspective, size, field-of-view and depth-of-field.* Perspective is the relationship among the sizes and spatial separations of image objects. There are several types of perspective, but eyes and most cameras produce "rectilinear perspective," where straight lines in the scene are straight in the image.[2] Perspective is a function of camera/eye location during photography and of viewing angle during inspection. Despite much myth, lens focal length has no effect on perspective. While perspective refers to relative size, image fidelity also requires correct absolute size (visual angle at the viewer's eye), which is a function of picture size and viewing distance. Field-of-view is the overall area covered by the image and depth-of-field is the area that is sharply in focus;
- *Photometric factors: intensity, contrast and wavelength.* Pictures should reproduce luminances, contrasts and "color" (wavelengths) of the original scene. Photometric fidelity here depends on the technological capabilities of the camera and display (photographs, electronic screens, etc.). Technology is improving but it is still limited; and
- *Viewing conditions: viewing location and adaptation level.* Both optical and photometric factors depend somewhat on viewing condition. Physical image size, viewing distance and viewing angle affect optical factors of size, field-of-view and to some extent perspective. Ambient light and background affect photometric fidelity by altering intensity, contrast and color.

The visually unschooled may naïvely assume that image fidelity is the only criterion for similarity. However, neither a picture nor a scene uniquely specifies the viewer's perception or even sensation. "Psychophysical fidelity" is the match between the sensations experienced by those viewing the scene and the picture. "Perceptual fidelity" is the match between their perceptions of the picture and the scene. Perceptual fidelity is the most critical factor because viewers will fall prey to naïve realism and believe that they are seeing an objective, complete reality, regardless of how the pictures are presented or what they are told. Psychophysical and perceptual fidelity depend on:

- *Non pictorial visual information.* Viewers may use visual cues such as retinal disparity, motion and oculomotor feedback. Still photographs fail to capture any of these cues while movies capture only motion;
- *Viewer psychophysical variables.* Sensation is a function of both retinal image and a set of psychophysical factors lying in the viewer's head or his behavior, i.e., age, arousal level, retinal location, viewing duration, and state of light and chromatic adaptation. These factors cannot be reproduced in the courtroom; and
- *Cognitive factors.* Perception is highly dependent on mental set, including the viewer's knowledge, expectations, mental schema, motor schema, attentional allocation, and goals and purposes at the time of the accident. Jurors *cannot* have the same mental set as the original viewer.

The list of criteria for psychophysical and perceptual fidelity exposes the limitations of pictures as evidence of viewer vision. It is extremely difficult, and perhaps impossible, to create a picture that is substantially similar to the original scene for many purposes, even if image fidelity were perfect. However, several factors usually prevent perfect image fidelity. Recent advances in camera and display technology allow imaging experts with properly calibrated equipment to produce increasingly higher image fidelity under proper viewing conditions, but the state of the art is still limited. Moreover, much, if not most, pictorial forensic evidence is created by people who lack expertise in imaging as well as in perception and who simply use low-tech, uncalibrated equipment. Lastly, creating proper viewing conditions may be difficult or even impossible.

This chapter begins with an analysis of image fidelity factors. It first discusses the nuances of capturing accurate size and perspective, which is theoretically simple but which has some practical difficulties. The ensuing discussion outlines the greater difficulty of capturing and then displaying correct scene intensities and contrasts, especially in nighttime photographs. It will be clear that dynamic range and exposure durations are prime problems and that photographers can easily manipulate scene brightness and contrast to create any impression. The chapter then switches to psychophysical and perceptual fidelity by describing the important visual information that is not captured by static and even moving pictures. Finally, the chapter briefly outlines the cognitive factors that cannot be reproduced in the courtroom and which make pictorial evidence so potentially prejudicial and misleading.

Before starting, however, I should clarify the chapter's scope. First, the discussion assumes that the pictures represent a faithful accident recreation. Obviously, changes in lighting or other environmental factors decrease a picture's validity. The chapter is not concerned with forgeries or any other purposeful misrepresentation. Second, I focus on still digital photography, which has largely replaced more traditional film technology. I will say nothing about simulations that are created entirely on a computer by means of a mathematical model. As both psychophysical and perceptual representations, however, they are usually inferior to the best possible photographic images. I only briefly mention movies. Third, the discussion focuses on visibility and conspicuity, especially in nighttime scenes. This makes contrast and brightness the primary photometric concerns. Color receives little attention, although it can be important in some circumstances. Fourth, the discussion focuses primarily on the most common form of pictorial evidence, LDR ("low dynamic range photography"), which comes in two varieties. In the more primitive case, the photographer snaps an LDR picture using the camera's automatic settings. A more sophisticated photographer might switch to manual control and take several photographs at different exposures and then chose the one that he deems most representative. The chapter only briefly mentions HDR ("high dynamic range") photography that mathematically combines multiple exposures of different duration into a single image. HDR avoids some, but not all, of the image fidelity problems that I discuss (e.g., see McCann, and Rizzi, 2007). However, it suffers from the same psychophysical and perceptual fidelity problems. Also, camera and display technology are improving rapidly and some comments may be somewhat outdated by the time this chapter reaches the reader's hands. Lastly, although the chapter focuses on pictures intended to portray some aspect of perception, the same issues arise when litigants use pictures as other forms of evidence. See Dellinger (1997) for more discussion.

## 18.2 Image Fidelity

Figure 18.1 schematically shows the image fidelity problem. The original viewer fixates a point in a scene, which casts an image on his retina. Later, a photographer (ideally) aims his camera from the same eye position at the same fixation point. The aperture opens, and light strikes the camera's photo-sensitive surface (film in standard photography or an electronic sensor in digital photography) which codes the light intensity and wavelength into "image data." The image data then produce a picture on a display, usually a photograph or an electronic screen, which is presented as evidence. Finally, a juror views the picture, which creates an image on the retina. In a perfect world, the retinal images generated by the scene and the picture are identical, resulting in perfect fidelity.

Perfect image fidelity is usually unachievable so a discrepancy between scene- and picture-generated retinal images occurs. The degree of its forensic significance varies greatly from image to image and with the intended purpose. The image fidelity requirements of pictures intended to represent what a viewer would see are very different from pictures that are introduced merely to demonstrate the extent of vehicle damage or of injury. If layout is the issue, then correct perspective is important but correct intensity/contrast may play a lesser role. Conversely, if visibility in a night scene is important, the correct size and intensity/contrast may be more critical than perspective. Lastly, motion is important for correct portrayal of dynamic events, such as impending collision or of movement/flashing conspicuity.

Image fidelity variables fall into two categories. The first is optical factors, perspective, size, field-of-view and depth-of-field. The second category is photometric properties, intensity, wavelength and contrast.

## A. Optical Factors

### 1. Perspective, Camera Placement and Focal Length

Incorrect perspective distorts relative object sizes and distances. The distortions appear as some object(s) being abnormally large compared to others. In addition, there is compression or expansion of the apparent distance between foreground and background. Incorrect perspective can also distort apparent speed and motion.

As usual, the best place to start is by dispelling a common fallacy. Many people mistakenly believe that perspective is related to lens focal length and that there is a "normal" focal length that captures what the eye sees. In this view, the use of other focal lengths, such as shorter, wide-angle lenses, changes perspective and distorts the image.[3] In fact, it has no effect on perspective. Rather, lens focal length determines only 1) field-of-view and 2) magnification.

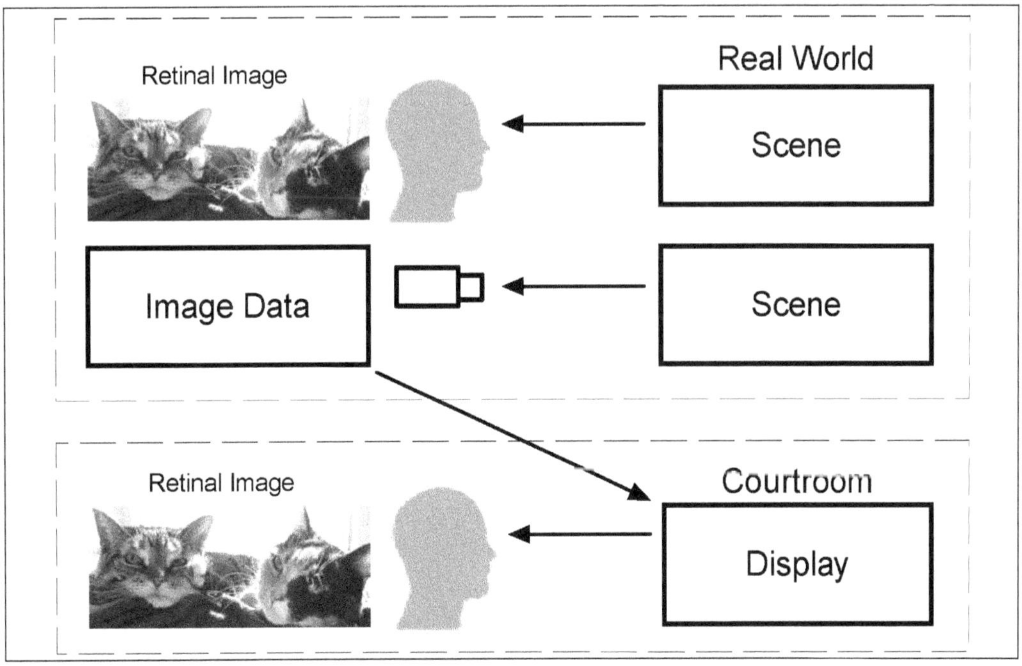


***Figure 18.1** The image fidelity problem has three transformations: 1) from scene to image data, 2) from image data to display and 3) from display to retina.*

**Table 18.1**
**Common lens focal lengths and their resulting fields of view in degrees**

| Focal Length | 18mm | 20mm | 28mm | 35mm | 50mm | 85mm | 105mm | 135mm | 200mm |
|---|---|---|---|---|---|---|---|---|---|
| Horizontal deg | 90 | 84 | 66 | 54 | 40 | 24 | 19 | 15 | 10 |
| Vertical deg | 67 | 62 | 46 | 38 | 27 | 16 | 13 | 10 | 7 |

The relationship between focal length and field-of-view size resembles the normal visual angle calculation:

$$\mathrm{FOV} = 2\arctan(\mathrm{x} / 2f)$$

where FOV is the field-of-view, x is the film/sensor dimension and $f$ is the focal length. Table 18.1 shows some values for common lenses with a typical film or consumer digital 35mm camera: the table assumes focus at infinity.

A normal 50mm lens provides a field size of about 40°×27°, covering most of focal vision but little of ambient vision. However, field-of-view also varies with sensor size, x. The normal 35mm format uses 36×24 mm sensors/film. Digital single lens reflex (DSLR) cameras have smaller sensors and produce smaller visual fields. A 50mm lens on a digital SLR might have a field size equivalent to an 85mm lens[4] on a consumer camera and create a small field size of only 24°×16° covering only 1 percent of the human visual field and less than the central 30° allotted to focal vision.

Given the small field-of-view created by 50mm lenses, photographers are apt to use a wider angle lens in order to capture a field size that better represents normal vision. A switch to a 28mm lens in a normal consumer camera increases the field to 65.5°×46.7°. While increasing overall field size, the wider lens shrinks individual objects, which become less distinct. The only way to increase field-of-view without shrinking individual objects is to move forward and closer to the main object. (Or to switch to a larger and more expensive sensor format.) This change in camera position alters the relative sizes and locations of objects in the scene. That is, it changes perspective.

Figure 18.2 demonstrates that focal length affects field-of-view size but not perspective. I shot picture A with a zoom lens set to about 35mm focal length and picture B with the same lens set to about 105mm, three times the focal length. The difference in field size is obvious. Picture C is picture A, the 35mm image, blown up by a factor of three. It is virtually identical (except for a slight difference in size and lateral change in camera position) to picture B, taken with a 105mm lens. Most importantly, there is no perspective distortion of the nearby tree limbs compared to the distant house.

In contrast, changing camera position will change perspective. Figure 18.3 depicts two people of the same size at distances of 300 and 600 feet. Assuming a 6 foot height, the near person has a visual angle of 69 minarc (arctan(6/300)) while the far person at 600 feet is 34 minarc (arctan(6/600)). Their image size ratio is 2:1, which is proportional to distance. Suppose the photographer wants to keep the same lens and field size but also wants to get a better picture of the nearer person. He moves forward, say to 150 feet, making both object images larger. The closer person's visual angle doubles to ~137 minarc while the more distant person, now at 450 feet, increases image size by 133 percent to ~46 minarc. The size ratio, however, has increased from 2:1 to 3:1, and the far image has shrunk relative to the near image. If the photographer moves to a 50-foot distance from the nearer person, then the visual angle ratio becomes 7:1.

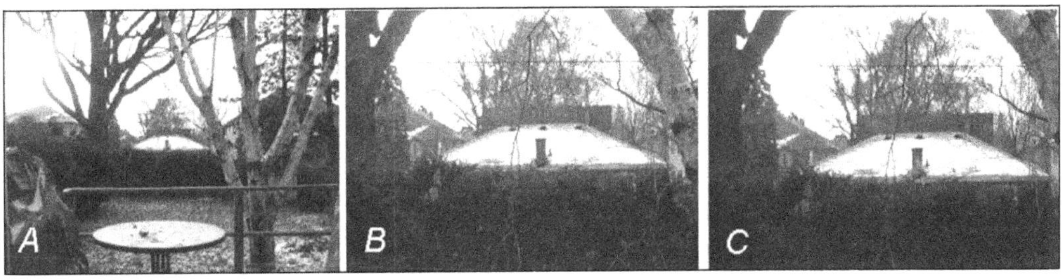


***Figure 18.2*** *Pictures taken with different focal lengths: A is 35mm, B is 105mm and C is 35mm blown up by 3. Despite using lenses differing in focal length by 3:1, correct perspective is maintained.*

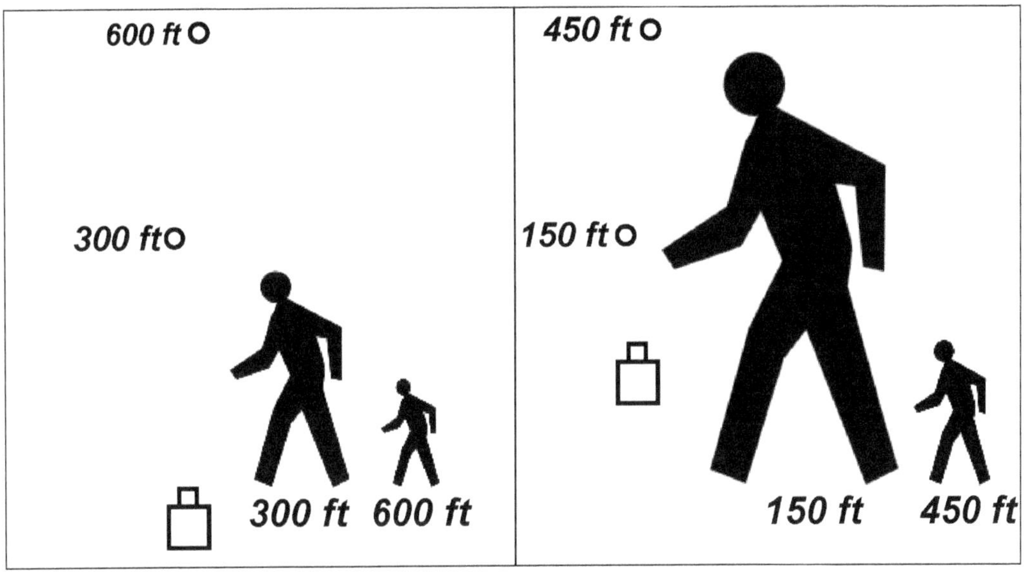


***Figure 18.3*** *Relative sizes of objects at two camera locations.*

This change in camera distance and visual angle ratio distorts perceived distance as well as size. Viewers intuitively know that more distant objects create smaller retinal images. Bigger size ratios mean greater relative distances.

Some experts produce photographs and proclaim that they have captured what the eye sees because they used a 50mm lens. The rationale for this statement varies widely. Some say that the focal length should be close to the diagonal dimension of the sensor, i.e., 43mm for the normal 24mm X 36 mm sensor/frame size. There is no obvious explanation for this explanation, so it's just another magic formula. A more frequent explanation is that a 50mm lens creates proper perspective. This, of course, cannot be correct because focal length only magnifies/minifies and has no effect on perspective. Camera/viewer position determines perspective, so a photographer with a 50mm lens can still move up closer to the subject and change perspective.[5] Lastly, "what the eye sees" is also a function of picture size, viewing distance and viewing angle. Obviously it is false to say that 50mm, or any other specific focal length, captures what the eye sees.

In sum there is no single focal length which "captures what the eye sees." Choice of focal length does not change perspective, but camera position does. On the other hand, focal length choice determines field-of-view, and object size. In the end, choice of lens focal length is primarily a tradeoff between field-of-view size and image clarity. Short lenses create more realistic field sizes but smaller images for individual objects. Unless the photographer moves forward and changes perspective, he must enlarge the final image, a process that can make the objects low resolution, grainy, noisy and less distinct.

### 2. Size

Perspective specifies the *relative* sizes of objects in the image but not their *absolute* sizes, which means their absolute visual angles at the viewer's eye. Image fidelity requires a size match between objects in the scene and the picture. Fortunately, it is easy to equate retinal image sizes by simple visual angle calculations.

Suppose a viewer saw a 6-foot tall pedestrian at a distance of 100 feet. A photographer subsequently goes to the scene and takes a photograph of an exemplar pedestrian at the same 100 foot distance. The photographer makes a print of a given size, where the pedestrian measures .95 inches. In court, the juror is handed the photograph. The pedestrian's retinal image size depends on juror viewing distance—the closer to the eye, the larger the retinal image. What is the correct viewing distance for creating a retinal image that matches the viewer at the scene?

A 6-foot pedestrian at 100 feet is arctan(6/100)=3.4° in size. The question then becomes, "At what viewing distance does .95 inches equal 3.4 degrees?" The answer is 16 inches because arctan(.95/16)=3.4°. What about field-of-view size? It will be correct as well. Matching individual object size and field-of-view is the same problem, as long as perspective is correct.

### 3. Visual Field Location

In many cases, the critical information was located in the original viewer's peripheral field. For perceptual fidelity, the juror must then view the object in the same peripheral location. For example, suppose a driver failed to avoid a pedestrian who stepped off the curb and crossed the road. Assume that the pedestrian was located 12 feet to the left of the driver's sightline and at a distance of 100 feet (measured straight down the road). The pedestrian's image then falls 6.8° (arctan(12/100)) in the periphery. To have validity, the juror must 1) look straight ahead in the same direction as the driver and 2) view the image so that the visual angles of pedestrian size and distance from the sightline are both correct. The calculations show that:

- At 100 feet, pedestrian size is arctan(6/100)=3.4°;
- Viewing at 16 inches, each inch in the frontoparallel plane is arctan(1/16)=3.6°;
- Viewing at 16 inches, 1.9 inches is 6.8°

The pedestrian must then be located 1.9 inches laterally to the sightline with a viewing distance of 16 inches. This is no problem because all sizes vary together in proportion. If the 6 foot tall person has the correct visual angle, then the 12-foot distance from the sightline and location in the visual periphery will also have the right visual angle.

If the viewer moved the picture closer or farther than 16 inches, however, then peripheral angle and size would change and ecological validity[6] would decline. Greater viewing distances bring the pedestrian closer to the fovea and more visible or at least more conspicuous but also smaller. Closer viewing distances push the pedestrian farther into the periphery while making him bigger. The main point is that an attorney could not simply place a screen in front of the jury and hope for the best. Even if the visual angles were correct for one juror, they would be incorrect for the rest. Each juror should view the picture from exactly the correct distance and angle.

Lastly, each juror would have to look straight ahead at the road and avoid looking directly at the pedestrian at any time. This, of course, is simply not going to happen, so the jury will be misled about visibility and conspicuity. As the dog example in Figure 1.5 showed, once a viewer knows what is in the image, he cannot remove the knowledge from his mind.

### 4. Depth-Of-Field and Blur

When an optical system focuses a 3D scene, it creates sharpest focus for objects located at a particular distance in space. When taking a picture, for example, the photographer typically focuses on the principle subject in order to create the clearest image on the sensor. All farther or nearer objects are relatively defocused, creating blurred images. The farther in front or behind the focal point, the greater the misfocus and blur. For short distances, however, the blur is small and is not perceptible. As distance increases, the blur increases. At some point the blur is so great that it becomes clearly perceptible. In non-technical terms, depth-of-field is the range, extending from near to far around the focal plane, where objects are acceptably sharp. The depth-of-field decreases with shorter focal distance and with increasing aperture size. Since wide apertures are needed in low light, nighttime photographs are likely to exhibit very little depth of field. As with perspective, lens focal length has no effect.

An unnaturally narrow or wide depth-of-field distorts perception because humans use blur to interpret scenes. Blurred objects have higher contrast thresholds and appear less contrasty even when visible. Blurred objects also appear farther away due to aerial perspective. Since apparent distance affects apparent size, blurred objects will appear larger. (The same visual angle at an apparently greater distance is interpreted as a larger object.) Further, blur affects conspicuity. Sharp images in the focal plane standout against blurred backgrounds. In movies, blurred objects appear to move faster and more smoothly.[7]

### 5. Size and Perspective Effects On Motion

Movies should depict correct size in order to avoid distorting perception of speed and distance. In looming, for example, retinal image size is a factor in angular velocity and time to collision. Assume that a train and vehicle collided at a crossing. The driver was stopped and looked straight down the tracks as the train approached at 50 mph (73.5 ft/sec). An attorney wishes to show the jurors how quickly the train came upon the unfortunate driver, who presumably had no time to respond. The photographer visits the scene and makes a movie of an approaching train.

The jurors later see a video of the looming train projected onto the screen. Their impressions, however, will depend greatly on their viewing distance, as Table 18.2 demonstrates. Recall that distant objects appear stationary because their motion is below looming threshold. As the object approaches, angular velocity increases at a rate that is dependent on size. At 500 feet, the 10-foot wide train has a visual angle of 1.15° and angular velocity of .0029 rad/sec. Assume that looming threshold is .0082 rad/sec. The viewer initially sees the train as stationary for 2.7 seconds. It approaches with increasing angular velocity and reaches a looming threshold of .0082 rad/sec at a distance of 300 feet, which is 4.1 seconds from collision.

To achieve correct size, the viewer must sit at a distance that renders the train at a visual angle of 1.15° when the movie begins. Assume that the train is 1 inch wide on the screen. The correct viewing distance is about 50 inches because arctan(1/50)=1.15°.

Now, suppose the jurors actually view the screen at a distance of 100 inches which halves the train starting visual angle to .057°. This is the equivalent of looking at the approach of a 5-foot wide train. The smaller size translates to a lower angular velocity. As Table 18.2 shows, the looming threshold moves closer to 200 feet. Actually, .0082 rad/sec is achieved at a distance of 212 feet and a TTC of 2.9 seconds. The juror will now see a stationary train for 3.9 seconds that then suddenly explodes in speed closer to the time of collision. The impression is that the driver had less time to respond that he actually had. The video also does not permit viewer use of retinal disparity and stereopsis. As explained in Chapter 16, lack of relative disparity can decrease looming thresholds significantly. The optical information will then foster an impression of less time to react.

Changing camera location also changes perspective and motion perception. At a shorter viewpoint distance, near objects grow relative to distant ones. The final image of the train will be magnified compared to the original distant image. Since the size difference and perceived distance are greater but motion duration is the same, speed and growth rate will appear greater. It will seem that the train suddenly arrived at a very high rate of speed. The camera placement determines perspective, so this distortion occurs even if the movie is viewed at the correct distance and viewpoint.

## B. Photometric Factors

The next problem is to match corresponding scene and image intensities and contrasts. Success depends on two distinct technologies, the camera that records the image and the display that presents the image to the viewer.

In digital cameras, the key recording element is the sensor, the device which transforms light energy into electrical energy. Cameras then process the sensor output before digitizing it into bits for the final image data. This process is characterized by two key variables: dynamic range (contrast ratio) and gamma. In accordance with Judkins' Law, it is helpful to know some digital camera basics in order to understand these variables.

### 1. Digital Camera Technology

Digital cameras vary considerably in design, but can be roughly divided into two categories: standard consumer models (also called "point and shoot" or "P&S") and digital single lens reflex (DSLR) models which are more sophisticated and more expensive. While the eye has the retina comprised of photoreceptors, the digital camera sensor contains an array of "photosites" (sometimes confusingly called "pixels"). Photosites are analogous in some ways to photoreceptors because they capture quanta and transduce the light energy into an electrical signal.

The photosites are arrayed in a regular rectangular grid. The size of the individual photosites, the number of photosites in the grid, the spacing between photosites and the total sensor area vary with the camera. Photosite size is an especially important variable. The smaller the photosite, the more that can fit on a sensor of a given dimension and the higher the resolution. On the other hand, smaller photosites have less ability to portray high contrast.[8] There is an inherent trade-off between contrast and resolution.

**Table 18.2**
**Train looming rates for a video viewed at different distances**

| | | | Viewing Distance = 50″ | | | Viewing Distance = 100′ | | |
|---|---|---|---|---|---|---|---|---|
| Distance | V | TTC | "Width" | VA | Rad/Sec | "Width" | VA | Rad/Sec |
| 100 | 73.5 | 1.4 | 10 | 5.71 | 0.0735 | 5 | 2.86 | 0.0368 |
| 150 | 73.5 | 2.0 | 10 | 3.81 | 0.0327 | 5 | 1.91 | 0.0163 |
| 200 | 73.5 | 2.7 | 10 | 2.86 | 0.0184 | 5 | 1.43 | 0.0092 |
| 250 | 73.5 | 3.4 | 10 | 2.29 | 0.0118 | 5 | 1.15 | 0.0059 |
| 300 | 73.5 | 4.1 | 10 | 1.91 | 0.0082 | 5 | 0.95 | 0.0041 |
| 350 | 73.5 | 4.8 | 10 | 1.64 | 0.0060 | 5 | 0.82 | 0.0030 |
| 400 | 73.5 | 5.4 | 10 | 1.43 | 0.0046 | 5 | 0.72 | 0.0023 |
| 450 | 73.5 | 6.1 | 10 | 1.27 | 0.0036 | 5 | 0.64 | 0.0018 |
| 500 | 73.5 | 6.8 | 10 | 1.15 | 0.0029 | 5 | 0.57 | 0.0015 |

When a photosite catches quanta, it produces an analog[9] electrical signal. The signal is proportional to the number of quanta, so it represents the relative light intensity. The camera then uses an analog/digital (A/D) converter to quantize the analog voltage into a digital value for storage. Consumer cameras typically use 8 bit A/D converters, which can represent 256 ($2^8$=256 or a dynamic range of 2.4 log units) intensity levels. This coding has several problems. The steps are too large at the low end and too small at the high end, so it captures far fewer than 256 JNDs. It also causes banding artifacts, where low smooth gradients appear blocky. The amount of banding depends on dynamic range, the difference between the highest and lowest intensities. If this range is only 50 and viewer contrast sensitivity is 1 percent, then the display would require 390 levels or 8.6 bits ($1.01=50(^{1/390})$) to create smooth images. If the dynamic range is 500, then the number of required levels is about 630 or about 9.3 bits. DSLR's theoretically capture much more accurate images because their A/D converters have at least 12 or 14 bits (4096–16384 levels or 3.6 to 4.2 log units). DSLR's also usually have the option to save 8 bit data; they can produce pictures of different quality.

Both consumer and DSLR cameras have three separate sets of photosites, one for each of the three primary colors. The total number of bits stored is actually 24 (for 8 bit A/D) or 36–42 (for 12 and 14 bit A/D). Lastly, digital cameras are not passive light recorders. At several stages, cameras process the image data to reduce several types of artifact. For example, the perfectly rectangular grid arrangement creates sampling artifacts that most cameras attempt to remove.

## 2. Gamma, Dynamic Range and Contrast Ratio

Gamma is the function describing the relationship between input and output. Recall from Chapter 2 that Stevens' psychophysical law has an exponent for each sensory input-out relationship. A version of the same function applies for specifying the light intensity- electrical output photosite response:

$$\text{Output} = \text{gain} * \text{input}^{\gamma} + \text{black level}$$

The $\Upsilon$ is the exponent, gamma, black level is the output value created when input intensity is 0 and gain is a multiplier. The gamma changes relative intensities of midtones (Figure 18.4). As gamma rises, intensity in the low range increases very little, so contrast and visibility are depressed. In the high range, intensity increases rapidly, causing steep contrast increments.

Gamma is a minor issue for digital cameras but is a major issue for displays. Figure 18.5 schematically shows the reason: the response of a camera photosite theoretically has a gamma of about 1, the ideal value. (In contrast, the input-output function for photoreceptors approximates the logarithmic Fechner's Law.) The main limitation is that the camera does not capture the entire "dynamic range" (DR), the span from lowest to highest scene intensities. If the scene has a greater dynamic range and contrast ratio than the camera can capture, then the camera loses some of the contrast. At low and high levels, the camera's response is flat. All low light intensities are coded with the same value so scene contrast is lost. For example, all dim areas will be coded with the same dark intensity so any contrast variation is thrown away. Similarly, all high intensities are coded with the same value, so their contrast is also lost.[10]

Physical factors limit a camera's dynamic ranges. At the high end, photosites saturate or "overflow." They reach an upper limit, so that all intensities generate equal outputs. They may also literally overflow into neighboring photosites creating the blurry, oversized quality of bright lights in nighttime photographs. The saturation point is partly a function of size because large photosites can catch more quanta, giving them a higher saturation point and higher top end of the dynamic range.

Larger photosites might seem desirable, but there is a cost—lower resolution. This is exactly the same tradeoff that exists in the visual system. In low light, the eye becomes more sensitive to illumination but objects appear less distinct due to "convergence," the increasing area of retinal photoreceptors that contribute to each post receptor nerve cell. Unlike camera sensors, the eye can vary its "photosite"[11] size, sensitivity and resolution by adaptation.

At the low end, the blackest black is limited by several factors, including sensitivity, noise and stray light. Ordinary consumer cameras are limited in sensitivity—they have smaller photosites and so they don't respond to very low numbers of quanta. Noise, spontaneous activation of the sensor, is also a key factor limiting dynamic range and contrast ratio. Just as the eye's sensitivity is limited by photon noise and internal "dark light," "dark current," photon noise and other sources add background noise to photosite response. In the extreme, the noise may even appear as a cloud of small dots that cause graininess and masking. Systems are often characterized by the "signal-noise ratio" (SNR), the degree to which the signal is above the background. If this sounds familiar, Chapter 2 discussed the same concepts in terms of Signal Detection Theory, which shows how low SNR creates poor detectability.

The ordinary consumer camera has smaller photosites but also more noise that offsets any gain in resolution. Visible noise is most apparent when the image is displayed in a large size, such as a projection or a photographic blow up. The amount of noise also varies across cameras and even temperature when the picture was taken.

Stray light is another variable limiting the dynamic range floor. Sensors live in a camera with an optical system, which limits their performance. Camera optics scatter light and cause veiling similar to glare created by the eye's optics. The sensors are then activated by this scattered light and do not signal their best, noise-limited black levels. Depending on the brightness of various objects and scene areas, the amount of scatter and effect on black level can be substantial. Of course, optical image quality always limits image sharpness, too.[12]

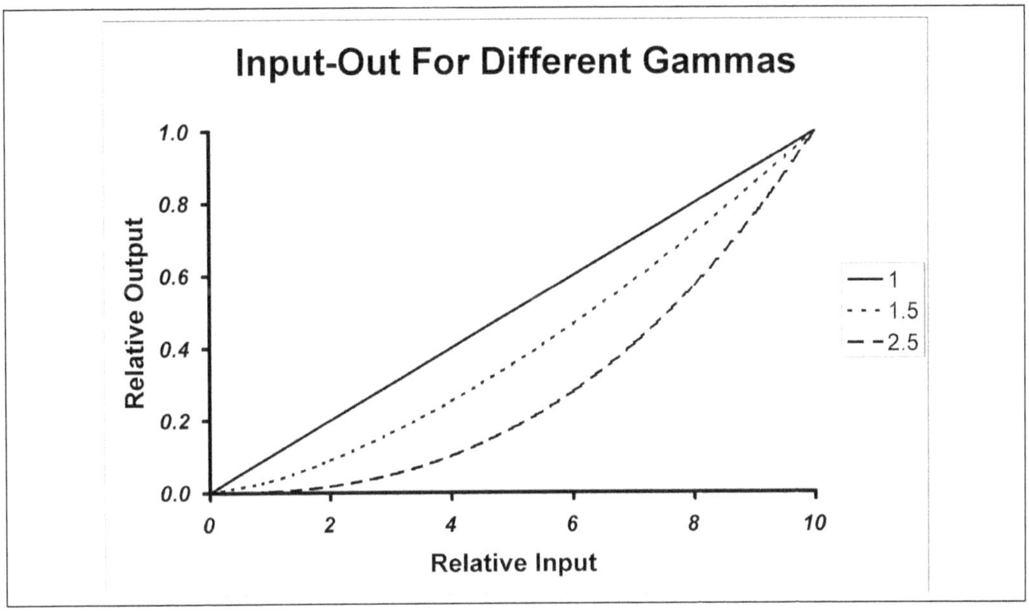


**Figure 18.4** *Relative response as a function of three different gammas. Gain is 1. If the gain is greater, then contrast is exaggerated.*

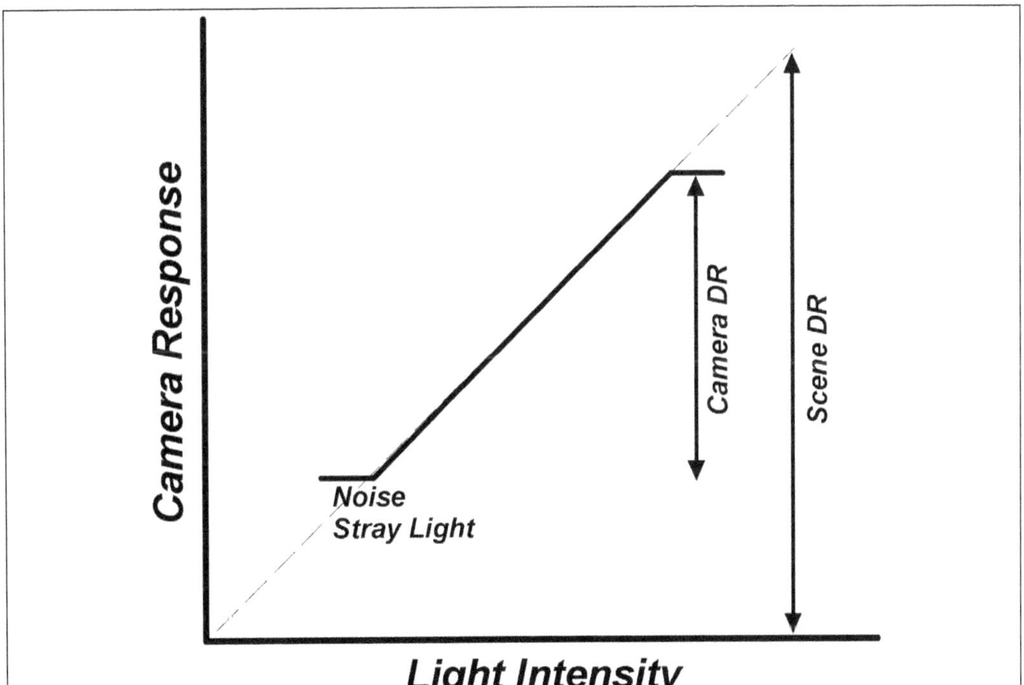


**Figure 18.5** *Scene intensity and camera responses to light. The camera gain is 1—the slope matches the real world.*

Lastly, dynamic range also depends on camera ISO, a measure of the overall light sensitivity. The term is borrowed from photographic film and strictly speaking doesn't apply, but digital cameras are often rated by their ISO film equivalent. An ISO of 400 is twice as sensitive as an ISO of 200, four times as sensitive as an ISO of 100, etc. Digital camera settings with higher ISO have greater sensitivity and presumably better ability to accurately portray low intensity scenes. However, they are subject to more noise. As with high ISO film, there is a strong tendency for images to be grainy and to lose resolution. In nighttime photography where light levels are low, both film and digital photographers are prone to use the more sensitive high ISO's that produce poorer quality images.

### 3. Eye vs. Camera

The central question in evaluating image fidelity is whether a human viewer would have perceived the lost contrast and dynamic range. If the lost contrast and brightness were outside the range of human vision, then the picture's intensity/wavelength/contrast limitations are visually irrelevant.

A comparison of cameras to eyes shows that the viewers can see over a far greater dynamic range and contrast ratio than the camera sensors can capture. The human eye has a huge dynamic range of $10^{14}$ (Hood, 1998; see also Figure 3.11). Eyes create the large dynamic range by adapting to prevailing light level and adjusting sensitivity and gain. At any given moment, the eye has a dynamic range much smaller than $10^{14}$. The range is roughly centered around the prevailing light level, although it may be influenced by recent exposure to higher or lower intensities.

At a given adaptation level, the dynamic range varies with scene properties and stray light. Light from one part of a scene scatters in the ocular media and creates a veiling glare in the same way oncoming headlamps create veiling glare. In fact, the headlamps are actually just adding veiling glare to what is already produced by the scene itself. In scenes of relative uniformity, where there are equal amounts of light and dark area spread throughout the image, the eye can respond to a range of 1000:1 (Rizzi, Pezzetti and McCann, 2007), although others (e.g., Sharp and Phillips, 1997) have put the number at 10,000:1. The dynamic range of individual cones is about 50,000:1 (Rodieck, 1998).

Consumer digital cameras only have dynamic ranges of about 80–90:1 while typical DSLRs contrast ratios are about 600–700:1. This may seem to conflict with the statement that consumer cameras digitize data to 8 bits (256 levels) and DSLRs 12–14 bits (4096–13384 levels), but much of the theoretical capacity is unused in real application. I expand on this below when talking about display devices.

However, the eye codes contrast rather than intensity. Recall that white paper in dim illumination looks white, although its intensity may be lower than a piece of coal in the sunlight. The human eye can see details far better than its dynamic range suggests because it cares about local contrast and not about intensity. Figure 18.6 shows more proof, some classic demonstrations that contrast, not intensity, is what matters.

In sum, there are several fundamental problems with images captured by digital cameras.

- They can only capture a compressed range of scene intensities and contrasts;
- Consumer cameras quantize the range into 256 steps, which is so coarse that it loses contrast at the low levels;
- Sensors have noise which increases black level, and can cause graininess and masking;
- Stray light further limits the ability to portray blacks and low contrasts;

- Cameras with larger pixels have better dynamic range and less noise but have poorer resolution;
- Different cameras will produce different images. Cameras vary in overall sensor size, photosite size, grid dimensions and spacing, sensor technology and, as explained below, different metering systems. Moreover, they use different image processing algorithms to remove artifacts, making the final image outputs unpredictable; and
- Camera images may also distort color. Cameras must be "color balanced" for the wavelength spectrum of the incident illumination. This is usually not critical for visibility at nighttime, but it is worth remembering should color be an issue.

While these problems limit the fidelity of camera image capture, further problems lie in exposure metering. Other problems exist in displaying image data because media, photographs and electronic screens usually have lower dynamic ranges and contrast ratios than good cameras can capture.

### 4. Exposure

Different exposure durations and metering methods can drastically alter brightness and contrast and, give a false impression of visibility and conspicuity, and distort apparent size and distance. In daytime, the problem most commonly arises when the camera cannot capture the entire dynamic range of the scene. In this case, the camera chooses an exposure that sets the dynamic range at an optimum value, trading off the ability to portray contrast in dim and bright areas of the scene. In nighttime scenes, the vast dominance of dark areas over light areas compounds exposure problems. Camera exposure metering systems operate on assumptions that are invalid under these conditions.

The term "exposure" actually has two distinct meanings that are often confused. In one sense, exposure is a particular combination of aperture size ("f stop") and opening time at a given ISO. In another, it is the total amount of light received by a photosite. Unlike the first definition, it also depends on light intensity. Metering systems attempt to set exposure (in the first sense) to optimize the range of exposures (in the second sense) for different objects.

Cameras set exposure by sampling scene intensities and then making assumptions. First, the camera uses some method of estimating average scene luminance. Next, taking ISO into account, it then sets an exposure time and aperture based on assumptions about scene reflectance. The camera wants to set a dynamic range that prevents saturation of the brightest areas. The camera assumes that the brightest point represents 100 percent reflectance which is some multiple of the average. If the multiple is 7.8, the common value, then the camera is essentially assuming that the average scene reflectance is 12.8 percent ($7.8 \times 12.8 = 100$ percent). Said another way, the exposure scheme assumes that all scene contrasts result from uniformly illuminated objects with average reflectance of 12.8 percent. A slightly different way of figuring saturation level would calculate the assumed reflectance as 18 percent.[13]

Errors occur when the actual average scene reflectance differs from the presumed average. If most of the scene has very high intensity, the camera assumes that 12.8 percent reflectance is represented by a very bright value. The result is that bright areas become gray. Otherwise, daytime exposure metering is only a problem when a scene has a large dynamic range—i.e., both direct sunlight and deep shadow.

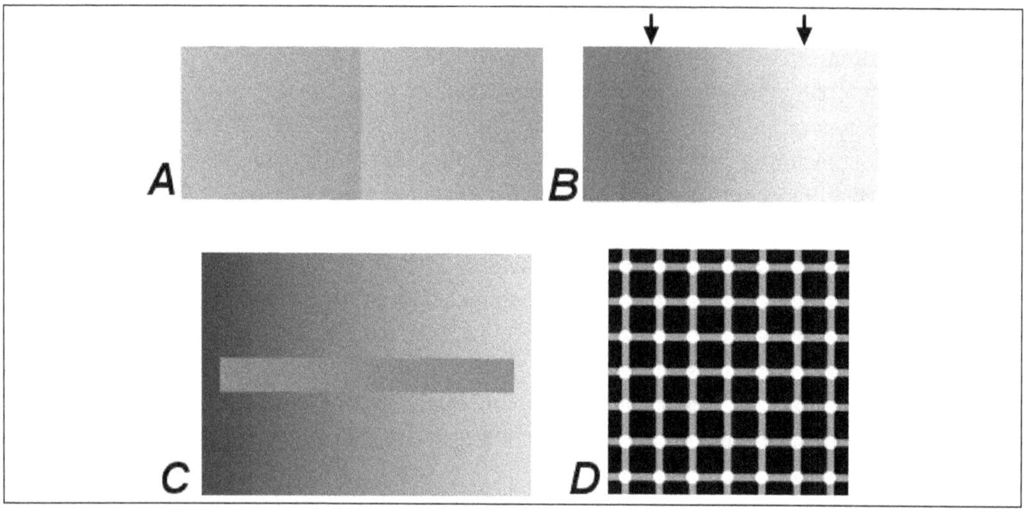


***Figure 18.6*** *Examples of the dissociation of intensity with brightness and contrast.*
*A. The left side appears darker than the right, but the two sides of the rectangle have the same luminance. Place a finger over the middle border to confirm. (Craik-Cornsweet edge.)*
*B. There appears to be a dark vertical band at arrow location 1 and bright vertical band at location 2. These are illusory. (Mach bands.)*
*C. The bar in the middle appears to become darker from right to left. In fact, it does not change intensity. Blot out the surround to confirm the illusion. (Simultaneous brightness contrast.)*
*D. The dots at the intersection appear to turn from white to black to white, although intensity is constant at a high level. (Modified Hermann grid.)*

In nighttime scenes, exposure is a greater problem because most scene areas are very dark. The camera assumes that the dark areas are about 12.8 percent reflectance and that the intensity range depends on uniformly illuminated surfaces of different reflectance. However, nighttime scenes do not meet the camera assumption. Many nighttime objects are self-luminous bright spots, such as warnings signals, traffic lights, or headlamps, that become drastically overexposed and over saturated.

Cameras vary in their methods for determining average intensity (location of the 12.8 percent reflectance level) and produce widely different exposure results. Moreover, most individual cameras offer several methods for determining average scene intensity, with the range of choices and exact methods varying across cameras. The most common method samples the entire scene and then combines samples to arrive at a weighted value. A camera will typically allow the user to choose the weighting of central vs. peripheral image areas. In one extreme, the photographer might be shooting a landscape, so he wants the entire visual field about equally weighted. At the other extreme, he might be shooting a portrait and want the visual field's center very highly weighted. Left on its own, the camera will likely choose a compromise, where the weighting is biased somewhat but not overwhelmingly toward the center.

The pictures in Figure 18.7 demonstrate some effects of varying exposure algorithm on my Canon A70 camera. The scene is much like a nighttime road environment that is dark with a few bright points. The left image shows a metering that only moderately center-weights, so the large dark area essentially determines the overall exposure. As a result, the camera sets the exposure to a long duration and large aperture. Bright areas, such as the computer screen, are overexposed and have exaggerated brightness. The long exposure also caused the sensor overflow and over saturation problem described above. Anyone who has seen many nighttime photographs will instantly recognize this artifact. However, some contrast is visible in the darker areas, such as the horizontal edge at the top.

Figure 18.7 (right) shows a photograph of the same scene with the exposure mode changed. Now the camera is on "spot metering," which weights the center much more heavily. The dark areas have little influence on the setting. The computer screen and the vertical thin light are more properly exposed but now the rest of the scene is underexposed and contrast in dark areas is completely lost.

I could easily produce any intermediate result by simply aiming the camera slightly to the left or right of the computer screen. Since the center is more heavily weighted, the farther I aim from the bright screen, the longer the exposure and the higher the overall scene brightness. However, this is only a tradeoff in whether the top or the bottom of the scene brightness range loses contrast. Lastly, the difference between the two pictures is entirely due to the use of different metering methods. If I had made a conscious effort to change aperture size or exposure duration, I could have produced much greater differences.

In sum, these pictures demonstrate the limitations and arbitrariness of nighttime photographs. A photographer can easily alter brightness and contrast and enhance or degrade visibility and conspicuity by:

- Using different metering modes on a single camera;
- Using cameras with different metering algorithms;
- Using different ISO settings;
- Changing the aim of the camera;
- Changing the exposure duration;
- Changing the aperture setting;
- Adding or removing bright objects from the scene;
- Changing the print development time; or
- Changing the photographic print paper.

The last two points refer to the image alteration occurring during the printing process. Development time changes contrast and brightness. Automatic systems change development settings in order to brighten dark prints and darken light ones and to perform color correction. Lastly, photographic print paper varies wildly in contrast and color response.

Some people attempt to circumvent the exposure problem by setting the camera to manual and taking a series of photographs at different exposure durations. The photographer then chooses the print that best represents the scene and then presents it as an accurate depiction of what the viewer would have seen. This sounds reasonable, but it is totally impractical. I have already described photography's inherent limitations in portraying dynamic range and contrast. Some photographs may be better than others, but none has complete fidelity. Next, human memory, especially for brightness, is extremely poor, so it is highly unlikely that a person could remember a previously viewed scene with much precision. Viewers also have a bias to remember colors as brighter and more saturated than they actually were. Even if it were possible to create a match in one set of viewing conditions, the jurors see the photographs/display under daytime illumination and are in a different state of adaptation. (See below.) Lastly, eyes and camera fundamentally set "exposure" in different ways. Both eyes and cameras can alter "exposure" by changing aperture size. However, cameras can change exposure duration over a wide range, but the eye has a limited ability to sum light over time. The longer photosite summation time permits greater accumulation of quanta, so that the camera can "see in the dark" better than a real viewer. Moreover, the camera sets a single overall exposure level for the entire scene. The eye adapts to the local intensity at each point on the retina, so there isn't a single "exposure" set for the entire image.

A simple afterimage demonstration proves the point. If you look at a black dot on a white background and then at a uniform gray surface (Figure 18.8), you see the white afterimage of the dot. The area of retina being stimulated by the dot was adapting to black while the rest of the retina was adapting to white. The gray would then look bright to the dark adapted area and dark to the white adapted area.

***Figure 18.7*** *Photographs of same scene taken with two different metering methods.*

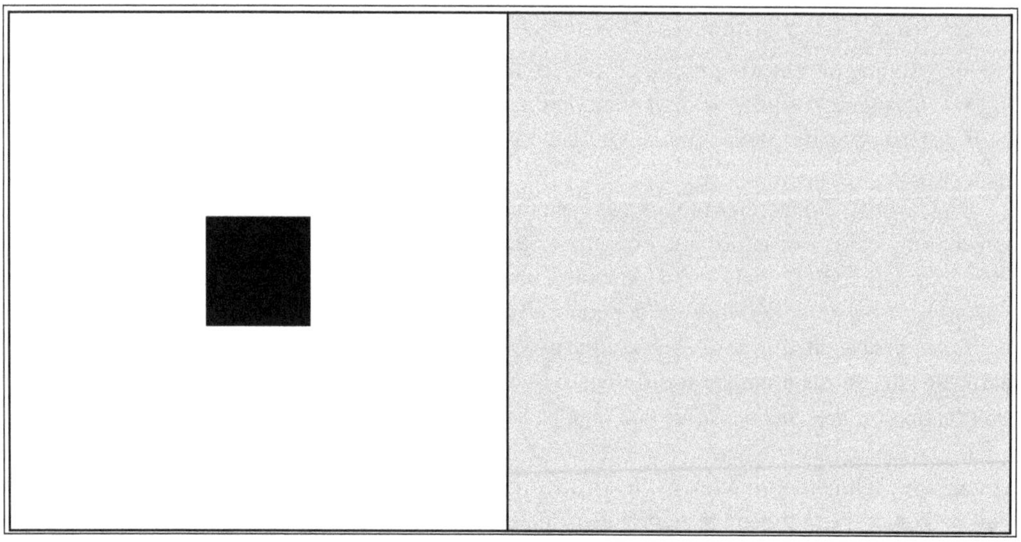

***Figure 18.8*** *Afterimages demonstrate local retinal adaptation.*

Similar effects occur in the real world. A driver traveling a dark road at night will likely fixate the point on the road where the headlamp beams hit the ground. The foveal area adapts to a relatively high light intensity. Meanwhile, the visual periphery sees the dark roadside and adapts to a very low level. The driver's eye simultaneously has two different adaptation states and two dynamic ranges. If the driver makes an eye movement to foveate the roadside, he will be foveally mis-adapted and have low sensitivity to objects such as a pedestrian in dark clothes. The juror in the courtroom can examine the picture as long as he likes until he is correctly adapted for image area.

Lastly, the eye can also be mis-exposed due to prior events. While a photographer can alter exposure at will to produce a desired result, a viewer who just experienced glare from oncoming headlamps will have his "exposure setting" incorrect for several seconds. Pictures do not capture these effects.

In sum, exposure variations allow creation of many different pictorial versions of the same scene. Exposure varies with camera algorithm, aim, ISO and location and brightness of all objects, even irrelevant ones. Taking a series of pictures of different exposure does not solve the problem because memory is poor, adaptation state cannot be easily replicated, and cameras have inherent limitations. Further, cameras set an exposure for the entire scene while the eye sets exposure locally. The eye's exposure, unlike cameras, is affected by prior light levels and by transient adaptation effects. Lastly, display nonlinearities, as discussed in the next section, tend to limit contrast.

## C. Display Media

To create a visual image, the camera data must be depicted in a display medium, usually photographs or electronic displays such as a CRT or LCD. The ability of cameras to capture images is usually better than the ability of displays to show them. Photographs and CRT screens portray very limited dynamic range and contrast ratio. This has led to extensive work on "tone mapping," the problem of rendering image data onto displays with smaller dynamic ranges. Recent advances in display technology, LCD and plasma screens with larger dynamic ranges, are lessening the difficulty of rendering the full image data.

The ensuing section briefly discusses the performance of various display media. Each is characterized by the same variables; gamma, dynamic range, contrast ratio and resolution that define camera capabilities.

### 1. Gamma

*CRT Screens.* All display media are nonlinear, i.e., they have gammas departing from one. For example, CRT screens typically have gammas of 2.2–2.5[14]. Figure 18.4 showed how gamma affects images. The major drawback is that higher gammas lose details in dimmer areas of the image and exaggerate contrast in brighter areas. Note in Figure 18.4 that the slope in dim areas is shallower when gamma is 2.5, so that intensity and contrast increase slowly.

It is possible to gamma-correct the images shown on CRT screens. Correction may require extra programming and possibly light measurement. The monitors must be set so that contrast and brightness controls are adjusted perfectly. Unfortunately, this can be tricky because CRT controls cause interaction among gamma, brightness and contrast. The "contrast" control on a CRT is actually brightness, and the "brightness" control is black level. Increasing brightness decreases gamma, so it may not be feasible to set the display to produce high contrasts, which require low black levels. The contrast control also has some effect on gamma.

*LCD screens.* LCD input-output curves have a different shape, somewhat resembling an ogive, and not readily described by a single gamma number. LCD displays typically have software to correct the nonlinearities, and the actual output gamma approaches 1. However, gamma can change severely with viewing angle, so jurors sitting in different positions will see different brightnesses, contrasts and colors.

*Photographs.* The paper used in prints also has an ogive-like shape, although there is usually a subrange where the input-output relationship is linear. However, different papers vary greatly in their linearity and their ability to portray contrast, but all have relatively low dynamic range. Correction is difficult and, unlike electronic displays, the camera image data would have to be preprocessed since prints themselves cannot be readily gamma-corrected. The expert would then have to admit to manipulating the image to get the results he wants.

## 2. Dynamic Range and Contrast Ratio

For camera sensors, "dynamic range" is the gamut of intensities from first response to saturation. For output displays, it is the range of intensities that can be produced. The final image's dynamic range depends on the weaker link, camera or display. If the dynamic range of the camera is lower than that of the display, the camera determines the final image quality. If the display has a smaller dynamic range than the camera, then the display is the bottleneck.

Table 18.3 shows some typical contrast ratios for various cameras and display media in normal viewing conditions. A scene with sunlight might have a range of 10,000:1 from bright highlights to shadows. Obviously, both cameras and display media produce contrast ratios far below both scene and eye.

Photographs will just about display the same contrast ratios of consumer cameras but not of DSLR's. CRT's typically have a lower contrast ratio and suffer greatly from the screen reflection problems discussed below. Pictures taken on a consumer camera and shown as photographs or CRT images are by far the most limited. Pictures taken by a consumer camera and displayed on an LCD screen will be limited by the camera rather than by the display. Finally, DSLR images will suffer badly unless viewed on a good LCD screen.

*CRT Screens.* The low quality of CRT images may surprise people who hear the common statement that they can create 16.7 million colors.[16] This is pure fiction. The misunderstanding lies in the confusion between the internal machine state (a number), the CRT output (a set of wavelengths) and the perceived colors. A 24-bit RGB system does not create 16.7 million colors; it simply creates 16.7 million (256 × 256 × 256) different machine states. Color is manufactured in the head, not the machine. Many of the machine states create the same, or at least indistinguishable, outputs to the screen. Further, the eye does not distinguish anything near 16.7 million colors, even in optimal conditions. In the real world the number is in the thousands, not millions.

In addition, a CRT monitor (and LCD screens) can't produce all of the colors that the eye can distinguish. Specifically, both computer and LCD screens can't produce the most saturated colors, so images are somewhat washed out. All image capture and display devices create color by mixing three primaries. The gamut of possible colors is determined by location in color space of these primaries. Both CRT and LCD displays use primaries that are not fully saturated, so they cannot produce highly saturated colors. The green primary has especially low saturation and makes greens appear washed out. The "red" primary is located closer to orange, so good reds are not possible. Look closely at a CRT red, and it is really reddish orange, at best. Moreover, ambient light falling on the screen further lowers saturation and shrinks the number of colors which the display can produce. Even within the range of color that it can produce, 24 bits still quantizes the color space too coarsely in some regions. Colors may jump by more than one JND (just noticeable difference step) because discriminability is not uniform throughout the RGB color space of monitors.

**Table 18.3**
**Typical contrast ratios under normal viewing conditions**
**These are rough values only, and there is wide variation**

| Factor | Medium | Dynamic Range |
|---|---|---|
| Environment | Daylight Scene | 10,000:1 |
| Record image | Eye | 1000-10,000:1 |
| | Consumer camera | 80-90:1 |
| | DSLR camera | 600-700:1 |
| Display image | Photograph print | 80-100:1[15] |
| | CRT display | 70:1 |
| | LCD display | 500-600:1 |

The same confusion exists in the assertion that DSLR cameras have 12–14 bits/color. This is a theoretical limit of the number of machine states inside the camera. It does not necessarily reflect the actual number of intensity levels or dynamic range captured. In sum, don't confuse the numbers inside a machine with anything in the real world. They are different domains that may or may not correspond.

*LCD Screens*. CRT's are losing popularity as the newer, superior LCD technology has improved in price and quality. However, creation of high LCD contrast ratios in the courtroom is difficult due to inherent tradeoffs among ambient illumination, background darkness and light adaptation.

Beware the extreme advertising claims. First, LCD screens have the same limited color rendering ability as CRT screens. As for contrast, LCD black level is limited by the technology, which uses a "back light" that always operates during operation. Some of the light leaks through the pixels preventing the black level from being low. LCD manufacturers also vastly exaggerate what is achievable in normal viewing. Manufacturers state specifications in terms of "full on/off" contrast, the difference between the screen being completely off and full on. The more realistic contrast is "ANSI" contrast, which uses a checkerboard of highest and lowest intensities to measure contrast. This better represents the contrast achievable with a real image, but it is lower than on/off contrast. Manufacturers are also known to fiddle with the setting between the off and on tests to minimize the difference. The message is clear: displays must be calibrated and manufacturer statements have little validity.

Manufacturers also give contrast ratios for displays seen in completely dark environments. Any ambient illumination lowers actual contrast by increasing intensity of the black level. Simple calculations show the great sensitivity of contrast ratios to ambient illumination. Consider an LCD display that claims a 2000:1 contrast ratio and a peak intensity of 500 cd/m$^2$. Assume that the ANSI contrast is 25 percent[17] lower at 1500:1. The black level must then be .333 cd/m$^2$ (500/.333=~1500). A typical TV LCD might have about 5 percent reflectance, although some LCD's have reflectances exceeding 10 percent. If the ambient room lighting is 100 lux, well below recommended courtroom levels, then the screen reflects 100×.05/3.14 = 1.592 cd/m$^2$. Add the intrinsic black level of .333, and the real black level becomes 1.925 cd/m$^2$ and real contrast ratio only ~260:1 (501.592/1.925) rather than 2000:1. The actual contrast is 13 percent of the manufacturer specifications.

The obvious solution is to use an LCD screen with a higher advertised contrast ratio. Figure 18.9 shows that this produces surprisingly little benefit. A 400 percent increase in advertised contrast from 2000:1 to 8000:1 improves contrast only from 260:1 to 299:1, an increase of only 15 percent. The improvement is small because contrast ratio depends primarily on the black level. When the reflected ambient light is the major factor limiting black level, then higher intrinsic screen contrast ratios make little difference. Figure 18.9 shows that when the ambient illumination is lower (50 lux) and a smaller determinant of black level, then higher intrinsic contrast ratios produce more gain.

Figure 18.9 suggests that the solution to creating high contrast courtroom displays is elimination of as much ambient light as possible by sealing the windows and extinguishing room lights, etc. Even if possible, however, this is a partial solution at best. First, the LCD screen itself creates light which reflects off the walls and ceiling back to the screen as ambient illumination. Incident illumination of only 1 lux would cut contrast by a quarter. Second, turning off the lights puts the juror in a lower adaptation state. Depending on circumstances this could cause viewers to become mis-adapted.

In addition, images viewed on a dark background of a dark room have significantly lower apparent contrast. The visual system has a mechanism called "contrast gain control," that helps it cope with the large dynamic range of natural scenes. When the difference between light and dark is very great, it turns down the gain so that the system doesn't saturate. The dark background border with the bright screen kicks in the gain control, so the image loses apparent contrast even though the physical contrast is unchanged (or even improved because of less stray light from ambient illumination). This effect is well known[18] and is one reason that the Illuminating Engineering Society advises that a display screen and its background should not differ in luminance by more than a 3:1 ratio. Similarly, studies of computer users shows that they prefer surrounds that are just slightly darker than the screens themselves. Eye movements back and forth across strong light/dark edges are very disrupting, causing discomfort glare and changing adaptation level. In nighttime scenes where the screen is most dark, however, this may be less important.

*Photographs.* As Figure 18.7 shows, photographic prints have a far lower dynamic range than scenes or eyes. However, they are relatively resistant to change due to ambient illumination in the photopic range. They create contrast by reflecting different amounts of light from various areas. If Weber's Law holds, then this should have little effect on apparent contrast, although they are subject to stray light. However, detection of small details does not follow Weber's law.

## D. Image Fidelity Summary

For perfect image fidelity, the following are necessary:

1. Image properties
    a. Perspective: correct the portrayal of object sizes and relative positions;
    b. Intensity: correct the mapping of scene point intensity to the picture points with the same relative location;
    c. Wavelength: correct the mapping of scene point wavelengths to the picture points with the same relative location;
2. Viewing conditions
    a. Viewing location: correct viewing distance and viewpoint;
    b. Ambient light: no extraneous light should be reflected from the picture; and
    c. Surround: should be close in luminance to the picture average with no distractions.

Producing correct perspective within a limited field-of-view is, in theory, not especially difficult. During photography, camera position is the key to capturing correct perspective. Lens focal length is primarily important in directly determining visual field size and indirectly determining resolution and image quality; images that are blown up will have more grain and noise. During display, viewers should see the picture from the correct viewing distance at the center of projection. However, controlling viewing conditions can be difficult. If the entire jury views a single screen, for example, both viewing distance and angle will vary, causing perspective and possibly contrast distortion. If a picture is passed around to jurors, they may hold it in the wrong position.

Creating correct image intensities and wavelengths is more problematic. Both camera and display media have limited dynamic range, contrast ratios and resolution and both are subject to various artifacts. Careful gamma correction is critical, but complex because gamma may interact with other variables that limit contrast and brightness. For photographs, brightness and contrast are readily manipulated by the printing process: longer development times increase photographic contrast, so some papers have more contrast than others, etc. Exposure, especially in nighttime photography, is perhaps the biggest problem. It is very difficult to determine, and it is essentially impossible to recreate the eye's exact light adaptation state.

Given the sensitivity of image fidelity to so many variables, an expert introducing pictures as evidence of perception should state quantitatively what the images actually represent. He should minimally be prepared to present:

- calibration data on both camera and display;
- luminance (and possibly wavelength) measurements of the actual scene; and
- luminance (and possibly wavelength) measurements of the displayed image under courtroom viewing conditions.

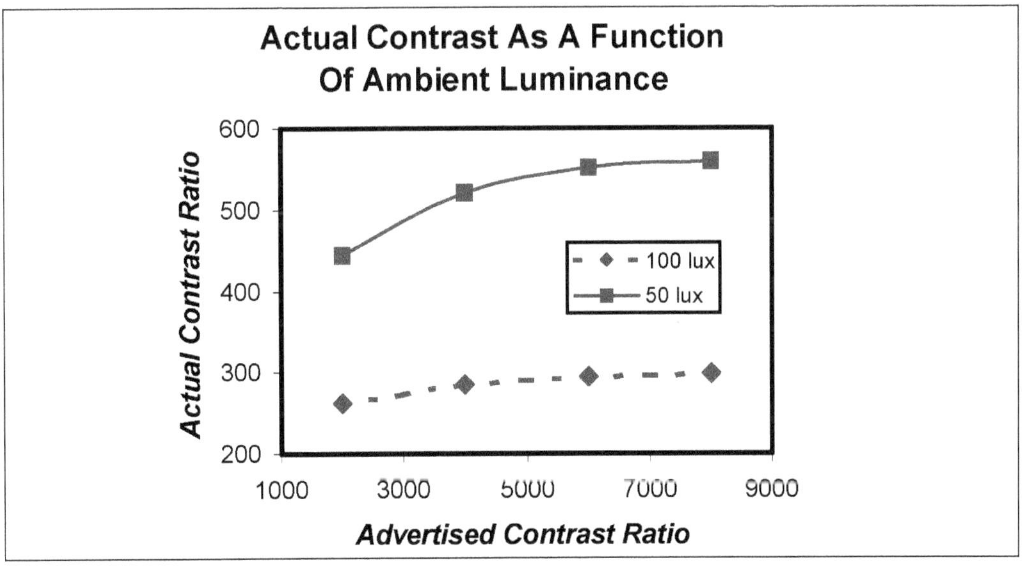


***Figure 18.9*** *Advertised vs. actual maximum contrast ratio as a function of ambient illumination, assuming a 25 percent difference between on/off and ANSI contrast.*

These requirements are similar to those that would be expected of any expert who testifies on scientific or technical research. Without this information, there is no way to tie the picture to the scene, to verify image fidelity and to evaluate similarity.

The final issue is whether the inevitable failures of image fidelity matter. There is no single answer since it depends on the nature of the scene, the limits of the particular technology used to record and to display the picture, the viewing conditions and perhaps, most important, the intended purpose. In the end, however, the intentions may not matter. Jurors are likely to accept the picture as an objective reality of what they would have seen if they were at the actual scene. They will fail to grasp that they are not "seeing" intensity, wavelength, size, distance and speed but rather that they are seeing brightness, color, *apparent* size and *apparent* distance and *apparent* speed. Even these are controlled by goals, expectations, etc. Said in a different way, there is no single, objective view of the picture or scene that is independent of the viewer. This is why psychophysical and perceptual similarity criteria are crucial for assessing similarity.

## 18.3 Psychophysical and Perceptual Fidelity

Let's assume for the moment that it were possible to overcome all limitations of perspective, dynamic range, gamma, viewing conditions, etc. and to create a picture with perfect image fidelity. What would be the justification for introducing the picture? Presumably, jurors could see the scene as it was and make their own judgments of reasonable behavior. There is a problem with this justification: it assumes that there is such a thing as an objective perception of an image. In fact, all image perception is subjective. Pictures cannot recreate either the sensation or the perception of the original viewer of the original scene. The reasons fall into three categories.

- Pictures don't capture all psychophysical information, e.g., disparity and motion parallax;
- Psychophysical viewing and viewer variables cannot be duplicated in the courtroom, e.g., fixation, viewing duration, age, and arousal; and
- There are cognitive variables such as expectation, goals, attention, concurrent tasks, uncertainty, etc.

### A. Psychophysical Information Not Captured By Pictures

Pictures fail to capture important visual information used by normal viewers. Perception is automatic, so jurors seeing the picture will then be unaware that their perception is impoverished and that they are not seeing the information available at the actual scene. There is no way to supply this missing information by instructions, description or by any verbal means. Psychophysical sensations are experiences that are largely cognitively impenetrable.

The following is a partial list of visual cues that pictures do not contain. Some are static cues, such as disparity, while others are dynamic, changes over time and space. Static pictures do not portray any of this information while movies have some ability to portray dynamic events. Although not discussed here, pictures also lack nonvisual sensory information, such as sound and vibration, that drivers incorporate into their perceptual judgments.

#### 1. Disparity

People perceive scene layout, objects distances, sizes, etc. using two general types of depth cues. One is "monocular" or "pictorial" because it can be viewed with one eye and/or seen in a picture. These include interposition, size, linear perspective, aerial perspective, texture gradient, brightness, shadowing height in the visual field and angle of declination. In movies, there is also motion parallax. The other class is "binocular" because it requires the use of both eyes. A person with one eye or a person with two eyes looking at a picture cannot use stereopsis.

Stereopsis is the perception of relative depth based on disparity, the position of images in the two eyes (see Chapter 3). It plays much the same role as brightness and color contrast in helping the viewer quickly decompose the scene into distinct objects and surfaces and to perceive scene layout. Without stereopsis, viewers will be slower to perceive depth, to recognize objects and to gain situation awareness, especially at night when there are fewer other cues. Stereopsis further separates foreground from background, allowing attention to be directed toward nearer, and presumably more important, objects. As discussed in Chapter 16, disparity also aids in looming detection.

### 2. Motion

Motion can serve as important visual information in a wide range of visual judgments. Motion naturally plays a key role in situation awareness for collision events. A viewer looking at a static picture, for example, cannot make an accurate assessment of time-to-collision. Further, motion can either increase or decrease conspicuity, depending on circumstances. Pedestrians, for example, are more visible when they are moving, especially if they are swinging their arms and signaling biological motion (see Chapter 15). Conversely, motion can mask and distract. Raindrops on windshields and traffic in the background cause movement that make road objects less conspicuous. Lastly, motion can lower visibility, since rapidly moving objects have higher detection thresholds.

"Motion parallax," is a particular type of motion cue, the relative movement of one object to another. A simple demonstration shows how it works. Hold up the index finger of each hand in front of your face with one finger farther away than the other. Move the head back and forth and note that the two fingers move relative to one another. The amount of this motion parallax is a cue to distance and size. (Alternately open and close each eye to reveal the different image seen by each eye. This is the retinal disparity that creates stereopsis.)

In the real world, motion parallax can be a critical cue for conspicuity, for distance judgments and for perceiving affordances. Brady (1992), for example, describes the problems of navigating safely and perceiving scene layout with only one eye and no stereopsis. He has problems seeing curbs and stairs unless he notes the motion parallax. As he moves toward a curb, the nearer pavement moves faster (on the retina) than the distant road, creating a sharp discontinuity in the motion field. The difference in motion rates alerts him to the step and tells him how far the road is from the pavement. A viewer looking at a picture is in Brady's shoes because he also has no stereopsis or motion parallax.

Optic flow is related to motion parallax, as it is the relative motion of different objects. As viewers move through the environment, objects move outward from the focus of expansion at rates dependent on location and distance. (See Figure 3.9.) Optic flow provides a rich source of visual information for a wide variety of perceptions, including object scene layout, object distance and heading. With reduced optic flow, viewers are more likely to have visual and heading errors, causing phenomena such as the "moth-effect" (Green, 2006). For example, pilots frequently become disoriented and misjudge landing. Optic flow supports ambient vision, which viewers use to maintain their orientation in space.

Lastly, a driver in motion experiences several visual effects that are absent from the juror sitting in a stationary chair viewing a static picture. The optic flow creates image motion that makes moving objects less conspicuous. The driver also experiences vibration that jiggles the eyeball and smears the retinal image, causing visibility to decline. Movement through the environment also narrows the field-of-view (e.g., Gibson and Crooks, 1938), controls concentration, and directs attention (Chapter 15).

#### 3. Field-of-view

The human visual field is 200° wide, with the central and peripheral visual areas having functional differences. People use only part of the visual field, about the central 30°, as focal vision for detecting and recognizing objects and scenes. The remaining outer peripheral field serves as ambient vision for orienting in space. In theory, a picture capturing at least 30° would be sufficient to portray the focal area that a viewer might use to scan the road. However, loss of the peripheral field produces subtle perceptual deficits.

First, small fields decrease optic flow information, creating the impaired orientation and ambient vision as already described. Second, field size changes distance judgments. When a viewer looks at a picture, he sees a representation of visual space. He must place himself in space relative to the scene in order to judge distance of objects in the picture. Field-of-view size affects this self-placement and the resulting distance judgments. For example, Psotka, Lewis, and King (1998) had viewers judge object distances in pictures containing correct "life size" visual angles and perspective. Viewers looking at smaller field sizes judged themselves closer to the scene and distances as shorter than those viewing the same picture through a larger field.

Small fields-of-view decrease contrast on dark backgrounds. As noted above, perceived contrast is lower when an image is viewed against a dark surround. The effect lessens at greater object distance from the edge. Smaller fields-of-view increase edge effects because objects are closer to the contrast edge.

### B. Viewer and Situational Variables

Sensation is also a function of many psychophysical variables that is not readily reproducible in a courtroom. Chapter 14 discusses these variables in detail, so the ensuing section only provides a brief refresher.

#### 1. Fixation and Visual Field Location

Visibility and apparent contrast depend on retinal location. The courtroom viewer must then look in exactly the correct location, so that scene objects fall at the correct retinal eccentricities. This is virtually impossible to enforce. Suppose the picture shows a pedestrian in the edge of the image. Once the juror knows that the pedestrian is in the image, he will fixate it. Once that knowledge is gained, it cannot be lost. Even if the juror then attempts to look at the center, the certainty of the object's presence increases its visibility and conspicuity.

#### 2. Viewing Time

Viewing time is one of the main factors separating the original viewer from the juror. The original viewer may have had only fractions of a second to detect, recognize, gain situational awareness, decide upon a response and program the motor command. Courtroom viewers can sit at their leisure and view the picture at length.

#### 3. Arousal and Stress

Jurors are not experiencing fatigue (hopefully), operating at 2 a.m. in the morning or suffering vigilance decrement. They are not confronted with a sudden emergency that distorts perceived space and time. They are not in a high stress situation that causes perceptual narrowing, a visual field shrinkage and general cognitive reduction in the amount of information processed.

### 4. Oculomotor Information: Vergence and Accommodation

When a viewer fixates an object in the distance at the scene, the lens thins, accommodating to create a sharp retinal image. In addition, the inward vergence angle between the two eyes becomes shallower. Conversely, examining a nearby object, such as a photograph held in the hand, causes lens thickening and sharper vergence angle.

Viewers use these oculomotor signals to judge depth, at least for short viewing distances. The thickened lens and sharper vergence angle tell the viewer that the objects are actually very close. Viewers then incorporate the oculomotor signals with other depth information to judge size, distance and scene layout. As a result, viewing a picture at a short distance causes an underestimation of depth. Objects then appear smaller when fixation is nearer (e.g., Heinemann, Tulving, and Nachmias, 1959). This is another example of the psychological size-distance tradeoff. If two objects have the same size retinal image and appear at different depths, then the near one must represent a smaller object—otherwise it would have a larger retinal image. Size and distance judgments are inextricably bound together. Distort one and the other is also usually distorted.

### 5. Viewer Age, Optical Correction, etc.

If the original viewer were old (and possibly had an eye disease) and the juror were young, then the juror will see the picture too well. The converse is also true, and an older juror may see the picture too poorly. Similarly, jurors should match the original viewer's eyesight. Lastly, differences in optical correction may also be significant. Recall from Chapter 14 that strong lenses can magnify or minify retinal images. If there is a large mismatch in correction among viewers, viewing distance may have to compensate for lens-induced variation in retinal image size.

### 6. Adaptation Effects

Real viewers adapt to environmental conditions such as light and motion. In order to create the same light/dark adaptation state in the juror, the picture must have the same overall intensity as the scene. Further, a juror would have to fixate the same objects for the same durations. The most likely problem is that jurors inspecting a nighttime image will be adapted to daytime light levels. Moreover, pictures cannot capture light/dark adaptation effects arising from events occurring in the past. An oncoming vehicle headlamp can produce glare that lowers sensitivity for several seconds or even minutes after the event. The jurors cannot see or adapt to anything occurring before or after the picture's instant in time.

Most drivers adapt to motion. The eye's motion sensors fatigue, making motion appear slower after prolonged viewing. The result is a deficit in looming perception and errors in obstacle avoidance and lane changing. Further, drivers "velocitate" to their own speed and gradually lose the sense that they are moving rapidly. Even movies cannot replicate these motion adaptation effects because the jurors do not watch the motion for long, uninterrupted, periods and because the movie field size is relatively small.

## C. Cognitive Variables

The previous discussion in this chapter is largely foreplay because now we come to the crux of the problem with pictorial evidence. These are the most important psychological factors and the principal reason that even high image fidelity cannot ensure substantial similarity. Vision = sensation + perception, and perception is largely a cognitive process. Since jurors cannot share the same cognition, they cannot perceive what the original viewer saw. I have previously explained cognitive influences on vision, so the following is just a brief review of factors that separate the original viewer from the juror. See Marshall (1966) for additional discussion.

### 1. Expectation, Attention and Goals

Chapter 1 discussed the essential nature of vision; sensation and perception are different processes; vision is largely cognitive; conscious perception of sensation is selective and a process that is inherently subjective and interpretive; and naïve realism makes commonsense understanding of vision largely incorrect. By now, I hope that the reader understands why these apparently theoretical and academic points are actually of great practical importance and why this book began with the quote:

> We see our world of organized scenes and moving objects by combining information from the light which reaches our eyes with knowledge stored in memory about the structure and identity of objects and scenes. We understand our surroundings partly by seeing them but also by inferring what is there…Vision is therefore a genuine cognitive function, not merely a sensory one. (Hampson and Morris, 1996)

These ideas are not new but rather basics that underlie the scientific understanding of vision. As early as 1890, vision experts already knew that:

> Whilst part of what we perceive comes through our senses from the object before us, another part (and it may be the larger part) always comes out of our own mind. (William James, 1890)

In other words, there is a large gulf between the retinal image and perception. Jurors, even if viewing an image with perfect image fidelity, will not have the same perceptions as the original viewer because *vision is as much a function of the contents in the viewer's head as the contents of the image*. The inattentional blindness, change-blindness and other research described in Chapter 4, Figure 1.5 and the Chase and Simon (1972) chess research in Chapter 1 and thousands of other scientific studies have dramatically made this point. Moreover, people are unable to separate sensation from perception. They assume that their subjective perceptual interpretation of the scene represents a fixed, objective reality. In other words, they suffer from naïve realism.

For people to act intelligently, they need information, which can come from two sources, perception and memory. People form memory structures called schemata and scripts that create expectations about the world and about appropriate behavior in different situations. This frees viewers from having to spend the time to stop, scrutinize, and consciously examine every detail of every new situation. However, the juror is not driving a car, trying to cross the street or doing anything other than passively examining a picture. He does not have either a memory or motor schema operating, and is not trying to perform a task or achieve a goal. He does not watch as the scene unfolds over time, updating his understanding and interpretation of events. He does not have any concurrent tasks (steering, watching for traffic, etc.) or distractions and can focus all attention on the picture. He has no payoffs to consider and no need to assess probabilities. Further, jurors have no uncertainty. They know not only where to look and what to look for, but also what will happen next. Once they know, they cannot ignore the information and put themselves in the mind of the original viewer.

Jurors also have an entirely different set of goals, which greatly affect perception, especially attention and conspicuity. The research reviewed by Land (2006), for example, describes how the attention and eye movements of a viewer are strongly determined by the task. Objects that are not task related go unnoticed, even if they have high sensory conspicuity. Seeing is a matter of experience, task relevance and goals.

Viewer perception and action are also closely connected. Jurors are not performing a task, so they do not see the same stimulus-response compatibilities. They do not see the same affordances, which depend in part on individual characteristics such as age, gender, physical abilities and risk tolerance. For example, determining whether there is an affordance (a safe gap) for crossing the street or making a turn depends in part on your own walking or driving speed. A juror who is merely looking at a picture will not make the same judgment as an actual pedestrian or driver. (Of course, the juror also has no motion information to judge time gap, either.) To re-quote from Chapter 1, "perception and movement are mutually dependent: perception requires movement and movement requires perception" (Lee, 2006).

### 2. Automatic Behavior

Humans can act in either a conscious and deliberate controlled mode or in an unconscious, automatic mode. The vast majority of behavior occurs automatically and without awareness. Experience forms expectation, narrows attention and transforms controlled behavior to automatic mode so that we can perform more efficiently and skillfully. People, however, are not aware that they are unconscious of most of their actions or how they have controlled their attention, etc. Remember, people performing routine and skilled tasks don't make conscious decisions; they just do what works. In contrast, jurors make conscious, controlled observations and decisions based on logical, deliberate reasoning and based on a knowledge of the outcome. The original viewer operated quickly, largely automatically and/or under stress, and without certain knowledge of the outcome.

### 3. Visuospatial Maps

The cognitive factors covered so far are the most important for visibility, conspicuity and recognition, but several others are important for perception of scene layout and situation awareness. The visuospatial mental map is another form of memory that contains the presence and location of objects in the scene. It extends direct vision, because the viewer can in a sense perceive parts of the scene falling outside the visual field or areas that are not receiving attention.

The existence of visuospatial mental maps is easy to demonstrate. A person can close his eyes and still navigate a familiar environment with some degree of accuracy because he carries around this mental map of where objects are. Visuospatial maps are also evident when people perform routine activities because they know in advance where to make the next eye movement and where to reach for the next object (e.g., Land, 2006). Visuospatial maps are useful even in unusual circumstances; a person who starts to fall can reach for the handrail even if he is not looking at it because it is located in his mental representation of the scene.

Experts know that there can be a big difference between visiting the accident scene and simply looking at photographs. Although the reason is often difficult to put into words, appreciation of space and scene layout cannot be fully transmitted in a photograph or even in a video. I suspect one of the main reasons is that pictures of unfamiliar locations are insufficient to create a visuospatial map. The map is formed in part by viewers moving around the scene, observing it from different distances and viewpoints, observing the motion parallax, etc. to gain a mental representation of layout. Pictures show scenes from a single viewpoint with no motion, which provides limited opportunity to form the map. The juror has no mental map and does not fully appreciate the scene 3D spatial relations. He does not see what is outside the range of the photograph and cannot put himself in the place of the original viewer.

### 4. Inherent Distortions In Picture Perception

In picture perception, the viewer must recreate the 3-D scene from the limited field 2-D image without the help of familiar disparity and motion cues, a visuospatial map, etc. Research has shown that in forming the reconstruction, viewers make errors and indulge in some innate biases and heuristics. I've already noted that viewers must place themselves in space relative to the scene and that even correct perspective does not insure accurate perception. Other studies have reported a wide range of perceptual distortions of shape, size and distance (e.g., Bartley and DeHardt, 1960; Hecht, van Doorn and Koenderink, 1999).

Interestingly, viewers seldom notice that they are making all these perceptual errors when looking at pictures. The same phenomenon occurs in memory, where people seldom notice errors and generally have great faith in their accuracy, although memory is highly unreliable and error-prone. In both cases, people don't notice because the errors usually don't matter and because they seldom receive feedback that their perception/memory is incorrect.

## D. The Psychologist's Fallacy: The Harmful Effects Of Pictures

Misleading pictures have harmful effects that go beyond the misleading appearance of visibility, conspicuity, etc. Juror perceptions instantly create inferences and extrapolations that affect their entire viewpoint on blame attribution. The most obvious effect is the "psychologist's fallacy."

William James (1890) coined the term "psychologist's fallacy" to note that many in his profession made a common mental mistake: they confused their own reality after an event had occurred with the reality of the person prior to the event. This reasoning error is now more descriptively called "hindsight bias." It is a general, powerful and almost inescapable influence on blame attribution. Jurors sitting in a courtroom view events occurring at the time of an accident very differently than the actor at the time (Green, 2002a)

Images presented as evidence of visual circumstances contribute greatly to hindsight bias. The link lies in the "counterfactual thinking," the imagination of what-if scenarios. What if the driver had turned left rather than right? What if the driver had been traveling 10 mph slower?, etc. Once it becomes clear that the user could have changed the outcome by different behavior, he is firmly fixed as the cause. People tend to place causation on mutable, i.e., changeable, aspects of an event. If a person slips and falls, for example, the cause cannot be gravity because it is immutable.

When jurors see a picture presented as "what there was to be seen," they will accept the image as what they would have seen at the time and ignore their advantages, such as knowing where to focus attention, unlimited viewing time, etc. They apply counterfactual reasoning and think, "the driver could have seen the pedestrian, so he must be the accident's cause." *Could have seen* quickly morphs into *should have seen.*

### E. Psychophysical and Perceptual Fidelity Summary

Even with perfect image fidelity, a picture does not represent a scene. *There is no such thing as an objective perception of an image.* Pictures do not capture all the visually useful information in a scene. Next, viewer and psychophysical variables prevent the reproduction of the sensations experienced by the original viewer. Lastly, naïve realism leads virtually all laypeople to make the fundamental error of believing that we see some fixed reality that is both objective and complete. Quite the contrary, perception is selective and a subjective interpretation dependent on viewer cognition, which is in turn a function of knowledge, expectations, goals and actions.

Table 18.4 summarizes the difference between a real driver viewing a scene and a juror viewing a picture. At each stage of the behavior sequence outlined in Chapter 1, the jurors has the advantage.

Table 18.4 distills the results from vast quantities of scientific research. Some readers may agree with the table but still find it difficult to accept that viewer-juror vision could be so different. After all, vision is so effortless that it must be simple with few variables at work. Those who have read the preceding chapters and who have learned to beware naïve realism should no longer believe this. However, they still may be wondering, "If cognition governs perception and everyone has different cognitions, then why do we generally agree about what we see?" The general agreement is hardly surprising because we are all wired-up roughly the same and to a large extent share similar cognitive processes and experience similar environments, and perform similar tasks with similar goals. However, our experiences and cognitions are not identical and are situation, activity and goal specific. Moreover, most of our cognitive processing operates automatically and by habit with little or no conscious supervision. However, the juror who consciously and deliberately views a picture about an event whose outcome is known simply cannot share the cognitions of a person who is guided by unconscious schema and habit and who is actively engaged in attempting to achieve a goal. There is a huge cognitive gap, for example, between looking at a picture and consciously thinking about driving and actually automatically driving. As Chapter 1 hammered home, vision is highly contextual.

Further, viewers' perceptions differ much more than people might suppose. As discussed above in picture perception and memory, most perceptual disagreements and memory errors don't matter and don't elicit any feedback that makes us aware of the disparities. If perceptions are closely examined because they matter, as in court proceedings, then the high degree of perceptual disagreement among viewers becomes apparent.

## 18.4 Conclusion

This chapter has examined the visual properties of pictures that are introduced as evidence of a visual scene's perception. Virtually all companies that create such pictures, animation and simulations for courtroom use proclaim that their service is important because "seeing is believing." This is undoubtedly true. It is also the danger of allowing jurors to see the pictorial evidence. The power to persuade is also the power to mislead.

The presumed justification for introducing pictorial evidence is that the jurors can see for themselves how the scene appeared. The underlying assumption is that scene perception is nothing more than registration of an image on the retina. If this were true, then image fidelity would be the only factor that determines substantial similarity. At this point in technology, the ability to correctly portray brightness, color and contrast limits image fidelity. Correct rendering of brightness, contrast and sharpness is limited by dynamic range, contrast ratios and gammas of cameras and especially of displays as well as by viewing conditions. Pictures taken on consumer, and even DSLR, cameras and shown as photographs are particularly poor representations. While it is theoretically possible to create proper perspective in a small visual field, it may be practically difficult to achieve in a courtroom setting.

However, there is much more to vision than image fidelity. A static picture does not capture visual information such as disparity and motion cues such as parallax and optic flow. Moreover, recall from the Chapter 14 discussion of visibility that multipliers of 5–20 are needed to reflect the vision of viewers in the real world. Jurors closely resemble the experimental subjects. They already know the outcome. There is no uncertainty.

**Table 18.4**
**Driver vs. juror in the behavior sequence. See Chapter 1 for more details**

| Information Processing | Original Viewer | Juror |
|---|---|---|
| 1. Search and Vigilance | Unconsciously and automatically employs expectation, habit, goals, concurrent tasks, affected by arousal state. | Consciously employs knowledge of the outcome. Moderate arousal state. |
| 2. Detection and Visibility | Detects contrast of an uncertain target located in uncertain part of the visual field viewed for a limited time. | Detects contrast of a known, fixed target seen for an unlimited time. |
| 3. Attention and Conspicuity | Unconsciously and automatically employs expectation, habit, goals, concurrent tasks, arousal. Spatial and object uncertainty. | Consciously employs knowledge of past events and outcome. Looks at known place for known object. |
| 4. Recognition | Controlled by expectation, habit, goals, concurrent tasks. Object uncertainty. | Controlled by knowledge of past events and outcome. Knows what the object is before looking. |
| 5. Situation awareness | Based on expectation, habit, goals, visuospatial map. Limited by perceptual narrowing. | Based on knowledge of the outcome. No stress and no perceptual narrowing. |
| 6. Response Selection | Uses all of the above, plus affordances, risk assessment, stimulus-response compatibilities. | None in reality. Mentally may think of response, which is determined by knowledge of the outcome. No risk, no stress and no perceptual narrowing. |
| 7. Response | Responds under stress. | None |

Further, vision is a function of many cognitive variables which cannot be readily duplicated in a courtroom. As explained in Chapter 1, people perceive and act based on the distant past (expectation) and recent past (the unfolding event) and on the future (goals), but pictures are at best a snapshot of the present. The juror sees the image completely disembodied from context.

Despite all the clear scientific evidence, some courts persist in allowing the presentation of pictures as evidence of what a viewer could see. This practice can be highly misleading and destroys any attempt to judge the case based on scientific evidence and analysis. Once jurors view the picture, they form a gut reaction that is largely resistant to any attempts at verbal qualification or rational refutation. "Photographs and images on video are typically seen as direct copies of reality" (Messaris, 1997). Humans almost invariably attempt to reduce the cognitive complexity of a situation. Few jurors will care about contrast threshold calculation, mental models, schemata, motion adaptation, glare, etc. when they can simply look at an image and decide for themselves using commonsense, which is wrong in fundamental ways. Moreover, jurors cannot appreciate how an image differs from a scene that they have never viewed. As Kanazawa (1991) notes, "If the lawyer does not **SHOW** them reasons for not believing what they see, they will believe what they see along with all the extrapolations they place on the visual images." Kanazawa bolded and capitalized the word "**SHOW**" to emphasize that verbal argument will have little effect. He also correctly notes that the viewer superimposes assumptions and forms extrapolations that go far beyond the actual image content.

Perhaps the best way to summarize the misleading effects of pictorial evidence is by the example of a common accident type and subsequent attempt to create and introduce pictorial evidence. The example ignores image fidelity problems and focuses on cognitive factors:

> A driver failed to see a pedestrian at night and struck him with his vehicle. The plaintiff's attorney hires a photographer to take pictures at the accident scene recreation with an exemplar pedestrian. The plaintiff's attorney then shows the pictures to the jury with the intent of proving that the pedestrian was highly visible and conspicuous. However, conspicuity is largely a function of attentional set and cognitive factors. The jurors do not share expectation, goals, tasks, etc. with the original viewer. Moreover, the jurors know what has happened and know exactly where to look, what they will find. They have unlimited time to look and to recognize. How can the jurors make a fair assessment of conspicuity? By its very definition, conspicuity is the attraction of attention to unexpected objects at unexpected locations. Further, the jurors suffer naïve realism, so they believe that their vision is complete and objective. Each juror will almost certainly ignore all scientific evidence about the limited image fidelity and about the psychophysical and cognitive differences between himself and the defendant and conclude, "If I can see the pedestrian, the driver should have been able to see him, too." *Seeing is believing*. Jurors will engage in hindsight bias.

This scenario is not hypothetical. I have frequently been asked by attorneys to vouch for the validity of similar pictures and videotapes but have declined every time. However, such pictures frequently appear as evidence of vision despite their flaws. Some make claims about the pictures representing vision. Other experts use a more sophisticated tact by calling the picture a "visibility analysis." They go through all the steps that they believe necessary to render a picture with best image fidelity. However, there is no specific claim that the picture represents what the original viewer would have, could have or should have seen. The expert may even agree that the picture does not necessarily recreate real viewer perception. It is merely "what there was to be seen."

The term "visibility analysis" is both misleading and disingenuous. Visibility is inherently a psychology concept and does not exist independently of the viewer. Moreover, once judges and jurors see realistic-looking pictures naïve realism takes over and the jurors will implicitly believe that pictures represent what the original viewer perceived or should have perceived. They will behave exactly like the jurors in the hypothetical example above. They will unconsciously extrapolate beyond the pictures and draw a host of inferences. They are not trained visual scientists and cannot separate the image from the percept. The pictures undermine any attempt to present a scientific analysis of visibility and perception.

Lastly, even pictures introduced for other purposes can unduly mislead and bias jurors. Suppose an animation provides an overhead view of a collision between vehicles. The intent may merely be to provide a visual representation of events. However, jurors may easily confuse *their perspective and perception* of speed and location of objects seen in the animation with the *driver's perspective and perception* of location and speed at the time of the accident. The jury may draw incorrect inferences from the animation about the visibility of vehicles, perceived speed, time to respond, etc. For example, the animation may show a truck rear-ending a small car stopped on a roadway. An overhead view shows frontoparallel motion, so it may appear that the truck driver should easily have seen the car and braked in time. The actual driver had only looming, which is far more difficult to judge. Recent research (Roese, Fessel, Summerville, Kruger and M. Dilich, 2006) of such an animation found increased "juror" bias toward blame assignments. Regardless of a picture's intended purpose, viewers may use it for other cognitive purposes.

In sum, the assessment "substantial similarity" requires both an analysis of image fidelity and a careful examination of psychological differences between jurors and original viewers. It is hardly surprising that judges, attorneys, forensic photographers and even most experts seldom consider them in any depth. They don't have the psychological viewpoint that appreciates vision as an integration of eye and mind, of sensation and perception and of past, present and future.

## References

Bartley, S. H., and D. DeHardt. 1960. A further factor in determining nearness as a function of lateral orientation in pictures. *Journal of Psychology* 50, 53-57.

Brady, F. 1992. *The Singular View: The Art of Seeing With One Eye*. Canadian Edition. Toronto: Edgemore Enterprises.

Dellinger, H. 1997. Words are enough: the troublesome use of photographs, maps, and other images in Supreme Court opinions. *Harvard Law Review* 110.n8, 1704-1753.

Evans, R. M. 1976. Using photography to preserve evidence. *Kodak Publication M-2, 1976.*

Gibson, J. J., and L. Crooks, 1938. A theoretical field analysis of automobile-driving. *American Journal of Psychology* 51, 453-471.

Graham, M. 1982. Evidence and Trial Advocacy Workshop: Relevancy and Exclusion of Relevant Evidence-Real Evidence, *Criminal Law Bulletin* 18, 241.

Green, M. 2002. Inattentional Blindness, *Occupational Health and Safety Canada* Jan/Feb, 23-29.

Green, M. 2006. Is the moth-effect real? *Accident Reconstruction* May/June, 18-19.

Hampson, P., and P. Morris. 1996. *Understanding Cognition.* Oxford: Blackwell.

Hecht, H., A. J. Doorn, and J. Koenderink. 1999. Compression of visual space in natural scenes and in their photographic counterparts. *Perception and Psychophysics* 61, 1269-1286.

Heinemann, E., E. Tulving, and J. Nachmias. 1959. The effect of oculomotor adjustments on apparent size, *The American Journal of Psychology* 72, 32-45.

Hood, D. 1998. Lower-level visual processing and models of light adaptation. *Annual Review of Psychology* 49, 503-535.

James, W. 1890. *The Principles of Psychology.* New York: Henry Holt & Company.

Kanazawa, S. 1991. Seeing is believing – Or is it? Attacking video and computer reconstructions. *Emerging Issues In Automobile Product Liability Litigation.* American Bar Association Meeting: Tucson, Arizona.

Land, M. 2006. Eye movements and the control of actions in everyday life. *Progress in Retinal Eye Research* 25, 296-324.

Lee, D. 2006. How movement is guided. http://www.perception-in-action.ed.ac.uk/PDF_s/Howmovementisguided.pdf. Downloaded 30 May 07.

Marshall, J. 1966. *Law And Psychology In Conflict.* New York: Bobs-Merrill.

McCann, J., and A. Rizzi. 2007. Camera and visual veiling glare in HDR images, *Journal of The Society For Information Display* 15, 721-730.

Messaris, P. 1997. *Visual persuasion: The Role Of Images In Advertising.* Thousand Oaks, Ca: Sage.

Psotka, J., S. Lewis, and D. King. 1998. Effects of Field-of-view on Judgments of Self-Location: Distortions in Distance Estimations Even When the Image Geometry Exactly Fits the Field-of-view. *Presence: Teleoperators and Virtual Environments* 7, 352-369.

Rizzi, A., M. Pezzetti, and J. McCann. 2007. Measuring the range of high dynamic range images. *European Conference on Visual Perception.*

Rodieck, R. 1998.*The First Steps in Seeing.* Sinauer Associates, Massachusetts.

Roese, N., F. Fessel, A. Summerville, J. Kruger, and M. Dilich. 2006 . The propensity effect: When foresight trumps hindsight. *Psychological Science* 17, 305-310.

Sharp, P., and R. Phillips. 1997. Physiological Optics. In W. Hendee and P. Wells (eds.) The *Perception Of Visual Information* (2nd Ed.) Springer Verlag: New York.

## Endnotes

1. Some call this property "visual realism," but this is not a good term because it confuses several distinct concepts, image fidelity, sensation with perception. The term "photorealism" is better. Another common term is "life-like."

2. Do not confuse object perspective with image perspective. If I place my eye 1 inch from my cat's face, the nose looks huge and the eyes relatively small. This a distortion relative to the actual object sizes created by my viewpoint. However, the discussion here has nothing to do with such object distortion but rather with image distortions. The image on my retina has proper perspective on my cat's face *for that particular viewpoint.* A picture has the correct image perspective if it produces the same retinal image, including any object distortions.

3. Very short focal lengths, however, can introduce some types of aberration, such as "barrel distortion," where lines in the image periphery appear curved. These are ignored.

4. The actual difference between standard and DSLR field-of-view is determined by the "crop factor," which is usually 1.5–1.7.

5. The statement is inherently misleading because cameras don't see anything. They record images. Seeing involves much more than this, as I have discussed in earlier chapters and will repeat later. Further, even at a very basic level, the eye-camera analogy is limited. The eye has super large format and has a curved sensor surface, unlike the flat surface of camera sensors.

6. Ecological validity is the degree to which a concept matches the real world.

7. Image blurring is an old trick to create better motion in movies and in TV. Once upon a time, for example, TV cameras at NBA games blurred the basketball, so that it moved more smoothly.

8. Note to the mathematically inclined: when an image is sampled, the crucial variable is the sampling rate. For digital camera sensors, this is a function of both photosite size and spacing. Ideally, the sampling rate will exceed the Nyquist rate, minimum sampling rate required to avoid "aliasing," which in linear systems terms is the creation of the spurious spatial frequency replicas of the Fourier spectrum. The sampling rate must be high enough to drive the replicas outside of the 60 cycle/degree range of human vision. Otherwise, they create image artifacts.

9. Analog means that it can take on any value, 1.5, 1.6, 3.3, etc. This contrasts with digital values, which are only whole numbers, 1, 2, 3, 4, etc. "Quantization" is the conversion of analog to digital values.

10. In HDR, the photographer takes a series of shots with increasing exposure duration in order to move the dynamic range downward. Software then sews the individual images together to create one big dynamic range. However, exposure duration must be carefully calibrated. My experience measuring actual camera exposure times has shown that camera setting and actual durations often differ.

11. In one sense, photosites are analogous to photoreceptors but in another they are analogous to "receptive fields," the area of retinal photoreceptors that contribute to the postreceptor cell's response. In dim light the area grows, favoring sensitivity but losing resolution. In bright light, the area shrinks and inhibition further sharpens resolution and decreases sensitivity.

12. One line of psychophysical research uses laser interference fringes to create images directly on the viewer's retina without the usual optical degradation created by the lens and cornea. The results showed that the eye's neural components and optical components are perfectly matched and that humans have evolved the best possible visual system given the limitation of our optics. That is, even if the eye's optics could create a sharper image, there would be no improvement in contrast sensitivity or acuity. Of course, what would be the point of having a neural acuity capacity that could never be realized due to limited optics?

13. This is why photographers often use the "standard" 18 percent gray card to set exposure—the camera presumably meters on exactly the assumed reflectance.

14. Many discussions of CRTs state that having a nonlinear gamma of 2.2–2.5 is a good thing because the eye's response to light is also nonlinear. Recall from Chapter 2 that brightness is a compressive function which rises quickly from 0 and then begins to level off. In contrast, the CRTs' gamma causes the output to rise slowly at first and then to accelerate. By a quirk of fate, the CRT gamma nonlinear roughly compensates for the eye's nonlinearity, so the combination of the two comes out linear. This is nice but irrelevant to the current discussion, which is concerned with reproduction of scene luminances directly to an image. Here, any nonlinearity is bad.

15. Photographic negatives can capture a much larger dynamic range, but the printing process limits the final picture to the small range.

16. 8 bits of each primary = 256 reds × 256 greens × 256 blues = 16.7 million.

17. The exact number depends on room luminance. It will be greater in darker rooms because the effect of scatter light from the white checks is larger.

18. TV signals are processed to create an input-output gamma of about 1.2. Slide film (remember that?), which was designed for viewing in the dark, had a gamma of 1.5.

# Chapter 19

# Forensic Vision Toolkit

Bernard S. Abrams, O.D.

***Synopsis***



## 19.1 The Practice of Forensic Visibility

### A. Introduction

The practice of forensic visibility by a vision specialist is, relatively speaking, in its infancy and growing with the general recognition that vision is of major importance, primarily in vehicular accidents. When litigation results from those accidents with a resultant question of fault, human visibility expertise is needed to understand what happened and why. Night visibility, in particular, has gained prominence due to the high injury and death rates related to vehicular accidents at night.

Forensic practice is distinguished from other areas of consultation largely by the system (legal) in which one works. Most practice is in the civil, as opposed to the criminal system (however, this author has worked in both areas), so most of what is important to the forensic consultant does not appear on L.A. Law! Most cases are settled before trial primarily as a result of the fact that both sides will know the theories, opinions, and basis for these opinions well in advance of trial through a "discovery" process.

For visibility experts the important parts of discovery are our depositions and/or written reports. A deposition is composed of questions asked of the vision specialist practitioner by the opposing attorney, answered under oath, and recorded for later typing by a court reporter. The practitioner's client (the attorney) will play a minor role here, possibly objecting (for the record and possible later ruling by the judge) to improper or confusing questions, or simply alerting the witness to a specific word in the question that might change its meaning. The expert witness might be asked his or her opinions, the analyses behind those opinions, his or her qualifications to render such opinions, and even questions concerning fees and other cases on which he or she has worked. Part of the deposition also examines a witness' communication style and evaluates how well the expert witness might impress a jury and stand up under cross-examination.

In the experience of this author, written reports are frequently called for; if they are, they are "discoverable" by the other side. Strong and well-presented reports and/or depositions may be used by one's own side to attempt a favorable settlement.

Trial testimony consists of direct examination by one's own attorney, followed by cross-examination by the opposing attorney (and occasionally redirect, recross, ad nauseam). "Direct" includes the expert witness' qualifications, work performed, and opinions formed. Because the witness can respond only to questions asked, it is important that direct be carefully worked out in advance with the attorney. One of the worst moments in court is when the employing attorney asks the expert witness a question to which the attorney really doesn't want the answer. Experienced, knowledgeable attorneys will need preparation, even if the expert's deposition or report and curriculum vitae (CV) are fairly complete. This expert has found it useful to discuss a specifically exemplar case(s) with the retaining attorneys, outlining strengths and his experiences that might be related to the specifics of that case.

The visibility forensic practitioner has only one opportunity to communicate effectively to the judge and jury. A frustrating aspect of this occurs when objections are raised by the opposing attorney and ruled on by the judge. Although the jury will make the ultimate decision, the judge will make many decisions along the way in response to objections and motions. Sometimes the clear and complete analysis that had been prepared will not be allowed to reach the jury. If the jury doesn't understand what is said or doesn't believe it, then all of the expert witness' efforts may be for naught.

During cross-examination the visibility practitioner attempts to defend his or her credentials, opinions, analysis, and general credibility before the judge and jury. All manner of trick questions and emotional ploys might be used in an attempt to discredit the witness. He or she will be asked yes/no questions when either response would be misleading to the jury, and skill at squeezing in explanations around objections may be critical. The practitioner's decision to continue or no continue forensic practice will probably be made during cross-examination.

## B. A Hypothetical Case

Consider an accident involving a small vehicle that during darkness went off a two-lane rural road onto the shoulder after swerving to avoid a nonlighted, stopped tractor/trailer. The vehicle then went out of control when its driver tried to re-enter the roadway. The tort liability against both the highway department and the tractor/trailer was based on improper road design and failure to place a retroreflective triangle, respectively. A civil engineer in road design presented analyses and opinions on these issues for the plaintiff.

The defense involved not only arguments about the roadway, but also the fact that the driver had sufficient time to avoid the crash based on .75 second alert reaction time. A visibility expert was retained by the plaintiff's attorney to assist in examining evidence, and analyzing the reaction times and visibility distances available to the driver.

The expert's testimony would be used chiefly in the direct testimony of the plaintiff's case, and/or in rebuttal of the defense's position, or not at all if analysis showed the driver had, in fact, had time to avoid the crash. (The various experts base their analyses on the accident site, the plaintiff's deposition, the police accident report, engineering reports, reaction time, light levels, and road drawings.)

The site in the hypothetical case was on a dark, nonlighted road which was curved and lined with trees and brush to create a "dark hole." Given this complexity of night visual observation of the scene and assuming the speed of the vehicles, the visibility expert should be able with headlight profiles to calculate a point of sighting, then explain to the jury when the cone of vision of the driver directly encompassed the other vehicle and the approximate time it appeared. Assuming this ideal, one estimates the distance of the first step of visibility between the vehicles and the perception/reaction time available for the vehicle to avoid the tractor/trailer. This perception/reaction distance at night in an unexpected situation would be, in this author's opinion, between 2.5 seconds to 3.5 seconds.

The four steps are detection, identification, perception, and reaction. Based on the plaintiff's testimony, the vision expert then divides this time (2.5 to 3.5 seconds) into four segments:

1. Detection: of the parked object and its position.
2. Identification: of the object as a parked tractor and the danger due to its inability to move.
3. Decision: that a danger or hazard condition existed due to the fact that movement of the object stopped, recognized that it is necessary to attempt an avoidance or evading maneuver.
4. Reaction: by sending a message to the muscular skeleton system to leave the road.

A chart was drawn for the jury showing these categories and the processes of visual and human factor detection, identification, decision making, and reaction with both estimated average and complex times and distances at the end of the four stages.

A critical question would be why the vehicle driver did not apply his brakes before going off the road. By entering this possible perception/reaction time into the analysis, the visibility expert was able to estimate that under the best reaction conditions, the distance between vehicles would have been only forty feet when the brakes could have been applied. The opinion of the reconstructionist was that had braking been selected, a head-on or out-of-control collision might have occurred. The visibility expert also gave opinions regarding factors that would increase processing time, such as non-expectancy or surprise.

Experience suggests that the jury's acceptance of opinions of vision experts is based on credibility in structuring four issues:

1. Estimates of the discernibility related to sight distance.
2. Explanation why 2.5 to 3.5 seconds for perception reaction was valid and .75 seconds was in error.
3. Explanation of what steps the driver had to accomplish within this critical period when 90 percent of the information necessary to guide a vehicle to a safe stop is processed.

## C. The Practitioner's Role

Accident causation and the surrounding technical and social systems and environment are often complex. Ideally, it might be desirable to have many experts. As in any field of practice, however, resources of both time and money are limited, so the attorney might employ, in addition to a night visibility specialist, a reconstructionist to cover all of the issues that the many experts might have addressed.

The practitioner must look at this from two opposing perspectives. The obvious primary perspective is one's ethical and professional responsibility not to offer opinions outside one's knowledge and experience. The other perspective is the difficult one. If the practitioner chooses not to express an opinion in some area, how will the judge and jury pursue questions related to that area?

Either another, possibly less qualified expert fills in, or the judge and jury base their decisions on prior learning. Thus, the training, experience, education, background and research, if any, come into play.

Probably the clearest example is in the night vision area as related to visibility, discernibility, and reaction times, where so-called experts, lacking valid scientific training or experience, have been expressing opinions for many years. In today's world, these tests are the "Frye rule" or the "Daubert rule."

Forensic visibility, in particular, is an important area for the professional who understands illumination, diseases, and vision. It has high visibility for both the practitioner and the profession. However, the forensic area is also fraught with difficulties and dangers ranging from procedural complexities and subtleties to ethical dilemmas. It is a challenge that can be worthwhile but should not be taken without forethought and preparation.

This introduction is a composite of the thoughts of many distinguished practitioners in the field of forensic human factors, visibility, and the jurisprudence system.

*I am particularly indebted to the following individuals: Dr. Gordon H. Robinson, Dr. Merrill J. Allen, and Lyman Brownfield, Esq., from whose writings and thoughts I have borrowed liberally for this chapter.*

## 19.2 Questions

### A. Work/Note Questions You May Be Asked to Answer in Order to Qualify As a Nighttime Visibility Expert

1. Any formal training in the visual function of the human eye?
2. Any formal courses or degrees in physiological optics? Please describe your understanding of physiological optics.
3. Are you a member of the Illuminating Engineering Society of North America?
4. Are you a member of the Human Factors Society?
5. Are you a member of the National Safety Council?
6. Are you a member of the International Traffic Engineers Society?
7. Are you a member of the Forensic Engineers Society?
8. Are you a member of the American Institute of Physics?
9. Are you a member of the Optical Society of America?
10. Have you ever been qualified as an optical or visibility consultant? Do you consider yourself an expert in visibility?
11. Have you ever been certified as an accident reconstructionist?
12. Have you ever been qualified as an accident reconstructionist?
13. Have you ever read the nighttime concepts of traffic reconstruction issued by the University of Michigan Transportation Institute?
14. Is it your testimony that you performed a nighttime accident reconstruction of this accident including a nighttime visibility reconstruction?
15. Isn't nighttime visibility reconstruction more effective when accomplished by one trained in physiological optics?
16. Have you ever written any books, articles, or papers on nighttime visibility? Discernibility? If not, what learned treatises have you read?
17. What is the difference between visibility and discernibility?
18. Have you ever heard of Dr. Merrill Allen?

19. Have you read his book? Papers? If so, which?
20. Have you ever heard of Dr. Herschel W. Liebowitz? In what respect?
21. Have you ever taught courses related to accidents? What subjects? Any visibility? Any visibility human factors? Have you attended such courses? Full-time or single lectures? Name instructors.
22. Define human factors.
23. Are you familiar with the terminology "perception/reaction"? Explain.
24. What steps are involved in perception/reaction?
25. Can you explain the visual pathway components from visual stimulus to discernment?
26. Do you have formal training in human factors?
27. Do you know of Dr. Paul Olson?
28. Have you read any of his treatises? Do you agree with them?
29. Is he an expert in perception/reaction? Was his training as a visibility professional?
30. Are you familiar with the theory of veiling glare? Disability glare? Discomfort glare? If so, describe.
31. Do you know the definition of low luminance acuity?
32. Do you know the definition of low contrast acuity?
33. Do you know the definition of glare susceptibility?
34. Do you know the definition of glare recovery?
35. Do you know the definition of low contrast target detection threshold?
36. Do you know the definition of photopic vision? If so, describe.
37. Do you know the definition of scotopic vision? If so, describe.
38. Do you know the definition of mesopic vision? If so, describe.
39. What cellular tissue of the eye is used in each (Nos. 36, 37 and 38 above)?
40. Do you know what the fovea is? Describe.
41. What is foveal cone of vision? Can you calculate foveal cone at 200 feet?
42. Do you know what rods and cones are? Define the function.
43. Define illuminance. How is it measured?
44. Do you know the patterns or isocandela of headlights? Low-beam? High beam? What are SAE recommendations?
45. Do you have any idea whether visual function declines as illumination declines? At what light levels does function change?
46. Have you done research work in reaction time? In automobile accidents?
47. Can expectancy affect reaction time?
48. What is positive guidance?
49. Who is Hal Lunenfield?
50. Have you done any studies dealing with how driving at night differs from driving in the day time? Research? Do you research?
51. In reaching your conclusions, did you take into account any optical factors?
52. In reaching your conclusions, did you take into account any vision factors?
53. What is a vision time line?
54. Do you consider yourself an expert in the field of driver response time? Visual pathway? Nighttime visibility?
55. In your calculations did you use perception and reaction times? Before or after motor reaction?

56. Isn't the standard perception/reaction time used in highway design 2.5 seconds (AASHTO)?
57. If it takes a driver longer to perceive and react, is it going to take him longer to stop his car?
58. Does expectancy enter into your calculations?
59. Have you ever done any research yourself into perception/reaction time as applied to automobiles?
60. Are you familiar with the term "surprise intrusion"?
61. Are you qualified to formulate opinions about properties and characteristics of light?
62. Do you have sufficient training expertise to give opinions about light properties? If so, explain.
63. Do you know the meaning of scientific terms related to light? Lux?
64. Are you or have you been licensed in this or any other state as an eye doctor? Optometrist? Ophthalmologist?
65. What degree do you have?
66. Do you consider your visual background to qualify you in the same manner as a trained eye doctor?
67. Can you define Snellen acuity? (quantity)
68. What is the formula?
69. If an object is 40 feet by 5 feet, what acuity is required at 1000 feet?
70. What is static acuity? How is it measured? What is 20/20?
71. What is dynamic acuity? What happens at night when it is used?
72. What is contrast sensitivity?
73. What articles have you reviewed on contrast? Have you ever been tested for contrast sensitivity?
74. What is the formula for contrast?
75. What was contrast at the scene? How did you measure it?
76. Have you taken courses relating to human factors? Vision?
77. When? Where?
78. Who were the instructors?
79. Have you heard of Dr. Bernard Abrams?
80. Have you read any of his articles? Attended his courses?
81. Do you recognize him as a visibility consultant?

## B. Questions You May Be Asked Relating to Nighttime Accidents on Cross-Examination

1. Please give a brief description of your former subspecialty in nighttime visibility as related to vehicular accidents.
2. What training and studies have you had in the area of nighttime vision?
3. Have you been qualified as an expert in other cases? If so, what percentage for plaintiffs and what percentage for defendants?
4. Are you being compensated for your time here today based on your knowledge of the human eye?
5. Can you describe briefly for us how it is that we see? Do you wish to use diagrams or exhibits?

6. What is it that enables us to see and recognize objects at night?
7. How does the eye work?
8. Function of cones.
   a. Day or bright conditions
   b. Produce clearest image
   c. Able to perceive color
   d. Area of foveal cone
9. How do the following aspects of vision form what we see and how well we see?
   a. Visual acuity-clarity and sharpness
   b. Depth perception
10. How many vision systems does a human have?
11. What are these systems?
12. How do they differ?
13. According to your research, the use of which vision system is found in most accidents during scotopic, mesopic, and photopic conditions?
14. What is required for an object to be discernible at night?
15. What visual conditions are important to the nighttime driver?
16. Can you explain to the jury what is meant by the term "human factors"?
17. Can you explain some of the human factor considerations applicable to motor vehicle collisions and nighttime driving?
18. What four steps of driver information processing are important to you in evaluating a case?
19. Is driver response time different in daylight hours as opposed to when it is dark? If so, why?
20. Can you explain to the jury the meaning of the following terms?
    a. Illumination
    b. Luminance
    c. Reflectivity
21. Can you explain what the term "visibility" means?
22. Can you explain what the term "cognitive discernibility" means?
23. Can you describe nighttime visibility with headlight illumination?
24. What is it that enables us to see and recognize objects at night?
25. At the scene, did you conduct any of the following testing?
    a. What sources of light are available at this nighttime scene? Did you take into account the following:
       1) Environment?
       2) Luminaires?
       3) Headlights?
       4) Signs?
    b. What about the moon?
       1) What effect did it have on your analysis? How did you arrive at your conclusions?
    c. What is "valley of darkness" or "black hole"?
       1) Where can you find "black hole" literature?
    d. What readings were taken?
       1) Ambient light?
       2) Reflectivity?

26. What steps in your analysis have you done as it relates to vision?
    a. Review data.
        1) Transcripts of depositions?
        2) Summaries of depositions?
        3) Discuss case with counsel?
        4) View state highway patrol photographs and reports?
        5) Review learned treatises?
        6) Site visit?
    b. When did you visit the accident scene?
        1) Dates: day/night?
        2) What did you do at accident scene?
        3) Take any measurements?
        4) Consult photographs/deposition transcript?
        5) Describe the road at the scene of the accident?
    c. Have you had an illumination map prepared to show lighting conditions at night on the scene?
    d. Third step in your analysis-weather report.
        1) Why is it important?
        2) How do you check the weather?
        3) What assumptions were made about weather at the time of the accident?
27. Will your testimony help the jury in understanding how this incident took place?
28. Unless otherwise indicated, will you state all of your opinions today with a reasonable degree of professional and scientific probability based on your experience, training, background, and research?
29. What makes your knowledge and expertise different from:
    a. an accident reconstructionist?
    b. a mechanical engineer?
    c. a photographer?
    d. a state trooper?
    e. a visibility expert?
    f. a human factors expert?

## 19.3 Nighttime Visibility Expert on Direct Examination

### A. Hypothetical Case Review and Decision

IN THE COURT OF APPEALS, COUNTY OF UNKNOWN
George H. Ogle, et al.
Plaintiff: No. 33XY-196-53
v.
Arthur Greene
Defendant
Jonathan Edwards, L.P.A., for the Plaintiff
Smith, Smith & Smith, for the Defendant

Plaintiff George Ogle, on August 13, 1983, at approximately 10:30 p.m., was walking along the right edge of State Route 631. His car had broken down and he was walking to the nearest town or village to seek assistance. As he was walking along the roadway, he was struck from behind by a vehicle driven by Arthur Greene, the defendant, who was traveling southbound on State Route 631, an unlit, rural, two-lane highway with rolling hills. It was a clear night.

Ogle alleges that defendant Greene negligently operated the motor vehicle he was driving by failing to maintain assured clear distance ahead.

The plaintiff, Ogle, a dentist, age 40, said the personal injuries he sustained had required multiple surgeries and lengthy therapy and that said injuries and resultant handicap made it impossible for him to return to work for his lifetime.

The plaintiff seeks compensation for personal injury, pain, and suffering in the amount of $4 million. Additionally, he seeks compensation for hospital, medical, and therapy expenses incurred during his recovery from said injuries in the amount of $178,365.33. The plaintiff also seeks compensation for loss of wages, both past and future, in the amount of $2,500,000.00 (25 years × $100,000.00).

Additionally, the plaintiff's spouse, Mary Ogle, joins in the suit, seeking compensatory damages for mental anguish plus loss of services and, on behalf of the plaintiff's children, seeking compensatory damages for mental anguish and loss of society with the plaintiff in the amount of $2 million.

The defendant Greene was driving at approximately the posted speed limit of 35 miles per hour with his headlights on low beam. Greene said that as his vehicle approached a small crest in the road, he saw Ogle just before he struck him with the right front fender of his vehicle, knocking him to the pavement.

Green stopped his vehicle immediately and went back to assist Ogle who was unconscious and appeared to be severely injured. After putting a blanket over the injured man, Greene called for assistance on his cell phone.

The defendant, Greene, claimed that he saw Ogle just before impact and did not have enough time to stop or swerve out of the way. Greene claimed that he had no control over the circumstances as he was confronted by a sudden and unforeseeable emergency which made compliance with statute impossible.

Greene stated that the plaintiff was dressed in dark clothing and was walking on the right side of the road with his back to traffic, which is contrary to the State Revised Code. This requires that a pedestrian on a highway, where neither sidewalk nor a shoulder is available for use, must walk as near as he can to the outside edge of the roadway and on the left side of the roadway, facing oncoming traffic.

Defendant further claimed that the plaintiff was wearing dark clothing which made him difficult to discern. Under State Revised Codes, a "discernible object is a reasonably visible object. An object is discernible when it is visible or can be detected or perceived." Ogle contended that the plaintiff was nondiscernible until just before the impact, and therefore, the plaintiff committed an act or acts of negligence which directly and proximately caused his injury.

The plaintiff, Ogle, called Paul Jones, an expert in accident reconstruction, to discuss the issue of driver sight distance and reaction time. Quoting from a manual for drivers, Jones stated that visibility distance with low beams is 350 feet. Mr. Jones points out that on that basis, in his opinion, the driver should have had plenty of time to detect the plaintiff and avoid the impact. He further quoted numerous articles that stated perception reaction time was 1.5 seconds. Therefore, at 35 miles per hour (1.46 × 35) Green would need only to travel approximately 80 feet in 1.5 seconds and, with 350 feet sight distance, should have been able to view the plaintiff in time to avoid a collision.

Counsel for the plaintiff cited the statute relating to assured clear distance where there is a curve, hill, or an obstruction of view in the highway, the assured clear distance is that distance between the driver of a vehicle and the point where his vision ends or is cut off. The driver must drive at such a speed that he can stop within the distance between him and the point where his vision ends. The plaintiff alleged that the defendant was negligent in not maintaining assured clear distance ahead as defined by the State Revised Code.

The plaintiff's counsel also cited the State Revised Code referring to light. "Distribution of lights must be high enough to reveal persons, vehicles and substantial objects on the highway at a safe distance in advance of his moving vehicle." Plaintiff alleges that the defendant is negligent for not providing adequate illumination for the section of highway he was traveling.

In charging the jury, the judge explained to the jurors that the element of discernibility is at issue in the case and that in the statute, "discernible" implies something more than "visible." "Visible" means perceivable by the eye, whereas "discernible" means mentally perceptible or distinguishable; capable of being discerned by the understanding, not merely by the senses. Reasonably modified, "discernible" in this statute means an object which the driver should or could have seen if he was operating his vehicle at a speed which would have permitted him to bring the vehicle to a stop within an assured clear distance.

The judge further explained that the fact that some other cause concurred with negligence of the defendant in the production of an injury does not relieve him from liability, unless it is shown such other causes would have produced the injury independently.

The judge charged the jury to determine if the car driven by the defendant did strike an object-to wit, the plaintiff-that the object was ahead of the driver in his path of travel, that the object was stationary or moving in the same direction as the driver, that the object did not suddenly appear in the driver's path, and that the object was easily discernible.

Comparative negligence also was explained to the jurors. They were told that if comparative negligence was found to be involved, they would have to determine to what degree each party was at fault.

The jury rendered a verdict in favor of the plaintiff, against Greene. The jury found the defendant, Greene, 51 percent negligent and the plaintiff 49 percent negligent.

The Ogle v. Greene case is hypothetical and is an atypical conclusion to the vast number of night pedestrian traffic accident cases argued before juries all over the country. Most cases of "assured clear distance" and/or discernibility are found for the defendant.

The cases always involve questions of driver visibility and discernibility or when a driver could have or should have seen, or at what distance the driver should have discerned something, and what reaction time is involved.

Prior to the introduction of visibility experts, a common practice is for an accident investigator, usually a former police officer or possibly an engineer, to prepare a reconstruction of the event in an effort to determine answers to the questions. In the past, reconstructionists of night accidents, however, had some distinct limitations. They were not trained in accident reconstruction to understand how human factors and the visual information gathering system interact under nighttime conditions.

A paper by Olson (SAE 870600)[1] titled "Visibility Problems in Nighttime Driving" states that:

> Estimating something like nighttime detection distance for an object by measuring the distance at which one or even several persons can see it in a daylight reconstruction is like trying to estimate the stopping distance of a large truck by using a sports car. No judge would allow the latter type of evidence to be introduced. No judge should allow the former evidence to be introduced either.

There are visibility experts with backgrounds in vision, human factors, and a vast body of literature. In addition, Abrams[2] is conducting classes across the land for reconstructionists, engineers, and other interested parties.

This chapter is intended to summarize information on the question of driver visibility and discernibility under nighttime operating conditions and not to state a case for the defendant or plaintiff. The hope is that it will aid individuals involved in accident cases to better understand the information-gathering process. Then, with this knowledge each case can be judged on its own merits and an equitable decision can be rendered after a full disclosure of all of the facts to the jury.

It is absolutely essential for those who are involved in accident analysis to understand that 90 percent of all information-gathering is over the visual pathway and to be able to qualify as an expert who can assist the jury in understanding how the collision occurred.

Vital to that understanding are the steps in driver information processing. This is a four-step process that takes time, and that time varies from person to person. The four-step process involves detection, identification, decision, and response.

This multistep process is a general rule that applies to every driver. It means that before a driver can be expected to make an appropriate response to any roadway situation, four things have to happen: detection, identification, decision, and response. Detection is the conscious awareness that something is present in the roadway. Identification is the process of gathering information about the object in the road until enough information is gathered that the driver can make an appropriate decision as to what it is, whether it poses a threat, and whether its existence calls for some responsive action. The next step is decision, and this is the process of the driver's deciding on a response to the condition which has been identified. Then, finally, we have response. This occurs when orders are issued by the driver's brain to the appropriate muscle groups in order to initiate the responsive action decided upon.

## B. Use of Qualified Expert Witness with a Visibility Background

The previously discussed hypothetical case was a close decision for the plaintiff; however, let us now inject an expert on vision and associated human factors.

Let's presume in the testimony of the Ogle v. Greene case that the defendant, Greene, calls in visibility expert Tom Jackson who on direct examination can discuss such concepts as how we see and the average driver's night visual capabilities. He also defines what are reasonable response times to either an expected or unexpected object in the roadway ahead:

Tom Jackson-Direct Examination
Section II
(After qualifying as an expert)

*Mr. Jackson, will your testimony and your opinions assist the ladies and gentlemen of the jury in understanding how this collision occurred? And why?*

Jackson: It is a well-known fact that a disproportionately greater number of U.S. traffic fatalities and injuries occur at night. He points out that night vision is distinctly different from day vision (photopic) and that these different factors involved in night (scotopic) visibility need to be given consideration by the court as do the questions of what are reasonable responses. Understanding how humans function visually at night is a missing piece in case law and in sections of various State Revised Codes.

*Can you describe for us how it is that we see?*

Jackson proceeds to present basic information concerning visual perception to provide the jury with a foundation for understanding how the visual system works under nighttime driving conditions.

Jackson: Vision begins with the energy of electromagnetic radiation reaching the eye-that is, light that is either emitted or reflected from things.

Before seeing is possible, however, a new form of energy called a nerve impulse must relay the image message to the brain. It is within the dark confines of the skull where vision is created. Thus, it becomes evident that visual perception is the final outcome of a long chain of complex events.

It is dependent upon light rays that come into the eyes and form retinal images. It is further dependent upon the complex physiological process that takes place from the retina to the occipital lobe in the brain. Finally, it is directly dependent upon the brain activity itself. The termination of the impulse from the eye is in the occipital lobe of the brain along what is known as the optical pathway. This traveling of impulse can be measured by noninvasive technology and renders great information about what one is seeing, plus how one is thinking.

The cornea is the transparent front surface of the eye through which light enters. This lens helps bring light to focus on the retina while the iris controls the size of the opening in front of the lens (the pupil).

The retina is the light-sensitive layer of the eye which covers about two-thirds of the interior of the eye. The central portion of the retina is the fovea which plays a central role in visual acuity. The fovea is an area about two degrees in size where vision is the sharpest. Only five degrees to the left or right of the fovea, visual acuity is only half as much.

The retina contains two different types of cells-the rods and the cones. These cells differ functionally as well as in their distribution throughout the retina.

The cones function at higher (daytime) light levels, providing what is call photopic vision. They are wavelength sensitive, producing the sensation of color. Cones have far fewer neural interconnections and are hence capable of finer discriminations. Cones are found exclusively in the fovea and in rapidly diminishing numbers as one moves away from the fovea.

At low light levels (darkness or nighttime) the eye relies chiefly on a set of about 125 million cells called rods that are sensitive to small amounts of light and provide what is called scotopic vision. Rods are found throughout the retina with the exception of the fovea. They are not wavelength sensitive. Hence, a pure rod vision is in shades of gray.

There is a middle range of light levels in which both rods and cones function. This is called mesopic vision. Typically, night driving is done under mesopic conditions, depending on the amount of light available.

*How is nighttime defined?*

Jackson: Here is the definition of nighttime illumination as stated in the Illuminating Engineering Society Lighting Handbook, 1987 Reference Volume:

Nighttime: those hours between the end of evening civil twilight and the beginning of morning civil twilight when auxiliary illumination is needed to perform a task, such as driving.

Note: Civil twilight ends in the evening when the center of the sun's disk is six degrees below the horizon and begins in the morning when the center of the sun's disk is six degrees below the horizon.

*Can you explain why and how low-beam headlights are used?*

Jackson: Because of the limitations imposed by traffic flow and highway design, we primarily must use low beams to guide vehicles at night even though all vehicle headlamps offer two beams: a low-beam and a high-beam. However, drivers must use the low-beam headlight the vast majority of the time. The object of a low-beam headlight design is to get as much of the illumination below the horizontal axis (that is, approximately thirty-six inches above the ground) to reasonable levels, because it causes glare for other drivers. Typically, low-beam headlamps in automobiles produced for use in America illuminate an area between 150 and 175 feet in front of the automobile. They attenuate rapidly as they leave the headlamp, and at 175 feet the light drop off is approximately .3 foot candles or darkness by definition.

*Can you explain to me the meaning of the terms: illumination, luminance and reflectivity?*

Jackson: Illumination is the measure of the amount of light falling on a surface without respect to the direction from which the light comes, the type of light source, or the type of surface upon which it falls. The illumination will be the same whether the surface is a polished steel plate or a piece of black felt cloth. Luminance, on the other hand, is the measure of the amount and concentration of light leaving a surface. It is luminance that controls the magnitude of the sensation that the brain receives off an object. In other words, luminance is the amount of light reflected or "thrown off" by the object and is a key factor in how well we can see the object. The luminance of a surface depends upon the direction from which it is viewed and the reflective properties of the surface itself.

*What is it that enables us to see and recognize objects at night?*

Jackson: There are a number of factors that determine whether we will be able to observe and recognize an object at night. One of these is "conspicuity." Conspicuity (stemming from the word "conspicuous") is the sum of the characteristics of an object that determines the likelihood that the object will come to the attention of the observer. The fact that something may be present in the visual field does not necessarily mean that it will be detected because it may have less conspicuity than other visible features. Another important concept is that of "visibility." Visibility refers to how well something can be seen by the human eye. Visibility, therefore, involves human judgment. There is no device that can measure visibility directly. However, one key factor influencing visibility of an object is "contrast." Contrast refers to characteristics of an object that cause it to appear different or separate from something else. The eye responds to contrast. Under daylight levels of illumination, there are a variety of forms of contrast available-for example, color, texture, brightness. In addition, during daylight the visual system is operating at the highest level of sensitivity and has the greatest capability of distinguishing differences between objects in the visual field. However, at night, brightness contrast is generally the only form of contrast of any consequence and the visual system has a reduced capability for distinguishing differences between objects in the visual field. Thus, in order to be seen at night, objects must be sufficiently brighter or darker than their backgrounds. Specifically, in nighttime driving conditions, an object will be discernible in the forward visual field if it is illuminated by the headlights of an approaching vehicle until it is sufficiently brighter than the background to be seen. White or reflectorized objects are discernible at approximately twice the distance as dark objects.

*Why is it that sometimes we humans do not see an object?*

Jackson: Because the foveal area or cone of vision of the retina is so small relative to the entire visual field, detection typically occurs in the periphery. It may take several "glimpses"-combinations of eye movements and fixations-before an object, depending on reflectivity, in the peripheral visual field can be recognized. However, in order to be detected, an object in the periphery must be much more conspicuous than if its image had fallen on the fovea.

This multiple-glimpse requirement for recognition is one reason why accepting a "standard human reaction time" of 0.75 seconds for response often is not applicable in non-laboratory settings and tasks.

This presents a simple scientific fact: The variation of object reflectivity accounts for why people, even careful observers, sometimes don't see what is there to be seen.

Responding to what is seen takes time. The time for a driver to respond to the stimulus of a traffic situation or hazard equals the time it takes for the driver to recognize the situation, understand the situation, decide to take action, and take that action. In brief, that four-step process, as mentioned above, is detection, identification, decision-making, and reaction.

*Why are the four steps of driver information processing important to us in this case? And why is expectancy a factor?*

Jackson: They are important to us, quite simply, because taken together, they constitute "driver perception/reaction time." These four steps, which will always occur in sequence, require time to accomplish. How much time varies, depending upon the circumstances, and that is very important to our understanding of the collision we are concerned with here. In order to fully appreciate the concept of driver response time, it is necessary that we consider one other fact, and that is driver expectancy.

Based upon their driving experience, people develop expectations about matters such as traffic control devices, roadway design, and driver behavior. This is true for both night and day driving although it becomes more important at night because so much of the information available during the day is lost when it becomes dark. Accordingly, a driver's response time will be affected by his expectations of the environment. For example, in a school zone, one is cautioned to expect children. Most drivers know that children are sometimes unpredictable. Hence, a driver will be alert to a child's darting out into the street after a ball or otherwise in the furtherance of some childhood endeavor. Because the driver has been alerted to expect such an occurrence, his or her response time will be less.

Likewise, if a driver is cautioned to be alert to falling rock and the driver rounds a curve to find a boulder in the roadway, his or her response time will be less than if he or she had not been warned of the possibility of such an occurrence. The important points to be made are that all drivers have expectations, and these expectations are based on general experience. When these expectations must be violated, great care should be taken to alert approaching drivers to the condition in sufficient time so that they can make the necessary adjustments. It is very important to understand that this is not a question of whether a driver is paying attention or not. It is a question, rather, of how long it takes the driver to process information that comes to his attention in order to create object discernibility.

At any given point in time there may be a great deal of information imaged on the retina. However, while the brain handles information very rapidly, it also handles it serially. At night new information is most likely to appear on the retinal periphery where it is less well seen, and it must be strong enough to capture the attention of the observer. In motor vehicle operation, the time available for this to happen is typically fairly short.

In recent years, it is generally accepted in the field that driver response time is "elastic," and during non-daylight hours the time is between 2.5 and 3 seconds. It is important to understand, however, that perception reaction time begins when the driver becomes aware of an object in his field of vision.

*What does the term peripheral filter mean to us? And how does it affect conspicuity?*

Jackson: The peripheral filter is a mechanism which determines what will come to the attention of the observer. While the way the filter works is not yet understood, the types of stimuli that are likely to create a foveal fixation or saccade are known. In general, they are objects that differ greatly from their backgrounds in terms of brightness, texture, and color; objects that are flickering or flashing; objects of large size; and object that are moving.

The fact that something may be present in the visual field does not necessarily mean that it will be detected because it may have less conspicuity than other visible features.

*What is visual acuity?*

Jackson: The measure of visual performance at a doctor's office which most people are familiar with is called static acuity, or a measure of the ability to distinguish fine detail in a high contrast stationary target and generally represented as a comparative figure-for example, 20/20. This is the standard test used for obtaining a driver's license. A number of other measures of visual acuity are more meaningful in the night driving such as low-luminance acuity, low-contrast acuity, glare susceptibility, glare recovery time, and low-contrast target detection threshold.

*Why is driver response different during nighttime as opposed to when it is daylight in this case?*

Jackson: Things become even more complicated with night driving because of low light and low contrast. They are important elements in being able to discern various objects, including pedestrians from their background.

"Contrast" is defined as those characteristics that cause something to appear different or separate from something else. The eye responds to contrast. Contrast is far more important in determining whether something will be visible and depends primarily on illumination-incident lighting on an object-and the luminance-reflected light of an object.

For example, a person with a white shirt has a reflectance factor of 80 percent and will stand out from a darker night surrounding while a person wearing blue jeans has a reflectivity of 6 percent and will be difficult to distinguish at nighttime.

During daytime levels of illumination, due to the photopic eye functioning, there are a variety of forms of contrast available-color, texture, brightness. In addition, the visual system is operating at its highest level of foveal sensitivity and has its greatest capability of distinguishing differences and finite details.

However, under nighttime driving conditions, when this accident occurred, due to the scotopic eye function, the visual system has a significantly reduced capability of distinguishing differences. Brightness contrast is generally the only form of contrast of any consequence. The job of the headlights is to provide the necessary illumination to create object brightness contrast from its background.

*Why is your opinion different than Mr. Jones'? (Plaintiff's expert)*

Jackson: The setting in which the accident involving Ogle and Greene took place was a rural area with many trees at both sides of the roadway creating a black tunnel effect. There were no streetlights and no ambient lighting. The plaintiff was wearing low reflective (6 percent) dark denim clothing which, due to its low contrast, blended into the background making him difficult to discern.

*Why do you feel Mr. Jones' opinion of low beams 350 feet sight distance at night is in error?*

Jackson first points out 350 is an error and is used for high beams which, due to opposing traffic, were not permitted. In addition, this State Code requires object visibility at 175 feet but does not specify object color.

Jackson then proceeds to introduce results of a field test of different head-lighting systems and four possible pedestrian targets wearing various types of clothing-three clad in various denim and one in a white vest.

Jackson: The analyses suggest that when confronted with a low-contrast object, such as an unexpected pedestrian wearing dark clothing in a rural setting, low-beam headlights will not provide adequate detection-identification distance at speeds in excess of 35 mph. If the pedestrian is approaching from the left side of the vehicle, with most of the energy from headlights focused on the right, the detection-identification problem became more pronounced.

The data indicated that pedestrians who must venture forth at night can make themselves much more likely to be seen by wearing light-colored garments and/or reflective tapes; otherwise, they are laying a trap for approaching drivers.

Additionally, there is evidence (Allen, Hazlett, 1970) that indicates that individuals who walk in traffic at night overestimate by a factor of two the driver visibility distance provided by the oncoming vehicle's lighting system.

*Assuming all of the facts you have stated to be true, and based upon your education, training and experience, as well as your investigation of this occurrence, do you have an opinion, which you can state with a reasonable degree of professional and scientific probability as to the visibility of Mr. Ogle on the roadway at the scene of this occurrence?*

Jackson: Yes.

*In your opinion, was Mr. Ogle discernible to Mr. Greene in time for him to avoid or evade this incident? And what facts do you base your answer on?*

Jackson: Based on the facts presented in this case, in my opinion, the plaintiff, Ogle, was non-discernible to the defendant, Greene, in sufficient time to avoid or evade a collision. I base my opinion on the following facts:

1. Low contrast factors of pedestrian and background
2. Headlight profile
3. Perception/reaction times
4. Distances at which the prior three items occur
5. Time required to avoid prior to maneuver

*...Now, with this new information, you be the judge and jury and decide if the original decision was correct or in error in this case.*

## 19.4 Suggested List of Documentation Which May Be Needed for Visibility and Human Factors Evaluation

All accidents require pre- and post-impact data. The sensory mechanism most basically involved is vision. It is essential to comprehend the physiological visual functions in order to assess the human factors that guide a driver's response.

From the case studies, it is relatively easy to infer the kind of evidence that will be needed in a given type of accident. For example, in a simple skid to a stop with no collision, the key elements are length of skid, slope of roadway, type of road surface, and condition of road surface. The vehicle weight is irrelevant in this case.

For collisions, in addition to the evidence cited above, vehicle weights become important. In addition, it is important to determine exactly where the collision took place-the point of impact. Photographs or diagrams should document the precise angles that any skid marks have relative to each other and to clearly defined road directions such as center lines. Furthermore, any collateral damage to obstacles such as trees, fire hydrants, buildings, and the like should be documented as completely as possible. Photographs should be taken of each vehicle from angles such that the depth of crush can be estimated fairly accurately.

For accidents involving loss of control due to travelling around a curve, the exact shape of the yaw mark (assuming there is one) should be documented. The critical measurement is the radius of curvature of this mark and any bank angle of the roadway.

For accidents involving visibility/discernibility problems, it is important to determine the sight distance, lighting, and weather conditions at the time to name a few. If the accident occurred at night, then it is critical to determine the position of any lights that may have distracted or blinded a driver involved in the incident. If the accident occurred at dawn or dusk, then it is important to determine the exact time of the accident and the sky conditions that existed at that time-an overcast sky will greatly reduce light, while a sunset will greatly increase it.

For accidents involving an airborne object, it is important, if possible, to determine the point from which the object left the ground, the point at which it returned to the ground, and the point where it finally came to rest. Often the mistaken assumption is made that where the object finally came to rest is where it first hit the ground. This is not usually the case. However, it will require a careful examination of the ground to find where the object first struck.

The following pages list suggested information which you may need to document the forensic visibility aspects of this incident. The information obtained should be divided into two sections: (1) pre-impact and (2) post-impact.

**Vehicle at Scene Documentation**
**Visibility Aspects**
**Pre-Impact**

A. Minimum View 1000 Feet Prior to Impact

   1. Written Description

B. Obtain Light Level

   1. Time:________________ Environmental:_________

      Luminaire:____________ Other: _________________

   2. Sun Rise _______ Sun Set _______ Both ________

C. Obtain Vehicle Windshield Data

   1. Windshields: Clear _____ Tint _____ Color _____

      Dirty _____ Scratched _____ Sloped _____

      Other _______ Photo _____

D. Color of Car __________ Pantone ________ Y _____ X ______

   1. Sample Paint

   2. Percent Reflectance

E. Inspect Lighting System

   1. Headlight

      a. Lens: Dirty _____ Scratched _______

      b. Filament _________

      c. Low/High: ________

      d. Ground to Bulb: _________ to Center: _________

      e. Separation: __________

      f. Type: _______________

   2. Taillight

      a. Dirty _____ Pitted _____ Scratch _______

         SAE #________ Lens Color _________

         Stop _________ Turn _______ Regular __________

         Transmission % _____ Y _______ X ________ Each ________

         Other __________

F. Sight Distance/Site Distance

1. Day
2. Night
3. Obstruction-Describe

G. Road: Asphalt ____________ % Ref.

Concrete ___________ % Ref.

H. Background: Visual Clutter: ______ Clear ______

Luminance: Absolute _______ % ________

Other: ______________________________

I. Driver V-1

a. Wear Glasses ______ Tint

b. Age _____

c. Size _____

Driver V-2

a. Wear Glasses ______ Tint

b. Age _____

c. Size _____

J. Other Involved

a. Pedestrian

Clothes Color: _______ Pants _______ Shirt _______

Size _______ Shoes _______ Other _______

b. Locomotive (See Railroad Work Up)

c. Bicycle

Color _____ Headlamp ________

Reflector ________ % ______ Size ________

Location: ________________

K. Weather/Climatology

Rain ______ Estimate Light, Medium, Heavy

Fog ___ Estimate Light, Medium, Heavy

Snow ______ Estimate Light, Medium, Heavy

Mist ______ Estimate Light, Medium, Heavy

Condition: Wet ___ Dry ____ Snow _____ Ice _____

L. Road Design: 1000 Feet Prior to Scene

Draw Map

Items: Signs, Houses, Driveways, Contour, etc.

2 Lane ______ 4 Lane _______ Other _________

M. Visual Clutter-Describe

N. Traffic Controls/Location

1000 Feet Prior Signs ______ Road _______ Berm _______

Signals _______ Other _______

O. Special Conditions

a. Construction

Describe Controls ___________________________

b. School

c. Hospital

d. Urban _____ City ________ Township _________

e. Other/Describe

**Post-Impact Documentation**
**Visibility Aspects**
**Scene Data Required**

1. Moon Evaluation as to Light Quantity, Azimuth, Bearing.
2. Sun Evaluation as to Azimuth and Location.
3. Percent Transmission of Windshield
4. Taillight/Headlight SAE Number: _________

   Height/Ground Center Bulb _____________

   Angular Separation: Center to Center___________
5. Retro-Reflection Signs
   a. Age
   b. Type
   c. Condition
6. Truck Light/Lens Inspection
   a. Age
   b. Condition
   c. Emission
   d. Lens

7. Retro-Reflection Tapes
    a. Location
    b. Condition
    c. Type
8. Photographs
9. Dynamic Photo Documentation
10. Drivers Health Records
    a. Vision
    b. Medicine
    c. Height, Weight, Age
11. Contrast of Scene (Quality)
12. Geometric Optics (Quantity)
13. M.U.T.C.D. Requirements
14. Headlight Profile
15. Street Light Profile

## Endnotes

1. Dr. Paul Olson, U.M.T.R.I.

2. Dr. Bernard Abrams, Institute of Vehicular Safety.

# Appendix B

# Geometric Optics

Bernard S. Abrams, O.D.

*Synopsis*



## B.1 Sample Work Problems

### A. Retinal cells

**Problem**: Which retinal cells are activated?

Illumination: 5000 fc
Object reflectivity: 50%
Background reflectivity: 3%
.50 × 5000 = 2500 fl
2500 × 3.4 = 8500 cd/m$^2$

**Answer**: Photopic vision (3.4 cd/m$^2$) with pure cone cell = equal to normal day.

**Problem**: Which cells are activated?

Illumination: 1.5 fc
Object reflectance: 50%
Background reflectivity: 3%
.50 × 1.5 = .75 fl
.75 Fl × 3.4 = 2.5 cd/m$^2$

**Answer**: Mesopic vision (.34 cd/m$^2$) = dusk driving with combination of cone and rod cells.

**Problem**: Which cells are activated?

Illumination: .1 fc
Object reflectance: 50%
Background reflectivity: 3%
.50 × .1 = .05 fl
.05 × 3.4 = .017 cd/m$^2$

**Answer**: Scotopic vision (.034 cd/m$^2$) = night; rod cells.

## B. Time and distance required with 20/20 acuity

**Problem**: Time and distance required for driver with 20/20 acuity to read signs on highway.

| | |
|---|---|
| Sign letters: | 6” |
| Speed: | 60 mph |
| Driver visual acuity: | 20/20 |
| 20/20 = | 5’ of arc |
| tan = | side opposite/over side adjacent |
| 1 degree = | 60 minutes |
| tan 1 degree = | .017455 |
| 1 minute = | $\frac{.017455}{60} = .0002909$ |

5’ = 5 × .0002909 = .0014545

Distance

$$\tan 5' = .00145 = \frac{6''(\text{letters})}{X''(\text{distance})}$$

$$.00145X = \frac{6''}{.00145X}$$

$$\text{Distance required} = 4137'' = \frac{4137}{12} = 344.75 \text{ feet}$$

Time

feet per second:

1 hour = 60 minutes

1 minute = 60 seconds

1 hour = 3600 seconds

1 mile = 5280 feet

$$\frac{5280}{3600} = 1.466 \text{ feet per second} \times \text{mph} = \text{feet per second traveled}$$

1.47 × speed = distance traveled at known speed

60 mph = 1.47 × 60 = miles per second = 88.2 feet per second

$$\frac{344.75}{88.2} = 3.9 \text{ seconds}$$

Time required = 3.9 seconds

A driver with 20/20 visual acuity will have 3.9 seconds available to read the sign at 60 mph or 88 feet per second.

Commentary: Ample time for decision making.

## C. Read signs with reduced acuity

**Problem**: Read signs/time/speed with reduced acuity.

| | | |
|---|---|---|
| Facts: | Acuity: | 20/100 |
| | Letter/signs: | 6” (inches) |
| | Vehicle speed: | 60 mph |
| | Design used for 20/20 visual acuity (344 feet) | |

| | |
|---|---|
| Each 5’ arc = | 20/20 |
| 20/20 = | tan 5’ arc= .0014545 (See Section B.) |

20/100 = tan 25' arc= .0072729 (Calculated similar to Section B.)

Distance calculation 20/100 acuity to read sign

Tangent = $\frac{\text{side opposite}}{\text{side adjacent}}$

.0072729 = $\frac{6''}{X''}$

.0072729 X" = 6"

Distance

X" = 825" (inches) 825 ÷ 12 = 68.7 feet

X" = 68.7 (feet)

68 feet = .78 seconds time available to read a 6" letter/sign at 60 mph or 88 feet per second for driver with 20/100 visual acuity

A driver with 20/100 visual acuity will have only 0.78 seconds available to read the sign at 60 mph or 88 feet per second.

Comparison 20/20

20/20 visual acuity time = $\frac{344}{88}$ = 3.9 seconds

Time reduced 3.9 – .78 = 3.12 seconds shortage for 20/100 acuity

Commentary: Foreseeable driving errors.

## D. Read signs with minimum driver vision acuity of 20/40

Problem: Read signs/time/acuity/speed with minimum driver visual acuity of 20/40.

Facts: Acuity: 20/40
Sign/letters: 6" (inches)
Speed: 60 mph
Design time: 6" letter for 20/20 requires 3.95 seconds

Distance

20/40 = 10' arc (tangent)

tan 10' = 10 × .0002909 = .002909

.002909 = $\frac{6''}{X''}$

.002909X" = 6"

X = $\frac{6}{.002909}$

X = 2062"

X feet = $\frac{2062''}{12}$ = 171.8 feet

X = 171.8 feet required for 20/40 acuity to read 6" sign

Time

60 mph = 1.47 × 60 = 88.2 ft/sec

$\frac{171.8}{88.2}$ = 1.94 seconds

Available time = 1.94 seconds for 20/40 visual acuity.

**Answer**: 20/40 vision permits only 1.94 seconds to read a sign with 6" letters or 171.8 feet from sign at 60 mph.

Commentary: Signs of 6" are designed for 20/20 visual acuity and a time of 3.9 seconds. With 20/40 visual acuity there is still a time shortage of 1.95 seconds when compared to an individual with 20/20 acuity. Obviously, signs need to be larger for a licensed portion of driving population.

## E. Angular separation headlights

**Problem**: Angular separation headlights (Figure B.1).

Solve for: Time it takes for headlights to double and be resolvable for driver with acuity of 20/20 visual acuity.

Headlight separation = 5 feet

Dist: A) 1 mile = 5280 feet

B) .5 mile = 2640 feet

Vehicle speed = 60 mph

Acuity

A) Solve for angular separation and acuity at 1 mile.

tan a = $\frac{5\text{ (headlight)}}{5280\text{ (1 mile)}}$ = angular separation

tan a = .000946

tan 1' = .00029

tan a = $\frac{.000946}{.00029}$ = 3.2 minutes of 1 degree (angular separation)

$$\frac{20}{X} = \frac{5}{3.2}$$

Acuity required: X = 12 (20/12 visual acuity)

3.2' of arc = requires 20/12 visual acuity

Distance

Distance = 5280 feet

60 mph time = 88 feet per second

$\frac{5280}{88}$ = 60 seconds

Commentary: Nonresolvable separation for most individuals with 20/20 visual acuity at 5280 feet or 60 seconds away. Pair of headlights appear as a single point source of light.

B) Solve for angular separation and acuity at .5 mile (2640 feet).

$$\tan b = \frac{5}{2640} = .0018939$$

$$\tan 1' = \quad .00029 \quad \frac{.00189}{.00029} = 6.5$$

tan b = 6.5' minutes

20/20 = 5' minutes

Visual acuity required = $\frac{6.5}{X} = 1.3 \times 20 = 26$ or $20/26$ visual acuity at 2640 feet (.5 mile)

Time 60 mph = 1.47 × 60 = 88 feet per second

Distance traveled = $\frac{2640\ \text{(.5 mile)}}{88\ \text{feet per second}}$ = 30 seconds

Time = 30 seconds required to double angular separation of 5-foot headlight separation from 1 mile to .5 mile for person with 20/20 visual acuity

Commentary:

1. A 5-foot separation of headlights when dividing distance traveled by half doubles its angular separation.
2. As distance shortens, the brightness of each headlight increases.
3. As distance shortens, the visual stimulus requires less acuity to judge separation and indicates increasing closeness.

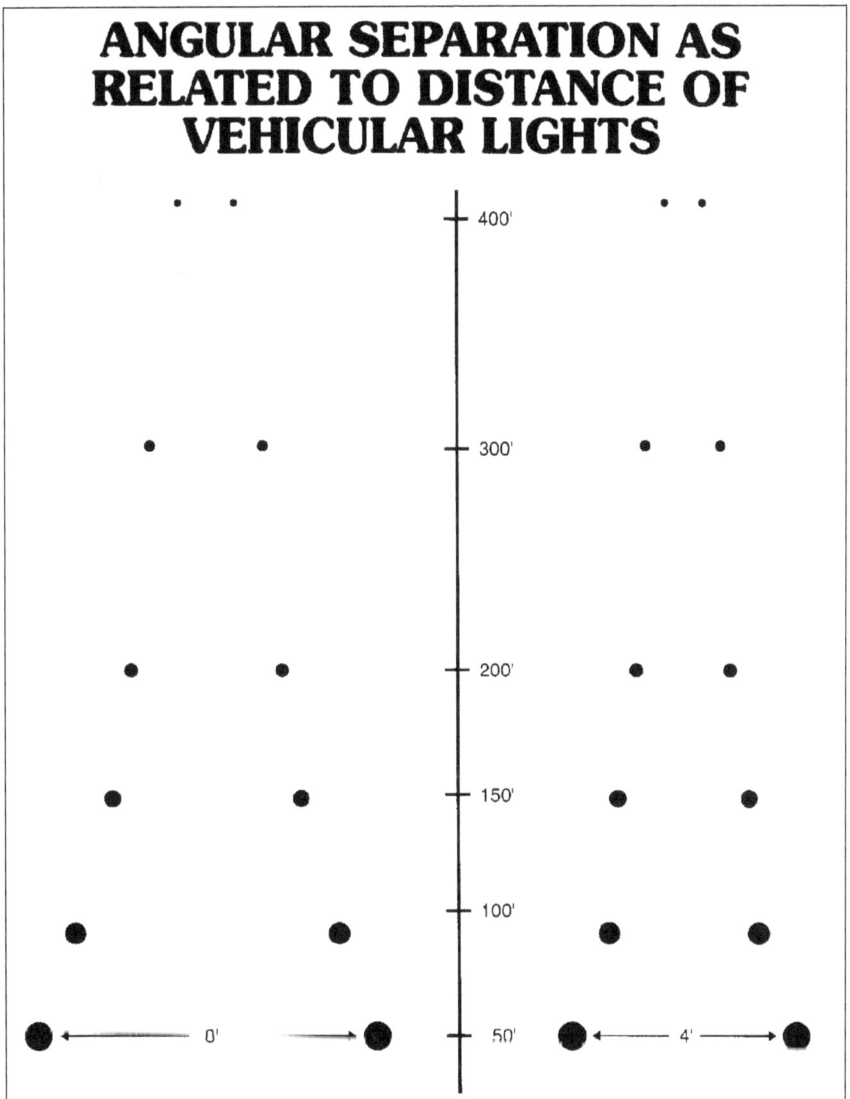


APPROXIMATE APPARENT IMAGE SIZE AND DISTANCE BETWEEN LIGHT (8 FOOT AND 4 FOOT) AT SIX RANGES TO OBSERVE

*Figure B.1*

## F. Visual acuity required to detect 5-foot object

**Problem**: What visual acuity is required to detect a 5-foot object at 500 feet [or tan X]?

Facts: 20/20 = tan 5' arc

circle = 360 degrees

1 degree = 60'

tan 1' = .017455

$$\tan 1' = \frac{.017455}{60} = .00029$$

tan 5' = 5 × .00029 = .0014545

Solve: $\tan X = \frac{5\text{ ft}}{500\text{ ft}} = .01$

tan 1' = .01745

$$\tan 1' = \frac{.01745}{60} = .00029$$

$$\tan X' = \frac{.01}{.00029} = 34.4'$$

5' = 20/20

$$X = \frac{34.4}{5'} = 7$$

Acuity required

**Answer**: Visual acuity = 7 × 20 = 20/140 visual acuity.

Proof: 20/140 = tan 34.4 minutes of arc

tan 1' = .00029

tan 35' = .01

$$.01 = \frac{5\text{ ft}}{500\text{ ft}} = \frac{\text{object}}{\text{distance}}$$

Commentary: By use of tangent formula, one can compute the Snellen visual acuity required to see an object of known size at a known distance.

## G. Visual acuity required to see a bicycle rider

**Problem**: What acuity is required to see a bicycle rider when the total object size is 6 feet high at 100 fc?

Facts: 1 mile = 5280 feet

bicycle and rider: 6 feet high

lighting: 100 fc [approaching sunset]

Acuity calculation:

1 mile

$$\tan X = \frac{6\text{ ft}}{5280\text{ ft}} = .0011$$

tan 5' = .00145 = 20/20

$$\text{Visual acuity} = \frac{.0011}{.00145} = .78$$

Visual acuity = .783 $.78 \times 20/20 = 20/16$ visual acuity
X = 20/16 visual acuity required
Commentary: Border line to distinguish object at 100 fc level due to size and amount of light.

## H. Telephone poles' size at various distances

**Problem**: Why do telephone poles of equal size appear smaller at various distances?
Facts: Each telephone pole is 40 feet high.
Distances: (a) 2 miles, (b) 1 mile, (c) .5 mile, (d) .25 mile

(a) 2 miles (10,560 feet):

$$\tan X = \frac{40 \text{ ft}}{10{,}560 \text{ ft}} = .003788$$

tan 1' = .00029

$$\text{Visual acuity } \tan X = \frac{.003788}{.00029} = 13 \text{ minutes of arc}$$

20/20 visual acuity = 5' $\frac{13}{5} = 2.6 \times 20 = 52$

20/52 visual acuity required

(b) 1 mile (5280 feet):

$$\tan X = \frac{40 \text{ ft}}{5280 \text{ ft (1 mile)}}$$

tan X = .00757
tan 1' = .00029

$$\text{Visual acuity } \tan X = \frac{.00757}{.00029} = 26 \text{ minutes of arc}$$

20/20 visual acuity = 5' $X = \frac{.01515}{.00029} = 52.2$ minutes of arc

20/104 visual acuity required

(c) .5 mile

$$\tan X = \frac{40 \text{ ft}}{2640 \text{ ft (.5 mile)}}$$

tan X = .01515
tan 1' = .00029

$$\text{Visual acuity } \tan X = \frac{.01515}{.00029} = 52.2 \text{ minutes of arc}$$

20/20 visual acuity = 5' $X = \frac{52.2}{5} = 10.45 \times 20 = 208 = 20/208$

20/208 visual acuity required

(d) .25 mile

$$\tan X = \frac{40 \text{ ft}}{1320 \text{ ft (.5 mile)}}$$

tan X = .03030
tan 1' = .00029

$$\text{Visual acuity } \tan X = \frac{.02985}{.03030} = 104.4 \text{ minutes of arc}$$

20/20 visual acuity = 5' $X = \frac{104.4}{5} 20.9 \times 20 = 417 = 20/417$

20/417 visual acuity required

Commentary: The angle subtended diminishes with distance. The pole at a distance of 1320 feet is equivalent 20/417. At a distance of 10,560 feet, the visual acuity is equivalent 20/52 or an 8:1 ratio.

## Endnotes

1. Fact. Miles per hour × 1.47 = feet per second
   60 miles per hour × 1.47 = 88 feet per second

# Appendix C

# Psychophysical Laws

Marc Green, Ph.D.

| | | |
|---|---|---|
| **Weber's Law** | $\Delta I = kI_B$ | $\Delta I$ = intensity change (JND)<br>$I_B$ = background intensity<br>K = constant |
| **Devries-Rose Law** | $\Delta I = k\sqrt{I_B}$ | $\Delta I$ = intensity change (JND)<br>$I_B$ = background intensity<br>K = constant |
| **Ricco's Law** | $\Delta IA = k$ | $\Delta I$= intensity change JND<br>A = area<br>K= constant |
| **Piper's Law** | $IA^2 = k$ | $\Delta I$= intensity change JND<br>A = area<br>K= constant |
| **Bloch's Law** | $\Delta IT = k$ | $\Delta I$= intensity change JND<br>T = viewing duration<br>K= constant |
| **Blondel-Rey Law** | $\Delta IT = \Delta I_\infty (T + a)$ | $\Delta I$= intensity change JND<br>$\Delta I_\infty$ = JND for steady light<br>T = viewing duration<br>a = constant (~.2 sec) |
| **Ferry-Porter Law** | $CFF = a \log L + b$ | CFF= critical flicker fusion<br>L = luminance<br>a & b constants |

| | | |
|---|---|---|
| **Stevens' Law** | $\psi = k\Phi^a$ | $\Psi$ = perceived magnitude<br>$\Phi$ = physical magnitude<br>k= constant<br>a=exponent |
| **Fechner-Weber Law** | $\psi = k\log\Phi$ | $\Psi$ = perceived magnitude<br>$\Phi$ = physical magnitude<br>k= constant |
| **Ekman's Law** | $\Delta\psi = k\psi_B$ | $\Delta\Psi$ = sensation change (JND)<br>$\Psi_B$ = background sensation<br>K = constant |
| **Koschmeider's Law** | $V = \frac{3}{\sigma}$ | V = visual range<br>$\sigma$ = extinction coefficient |

# Appendix D

# Recommended Sources

Bernard S. Abrams, O.D. and Marc Green, Ph.D.


1. *Adler's Physiology of the Eye*, Clinical Application, Seventh Edition, Edited by Moses.

2. *Auto Accident Checklist*, 1995, Jon Abele, Esq, Lawyers and Judges Publishing.

3. *Basic Collision Analysis and Scene Documentation*, 2000, Second Edition, David A. Casteel and Steven D. Moss, Lawyers and Judges Publishing.

4. Bruce, V. and P. Green. *Visual perception: Physiology, psychology and ecology*, 2nd ed. 1990. Hillsdale, Lawrence Erlbaum Assoc.

5. *Bus and Recreational Vehicle Accident Reconstruction and Litigation*, 2000, Dr. Roy Scitt Hickman and Paul F. Hill, Esq., Lawyers and Judges Publishing.

6. *Defensive Driving Course*, Professional Truck Driver, Driver's Notebook, National Safety Council.

7. Dekker, S. *The Field Guide To Human Error Investigations*. 2002. Bedfordshire Cranfield UK: University Press.

8. Engineering Data Compendium: Human Perception and Performance, 1988. Boff, K.R. and Lincoln, J.E., Sec. 1.235, AAMRL, Wright-Patterson AFB, OH, 1988.

9. *Federal Motor Carrier Safety Regulations*, July, 1990, U.S. Department of Transportation, Federal Highway Administration, American Trucking Association.

10. *Forensic Aspects of Driver Perception and Response*, 1996, Paul Olson, Lawyers and Judges Publishing.

11. Goldstein, E. B.: *Sensation and Perception*, 1999. Brooks/Cole Publishing Company.

12. *Handbook of Human Factors*, Gavriel Salvendy.

13. *Human Element-Proceedings*, Volume II, 1990 International Motorcycle Safety Conference.

14. *Human Factors in Engineering and Design*, 6th Edition, Mark S. Sanders, Ernest J. McCormick.

15. *Human Factors in Highway Traffic Safety Research*, Edited by T.W. Forbes, Michigan State University, East Lansing.

16. *IES Lighting Handbook*, 2000 Reference Volume, Illuminating Engineering Society of North America.

17. *IES Lighting Handbook*, 2000 Application Volume, Illuminating Engineering Society of North America.

18. Levine, M. and J. Schefner. *Fundamentals of Sensation and Perception* 1991. 2nd Edition Brooks/Cole.

19. *Low Speed Automobile Accidents: Accident Reconstruction and Occupant Kinematics, Dynamics and Biomechanics*, 1999, Second Edition, Alan J. Watts, Dale R. Atkinson and Corey J. Hennessy, Lawyers and Judges Publishing.

20. *Manual on Uniform Traffic Control Devices*, 1988 Edition for Streets and Highways, U.S. Department of Transportation. Available from Lawyers and Judges Publishing.

21. *Motorcycle Accident Reconstruction and Litigation*, 1997, Second Edition, Kenneth Obenski, P.E., and Paul F. Hill, Esq. Lawyers and Judges Publishing.

22. *Old Farmer's Almanac*, Annually.

23. *Pedestrian Accident Reconstruction and Litigation*, 1999, Second Edition, Jerry Eubanks and Paul F. Hill, Esq., Lawyers and Judges Publishing.

24. *Policy on Geometric Design of Highway and Streets*, 1990, American Association of State Highway and Transportation Officials.

25. *Roadway Defects and Tort Liability*, 1996, John C. Glennon, D. Engr., P.E., Lawyers and Judges Publishing.

26. *Roadway Through the MUTCD: Vision and Other Human Factors in the Manual on Uniform Traffic Control Devices*, 1998, Archie C. Burnham, Jr., and Bernard S. Abrams, Lawyers and Judges Publishing.

27. *SAE Ground Vehicle Lighting Manual. 1996.*

28. *SAE, CD-ROM, Database-2000.*

29. *Sensation and Perception* 2002. E. B. Goldstein, Wadsworth Group, Pacific Grove, California [Note: best beginner's textbook.]

30. *Taar Safety Engineering*, Accident Investigation Software.

31. *The ecological approach to visual perception.* 1979 James J. Gibson. Boston : Houghton Mifflin.

32. *The senses considered as perceptual systems.* 1966 James Jerome Gibson. Boston, Houghton Mifflin.

33. *Tractor-Trailer Driver Manual*, A Guide for Professional Drivers, Professional Truck Driver Institute of America, American Trucking Association.

34. *Traffic Accident Investigation and Physical Evidence*, D.R. McGrew, Certified Legal Investigator, National Director, National Association of Legal Investigators.

35. *Traffic Engineering Handbook*, Fourth Edition, Institute of Transportation Engineers.

36. *Train Accident Reconstruction and FELA & Railroad Litigation*, 1998, Third Edition, James Loumiet and William Jungbauer, Lawyers and Judges Publishing.

37. *Transportation in an Aging Society, Improving Mobility and Safety for Older Persons*, Special Report 218, Volume 2, Transportation Research Board, National Research Council.

38. *Understanding driving: applying cognitive psychology to a complex everyday task.* 2000. John A. Groeger. Psychology Press, Hove.

# Appendix E

# Cone of Vision

Bernard S. Abrams, O.D.

## Area the Eye Sees at Various Distances from the Fovea

Central visual acuity is measured by viewing targets (letters, numbers, etc.) at a fixed distance of 20 feet (or 6 meters). Targets of progressively smaller size are viewed, each of which subtends a smaller and smaller angle on the retina. Larger targets, for example, subtend a large angle and correspond to a visual acuity of 20/400 (or less) while smaller targets which subtend a smaller angle correspond to a visual acuity of 20/20 (or better).

The best visual acuity is obtained in the central fovea area.[1] If portions of the fovea or the macula are damaged, visual acuity will be reduced. Thus the visual acuity when viewing from the foveal area is 20/20. The fall-off in vision is rapid, thus when viewing from 10° from the fovea, visual acuity is 20/100 and falls off rapidly thereafter (refer to Figures 18.9 and 18.10 in Chapter 18). The high density of cones in the fovea accounts for the high degree visual acuity discrimination in this area of the retina. It has been shown that the density of cones in the fovea is approximately 18 times greater than anywhere else in the retina where they reach a density of approximately 1900 cones/mm$^2$. Within 5 degrees of the fovea there is a rapid fall-off to about 200 cones/mm$^2$. Rods, which are absent from the fovea, make their first appearance about 5 degrees from the fovea and reach their maximum density approximately 20 degrees from the fovea.

The cones which subserve the functions of sharp and color vision do not adapt to the low light levels of the rods. Indeed, the latter are a 1000 times more light-sensitive than the cones, and during the course of dark adaptation, the final lowest threshold for the eye takes about 25 minutes to achieve and is situated outside the fovea.

### Example

| | | |
|---|---|---|
| Problem: | Acute cone of vision at 150 feet | |
| Facts: | Foveal acute cone = | 3 degrees |
| | Distance = | 150 feet |
| | Visual acuity = | 20/20 |
| | Solve for: | area X |

Distance:

tan 1° = .01745

tan 3° = 3 × .01745 = .05236

$$\tan = \frac{\text{side opposite}}{\text{side adjacent}}$$

tan 3° = .05236

$$.05326 = \frac{X}{150 \text{ feet}}$$

X = 7.85 feet

## Commentary:

*This is the area that is considered the cone of vision and has the most acute vision.*

*If an individual has Snellen visual acuity of 20/20, said vision will cover a width of 7.85 feet at a distance of 150 feet.*

## Example

Problem: Sub-acute cone of vision at 150 feet

Facts: Sub-acute foveal cone of vision = 10°

| | |
|---|---|
| Distance = | 150 feet |
| Visual acuity at 10° = | 20/100 |
| Solve for: | area X |

Distance:

tan 1° = .01745

tan 10° = 10 × .01745 = .1745

$$\tan = \frac{\text{side opposite}}{\text{side adjacent}}$$

tan 10° = .1745

$$.1745 = \frac{X}{150 \text{ feet}}$$

X = 26.18 feet

Commentary:

*When viewing in the sub-acute retinal area or 10 degrees from the fovea, the area is 26.18 feet in width. At the periphery the vision is 20/100. An object to be seen would need to be 5 times larger to be equivalent to that in the cone of vision. The area between 3 degrees to 10 degrees has a visual transformation from 20/20 to 20/100.*

## Endnotes

1. The area varies with researchers; however, the standard conservative is 3 degrees in width.

# Appendix F

# Relationship of Visual Angles/Visual Acuity

Bernard S. Abrams, O.D.

## Visual Angles/Visual Acuity

An object subtends different visual angles at various distances. This visual angle may then be corrected to an approximate visual acuity level.

The standard equation used in these calculations is:

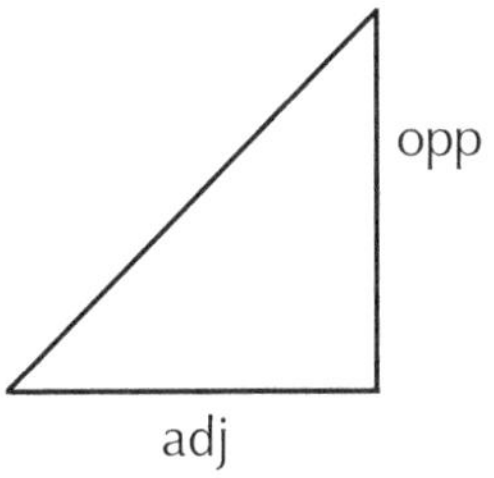


$\tan \theta$ = opposite/adjacent
$\theta$ will be in degrees
We change the value in degrees to minutes.

| Visual Acuity | Visual Angle (mins of arc) at 20 feet |
|---|---|
| 20/20 | 5 |
| 20/25 | 6.25 |
| 20/30 | 7.5 |
| 20/40 | 10 |
| 20/50 | 12.5 |
| 20/60 | 15 |
| 20/70 | 17.5 |
| 20/80 | 20 |
| 20/100 | 25 |
| 20/150 | 37.5 |
| 20/200 | 50 |
| 20/300 | 75 |
| 20/400 | 100 |

(a) The Snellen fraction is:

$$\text{Visual acuity} = \frac{\text{distance at which test is made}}{\text{distance at which the smallest letter read subtends an angle of } 5'}$$

If at 20 feet patient can read a letter “E” of a size .349” (inches), the fraction is recorded as 20/20.*

If at 20 feet patient can read a letter “E” of a size 1.392” (inches), the fraction is recorded as 20/80.**

* “E” subtends 5 minutes of arc at 20 feet.

** “E” subtends 5 minutes of arc at 80 feet (4 times taller letter/4 times the distance).

(See Figure F.1.)

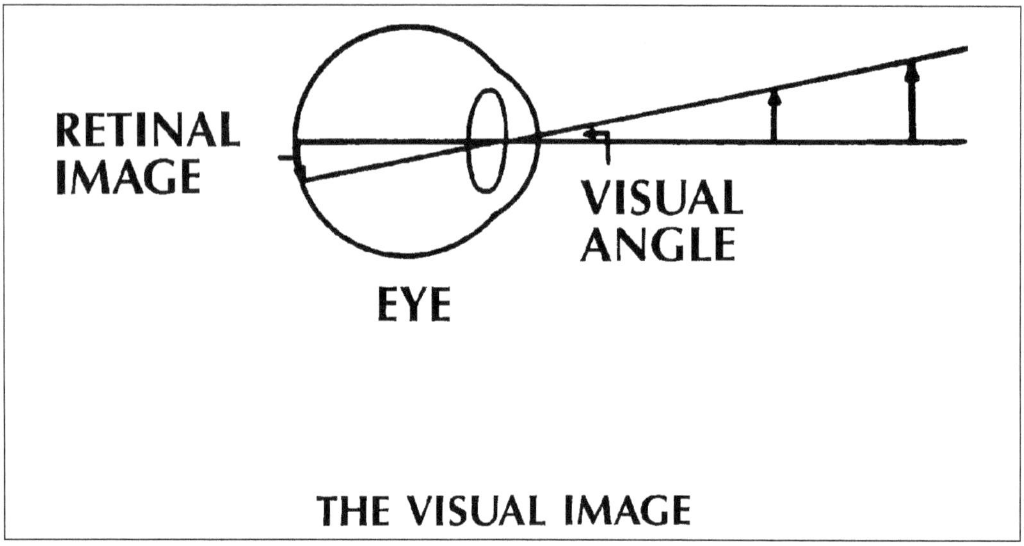


***Figure F.1***

# Appendix G

# Twelve Things You Should Know About Vision and Accidents

Marc Green, Ph.D.

1. "We are quickly brought to the conclusion that we shall understand accidents when we understand human nature."

—Kay (1971);

2. "Contrast detection is the basic task from which all other visual behaviors are derived."

—Kaufman and Hayes (1984);

3. "Only those items which I notice shape my mind—without selective interest, experience is utter chaos."

—William James (1890);

4. "We do not see what we sense. We see what we think we sense. Our consciousness is presented with an interpretation, not the raw data. Long after presentation, an unconscious information processing has discarded information, so that we see a simulation, a hypothesis, an interpretation; and we are not free to choose."

—Norretranders (1998);

5. "We see our world of organized scenes and moving objects by combining information from the light which reaches our eyes with knowledge stored in memory about the structure and identity of objects and scenes. We understand our surroundings partly by seeing them but also by inferring what is there... Vision is therefore a genuine cognitive function, not merely a sensory one."

—Hampson and Morris (1996);

6. "Vision is not merely a matter of passive perception, it is an intelligent process of active construction. What you see is, invariably, what your visual intelligence constructs. Just as scientists intelligently construct useful theories based on experimental evidence, so your visual system intelligently constructs useful visual worlds based on images at the eyes. The main difference is that the constructions of scientists are done consciously, but those of your visual intelligence are done, for the most part, unconsciously."

—Hoffman (1998);

7. "Perception is largely determined not by physical characteristics but by the perceiver's intentions and goals."
—Tijerina (2003);

8. "You don't see things as they are, you see things as you are."
—The Talmud;

9. "Oft expectation fails, and most oft there where it most promises."
—Shakespeare;

10. "Habit is the 6th sense that overrules the other 5."
—Arab Proverb;

11. "They're funny things, accidents. You never have them till you're having them."
—Milne (1995); and

12. "The law isn't justice. It's a very imperfect mechanism. If you press exactly the right buttons and are also lucky, justice may show up in the answer. A mechanism is all the law was ever intended to be."
—Raymond Chandler (1953).

## References

Chandler, R. 1953. *The Big Sleep*. New York: Random House.

Hampson, P., and P. Morris. 1996. Understanding Cognition. Oxford: Blackwell.

Hoffman, D. 1998. *Visual Intelligence: How We Create What We See*. New York: W. W. Norton & Company.

James, W. 1890. *Principles of Psychology*. New York: Henry Holt.

Kaufman, J., and H. Haynes. 1981. *IES Lighting Handbook*. New York: Illuminating Engineering Society of North America.

Kay, H. 1971. Accidents: Some facts and theories. In P. Warr (ed.) *Psychology at Work* 121-145. Baltimore: Penguin.

Milne, A. A. 1995. *Pooh's Little Instruction Book*. New York: Penguin.

Norretranders, T. 1998. *The User Illusion Cutting Consciousness Down to Size*. New. York: Viking.

Tejerina, L. 2003. Committee report: conspicuity enhancement for police interceptor rear-end crash mitigation. https://www.fleet.ford.com/showroom/CVPI/pdfs/CVPI_Conspicuity_Report.pdf. Downloaded 1 Nov 06.

# About the Authors

**Dr. Marc Green** has a Ph. D. in experimental psychology and 37 years of experience in basic and applied research in vision, cognitive science, and human factors design. He has served as an expert in matters related to road accidents, warnings, falls, police shootings, product design and other human factors issues as well as in matters related to intellectual property disputes.

Dr. Green is currently head of Visual Expert Human Factors Science and adjunct Professor of Ophthalmology at University of West Virginia Medical School. He was previously a postdoctoral fellow, faculty member at several universities, including Brown, Berkley, Indiana University, and Carnegie Mellon. His background includes 98 publications on topics including basic and applied visual science, warning effectiveness, road and other accident causation, and medical error. He has also given numerous presentations at scientific and professional conferences in the U.S. and abroad. Dr. Green has received research awards from the National Eye Institute, the National Science Foundation, the U.S. Air Force and the National Science Engineering and Research Committee. He has been interviewed by *The New Yorker*, *Los Angeles Times*, CTV National TV, the *National Post*, Canadian Broadcasting Company, IEEE radio, and National Public Radio.

**Merrill J. Allen, O.D., Ph.D., (1918–2003)** Professor Emeritus of Optometry of Indiana University, School of Optometry, Bloomington, Indiana, had been involved in vision research and teaching since 1941. He had over 200 publications and received 19 awards including the Research Medal Award from the British Optical Association (1970) and the Apollo Award from the American Optometric Association (1971).

He served as an expert witness in over 600 lawsuits, providing opinions on the role of visual factors and alcohol in the cause of motor vehicle accidents. He studied thousands of accident reports, performed accident reconstruction and studied other data in order to render his opinions.

Dr. Allen carried out government, industry and optometrically funded research projects and considered consulting on motor vehicle accidents to be attorney subsidized research. Many of his research publications were directed at improving motor vehicle safety by eliminating the design errors that kept showing up in accidents.

High-mounted brake lights were a direct result of a research study he did on the Indianapolis Speedway. Daytime running lights resulted from his research funded by the Indianapolis Star newspaper. A railroad crossing accident in Kalamazoo, Michigan, in which he testified, resulted in increasing the brightness of railroad signal lights across the U.S.

He believed that simple changes of the visual features of motor vehicles and the driving environment can reduce our accidents 80 percent or more and save over 30,000 lives per year.

**Bernard S. Abrams, O.D., (1929–2003)** was the founder of the Institute of Vehicular Safety. He received his B.S. in Visual Optics at Ohio State University. Dr. Abrams began pursuit of his lifelong interest in Traffic Safety in 1954 as a member of the Columbus Ohio Traffic Commission. Over the years, his interest in night vision and vehicular accidents was enhanced by his work in electrophysiological testing for the night vision of the aged. He lectured about vision on three continents, designed and built optical factories in several countries, and was Chairman of the Board of B.S.A. Industries. Dr. Abrams authored numerous papers and articles dealing with driver visibility, object conspicuity, and nighttime discernibility. He conducted research projects and served on committees related to the vision requirements of the older driver. Dr. Abrams served as a consultant to industries, attorneys, and governmental agencies. He was a nationally recognized expert witness in nighttime/daytime vehicular accidents.

Dr. Abrams also conducted classes at various universities, state patrols, and private institutions relating to the visibility aspects of vision in the courtroom.

**Leslie Weintraub, O.D.,** is a graduate of Cornell University School of Business and the University of Houston College of Optometry. She is currently in private practice in Tucson, Arizona, as a medical optometrist with an emphasis in pathology.

**J. Vernon Odom, Ph.D.** is Professor of Ophthalmology, Professor of Physiology and Pharmacology, and Adjunct Professor of Psychology at West Virginia University where he is research director at the WVU Eye Institute, heads the West Virginia Lions Visual Function Laboratory and formerly directed the Center for Vision Enhancement Technology. Dr. Odom has authored more than 200 articles, book chapters, and published abstracts. His research has centered on assessment of visual function using electrophysiology and psychophysics in normal and abnormal aging. Dr. Odom is the past editor in chief of *Documenta Ophthalmologica*, former member of the Board of Directors of the International Society for Clinical Electrophysiology of Vision (ISCEV), and chairs the ISCEV VEP standardization committee. He has served the Association for Vision and Ophthalmology on its program committee and on its long range planning committee. He was awarded the Francqui International Interuniversity Chair in 1996. Dr. Odom holds two patents and has three patents pending.

# Index

# E



# F

# G



# H



# I

## Q



## R



## S

www.ingramcontent.com/pod-product-compliance
Lightning Source LLC
LaVergne TN
LVHW081305021125
824697LV00003B/23
*9781933264547*